Global Health
and Global Health Ethics

Global Health and Global Health Ethics

Edited by

Solomon Benatar
Emeritus Professor of Medicine, University of Cape Town
Professor, Dalla Lana School of Public Health and Joint Centre for Bioethics, University of Toronto, Canada

Gillian Brock
Associate Professor of Philosophy, University of Auckland, New Zealand

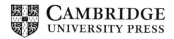
CAMBRIDGE
UNIVERSITY PRESS

CAMBRIDGE
UNIVERSITY PRESS

University Printing House, Cambridge CB2 8BS, United Kingdom

Cambridge University Press is part of the University of Cambridge.

It furthers the University's mission by disseminating knowledge in the pursuit of education, learning and research at the highest international levels of excellence.

www.cambridge.org
Information on this title: www.cambridge.org/9780521146777

© Cambridge University Press 2011

First published 2011
3rd printing 2012

A catalogue record for this publication is available from the British Library

Library of Congress Cataloguing in Publication data
Global health and global health ethics / [edited by] Solomon Benatar, Gillian Brock.
    p. ; cm.
  Includes bibliographical references and index.
  ISBN 978-0-521-14677-7 (pbk.)
  1. World health.   2. Public health–Moral and ethical aspects.   I. Benatar, S. R.   II. Brock, Gillian.
  III. Title. [DNLM: 1. World Health.   2. Healthcare Disparities.   3. International Cooperation.
  4. Public Health–ethics. WA 530.1]
  RA441.G566 2011
  362.1–dc22   2010042733

ISBN 978-0-521-14677-7 Paperback

....

Contents

Contents

Contributors

Isabella Bakker
Department of Political Science, York University, Toronto, Ontario, Canada.

David Benatar
Philosophy Department, University of Cape Town, South Africa.

Solomon Benatar
Bioethics Center, University of Cape Town, South Africa and Joint Centre for Bioethics, University of Toronto, Toronto, Ontario, Canada

Anne-Emanuelle Birn
Dalla Lana School of Public Health, University of Toronto, Toronto, ON, Canada.

Gillian Brock
Department of Philosophy, University of Auckland, Auckland, New Zealand.

Allen Buchanan
Institute for Genome Sciences and Policy, Duke University, Durham, NC, USA.

Colin Butler
National Centre for Epidemiology and Population Health, Australian National University, Canberra, ACT, Australia.

Justin Chakma
McLaughlin-Rotman Centre for Global Health, Toronto, Ontario, Canada.

Abdallah S. Daar
McLaughlin-Rotman Centre for Global Health, University Health Network and University of Toronto, Toronto, Ontario, Canada.

Norman Daniels
Department of Global Health and Population, Harvard School of Public Health, Boston, MA, USA.

Angus J. Dawson
Centre for Professional Ethics, Keele University, Staffordshire, UK.

Matthew DeCamp
Department of Internal Medicine, University of Michigan Ann Arbor, MI, USA.

Lesley Doyal
School for Policy Studies, University of Bristol, Bristol, UK.

James Dwyer
Center for Bioethics and Humanities, SUNY Upstate Medical University, Syracuse, NY, USA.

Sharon Friel
National Center for Epidemiology and Population Health, Australian National University, Canberra, ACT, Australia.

Stephen Gill
Department of Political Science, York University, Toronto, Ontario, Canada.

Jonathan Glover
Centre of Medical Law and Ethics, Kings College London, Strand, London, UK.

David Hunter
Centre for Professional Ethics, Keele University, Staffordshire, UK.

Samia A. Hurst
Institute for Biomedical Ethics, Geneva University Medical School, Switzerland.

Gerald T. Keusch
Department of International Health and Center for Global Health and Development, Boston University, Boston, MA, USA.

Arthur Kleinman

Department of Anthropology, Harvard University and Department of Global Health and Social Medicine, Harvard Medical School, Cambridge, MA, USA.

Meri Koivusalo

National Institute for Health and Welfare, Helsinki, Finland.

Ronald Labonté

Department of Epidemiology and Community Medicine, Institute of Population Health, University of Ottawa, Ottawa, Ontario, Canada.

Alex John London

Center for the Advancement of Applied Ethics and Political Philosophy, Department of Philosophy, Carnegie Mellon University, Pittsburg, PA, USA.

Salahaddin Mahmudi-Azer

Department of Medicine, University of Calgary, Calgary, Alberta, Canada.

Hassan Masum

McLaughlin-Rotman Centre for Global Health, Toronto, Ontario, Canada.

Alex Mauron

Institute for Biomedical Ethics, Geneva University Medical School, Switzerland.

Lynn McIntyre

Department of Community Health Sciences, Faculty of Medicine, University of Calgary, Calgary, Alberta, Canada.

Martin McKee

London School of Hygiene and Tropical Medicine, London, UK.

Anthony McMichael

National Centre for Epidemiology and Population Health, Australian National University, Canberra, ACT, Australia.

Nathalie Mezger

MSF-CH Administrative Board, MSF-Switzerland.

Tikki Pang

Research Policy and Cooperation (RPC/IER), World Health Organization, Geneva, Switzerland.

Sarah Payne

School for Policy Studies, University of Bristol, Bristol, UK.

Thomas Pogge

Philosophy and International Affairs, Yale University, New Haven, CT, USA.

Krista Rondeau

Department of Community Health Sciences, Faculty of Medicine, University of Calgary, Calgary, AB, Canada.

Jeff Rudin

South African Municipal Workers' Union, Cape Town, South Africa.

David Sanders

School of Public Health, University of the Western Cape, Bellville, South Africa.

Ted Schrecker

Department of Epidemiology and Community Medicine, Institute of Population Health, University of Ottawa, Ontario, Canada.

Michael J. Selgelid

Centre for Applied Philosophy and Public Ethics (CAPPE), The Australian National University, Canberra, Australia.

Peter A. Singer

McLaughlin-Rotman Centre for Global Health, University Health Network and University of Toronto, Toronto, Ontario, Canada.

Kearsley A. Stewart

Harvard Centre for Population and Development Studies, Cambridge, MA, USA and Department of Anthropology and Global Health Studies Program, Northwestern University, Evanston, IL, USA.

Ross Upshur

Joint Centre for Bioethics, University of Toronto, Toronto, Ontario, Canada.

Jonathan Wolff

Department of Philosophy, University College London, London, UK.

Anthony B. Zwi

School of Public Health and Community Medicine, The University of New South Wales, Lindfield, NSW, Australia.

Introduction

The *raison d'être* for this book is to draw attention to what we consider to be one of the largest and most important challenges facing humanity in the twenty-first century – to improve and promote global health. By global health we mean the health of all people globally within sustainable and healthy living (local and global) conditions. In order to achieve this ambitious goal we need to understand, among other things, the value systems, modes of reasoning, and power structures that have driven and shaped the world over the past century. We also need to appreciate the unsustainability of many of our current consumption patterns before we can address threats to the health and lives of current and future generations.

The world and how we live in it have been changing dramatically over many centuries, but in the past fifty years change has been more rapid and profound than ever in the past. Many positive changes have been associated with impressive economic growth, advances in science and medicine and in social policies regarding access to health promotion. These include more equitable access to primary care, greater focus on a primary health-care approach, expansion of social programs to improve living conditions and a welcome increasing emphasis on the rights of all individuals to be equally respected.

Sadly, emphasis on the exaggerated expectations of the most privileged people has resulted in neglect of a large proportion of the world's population with consequent widening disparities in wealth and health. In addition many of the world's health-care "systems" have become *distorted*, *dysfunctional*, and *unsustainable*. By *distorted* we mean that health-care services are not designed to meet the range of demands posed by local burdens of disease equitably. They are *dysfunctional* because they are driven more by adverse market forces and the requirements of bureaucracy, than by

emphasis on serving patients optimally and sustaining the professionalism required of health-care workers in the care of patients and the training of new generations of professionals. Finally, marginal benefits for a few are often prioritized while other cost-effective activities of potentially great benefit to many more people are ignored. Within limited resource environments, such strategies that contribute to costs of health care rising disproportionately are likely to prove *unsustainable*.

Disparities in health and in access to health care thus continue to widen globally. Such disparities, combined with population growth, unsustainable consumption patterns, the emergence of many new infectious diseases (and multi-drug resistance), escalating ecological degradation, numerous local and regional wars, a stockpile of nuclear weapons, massive dislocations of people and new terrorist threats (to list just a few relevant factors) have severe implications for individuals' and populations' health. Deeper understanding of the challenges we face and of the feasible changes that could be made to address these, are necessary first steps towards expressing better commitment to genuine respect for the dignity of all people (and, indeed, showing respect for everyone's dignity is an ideal our international agreements increasingly claim to embrace).

Adequate understanding of ethical issues concerning health requires that we extend our focus from the micro-level of individual health and the ethics of interpersonal relationships to include ethical considerations regarding public and population health, and justice concerns more generally. The domain of global health ethics provides a context within which the many relevant disciplines that have valuable insights to offer can usefully engage, and through that engagement promote better understanding of the extensive changes that are needed. Furthermore, developing a global state of mind about the world, and our place in it, is arguably

Global Health and Global Health Ethics, ed. Soloman Benatar and Gillian Brock. Published by Cambridge University Press.
© Cambridge University Press 2011.

relevant to making many of the necessary, progressive changes.

After noting the poor state of global health, there are three main issues covered by almost all contributing authors. They direct our attention to ways in which we exacerbate poor global health, what we should do to remedy the factors identified, and offer reasons why we ought to do something about the highlighted problems, thereby connecting global health issues more strongly with the domain of justice. Many of the chapters in this volume provide constructive suggestions about how national and global policy and institutional changes could function differently to make significant improvements. Together they contribute to a deeper understanding of the challenges we face in trying to improve global health and provide much practical and theoretical guidance, which builds a case for our ability to make a real difference if we so choose.

In what follows we give a brief synopsis of the chapters. A note about structure might be important here. Because almost all the authors cover the issue of responsibilities and global health, it has been difficult to impose a rigid structure on these chapters and the subsections of the book. Like the subject matter under investigation, several issues are intimately linked.

Global health, definitions and descriptions

Solomon Benatar and Ross Upshur pose many questions about the term "global health" and what it means to different people. They analyze various conceptions of, and perspectives on, global health, and show how these can influence the focus of action for improvements. They also draw particular attention to two human-created problems (drug-resistant tuberculosis and poor water management in the Aral Sea area) to show how the broad causal chain of health and disease goes beyond environmental and natural disasters to include avoidable problems directly attributable to acts of human omission or commission. So, while in the 1960s and 1970s we had the tools and resources vastly to reduce the global burden of mortality and morbidity from tuberculosis, we failed to do so and now face a future in which tuberculosis may become an untreatable disease in poor countries where the major burden of this disease is concentrated. The Aral Sea disaster provides an example at the micro-level of the irrevocable damage we may do to our global water supplies if lessons are not learned in good time

about the adverse effects of focusing on short-term economic gains.

Probably the most striking feature about the state of global health is that it is characterized by such radical inequalities. Here is just a sample of the more widely noticed and documented kinds. Life expectancy at birth varies enormously: from around 40 years in Sierra Leone or Afghanistan to twice that at more than 80 years for those lucky enough to be born in Japan or Australia. Similarly, there is huge variation in maternal mortality. A Canadian woman's lifetime risk of dying from childbirth or pregnancy complications is 1 in 11 000, whereas for a woman in the Niger it is 1 in 7. Whereas malaria is almost entirely absent in high-income countries, it kills around a million people each year elsewhere.

As Ronald Labonté and Ted Schrecker observe, a largely accurate explanation for these types of differences involves potentially avoidable poverty and material deprivation. However, these authors remind us that we should resist the inference that policies that promote economic growth are therefore the best way to achieve good population health. There is a threshold level, at about $5000 (US), beyond which the relationship between life expectancy at birth and per capita incomes breaks down. In addition we see many countries with very good life expectancies at birth despite quite low per capita incomes. For example in Costa Rica, with per capita income of about $10 500 per year, life expectancy is 79, notably more than the 78 years those who reside in the USA can expect to live, where per capita income is greater than $45 000.[1] Other social changes besides economic growth can have significant consequences for health. For example, improved female literacy and commitment to health as a social goal in Kerala (in India) have resulted in low infant and maternal mortality despite very low income (per capita income of about $3000). Another example is how increased urbanization and globalization have allowed the consolidation of power over food systems, which can lead to detrimental consumption patterns. (Consider, for instance, how Mexicans now consume 50% more Coca-Cola products per person than those who reside in the USA.)

---

[1] However, it should not be forgotten that economic growth remains important in countries with very low per capita incomes (for example, below $2000–3000), and that the extent of income disparities within countries is also important.

Some gains in the state of world health have been achieved through improved vaccination coverage and access to affordable antiretroviral therapies, but much work remains to amplify these meager gains. Providing extra resources for health care is at least part of what is needed. Jeffrey Sachs has calculated that a tax of 1 cent in every $10 earned by the wealthiest 1 billion in the world could provide the $35 billion required per year to give the poorest 1 billion people a $50 annual per capita health-care package.[2] Labonté and Shrecker conclude: "the fact that resource scarcities condemn millions every year to premature and avoidable deaths, and millions more to shorter and less healthy lives than most readers of this volume take for granted, must be understood as policy-generated, resulting from choices that could have been made differently and institutions that can function differently" (Chapter 2).

The distribution of power and of social, political, and economic resources is crucial in influencing and explaining population health. In her chapter, Anne-Emanuelle Birn analyzes the societal determinants of health: factors that shape health at various levels including household, community, national, and global levels. Living conditions both at the household and community level can cause numerous ailments including respiratory, gastrointestinal, or metabolic diseases. Availability of potable water and adequate sanitation are key factors. Though water is essential for life, more than a billion people (one-sixth of the world's population) have an inadequate supply. The facts about access to adequate sanitation are even more striking – almost half the world's population has inadequate access to basic sanitation facilities, which can result in soil contamination and increased rates of communicable diseases. The impact of other factors analyzed include: nutrition and food security (over 50% of child deaths are attributable to poor nutrition), housing conditions, public health and health-care services, and transportation. Social policies and government regulation (or lack thereof) can also affect health in dramatic ways through, for example, the domains of education, taxation, labor, and environmental regulations. Patterns of unequal resource distribution and political power play a fundamental role in the societal determinants of health. To address radical health inequalities

effectively means that we cannot ignore these other more basic factors.

Is all health inequality morally troublesome? We might tend to think it must be, but on reflection we see that matters are not straightforward here. Lesley Doyal and Sarah Payne explore some inequality and difference related to social gender and biological sex. They outline some important differences between male and female patterns of health and illness and offer various conceptual tools we need to understand the implications of these patterns, which patterns are objectionable, and what we should do about them.

Martin McKee presents an account of how health, well structured and integrated health-care systems, and economic growth can all co-exist and be mutually supporting. Health care, when appropriately delivered, can yield substantial gains in population health, which further reduces the demand for health care. Better population health can result in faster economic growth, through enhanced productivity. The additional economic growth can increase resources available for health care, and further investment in health care can also contribute to economic growth. None of this necessarily follows, however. Concerted action by governments is needed to ensure these relationships are mutually supportive and beneficial.

Global health ethics, responsibilities, and justice: some central issues

Angus Dawson and David Hunter explore the question of whether there is a need for global health ethics. They begin by examining different ways of understanding the term "global health ethics," and proceed to examine arguments that could be used either to support or rebut more substantive accounts of global health ethics, including those based on beneficence, justice and harm, and more cosmopolitan accounts. Some of the arguments they explore, that are used to resist more substantive global health ethics, include ones concerning the moral relevance of distance, property rights, and duties to prioritize the interests of compatriots. They argue that we need not take a stand on any of these arguments to make a convincing case for various global obligations we have with respect to health. Sometimes a case for global responsibilities pertaining to health can be marshalled via more self-interested concerns, such as with infectious diseases, or with the public goods nature of many global health issues (again, as is the case with infectious diseases).

---

[2] Jeffrey Sachs during a video conference presentation at the Canadian Conference on International Health. Ottawa, October 2009.

Indeed, infectious diseases are one of the most important areas for global concern. Historically, these have caused more morbidity and mortality than any other cause, including wars. Tuberculosis alone has killed a billion people during the last two centuries. But, as Michael Selgelid argues, infectious diseases do not affect us all equally. These primarily affect the poor and marginalized who are more likely to live in the kinds of crowded and poor conditions conducive to spreading infectious diseases, lack adequate hygiene provisions necessary to prevent or treat diseases, or lack access to adequate health care should they become infected, and are malnourished which also weakens immune systems. Infectious diseases therefore cause more morbidity and mortality in developing countries. However, since epidemics in one country can easily spread to others (and become more virulent and harder to treat in the process), rich countries have good self-interested reasons to be concerned about health-care improvement and poverty reduction in developing countries, in order to protect their own populations adequately. Michael Selgelid argues that wealthy developed countries also have ethical reasons to fund poverty and disease reduction in poor developing countries in virtue of other normative commitments, such as to equality, equality of opportunity, reducing injustices, or to promoting well-being.

International health inequalities are very often rightly disturbing, such as those concerning the differences in child mortality before age five or mothers' death rates during labor. Is it fair that there should be such clear losers in the "natural lottery," constituted by where one happens to have been born? Should such an arbitrary fact about one get to determine one's life prospects in such radical ways? Norman Daniels argues that "health inequalities between social groups are unjust or unfair when they result from an unjust distribution of the socially controllable factors that affect population health and its distribution" (Chapter 8). The sources of international health inequalities are explored more systematically and divided into three categories: some result from domestic injustice in the distribution of socially controllable factors (such as inequities experienced by different races); some result from international inequalities in factors not directly concerned with health such as natural conditions; while others result from international practices that harm health more directly, such as through our failure to build worker health and safety protections into our trade agreements. Since many of the causal

factors are socially controllable, it is in our power to remedy these.

Jonathan Wolff makes a case for the strategic value of a human rights approach in contributing to positive global health outcomes. Whatever concerns one might have about the philosophical or theoretical grounds for the approach, it does have an important advantage, namely that in many cases because human rights are objects of actual international agreements, there are some powerful mechanisms of enforcement available for protecting health in certain cases. Illustrating the approach with reference to case law, he shows how and when the approach might prove especially effective. Several other authors discuss the issue of human rights and health – its pitfalls and possibilities. Some are more skeptical about its current usefulness and draw attention to the fact that failure to meet human rights on a grand scale is predominantly the outcome of defects in global legal and economic structural arrangements (see Chapter 19 by Stephen Gill and Isabella Bakker).

The idea of who is responsible for doing what with respect to global health is a key issue and one touched upon by most of the contributors to this volume. Allen Buchanan and Matthew DeCamp offer some useful guidelines in translating our shared obligation to "do something" to improve global health into a more determinate set of obligations. They argue that states in particular have more extensive and specific responsibilities than is typically assumed to be the case, as they are the current primary agents of distributive justice, influential actors in the burden of disease, and indeed have the greatest impact on the health of individuals in our world. But non-state actors (such as the World Trade Organization and global corporations) have important responsibilities as well, which are discussed. Furthermore, institutional innovation is needed to distribute responsibilities more fairly and comprehensively, and to ensure accountability. Some of the determinate obligations they identify for states include avoidance of committing injustice that has health-harming effects, for example not fighting unjust wars abroad or assisting in training military personnel of states likely to use force unjustly. In supporting unjust governments and upholding the state system, we contribute to upholding unjust regimes that have health-harming effects. Simply refraining from such activities could do much to improve global health. As one example they point out that between 2000 and 2006 3.9 million people died in the Congo from war and that every violent death in that war zone was accompanied by no fewer than 62 "non-violent" deaths in the region, from starvation, disease, and associated events.

Solomon Benatar, Abdallah Daar and Peter Singer argue that improving health globally requires an expanded ethical mindset which appreciates that health, economic opportunities, development, peace, and good governance are all linked in our interdependent world. They suggest that such understanding, combined with a set of values that meaningfully respects the dignity of all people, could promote their flourishing more broadly construed than merely in economic terms. Five transformative approaches are outlined: (1) developing a global state of mind about the world and our place in it; (2) promoting long-term (rather than short-term) self-interest; (3) striking a balance between optimism and pessimism about globalization and solidarity; (4) strengthening capacity and commitment to broadening the discourse on ethics through global alliances; and (5) enhancing production and widespread access to public goods for global health. They argue that an expanded moral discourse that goes beyond the notions of individual freedoms and rights to include discourses that promote the idea of economic growth associated with fairer distribution, should comprise the agenda for ambitious multidisciplinary research and action.

Analyzing some reasons for poor health

In Chapter 12 Meri Koivusalo traces the many ways in which trade can and does affect health and vice versa. It is clear that robust interests in trade can undermine health-related priorities and practice. For instance, trade liberalization policies in agricultural products can affect price, availability, and access to basic food commodities that result in less healthy diets for local populations, and related issues of food security. Furthermore, trade liberalization has made available more hazardous substances such as tobacco and alcohol, leading to unhealthy consumption patterns. Poor, developing countries may be more vulnerable to adverse effects of trade liberalization than wealthier ones. We need improved global governance concerning health and trade, which better acknowledges and tackles the wide-ranging effects of trade on health. The call for better global governance in a variety of domains is one that is made by many other authors.

Jeff Rudin and David Sanders explore the origins and factors that perpetuate crippling debt poor

countries owe to the wealthy, focusing especially on structural adjustment programs. They also explore the connection between debt and health and note that the magnitude of the debt owed by poor countries is frequently unpayable, especially in the case of Africa (the poorest continent) and not least because of the ongoing extraction of resources from such countries that intensifies their poverty and reduces their ability to repay debt.

The link between international arms trading and global health is easy to appreciate. In his contribution to this volume, Salahaddin Mahmudi-Azer outlines the socio-economic impact of the global arms trade, with special attention to its undesirable effects on human health and the environment. These adverse impacts include death, injury, and maiming from weapons-use in conflict. There are massive opportunity costs to health, economic development, and human well-being when there is large-scale diversion of resources from health and human services into weapons expenditure. The impact of conflict can be far-reaching and includes important effects on children, such as psychological damage, loss of educational opportunities, destruction of families and nurturing environments, abuse, and the conscription of child soldiers. With trade in weapons growing fast and currently constituting "the largest economy in the world" the effects on human health and well-being are worrisome. He outlines some of the measures currently underway to limit the global arms trade and further measures that could be undertaken, including the role governments and bioethicists might usefully play.

The indirect effects of war on health are often unappreciated, and protracted health crises are often a festering feature of war-torn countries. Samia Hurst, Nathalie Mezger, and Alex Mauron describe the ethical challenges that face such organizations as Médecins Sans Frontières with humanitarian agendas that are driven by a rights-based view of international health. They illustrate how the challenges extend beyond meeting emergency needs to dealing with more protracted crises, and the implications these have for "propping up repressive and irresponsible governments" (Chapter 15). They focus on how resources could be fairly allocated when it is not possible to meet all needs, and they offer a variant of the Daniels and Sabin account of procedural fairness as a plausible option.

The high media profile of humanitarian crises in recent years has attracted resources from wealthy countries. While some of these resources are new, others represent shifts in allocations within only minimally increased Official Development Aid (ODA) budgets. Indeed there have been significant shifts away from projects that may contribute to structural developments with the potential to advance the economies of poor countries, towards humanitarian emergencies and specific health problems – for example HIV/AIDS. Whether or not such aid is effective has been a topic of great controversy in recent years. Overlapping and contesting views have been offered.[3] While it is clear that some impressive short-term gains have been achieved in focused areas (such as HIV/AIDS) it is generally agreed that for a variety of reasons little real development of infrastructure or of economies has resulted from ODA. Anthony Zwi reviews some controversial aspects of ODA, such as trends in the magnitude of such aid, the intentions that lie behind it, possible shortcomings (in particular as ODA relates to global health) and some emerging issues that require attention. He does so by considering the "seven deadly sins" associated with ODA described by Nancy Birdsall. These constitute impatience with institution building, envy among competing donors, ignorance as evidenced by failure to evaluate impact, pride (failure to exit), sloth (using participation to justify ownership), greed (stingy transfers), and foolishness (under-funding of public goods). He focuses his discussion on how these sins impact on health, and concludes with some recommendations for new approaches.

Moving towards macro scale considerations, Sharon Friel, Colin Butler and Anthony McMichael argue that although anthropogenic climate change will affect all human beings, it will affect the poorest and most disadvantaged much more intensely. Their chapter outlines the various ways in which this is likely to come about, and the implications for policy. Some of the pathways that will lead to health inequities include the fact that extreme weather events are likely to increase, resulting in more general destruction, flooding, infectious disease, or food shortages, all of which affect those with fewer resources much more than the better-resourced. Rising sea levels, drought, water insecurity, and human relocation are other mechanisms through which it can be predicted that the more vulnerable will suffer disproportionate effects. Considering that developed countries emitted much of the greenhouse gas that

caused the problem, they will have to take a lead role in solving it. Their inability (and perhaps unwillingness) to forge an agreement to reduce emissions fairly constitutes a major inequity. There is much developed countries can and should be doing here, such as assisting in the provision of affordable, clean household energy in developing countries.

David Benatar observes that concern with global health ethics is invariably limited to ethical issues that pertain to global *human* health, rather than a more expansive notion of global health that includes other species. He argues that this focus is unfortunate, and that we do have duties (whether direct or indirect) concerning non-human animals and the environment. He draws attention to the ways in which human and animal interests coincide and also the ways in which environmental degradation from our mass breeding and consumption of animal products threatens human health. While there is widespread awareness of how destruction of the environment can affect human well-being and health (through processes such as global warming, ozone depletion, and desertification), there is much less awareness of how connected animal and human interests are. Many infectious viral diseases have animal origins, including some of the most recent high-profile ones, such as SARS, HIV, and "swine influenza." Although some animal to human transmission of diseases is probably inevitable, much could be avoided through better treatment of animals, especially keeping them in less crowded, more sanitary conditions. Of course, if humans did not eat them in the first place, fewer animals would be bred for human consumption, and the risks would reduce.

Lying at the heart of many of these upstream causes of poor health is the way in which the global economy operates. Stephen Gill and Isabella Bakker describe three foundational political economy concepts (new constitutionalism, disciplinary neo-liberalism, and exploitative social reproduction) that correspond to some of the dominant historical structures of globalized capitalism. They also discuss three perspectives on capitalism and the current global economic crisis: pure neo-liberalism, compensatory neo-liberalism, and heterodox economics. They then argue that we currently face not only an economic or financial crisis but a more profound organic crisis which reflects the contradictions inherent in "market civilization" characterized as it is by individualistic, consumerist, privatized, and energy-intensive myopic lifestyles. Solving global health challenges will involve, in their view, addressing this more organic crisis. For instance,

---

[3] See, for instance, William Easterly (*The White Man's Burden* 2006), Paul Collier (*The Bottom Billion* 2007), Jeffrey Sachs (*The End of Poverty* 2005), and Dambisa Moyo (*Dead Aid* 2009) for some of this debate.

analyzing the global food crisis and resultant increased global malnutrition, we see multiple factors playing a part, including trends towards greater centralization of ownership and control in the agribusiness industry, and greater enclosure by corporations of food sources once held in common. Diversion of food resources, particularly grain, into biofuel production is of further significance. As with food markets, there is a similar shift to more market-based models in the provision of health care, where health becomes another commodity and there is continuing pressure to devolve the costs (and risks) of health financing, to individuals. They conclude with suggestions for reversing these trends and with the need to identify obstacles to realizing change – for example the tax system.

Shaping the future

As Thomas Pogge notes, about one-third of annual human deaths are traceable to poverty and these are easily preventable through such measures as safe drinking water, vaccines, antibiotics, better nutrition, or cheap rehydration packs. Is there an obligation to alleviate world poverty, and to prevent such deaths? Pogge argues that whatever the merits of the case that we should help more, there is much more clearly an obligation to harm less. How do we currently harm the poor? In multiple ways, he argues. One can challenge the legitimacy of our currently highly uneven global distributive patterns concerning income and wealth, which have emerged from a single historical process pervaded by injustices (such as slavery and colonialism). One might also criticize the dense web of institutional arrangements that we have created, and now fail to reform, which "foreseeably and avoidably" perpetuate poverty. Pogge has argued that the way in which we fail to reform these various institutional arrangements, which foreseeably and avoidably perpetuate massive global poverty, is morally culpable.

Notable among these arrangements are the international resource and borrowing privileges, referred to in several chapters in this volume, which allow whoever holds power to sell the country's resources legitimately (the international resource privilege) and borrow in the country's name (the international borrowing privilege), no matter how power was obtained. These privileges have disastrous effects for developing countries, especially in fostering corrupt and oppressive governments, as they incentivize the seizing of power through illegitimate means and enable the consolidation of that power by providing a steady stream

of resources helpful in maintaining corrupt and repressive regimes.

But these are by no means the only institutional arrangements that perpetuate poverty. The list would also include upholding grossly unjust intellectual property regimes that require all members of the World Trade Organization to grant 20-year product patents which effectively make new medicines unaffordable for most of the world's population. Reforming these unjust "TRIPS" arrangements are the focus of Pogge's chapter.

Advocates of these arrangements often argue that such patents are necessary to compensate innovators for the large investments necessary to develop new drugs. While Pogge is well aware of the need for incentives and rewards to compensate for research and development investment into new drugs, he presents an alternative proposal which can overcome at least seven failings of the present pharmaceutical regime. These include: high prices, neglect of diseases concentrated among the poor unable to afford the high prices for drugs (such as malaria or tuberculosis), a bias towards developing maintenance rather than curative or preventative drugs, massive wastefulness in policing patent law, the illegal manufacture of counterfeit and often ineffectual drugs, excessive marketing, and inattention to ensuring patients are using the drugs in beneficial ways.

The structural reform idea that Pogge offers is for a "Health Impact Fund" (HIF). Financed mainly by governments, this proposed global agency would present pharmaceutical innovators with an alternative option to participate during its first 10 years in the HIF's "reward pool," thereby being entitled to a share of rewards equal to "its share of the assessed global health impact of all HIF-registered products" (Chapter 20). The innovators would have to make the drug widely and cheaply available wherever it was needed, indeed, would be incentivized to do so. Pogge, and an interdisciplinary team, develop the details of the fund, so that it presents a clear alternative to the current regime and one that is not guilty of the seven main failings identified above. Importantly, it provides significant rewards for the development of drugs that would address some of the most widespread global diseases concentrated among the poor, who currently do not have the purchasing power to command the attention of drug developers. Since Pogge has presented a feasible alternative to TRIPs agreements for rewarding drug innovators, our imposition of these regimes on the world's poor is not only harmful but morally culpable, and our failure to reform current regimes is unjust.

Another high profile approach to improving global health is through the Grand Challenges supported by the Bill and Melinda Gates Foundation. These have a specific focus on technological solutions – for example vaccines for HIV and malaria, and new diagnostic technologies. While acknowledging that the role of advances in biotechnology may have been overplayed recently, to the neglect of other powerful determinants of health, Hassan Masum, Justin Chakma and Abdallah Daar credibly explore where and how advances in biotechnology might usefully assist in improving global health. They remind us that while many such advances take a very long time to improve the health of whole populations, the long-term potential of biotechnology should not be underestimated.

It is interesting to note that while massive attention has been directed to providing life-extending treatments to all with HIV/AIDS who need this, much less attention has been directed to the need to provide life-saving food for the millions of people who die from malnutrition. And indeed antiretroviral treatment works best in those who are well nourished.

Lynn McIntyre and Krista Rondeau address the issue of food security and argue for the important connection between food security and global health. They explore five challenges to food security, namely those presented by climate change, pockets of famine, population growth, agricultural production and sustainability, and dietary transition, especially as populations become more urbanized. They also discuss which interventions to address these challenges are likely to be most promising. Prominent among these strategies is the need for investment in agriculture, back to the levels previously common in the 1970s. Agricultural policies, research, and technology should aim to address productivity and poverty alleviation, to enhance capacity for food production. This broad strategy will have different implications for different economies. In middle-income countries this might translate into better integration into market chains while in low-income countries where more staple crops should be produced, the focus might be on more affordable inputs (such as seeds, fertilizer or credit) and improved access to technology.

In her chapter, Gillian Brock examines how reforming our international tax arrangements could be especially important in ensuring that everyone has the prospects for a decent life, which importantly includes enjoying access to decent health care. For every dollar

of aid that goes to assist a developing country, approximately $6–7 (US) of corporate tax evasion flows out. She reviews some current widespread practices that facilitate massive tax escape, such as the use of tax havens, transfer pricing schemes (that allow goods to be traded at arbitrary prices in efforts to suggest large, untaxable losses are being incurred), or practices of non-disclosure of sales prices for resources (that greatly assist corrupt leaders in diverting revenue from developing countries for their own private use). Ensuring adequate revenue collection and tax compliance is important for development and democracy, in addition to ensuring developing countries can adequately fund essential goods such as health care. She also considers some proposals concerning global taxes that have a reasonable chance of success and, in some cases, have already been implemented. The "air-ticket tax," operated by the WHO, which collects revenue to address global health problems such as malaria, tuberculosis and AIDs, is one example.

Tikki Pang draws attention to multiple problems that pervade health research, such as the fact that agendas for health research are largely uncoordinated, fragmented, and heavily influenced by donor agencies. He argues for the need to change the global health research agenda. Properly coordinated and harmonized health research could play an essential role in alleviating the massive problems currently facing the developing world. We need new strategic thinking and he argues that key elements to a new health research agenda would involve inclusiveness in defining priorities, ensuring more equitable access to the benefits of research, and ensuring better accountability in research activities.

An issue that troubles many in developed countries concerned with global health ethics is the way in which clinical research is being increasingly "outsourced" to poor countries with vulnerable populations. Does the severe deprivation in these countries render such activities exploitative? Or, alternatively, by providing some benefits (albeit sometimes small ones) to these people, are we assisting them? Under what conditions is research in developing countries morally defensible? Alex London investigates this issue in his chapter. By outlining his Human Development Approach to international research he argues for a position in which basic social institutions can be expected to advance the interests of all community members. Moreover on this approach, there are obligations to ensure that the results of the research are translatable into sustainable benefits for its population. This entails obligations either to build alliances with those able to translate the research into sustainable benefits or to "locate the research within a community with similar health priorities and more appropriate health infrastructure" (Chapter 25) Instructive examples of research that pass and fail the test are discussed.

Kearsley Stewart, Gerald Keusch and Arthur Kleinman note that debates shaping global health research, ethics and policy have developed along two tracks – one characterized by a neo-liberal approach and another that focuses on human rights, social justice and a broader, more inclusive model of the determinants of health. They argue that these two approaches are now converging around a focus on values. In their chapter they provide a synopsis of papers that emerged from a conference in which participants addressed such questions as: "What values are deeply embedded in the most important global health policies? How do we combine moral philosophy, applied (empirical) bioethics, economics and public health, and engage people in high income countries in work to improve the health of people in resource poor settings?" (Chapter 26) They argue that "an empirically based ethnographic approach may be the best way to effectively bridge local narratives of health with cosmopolitan global health values that shape macro-level policies." (Chapter 26) In support of this proposal they discuss the value of such an approach to resolving the problems that arose between local communities and global interventions in the WHO Global Polio Eradication Initiative in Nigeria.

Jonathan Glover examines the psychology of our attitudes to poverty and he explores some of the moral claims for why we should, but do not, more vigorously assist those in desperate need. In his examination of our tendency towards paralysis he examines the ideas of both physical and moral distance, and beliefs that the problem is insoluble or cannot be addressed by individuals. He rejects many common arguments used to rationalize not assisting, and reminds us of the power of collective action, for example the campaign for debt relief. In examining the moral claims of the poor on the rich he discusses humanitarianism, compensatory justice, and the moral scandal of extreme poverty. He concludes with an examination of how much is required of us and with a recommendation for a sustainable balance between the extremes of limiting our moral obligations to those

closest to us and excessive focus on unachievable moral maximums.

Jim Dwyer engagingly reflects on his experiences of teaching global health ethics. He reviews some of the content of his syllabus, the students' reactions to it, and his own reflections on these experiences. In a particularly useful section he explores a notion of responsiveness to global health injustices and offers guidelines for assisting students in thinking about morally appropriate responses to problems of global health.

In their second chapter, the final chapter in this volume, Bakker and Gill pose the challenge that new paradigms are needed to make the changes required for meaningful improvements in global health. They recommend at least three broad areas that need more attention. First, we should attend better to our interdependencies with each other and with nature. Second, we need to improve socialization of the risks experienced by the global majority. Indeed the public sector needs to be made more accountable to the needs of the public as a whole, and this should be connected to policies that also make private corporations more socially accountable and expects more of them in sharing the costs of the social goods and infrastructure from which many of their activities benefit. Third, we need to develop a new idea of "common sense" by nurturing progressive values. Some of the more particular ideas they consider include a call for new measures "to provide adequate financing to rebuild and extend the social commons with these resting upon a more equitable and broad-based tax system where capital and ecologically unsustainable resource consumption are taxed more than labor" (Chapter 29). The need for new media, more responsive to the diversity of public opinions, is also highlighted as is the need for more critical reflection on orthodox economic thinking.

To improve people's health globally and pursue the goals described in this book will require a considerable amount of collaborative multidisciplinary research and pervasive community engagement at many levels. It is arguable that this challenge is as great as, if not greater than developing an HIV vaccine. If equivalent research resources and intellectual attention were to be allocated to such research, significant progress is entirely possible. While we have considerable intellectual and material resources to improve global health, there is little reason to expect that major new initiatives, such as those envisaged in this text will be implemented without a great deal of effort in mobilizing the political will to do so.[4] However, like Jonathan Glover and others, we retain an element of hope that well-constructed arguments can, on occasion and in the right circumstances, play a significant role in influencing the future. To end on a more optimistic and inspiring note, as Nelson Mandela famously said: "It always seems impossible until it's done."[5]

---

[4] We note here that the topics covered in this volume are by no means fully inclusive of the numerous problems that undermine and aggravate conditions for overcoming global health challenges. For example we have not included chapters on such issues as child labor, use of children as soldiers, trade in sex and drugs, those cultural practices that have serious adverse health effects, pervasive corruption in business and in health care, and widespread Mafia-like organizations that increasingly influence (even control) the lives of many. All of these contribute to global injustices as well.

[5] Inaugural address, 1994.

References

Collier, P. (2007). *The Bottom Billion: Why the Poorest Countries are Failing and What Can Be Done About It.* Oxford: Oxford University Press.

Easterly, W. (2006). *The White Man's Burden. Why the West's Efforts to Aid the Rest Have Done So Much Ill and So Little Good.* Oxford: Oxford University Press.

Moyo, D. (2009). *Dead Aid: Why Aid is not Working and How There is Another Way for Africa.* London: Allen Lane.

Sachs, J. (2005). *The End of Poverty: Economic Possibilities for Our Time.* New York: Penguin Press.

Section 1

Global health, definitions and descriptions

What is global health?

Solomon Benatar and Ross Upshur

Introduction

To profess interest in global health is one of the latest trends in medicine, and many universities, especially in North America, are developing Departments or Centers of Global Health (McFarlane *et al.*, 2008; Drain *et al.*, 2009). The rapidly proliferating spectrum of new organizations, alliances and funds to address global health issues has generated a challenging new "global health landscape"(*Global Health Watch 2* – People's Health Movement, Medact and the Global Equity Gauge Alliance, 2008). But it is neither entirely clear what is meant by "global health," nor how this term is being used by a range of actors.

On the one hand we need to ask if it is: (a) a description of the medically measurable health status of all individuals globally (a medically defined state of affairs); (b) an assertion about (or aspiration to) the state of health of all throughout the world (an activist agenda); (c) about providing medical treatment to all globally who are suffering from medically defined diseases (an extended biomedical approach to health); (d) a description of how health services are, or should be, structured and governed worldwide (a governance of health issue); (e) about measures to improve health governance and reduce disparities in health and health care across the globe (a global social justice issue); or (f) reference to the quest to sustain a healthy planet (an environmental health concern).

On the other hand we could ask if it is merely a new "in vogue" term for what was previously called international health or whether it is truly a recognition of what global health means in a post-Westphalian world in which diseases know no boundaries and the lives of all people are of equal moral worth.

And then of course we need to ask who are the major players setting the agenda in the field – only academics and others in wealthy countries, or also those whose lives and health are adversely affected by unspeakable injustices driven by now recognized seriously flawed economic policies that have sustained and intensified poverty and miserable living conditions for so many?

In this chapter we highlight some of the key conceptual issues involved in situating our contemporary understanding of global health.

Some definitions of health

All definitions of health are potentially contentious. On the one hand such definitions may be too narrow, while on the other they may be too broad. However, some form of definition is required to frame clearly the object of inquiry. Although most definitions of health are contentious, inquiry in the absence of some definition leads to non-transparent reasoning and often fosters argument at cross-purposes. In order to mitigate this possibility, we explicitly provide selected definitions of health before proposing our candidate interpretations of global health.

Individual health. While many refer to individual health narrowly as the absence of disease (usually physical, but also mental), the Alma Ata definition of individual health is much broader (a state of complete physical, mental and social well-being, and not merely the absence of disease or infirmity) (Tejada de Rivero, 2003).

Public health. The definition of public health is also contentious, with some favoring a narrow perspective that "uncouples the etiology of disease from its social roots" Fee & Brown, 2000) and focuses on statistics, epidemiology and measurable proximal risk factors, while others prefer a broader view that does not separate public health from its broad socio-economic context. This broader view is considered to have "intellectual merit" because it identifies the

---

Global Health and Global Health Ethics, ed. Solomon Benatar and Gillian Brock. Published by Cambridge University Press.
© Cambridge University Press 2011.

fundamental causes of many public health problems, and provides more complete and concise explanatory models (Fee & Brown, 2000).

While Verweij & Dawson (2007) have been critical of making definitions of public health so broad that they are impossible to address, Powers and Faden, in their book on the foundations of public health and health policy (Powers & Faden, 2006), have offered an even broader perspective in arguing that:

> the foundational moral justification for the social institution of public health is social justice ... Our account rejects the separate spheres view of justice in which it is possible to speak about justice in public health and health policy without reference either to how other public policies and social environments are structured or to how people are faring with regard to the rest of their lives.

International health has its focus on health across regional or national boundaries and on the provision of health-care assistance in one form or another by health personnel or organizations from one area or nation to another, usually poorer nations (Birn, 2009a). Many of the new Departments and Centers of Global Health in North American universities are focused on such endeavors (Drain *et al.*, 2009).

Global health goes beyond international health to include acknowledgment of the lack of geographic or social barriers to the spread of infectious diseases, and indeed the interconnectedness of all people and all life on a threatened planet. A broad definition of global health could be offered by re-phrasing Winslow's 1920 definition of public health (the notion of which has been discussed in detail by Verweij & Dawson, 2007) and further expanding this.

> Global health is the science and art of preventing disease, prolonging life and promoting physical and mental health through organized global efforts for the maintenance of a safe environment, the control of communicable disease, the education of individuals and whole populations in principles of personal hygiene and safe living habits, the organization of health care services for the early diagnosis, prevention and treatment of disease, and attention to the societal, cultural and economic determinants of health that could ensure a standard of living and education for all that is adequate for the achievement and maintenance of good health.

Global health is thus about health in a world characterized by spectacular medical advances and amazing economic growth but also by aggravation of wide disparities in health and well-being by powerful social forces. Such a world is now under severe threat as evidenced by re-emergence of infectious diseases, resistance to drugs to treat infections that kill millions each

year and most seriously by environmental degradation and climate change that have profound implications for health (Garrett, 1994; Benatar, 2001, 2009; see Friel *et al.*, Chapter 17, this volume). Seeing global health as intimately connected to adverse social and economic forces requires a mind-set shift that seems to have eluded some (Koplan *et al.*, 2009).

Using Richard Lewontin's idea of "biology as ideology" (Lewontin, 1991) we can restate what he has said about science as follows in relation to "global health as ideology":

> Global health is a social concept about which there is a great deal of misunderstanding, even among those who are part of it. Global health work, like other productive activities (for example the state, the family, sport) is a social institution completely integrated into and influenced by the structure of all our other social institutions. Those who work on global health view the topic through a lens that has been moulded by their social experience. Global health work is a human productive activity that takes time and money, and so is guided by and directed by those forces that have control over money and time. People earn their living by "doing global health" and as a consequence the dominant social and economic forces in society determine to a large extent what global health is about and how it is pursued.

Stuckler & McKee (2008) have suggested that there are at least five metaphors that can be applied to global health. *Global health as foreign policy* is driven by political motives with a view to pursuing strategic interests and economic growth. *Global health as security* seeks to protect local populations against infectious diseases and bioterrorism. *Global health as charity* focuses on "victims" and addresses issues of poverty and disempowerment. *Global health as investment* is focused on those whose improved health could maximize economic growth. *Global health as public health* is aimed at decreasing the global burden of disease and focuses on those diseases that constitute the largest proportion of this burden. The authors acknowledge that while there is much overlap in how these are applied, the policies that will be pursued (by the USA and other powerful groups) crucially depend on which metaphor is dominant.

State of health globally

What is generally clear is that despite major progress in medicine and massive growth of the global economy there are wide and widening disparities in health as conventionally measured, with almost 50% of all people in the world lacking access to even the most basic health care, and living greatly deprived lives under conditions of severe poverty and environmental degradation in both rural and urban contexts (*Global Health Watch, 2005–2006*, People's Health Movement, Medact and the Global Equity Gauge Alliance, 2005).

Roughly one-third of all human deaths (18 million annually), are due to poverty-related causes (and 50% of these are children under 5 years of age). People of color, females and the very young are heavily over-represented among the global poor (Pogge, 2009). Life expectancy ranges from about 40 years in such countries as Sierra Leone, Angola and Afghanistan to over 80 years in others such as Japan, Switzerland and Australia.

Africa is the most severely afflicted region. Of over 800 000 deaths globally from malaria each year 91% are in Africa and 85% of such African deaths are in children under 5 years of age. Of 33 million people living with HIV in the world in 2007, 22 million were in Africa. Five million African children under the age of 5 die each year of preventable diseases. Of the estimated 536 000 annual maternal deaths globally, 99% occur in developing countries, including Africa. Globally, there are 963 million who are undernourished; 884 million who lack access to safe water; 2500 million who lack access to basic sanitation; 2000 million who lack access to essential medicines; 924 million who lack adequate shelter; 1600 million who lack electricity; 774 million adults are illiterate and 218 million children are child laborers – all of which are both indicators of poverty and directly or indirectly aggravate poor health. There are data showing that chronic diseases are also increasing globally bringing new challenges to health systems in both rich and poor countries, and there has been a call for a set of grand challenges in global chronic disease management (Daar *et al.*, 2007).

Concerns for the health impact of global warming and other associated dimensions of environmental degradation are increasing. The health of billions of people will be affected by climate change – through direct long-term effects on water security and food chain integrity, population migration and displacement, redistribution of vector-borne diseases, and significant short-term health impacts from catastrophic extreme climatic events (Costello *et al.*, 2009; see Friel *et al.*, Chapter 17, this volume). There are also significant environmental health concerns globally that are not directly associated with climate change such as chemical contamination of food and water supplies and the health effects of persistently accumulating toxic agents and deteriorating air quality. These are all global in nature, but may have differential health impacts worsened by systematic, often remediable, disadvantage of whole populations. Climate change together with competition for resources, marginalization of the majority of people in the world and global militarization have been described as the major threats to world peace (Abbott *et al.*, 2007).

Measuring health

How can we measure or quantify good or poor health? Can poor health be measured entirely through such quantitative metrics as life expectancy, or morbidity and mortality from various diseases, as so popularly portrayed in a succession of World Health Organization (WHO) Annual Reports? Alternatively, should the concept of health and disease also embrace qualitative assessments of the social suffering, for example of raped women, children who are orphaned or abused, those who are displaced refugees or homeless and those who suffer slow painful deaths without palliative care (Benatar, 1997)? How could such suffering best be documented?

Considerable resources have been devoted to the improvement of population-based metrics. The Bill and Melinda Gates Foundation has funded the Institute for Health Metrics and Evaluation at the University of Washington. The mission of this organization is to improve the health of populations by providing the best information. This is a key task. Important questions remain about what the most important health-related information is, who collects it, for what (or whose) purposes and to what ends.

The recently published WHO report on social determinants of health, *Closing the Gap in a Generation*, has many shortcomings (Birn, 2009b) but it does point the way to including several new measures such as access to land rights, social empowerment and gender equity that promise to move measurement beyond the confines of simple epidemiological indicators of morbidity and mortality (Commission on Social Determinants of Health, 2008).

It is essential, moving forward in global health, to engage a wide range of communities to determine what kinds of information they need to improve their health and well-being. The era of "data raiders," where researchers extract data, human tissue and other forms of information from communities for research purposes with no prenegotiated agreement on the ownership of the data, the purposes of its use and any benefits that may or may not accrue to the community should come to an end.

Improving global health

What could contribute most to improving global health? Should we focus on direct processes, such as biotechnological advances, philanthropically provided accessible medical care, improvements in nutrition and living conditions and vaccines? Alternatively, should we focus on indirect processes leading to sustainable improvements to living conditions and the quality of life through creation of a fairer global economic system? If we should include all of these then how could, and how should they be implemented and balanced to ensure optimal short-term and long-term improvements in health?

The problem is that many of these questions remain below our "horizons on health" in an era of high technology medicine accessible to, and desired by, the most privileged among us. Because of these confusions there is also no consensus or clarity regarding how to address the problem of what the goals of medicine, health care and global health should be.

Perhaps what is needed is a comprehensive philosophy of medicine and health care (Pellegrino, 1979). This could integrate at least four central components: (1) clarifying the ultimate purposes and goals of medicine and (2) the concept of agency of health carers, and of recipients of care (individuals, communities and whole populations) that would more easily yield (3) a progressive account of the rightness and wrongness of medical actions, by which we could evaluate (4) consequences, policies, and states of affairs concerning health. Such a new comprehensive philosophy of medicine and health care should also embrace the need for a new curriculum and training agenda for health-care providers in the twenty-first century, and engagement of a wider set of skills and professions in the field of global health in acknowledgment of the complexity of the challenges and the multidisciplinary approaches required to address these.

A range of perspectives on health care

Medicine and health care can be considered and viewed from many different perspectives, each of which may be relevant and necessary but none of which are sufficient on their own. In combination and with overlap they constitute a more nuanced whole.

A technological perspective

Within this notion of health the focus is on research, technological innovation, pharmaceuticals and an evidence-based approach to implementation. The attractiveness of this perspective is that it has contributed greatly to advances in medical practice with very significant advantages to individual patients – for example cardiac surgery, prosthetic joints, sophisticated radiological diagnostic methods, laparoscopic surgical treatments and much more. The disadvantages are that these are costly, they are often introduced before there is adequate evidence of their effectiveness and, more importantly, they are frequently overused and abused (Deber, 2008). As a result these advances are only accessible to a small proportion of people who could benefit, and their impact on the health of whole populations is minimal. Indeed excessive focus on high-cost technological advances can be counterproductive by deflecting attention away from less dramatic treatments and investigations to benefit many more patients.

Examples of the kinds of questions that need to be asked and answered within this perspective are: how many lives are saved by, for example, routine mammography, routine colonoscopy and routine screening for prostate carcinoma, and what are the opportunity costs of such activities in different countries? The emphasis placed on these and other technological innovations needs careful scrutiny.

It may also be time to consider integrating questions about the economic sustainability of new technologies into questions of technology assessment. This would entail incorporating aspects of social justice and priority setting into a new framework for the critical analysis of technologies by using methods akin to cost-effectiveness analysis, and cost–benefit analysis to evaluate the extent to which new technologies improve the welfare of those most disadvantaged as a condition of recommendation for their introduction into routine use.

An economic perspective

Here the focus is on medical care as a commodity predominantly available to those with resources, and within medical care systems driven by the profit motive by investors who view health care as a business. For example, pharmaceutical companies focus on development of new blockbuster drugs attractive to the wealthy or medically insured, while neglecting drugs for diseases of poverty. This perspective is closely linked to the technological focus. Remedies for this inadequate and damaging perspective would entail incorporating aspects of social justice and priority setting into a new framework. The recent work of Thomas Pogge (see Chapter 20, this volume) is an illustration of such innovative thinking and action.

A sociological perspective

Within this perspective, health care is viewed as a caring social institution access to which, like education, is necessary for achieving the human potential (intellectual and physical) and health status required to be satisfied and productive members of society. Here the emphasis is on global public goods (Kaul *et al.*, 1999) and is as much on prevention as on treatment. In relation to global health this perspective requires an understanding of the social determinants of health and disease (Commission on Social Determinants of Health, 2008; see Birn, Chapter 3, this volume) and of the links between the global political economy and health (Navarro, 2007; Benatar *et al.*, 2009; see Gill & Bakker, Chapter 19, this volume). The relevance of social conditions to health is well known from observations on the progressive decline in mortality rates from tuberculosis and other infectious diseases in the UK and the USA, consequent on improved living conditions, long before causative organisms were identified (Koch discovered the tubercle bacillus in 1882) or drug treatments became available (anti-tuberculosis drugs were introduced in 1944) (McKinlay & McKinlay, 1977; McKeown, 1979). Why do we fail to act on such knowledge?

A bioethical perspective

Bioethics focuses attention on the moral appraisal of actions affecting the lives of individuals and communities. It is a discourse devoted to reflection, argumentation and deliberation about the goodness, fairness and justice of human actions and interventions. It brings to bear concepts such as duty, obligation, reciprocity, caring and solidarity as important normative dimensions of any discussion of global health. Without a normative lens, that is a space for the consideration and weighing of what we (individually and collectively) ought to do to secure health goals, global health risks contraction into a simple exercise of measurement and comparison without regard to what possible standard we should seek to achieve for all humans. It is important to ground bioethics in the lives of individuals and communities, lest bioethics become an abstract and remote intellectual exercise of limited value to informing global health.

An existential perspective

Any illness is a potential threat to an individual's existence. As most people are incapable of differentiating mild evanescent illness from life-threatening disease, all illnesses generate anxiety and the need for access to affordable, competent evaluation and care either to restore patients to their normal life trajectory, or to optimize treatment for potentially disabling conditions. The existential threat of illness makes professional medical care a distinctly different need from access to other "commodities," and generates a unique professional role for physicians and health-care workers (Pellegrino, 1979). What illness means to individuals and how it affects their lives is neglected by modern medicine. Narratives of illness provide insights that medical descriptions ignore (Kleinman, 1988; Frank, 1995).

The medicalization and monetization of health

Much of the everyday focus on medicine and health care gives the impression that health is about making more modern medical treatments more widely accessible to more people. An example of this is most vividly illustrated by provision in the USA for anyone and everyone in renal failure to receive renal dialysis. This choice of one specific treatment for one particular human ailment that is made universally available to all within a nation, while other treatments are not, results in many people who are no longer able to enjoy any quality of life being kept alive indefinitely on renal support programs, while many with other diseases whose lives could be greatly improved are denied the basic health care required for productive and meaningful lives. The assumption is that only some forms of medical treatment (often technologically based or profitable) must be provided equitably. It is notable that such decisions, favoring technologically based treatments, are situated within a framework of medicine as a profitable endeavor (most especially to owners of, or investors in health-care facilities) and available predominantly to those who can pay – so equity in access gives way to privileging treatments that are remunerative.

When this value system is extrapolated to global health the goal becomes to increase access to whatever medical treatments are available. So we have a Global Fund focused on making drug therapy available to all who suffer from HIV/AIDS, malaria and tuberculosis, and a series of Grand Challenges with a (necessary but not sufficient) technological focus – but inadequate attention to lack of food, housing, clean water, etc. that drive the spread of such diseases, or to strengthening the infrastructure for providing basic primary health-care services.

In essence this segmented view of health being largely dependent on technological or pharmaceutical advancements is embodied in the latest Institute of Medicine (IOM) report on America's commitment to global health (IOM, 2008). This report makes it clear at the outset that it does not address such factors as food security (or sovereignty), clean water, sanitary measures or gender discrimination and their implications for health, or universal access to basic health care as essential for improved population health. The IOM focus is on American "foreign aid" for HIV/AIDS and other infectious diseases. So attention is drawn to those aspects of health that can be classified medically and treated with medications. It is regressive that a report from such a prestigious institution fails to examine the social determinants of health and disease at a time when the WHO is just beginning to do so – many decades later than it should have done!

This is just one of many examples of the medicalization of global health, increasingly associated with money as the most important bottom line in medicine. While such an approach has great potential to relieve the suffering of many individuals, it neither reveals insight into the extent that more technology and drugs fail to necessarily improve the health of whole populations, nor into knowledge that the global economy is structured to maintain the wealth and health care (often wastefully provided) of those with resources, while extracting human and material resources from poor countries and thus sustaining impoverished lives with little access to health care other than that provided philanthropically (Benatar, 2005).

Perpetuation of this medicalized (and monetized) view of global health while ignoring the powerful upstream forces that profoundly shape the health of whole populations (Sreenivasan & Benatar 2006; see Section 3 of this book) hardly does justice to human intelligence or to America's "vital interest in, or commitment to, global health" (IOM, 2008). Yet a provocative critique of American medicine and a challenge to the US medical establishment to set an example by addressing local and global health issues (Benatar & Fox, 2005) has received little attention.

Many short-sighted responses to the Obama administration's proposal for health-care reform in the USA illustrate the poverty of thought about, and lack of rational attention to, the limits of medicine and of human entitlement (Krugman, 2009; Reinhardt, 2009). Unless we can face up to the realities of life and squarely address what is required to deal with this intelligently, we are doomed to perpetuate old solutions (that do not work) for new problems which we do indeed have the ability to address constructively. The future is not what it used to be! As Benjamin Barber has so eloquently stated, "a revolution in spirit" is required (2009).

How should we think about global health?

In a world in which money is seemingly abundant, and we have so much knowledge that could be used widely to improve human flourishing, we are persisting with clearly failed ways of thinking and wasting limited resources. It would seem that medicine has lost its way as a caring social function, as health care and medical research are predominantly focused on those who can pay while diseases of poverty and affluence relentlessly undermine the lives of many. In the process we are losing the ability to sustain into the future the reproduction of health-care institutions capable of providing the care all need to achieve their potential and to lead decent human lives.

It is time to admit that we live in a world undergoing entropy. The global economic system is collapsing on itself – massive financial losses have severely jeopardized the lives and health of billions. The revealing lesson we learnt recently about our dominant value system and our "civilization," is that within months $17 trillion can be mobilized and pumped into rescuing banks and financial services, but that only $750 billion is pledged for the Millennium Development Goals (MDGs) over a 15-year period (it is unclear that these pledges will materialize) and the Global Fund has difficulty raising $15 billion per year.

Moreover, global security is failing due to an outdated focus on weapons as a means of protection, and neglect of the potential of infectious diseases and of spreading social disruption to cause havoc with the security of all. Finally the quality of our ecological environment is rapidly eroding due to irresponsible consumption patterns that are unsustainable. Within a few hundred years, humankind has moved from being limited by the forces of nature to learning to live with and control nature, and now into an era in which our destruction of nature and animal species seriously threatens future life and health on our planet.

Genuine interest in global health would extend to understanding our relationship with nature and developing a long-term view of human flourishing on a scale that would reflect insight into the need for the new complex goal of developing sustainability in place of the worn-out and failing agenda for sustainable development focused only on economic growth (Bensimon & Benatar, 2006). The central role of the way in which the global economy affects global health must surely now come to the forefront (Birn *et al.*, 2009; Benatar, 2009; see Gill & Bakker, Chapter 19, this volume).

What needs to be done?

Despite the magnitude of the task (seen telescopically) of improving global health it is necessary to concede the need to also see tasks microscopically and to work on solving many specific problems that have the potential to improve the health of whole populations. For example, the use of DDT to kill mosquitoes and the use of impregnated mosquito nets to prevent malaria have both been shown to be highly effective, and vaccines have been instrumental in eliminating smallpox and almost eliminating polio globally. The development of a vaccine to prevent cervical cancer has great potential to reduce morbidity and mortality from this dreaded disease. A malaria vaccine could be equally effective. So research, discovery and delivery through, for example the Gates Grand Challenges, the Malaria Vaccine Enterprise and Global Aids Vaccine Initiative (GAVI) and Global Fund also remain important.

Recent work on understanding the contribution of coordinated, integrated health-care systems to health, wealth and social well-being, provide a basis for evaluating and improving national health-care systems across the globe (see McKee, Chapter 5, this volume). Attention to health security will need to go beyond pandemic planning to include efforts to prevent the accidental release of toxins harmful to whole populations and efforts to combat bioterrorism. Finally much more attention should be directed to other vitally important humanly engineered disasters – to which we now turn.

Addressing human-created problems

One way in which global health can be seen as advancing beyond public health and international health is to engage seriously in addressing global health problems of human creation. Much praiseworthy humanitarian,

public health and international attention is devoted to responding to environmental and natural disasters and relief efforts from civil strife and war that arise from many causes. This type of emergency response is necessary and will no doubt be an important enduring demand-driver for global health efforts. Yet, global health should entail an enduring long-term commitment to redressing failures of human agency. In this regard two particular examples are worth exploring as a means of illustrating this: drug-resistant tuberculosis and water management.

Multidrug-resistant and extensively drug-resistant tuberculosis

Responding to drug-resistant tuberculosis is perhaps one of the most profound ethical challenges facing global health. Drug-resistant tuberculosis is not the result of catastrophic natural forces like earthquakes, tsunamis and hurricanes. It is not caused by malign human intent as are terrorism and war, nor is it fostered by our dysfunctional relationship with the animal kingdom, as are severe acute respiratory syndrome (SARS), and avian and swine influenza. The locus of risk and control is entirely within the human domain. Our response to the emergence of drug-resistant tuberculosis has profound ethical implications as it raises issues of how justice and human rights are realized in our collective response to a disease (Upshur *et al.*, 2009).

Although unpalatable to consider, we are at a watershed in the history of the control of tuberculosis (Fauci, 2007). The progressive worsening of resistance of tuberculosis to pharmacotherapy has raised the specter of a response to tuberculosis without a medical cure – in essence returning us to the situation as it was in the nineteenth century, or, as some have posited, the dawn of the "post-antibiotic age" (Benatar, 1995). Failure to implement a global program in the 1960s and 1970s to eradicate tuberculosis at a cost that was affordable thus accounts for tuberculosis remaining a major problem, with almost 2 million deaths globally every year, and emergence of multidrug-resistant tuberculosis (MDR-TB) costing up to 100 times more to treat per patient than those with drug-sensitive infections, and the possibility that tuberculosis may only be treatable in affluent countries. The combination of high rates of TB infection with high seropositivity rates for HIV in sub-Saharan Africa adds new levels of complexity to diagnosis and treatment and has enhanced the urgency of the need for global tuberculosis control.

It is instructive to note that from almost any perspective, tuberculosis is one of the most well-understood diseases in all of medicine. Understanding tuberculosis has been important historically in constituting the very notion of causality in biology and medicine. In the late nineteenth century, Robert Koch helped explain the concept of causation in infectious diseases, and stated his famous postulates largely on the basis of the study of tuberculosis. Our concept of clinical causality is rooted in randomized clinical trials, of which one of the first and most influential was the Medical Research Council of Britain's streptomycin trial for the treatment of tuberculosis. From Hippocrates to the present day, much of our understanding of clinical medicine, bedside lore and the signs, symptoms and phenomenology of disease arise from our collective experience of tuberculosis.

Our knowledge of the disease is extensive in a multitude of dimensions. We know its genetic fingerprints and its mechanism of resistance at the molecular level; and the social determinants rooted in poverty, adverse living conditions, and social disadvantage are not contested. The social consequences of stigma and how this varies from culture to culture are also well characterized (Verma *et al.*, 2004). There are ample literary allusions to the impact of tuberculosis on human life in the writings of Mann, Dickens and Dostoyevsky. The opera, La Bohème, and Susan Sontag's *Illness as Metaphor*, a significant work of literary criticism, feature tuberculosis prominently. Paleoarcheology has shown that tuberculosis has long been part of the human condition as witnessed in the bones of mummies. Thus, human interaction with the tuberculosis bacillus is long and devoid of mystery. Few other diseases can claim such abundance of human expression. Ubiquitous and well-attended diseases of modernity such as hypertension or cardiovascular disease can lay no such claim to accumulated science and art.

We know tuberculosis well indeed, yet knowing seems not to matter. Tuberculosis has transformed from a curable illness in the 1970s and 1980s to a difficult to treat but still curable condition with the emergence of MDR-TB followed by the WHO's declaration of a global emergency in tuberculosis control in the early 1990s. Now, the new millennium witnesses the emergence of extensively drug-resistant tuberculosis (XDR-TB), which may prove to be untreatable (Iseman, 2007).

The situation is, of course, considerably worse in situations of high TB and HIV burdens. As the recently documented outbreak in Tugela Ferry in South Africa demonstrated, the synergy between resistant TB and HIV is particularly deadly (Singh *et al.*, 2007). This outbreak has also raised some pointed and difficult questions concerning human rights and health as one looks to balance the mission of public health to prevent the transmission of infectious diseases and protect the health of communities against well-established liberties that may be derogated for those with persistent infection (Singh *et al.*, 2007). The initial report granted XDR-TB membership in an exclusive club of particularly deadly pathogens alongside rabies and Ebola virus (Ghandi *et al.*, 2006). Extensively drug-resistant TB has now been reported in over 40 countries, and in Tugela Ferry hospital cases of XDR-TB now outnumber cases of MDR-TB.

These trends are bitter news for those wedded to notions of medical progress and the efficacy of knowledge to control disease. Worse still is the recognition that XDR-TB is largely a human creation, and partly the result of the treatment itself. Pillay and Sturm (2009) demonstrated what many thought to be the case all along: the *Directly Observed Treatment, Short-course* (DOTS) strategy contributes to the development of drug resistance. Indeed, the development of XDR-TB is the predictable and logical consequence of treating TB inadequately in the first place. This merely underscores the existential tragedy that is unfolding every day. A similar fate could await HIV/AIDS treatments in the future (Benatar, 2001).

Our failure to prevent and manage drug resistance in tuberculosis should be transformed into a required lesson for all involved in global health. Reversing the trend of decades of neglect and worsening resistance patterns should be seen as one of the highest priorities of global health. There should be concerted efforts to develop measures across the broad spectra of the causal chains in tuberculosis, building on the substantial evidence base built from the human experience with mycobacterial infections to benchmark progress towards redressing past shortcomings. Failure to stem this regression will only secure the reputation of the global health endeavor as impotent and ineffectual.

Water management

While global warming has assumed precedence as the most significant issue of global environmental health, it should not distract us from collective failures to be good stewards for the most primordial resource crucial to human survival: fresh water.

The WHO estimates that better access to clean water could have dramatic impacts on improving health. A staggering 10% of the global disease burden could be prevented by simple measures such as increasing safe access to water, improving sanitation and hygiene. Currently 1.2 billion people lack regular access to clean drinking water. An additional 2.6 million lack adequate sanitation services. It is estimated that over 2 billion people will be affected by water scarcity by the year 2025 (WHO, 2009).

While there is room for innovation in new technologies to assure potable water, much of the knowledge required for wise stewardship of water resources is readily available. Water shortages, the product of mismanagement, are becoming a challenge in both wealthy and poor world contexts. Large urban centers are struggling to upgrade crumbling infrastructure, often the source of significant water loss. Agricultural and industrial processes lead to contamination of aquifers. Recreational and lifestyle practices divert fresh water to non-essential uses. Soft drink companies buy up water rights in poor countries and sell their products at prices much higher than fresh water.

Perhaps the most poignant, yet unappreciated lesson in water mismanagement has occurred in Central Asia with the disappearance of the Aral Sea. The Aral Sea was once the fourth largest body of water, larger than all of the North American Great Lakes except Lake Superior. In the 1960s Uzbekistan commenced a massive expansion in irrigation to grow cotton. As cotton growth expanded the amount of water withdrawn increased dramatically. From 1960 to 1980 the amount of irrigated land increased from 3 000 000 hectares to 7 600 000 hectares. Irrigation techniques were primitive. Canals were unlined, resulting in massive losses into the desert sands. Evaporative losses were also substantial. Consumptive withdrawals of water greatly exceeded the replacement from the rivers (Glazovsky, 1995).

In the last two decades the Aral Sea has largely disappeared as a body of water, creating a host of health issues and a situation of profound water scarcity for a population of over 5 million people. The Aral Sea disappearance has created an airborne hazard; specifically, the amount of particulate matter has increased. There is pervasive degradation of the physical environment and contamination of the food chain. High concentrations of persistent organic pollutants have been found in cord blood and breast milk. Dioxin levels in food are among the highest recorded. The result is a dystopic ecocide involving a diminution of all elements required for human flourishing, including social and cultural traditions. It should stand as a reminder of the immense fragility of the elements of human life (Small *et al.*, 2001).

What occurred in the Aral Sea region was deliberate and entirely the result of human volition. Similar water mismanagement is occurring globally.

The global political economy

Lying at the heart of all these adverse global health trends and the potential for their reversal is an understanding of how the global economy is structured, and could be modified (see Gill and Bakker, Chapters 19 and 29, this volume).

Conclusions

We return to our broad and ambitious description of global health defined as a social concept about which there is a great deal of misunderstanding, even among those who work on it. Global health work as a field of activity is a social institution that is integrated into and influenced by the structure of other social institutions in particular contexts. Those who work on global health issues tend to view the topic through a lens that has been molded by their social experience. Global health work is thus a human activity that takes time and money, and so is guided by and directed by those forces that have control over money and time. People earn their living by "doing global health" and as a consequence the dominant social and economic forces in society determine to a large extent what global health is about and how it is pursued.

As we outline in Chapter 11, the challenges we face in the twenty-first century are to explore the links between health, human rights, economic opportunities, good governance, peace and development; to understand the implications of how these are all intimately linked within a complex interdependent world. We surely have the responsibility to develop political processes that could harness economic growth to human development, narrow global disparities in health and promote peaceful coexistence globally. This multifaceted "grand challenge" agenda requires the cooperation of scholars from a whole range of widely diverse fields, and the active involvement of many sectors of society – academia, private and public organizations and the media, all working in a cohesive manner to comprehensively research and act to improve human lives globally. Such transdisciplinary processes are the key to success in seeking to improve complex systems.

References

Abbott, C., Rogers, P. & Sloboda, J. (2007). *Beyond Terror: The Truth about the Real Threats to our World.* . London: Random House.

Barber, B. (2009). A revolution in spirit. *The Nation.* January 22. www.thenation.com/doc/20090209/barber//print (Accessed May 7, 2009).

Benatar, S. R. (1995). Prospects for global health: lessons from tuberculosis. *Thorax* **50**, 489–491.

Benatar, S. R. (1997). Social suffering: relevance for doctors. *British Medical Journal* **315**, 1634–1635.

Benatar, S. R. (2001). South Africa's transition in a globalizing world: HIV/AIDS as a window and a mirror. *International Affairs* **77**, 347–375.

Benatar, S. R. (2005). Moral imagination: the missing component in global health. *Public Library of Science Medicine* **2** (12), e400.

Benatar, S. R. (2009). Global health: where to now? *Global Governance* **II**, (2). www.ghgj.org/benatar2.2wherenow.htm

Benatar, S. R. & Fox, R. C. (2005). Meeting threats to global health: a call for American leadership. *Perspectives in Biology and Medicine* **48** (3), 344–361.

Benatar, S. R., Gill, S. & Bakker, I. (2009). Making progress in global health: the need for new paradigms. *International Affairs* **85**, 347–371.

Bensimon, C. A. & Benatar, S. R. (2006). Developing sustainability: a new metaphor for progress. *Theoretical Medicine and Bioethics* **27**, 59–79.

Birn, A.-E. (2009a). The stages of international (global) health: histories of success or successes of history? *Global Public Health* **4**, 50–68.

Birn, A.-E. (2009b). Making it politic(al): closing the gap in a generation: health equity through action on the social determinants of health. *Social Medicine* **4**, 166–182.

Birn, A-E., Pillay, Y. & Holtz, T. (2009). *Textbook of International Health: Global Health in a Dynamic World.* New York: Oxford University Press.

Commission on Social Determinants of Health (2008). *Closing the Gap in a Generation: Health equity through action on the social determinants of health (final report).* Geneva: World Health Organization. Retrieved from: http://whqlibdoc.who.int/publications/2008/9789241563703_eng.pdf.

Costello, A., Abbas, M., Allen, A. *et al.* (2009). Managing the health effects of climate change: Lancet and University College London Institute for Global Health Commission. *Lancet* **373** (9676), 1693–1733.

Daar, A. S., Singer, P. A., Persad, D. L. *et al.* (2007). Grand challenges in chronic non-communicable diseases. *Nature* **450** (7169), 494–496.

Deber, R. B. (2008). Access without appropriateness: Chicken Little in charge? *Healthcare Policy* **4**, 23–29.

Drain, P. K., Huffman, A., Pyrtle, S. E. & Chan, K. (2009). *Caring for the World: a Guidebook to Global Health Opportunities.* Toronto: University of Toronto Press.

Fauci, A. (2007). Action now can halt new TB strains. http://new.tballiance.org/newscenter/view-innews.php?id=655

Fee, E. & Brown, T. M. (2000). The future of public health. *American Journal of Public Health* **90**, 691–692.

Frank, A. (1995). *The Wounded Storyteller.* Chicago, IL: University of Chicago Press.

Gandhi, N. R., Moll, A., Sturm, A. W. *et al.* (2006). Extensively drug-resistant tuberculosis as a cause of death in patients co-infected with tuberculosis and HIV in a rural area of South Africa. *Lancet* **368**, 1575–1580.

Garrett, L. (1994). *The Coming Plague: Newly Emerging Diseases in a World out of Balance.* New York, NY: Farrar, Strauss and Giroux.

Glazovsky, N. F. (1995). The Aral Sea Basin. In J. X. Kasperson, R. E. Kasperson & B. L. Turner II (Eds.), *Regions at Risk: Comparisons of Threatened Environments* (pp. 92–139). Tokyo: The United Nations University Press.

Global Fund to Fight AIDS, Tuberculosis, and Malaria. www.theglobalfund.org/en/

Institute of Medicine (2008). *The US Commitment to Global Health: Recommendations for the New Administration.* Washington, DC: Institute of Medicine, Committee on the US Commitment to Global Health. www.nap.edu/catalog.php?record_id=12506

Iseman, M. D. (2007). Extensively drug-resistant Mycobacterium tuberculosis: Charles Darwin would understand. *Clinical Infectious Diseases* **45**, 1415–1416.

Kaul, I., Grunberg, I. & Stern, M. A. (1999). *Global Public Goods: International Considerations in the 21st Century.* New York, NY: United Nations Development Project.

Kleinman, A. (1988). *The Illness Narratives: Suffering, Healing, and the Human Condition.* New York, NY: Basic Books.

Koplan, J. P., Bond, C., Merson, M. H. *et al.* (2009). Towards a common definition of global health. *Lancet* **373**, 1393–1395.

Lewontin, R. C. (1991). *Biology as Ideology: the Doctrine of DNA.* Concord, ON: Anansi Press.

MacFarlane, S. B., Jacobs, M. & Kaaya, E. E. (2008). In the name of global health: trends in academic institutions. *Journal of Public Health Policy* 19, 383–401.

McKeown, T. (1979). *The Idea of Medicine: Dreams, Images or Nemesis.* Princeton, NJ: Princeton University Press.

McKinlay, J. B. & McKinlay, S. M. (1977). The questionable effects of medial measures on the decline in mortality in the US in the 20th century. *Milbank Memorial Fund Quarterly* 55, 405–428.

Pellegrino, E. D. (1979). Toward a reconstruction of medical morality: the primacy of the act of profession and the fact of illness. *Journal of Medicine and Philosophy* 1, 32–52.

People's Health Movement, Medact and the Global Equity Gauge Alliance (2005). *Global Health Watch 2005–2006.* London: Zed Books.

People's Health Movement, Medact and the Global Equity Gauge Alliance (2008). *Global Health Watch 2: An Alternative World Health Report.* London: Zed Books.

Pillay, M. & Sturm, A. W. (2007). Evolution of the extensively drug-resistant F I5/LAM4/KZN strain of Mycobacterium tuberculosis in KwaZulu-Natal, South Africa. *Clinical Infectious Diseases* 45, 1409–1414.

Powers, M. & Faden, R. (2006). *Social Justice: The Moral Foundations of Public Health and Public Health Policy.* New York: Oxford University Press.

Singh, J. A., Upshur, R. & Padayatchi, N. (2007). XDR-TB in South Africa: no time for denial or complacency. *PLoS Med* 4(1), e50.

Small, I., Van de Meer, J. & Upshur, R. E. G. (2001). Acting on an environmental health disaster: the case of the Aral Sea. *Environmental Health Perspectives* 109 (6), 547–549.

Sreenivasan, G. & Benatar, S. R. (2006). Challenges for global health in the 21st century: some upstream considerations. *Theoretical Medicine and Bioethics* 27, 3–11.

Stuckler, D. & McKee, M. (2008). Five metaphors for global health. *Lancet* 372, 95–97.

Tejada de Rivero, D. (2003). Alma Ata Revisited. *Perspectives in Health Magazine.* The Magazine of the Pan American Health Organization 8 (2). www.paho.org/english/DD/PIN/Numberl7_articleI_4.htm

Upshur, R., Singh, J. & Ford, N. (2008). Apocalypse or redemption: responding to XDRTB. *Bulletin of the World Health Organization* 87, 481–483.

Verma, G., Upshur, R. E., Rea, E. & Benatar, S. R. (2004). Critical reflections on evidence. ethics and effectiveness in the management of tuberculosis: public health and global perspectives. *BMC Medical Ethics* 5, E2.

Verweij, M. & Dawson, A. (2007). The meaning of "public" in public health. In A. Dawson & M. Verweij (Eds.), *Ethics, Prevention and Public Health.* Oxford: Oxford University Press.

World Health Organization. *Ten Facts About Water Scarcity.* Geneva: World Health Organization. www.who.int/features/factfiles/water/en/index.html (Accessed August 10, 2009).

Chapter

2

The state of global health in a radically unequal world: patterns and prospects

Ronald Labonté and Ted Schrecker

Introduction

Sir Michael Marmot, who chaired the World Health Organization (WHO) Commission on Social Determinants of Health, has identified the need to seek "public policy based on a vision of the world where people matter and social justice is paramount" (Marmot, 2005, p. 1099). In this chapter, we ground this imperative in evidence of dramatic disparities in health status that are traceable, in large measure, to the globally unequal distribution of resources necessary for health. We further outline the contours of an international economic and political order that often magnifies those inequalities, and conclude that the imperative of mobilizing resources to protect health on a much larger scale than at present is central to any global health ethics worthy of the name.

"If living were a thing that money could buy"

Imagine for a moment a series of disasters that killed almost 1400 women every day for a year: the equivalent of four or five daily crashes of crowded long-distance airliners. There is little question that such a situation would quickly be regarded as a humanitarian emergency, as the stuff of headlines, especially if ways of preventing the events were well known and widely practised in some parts of the world. However, remarkably little attention is paid outside the global health and human rights domains to complications of pregnancy and childbirth that kill more than 500 000 women every year – a cause of death now almost unheard-of in high-income countries (HICs). A Canadian woman's lifetime risk of dying from complications of pregnancy or childbirth is 1 in 11 000. For a woman in Niger, one of the world's poorest countries, it is 1 in 7 and for the developing world as a whole 1 in 76 (Say *et al.*, 2007).

This is one example among many of the health contrasts between rich and poor worlds. Average life expectancy at birth (LEB) worldwide has been estimated at 28.5 years in 1800, much of the short average lifespan caused by high rates of death in the early years of life. By the end of the twentieth century, worldwide average LEB had increased to roughly 67 years (Riley, 2005), due in large measure to reductions in infant and child mortality. However, global progress conceals large variations between countries. For example, Canadians born today can expect to live to the age of 80, a figure that is among the world's highest. In countries classified by the World Bank as low-income, where nearly a billion of the world's people live, estimated LEB averages 59 years. In Zambia, one of several such countries ravaged by the AIDS epidemic, LEB has dropped to 45 years from a peak of more than 50 years in the 1980s (World Bank, 2009, accessed December 14, 2009).

Differences in the prevalence of specific diseases are even more dramatic. Although AIDS was first identified in HICs, more than 95% of new HIV infections now occur outside those countries, with the highest prevalence rates in sub-Saharan Africa, accounting for two-thirds of the world's infected population and an estimated 1.4 million of the 2.0 million annual deaths from AIDS (UNAIDS, 2009). Malaria and tuberculosis have been almost entirely vanquished in HICs. Elsewhere in the world they continue to kill almost a million and more than 1.7 million people per year, respectively (United Nations, 2009), despite the demonstrated effectiveness of relatively low-cost solutions.[1] Health disparities between rich and poor countries involve not only differences in

---

[1] An exception involves increasingly prevalent drug-resistant strains of tuberculosis in all countries of the

Global Health and Global Health Ethics, ed. Solomon Benatar and Gillian Brock. Published by Cambridge University Press.
© Cambridge University Press 2011.

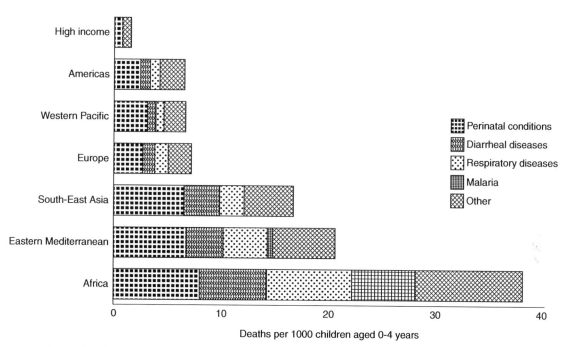

Figure 2.1 Annual deaths per 1000 infants and children (age < 5) by WHO region and major cause of death, with all high-income countries grouped separately.
Source: World Health Organization, Global Burden of Disease 2004 Update: Selected figures and tables (Powerpoint slides); www.who.int/entity/healthinfo/global_burden_disease/GBD2004ReportFigures.ppt. Used with permission.

the kinds of illnesses that affect their populations, but also the ages at which illness and death occur. Of the 49.4 million deaths in low- and middle-income countries (LMICs) in 2002, 21% occurred among children under 5 years of age; in the HICs, of 7.9 million deaths in the same year, just 1% occurred among children under 5 (Mathers, 2010). Although the worldwide statistical risk of child death declined steadily through the last decades of the twentieth century, far more substantial gains could have been achieved. In 2006 nearly 10 million children died before reaching the age of 5. All but 100 000 of these deaths occurred outside the industrialized countries, most of them from causes that are either extremely uncommon in those countries or rarely result in death there (Bryce *et al.*, 2005b; UNICEF, 2008b). Figures 2.1 and 2.2 show the far higher overall death rate among both children and adults outside HICs, but also the difference in causes of death.

world. However, the spread of those strains is itself largely attributable to a history of inadequate provision of the resources necessary for vaccination and treatment using first-line drugs in LICs (Coker, 2004).

Deprivation and economic gradients

The intuitive and largely accurate explanation for these differences involves poverty and material deprivation. On the best available estimates more than a billion people in the world were chronically undernourished as of 2009 (United Nations Food and Agriculture Organization, 2009); this figure refers only to long-term insufficiency of caloric intake, and not to a variety of micronutrient deficiencies some of which are even more widespread. According to one WHO estimate, underweight and other nutritional risk factors, including "suboptimal" breastfeeding, "were together responsible for an estimate 3.9 million deaths" in children under 5, and "[i]n low-income countries, easy-to-remedy nutritional deficiencies prevent 1 in 38 newborns from reaching age 5" (World Health Organization, 2009a, p. 13). This is a substantial underestimate of the overall contribution of inadequate nutrition to illness, since (for example) maternal undernutrition during pregnancy affects the health status of mothers as well as their children, and undernutrition almost certainly increases adult vulnerability to HIV infection and to a range of other

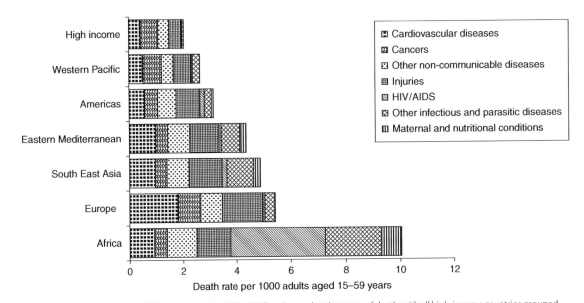

Figure 2.2 Annual deaths per 1000 adults (age 15–59) by WHO region and major cause of death, with all high-income countries grouped separately.
Source: World Health Organization, Global Burden of Disease 2004 Update: Selected figures and tables (Powerpoint slides); www.who.int/entity/healthinfo/global_burden_disease/GBD2004ReportFigures.ppt. Used with permission.

communicable diseases, as well as exacerbating their effects (Bates *et al.*, 2004; Stillwaggon, 2006).

Economic deprivation creates situations in which the daily routines of living are themselves hazardous. Charcoal or dung smoke from cooking fires is a major contributor to respiratory disease among the world's poor (Ezzati & Kammen, 2002). In the fast-growing cities of the developing world close to a billion people now live in slums, as defined by UN Habitat, with resulting exposure to multiple environmental hazards (Unger & Riley, 2007); the number will increase to 1.4 billion in 2020 in the absence of effective policy interventions (Garau *et al.*, 2005). Lack of access to clean water is a major contributor to infectious diarrhea and a variety of parasitic diseases (Prüss-Üstun *et al.*, 2008), yet an estimated 1.1 billion people lack access to clean water and 2.6 billion have no access to basic sanitation (United Nations Development Program, 2006). A further dimension of the role of material deprivation involves the lack of resources to access health care. At the individual level, the need to pay for health care pushes an estimated 100 million people into poverty every year (van Doorslaer *et al.*, 2006; Xu *et al.*, 2007); at the national level, many low-income countries (LICs) are simply unable to mobilize the resources needed for minimal health care from domestic sources. Ironically, both dynamics

have often been worsened by health sector "reforms" actively promoted by high-income countries (Lister & Labonté, 2009).[2]

In many respects, then, the words of the folk song "All My Trials" (made famous by Joan Baez) ring true: living is a thing that money can buy; the rich do live, and the poor do die. In addition to such national differences, socioeconomic gradients in health status – inverse correlations between health status and various indicators of socioeconomic status – are almost universal within national and subnational boundaries, in countries rich and poor alike. Figure 2.3 shows such gradients in mortality among children under 5 (U5MR): children in the poorest fifth of the population in five largely dissimilar developing countries are at least twice as likely to die before their fifth birthday, and sometimes three times as likely, as children in the richest fifth. In India alone 1.4 million child deaths would be prevented

---

[2] We recognize the importance of poor governance (including corruption) and low public spending on health in many LMICs, which compound the problems of medical poverty and inadequate health-care coverage; at the same time, these dynamics cannot be separated from those of globalization discussed later in this chapter.

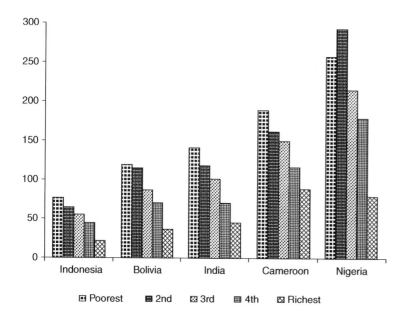

Figure 2.3 Under-5 mortality by income quintile, selected countries, c. 2000.
Source: Data from Gwatkin *et al*. (2007).

each year if U5MR for the entire Indian population were reduced to the level characteristic of its richest quintile (Commission on Social Determinants of Health, 2008, p. 29).

Socioeconomic gradients reflect not only daily conditions of life and work, but also economic influences on access to health services: for example, dramatic income-related disparities are observed in access to the skilled birth attendance that is critical to reducing maternal mortality and avoiding postpartum complications (UNICEF, 2008a). Socioeconomic gradients are widespread in high-income countries, as well. The "eight Americas" study in the USA, where racial and economic inequalities tend to be superimposed on one another, found that the life expectancy of African–Americans in "high-risk" urban counties is almost 9 years shorter than that of the mostly white residents of "Middle America" (Murray *et al*., 2006). In the words of the authors, "tens of millions of Americans are experiencing levels of health that are more typical of middle-income or low-income developing countries" (Murray *et al*., 2006, p. 9). This point was emphasized in a famous study (McCord & Freeman, 1990) that found young men in Harlem, an overwhelmingly African–American area of New York City, had a lower LEB than the national average for men in Bangladesh. Within individual metropolitan areas of the USA and the UK, even larger health disparities than those found in the eight Americas study can be

observed between rich and poor districts: close to 20 years in Chicago and Washington, DC and 28 years in Glasgow (Wang, 1998; Commission on Social Determinants of Health, 2008, pp. 31–32).

Growth (and wealth) are not enough

Discussions of global health ethics must avoid the simplistic leap from this set of observations to the conclusion that greater wealth through economic growth is the surest route to better health – and, therefore, that improvements in population health are best achieved by policies that promote economic growth. Superficial support for the growth → wealth → health causal pathway comes from a widely cited graph known as the Preston curve, after the economist who first drew it (Figure 2.4 shows the curve for the year 2000). The graph represents most of the world's countries with a circle, the area of which is proportional to the size of the country's population. The vertical axis shows average life expectancy at birth, and the horizontal axis shows the country's Gross Domestic Product (GDP) per capita, adjusted for purchasing power. The trend line on the graph shows the national average life expectancy that would be anticipated at a given level of GDP per capita, based on a population-weighted average of all the national data. The graph shows strong returns to economic growth in terms of LEB at low per capita incomes, up to about US$5000. Above that point, only a weak and inconclusive relation between LEB and

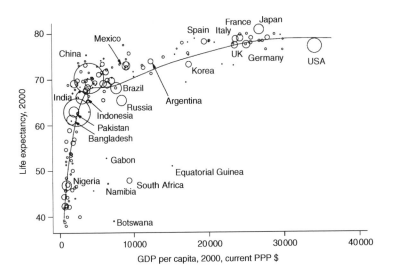

Figure 2.4 The Preston curve for the year 2000. Reproduced with the permission of the author and the American Economics Association, from Deaton (2003, p. 116).

wealth is evident.[3] However, wide variations exist in LEB among countries with comparable levels of GDP/capita. For example, in 2007 LEB in the USA, with a Gross National Income (GNI)/capita[4] of more than $45 000 was 78 years; it was also 78 years in Chile and 79 in Costa Rica, countries with GNI/capita of $12 280 and $10 510, respectively. Conversely, some countries do far less well in terms of LEB than one might expect given their income levels. The most conspicuous outliers in this respect are countries in sub-Saharan Africa where life expectancy has been drastically reduced by the AIDS epidemic. Thus, LEB in Zambia of 45 years in 2007 – a figure comparable to LEB in England in the 1840s – was more than 20 years lower than that in Bangladesh, a comparably poor country but one where AIDS is not a substantial contributor to the burden of disease; LEB in South Africa and Burundi was 50 years, despite the fact that South Africa's GNI/capita was 25 times Burundi's. Indeed, one of Preston's original conclusions was that "[f]actors exogenous to a country's level of income probably account for 75–90% of the growth in life expectancy for the world as a whole between the 1930s and the 1960s. Income growth per se accounts for only 10–25%" (Preston, 2007, p. 486; original publication 1975).

Medical advances and political choices

Two sets of factors explain much of the remainder. The first set comprises advances in medical treatment and preventive health measures: antibiotics, immunization, pesticides and bed-nets to limit exposure to mosquitoes that transmit malaria. In other words, the trend line of the Preston curve moves upward on the graph over time.[5] The second set of factors involves the extent to which countries use their available resources in ways that result in widely shared improvements in health status for their populations – including access to advances in treatment and prevention. At the high end of the national income spectrum, the USA not only is characterized by high and rising disparities in health status (Braveman & Egerter, 2008) but also underperforms in terms of national average LEB because of such inter-related phenomena as high homicide rates, high and rising rates of poverty and economic inequality, and a substantial proportion of its population that lacks health insurance. Conversely Sri Lanka, Costa Rica and the Indian state of Kerala are often cited as overperformers in population health status despite low GNI/capita and because of their provision of accessible primary health care and other social protection measures (Halstead *et al.*, 1985; Riley, 2008).

Based on such examples Deaton (2006, p. 3) concludes that: "Economic growth is much to be desired

---

[3] The same is not necessarily true for more nuanced indicators of health status such as chronic disease prevalence or limited functioning as a result of work-related disability (to give but two examples); mortality-based indicators are intrinsically crude.

[4] GNI is a measure now widely used in preference to GDP. All figures cited are adjusted for purchasing power.

---

[5] Readers can observe an animated demonstration of this effect, and of many of the variations discussed in this section of the chapter, in a graph generated on the Gapminder web site (http://tinyurl.com/ye7vhyb).

because it relieves the grinding material poverty of much of the world's population. But economic growth, by itself, will not be enough to improve population health, at least in any acceptable time … As far as health is concerned, the market, by itself, is not a substitute for collective action." That collective action pertains not only to the second set of factors (how countries allocate resource priorities and distribution), but also to the first set of factors (publicly financed or supported innovations in health knowledge, technology and global diffusion). Deaton points out that most health innovations that contributed to the global convergence in health in the last half of the last century, which has now been replaced by divergence (Moser et al., 2007), originated in wealthier countries. "In this sense, the first world has been responsible for producing the global public goods of medical and health-related research and development from which everyone has benefited, in poor and now-rich countries alike" (Deaton, 2004, p. 99). In the last 20 years, however, companies in high-income countries have led a push for worldwide expansion of intellectual property protection, notably in knowledge-based industries such as information technology and pharmaceuticals. This has led to the emergence of one of the most contentious issues in contemporary global health: that of access to essential medicines and other health technologies.

How health risks are distributed

A further complication of the relation between economic growth and health involves how growth influences the nature and distribution of risks to health. It was once argued that countries experienced a relatively standardized "epidemiological transition" as they grew richer, in which infectious or communicable diseases (disproportionately affecting children) declined while chronic diseases (disproportionately affecting adults) increased (Omran, 1971). Although still useful, the concept only partially captures a pattern in which LMICs are increasingly affected by a "double burden of disease," as persistent or resurgent communicable diseases coexist with rapid increases in non-communicable diseases such as cardiovascular disease, diabetes and cancer. Figure 2.2 shows that the combined death rate from cardiovascular disease and cancer in sub-Saharan Africa is comparable to that in the high-income countries; their proportional contribution to mortality in that region is lower only because of the toll taken by other causes of death.

On one estimate, 100 million men in China alone will die from smoking-related diseases between 2000 and 2050 (Zhang & Cai, 2003). Additionally, road traffic accidents kill an estimated 1.2 million people a year; WHO projects that the number will double by 2030 given current trends, mostly as a result of increases in LMICs (World Health Organization, 2009b). Ironically, those most likely to be injured are the poor, who are least likely to own a vehicle – a distribution of risks that is sometimes exacerbated by planning practices that favor high-speed roads for the emerging middle classes. In many cases, additional hazards are associated with exposures to industrial or motor vehicle pollution and dangers in the industrial or agricultural workplace. Birn et al. (2009, chapter 6) have suggested that it may be useful to replace the familiar categories of communicable and non-communicable diseases with a threefold typology: diseases of marginalization and deprivation, such as diarrhea, neglected tropical diseases, malaria, respiratory infections; diseases of modernization and work, such as cardiovascular disease, cancer, road traffic injuries; and diseases of marginalization and modernization, such as diabetes, chronic obstructive pulmonary disease (COPD), tuberculosis, HIV/AIDS. Socioeconomic gradients are observable with respect to all three categories of disease, including those widely regarded as "diseases of affluence" (Ezzati et al., 2005).

The significance of the double burden of disease concept is illustrated by the coexistence of undernutrition with rapid growth of overweight and obesity in LMICs: indeed, in some instances, of undernutrition and overnutrition in the same household (Popkin, 2002). Reflecting a "nutrition transition" involving a rapid shift to diets higher in fats, caloric sweeteners and meat coupled with reductions in physical activity (Popkin, 2009), overweight and obesity in several middle-income countries are approaching the levels seen in countries like the USA. An especially striking study involves a sample of women in regions that account for more than 70% of Brazil's population. In 1975, almost twice as many Brazilian women were underweight as were obese; by 1997, the proportions had reversed, with the increases in obesity concentrated among low-income women (Monteiro et al., 2004). The emergence of this socioeconomic gradient is a broader trend in Brazil (Monteiro et al., 2007) and in many other LMICs (Popkin, 2008).

An equally disturbing observation is that the prevalence of overweight and obesity in many cases is increasing far more rapidly than it did in the high-income countries decades earlier (Popkin, 2006), setting the stage for future increases in cardiovascular disease and diabetes that will widen existing health disparities. These developments, in turn, must be understood with reference to urbanization and its effects on dietary choices and physical activity (Mendez & Popkin, 2004) and various aspects of globalization. The lowering of barriers to trade and cross-border investment has facilitated consolidation of power over food systems in the hands of supermarkets at the top of global commodity chains; led to increased foreign direct investment in supermarkets and fast-food chains; and lengthened the reach of transnational marketing campaigns featuring brands such as McDonald's and Coca-Cola (Hawkes, 2005; Hawkes *et al.*, 2009). Mexicans are now the world's leading consumer of Coca-Cola products, drinking roughly 50% more per person than people in the USA (The Coca-Cola Company, 2009).

Globalization, markets and health in an unequal world

Globalization, defined here as "[a] pattern of transnational economic integration animated by the ideal of creating self-regulating global markets for goods, services, capital, technology, and skills" (Eyoh & Sandbrook, 2003), presents broader challenges as well, starting with the "inherently disequalizing" character of global markets (Birdsall, 2006): they reward those

countries, and economic elites within them, already well endowed with financial assets and economically productive factors while operating according to rules that are shaped to magnify these advantages.

The first dynamic is exemplified by the fact that hedge fund managers, the quintessential players on global financial markets, now draw multibillion-dollar annual incomes (Taub, 2008) against a background of only modest reductions in global poverty rates over three decades during which the value of the world's economic product quadrupled (Chen & Ravallion, 2008). Descriptions of global economic inequality tend to be highly abstract; Figure 2.5 is a visual presentation of the distribution of income within and among the world's countries. In Figure 2.5, countries are allocated a number of rows of columns based on their population; so each column represents approximately one million of the world's people. Countries are ordered from poorest to richest along the left-to-right axis; for each 10 million people, income is ordered in deciles (10 columns of one million each) along the front-to-back axis. The vertical axis shows income per capita, after adjustment for purchasing power. Although intracountry income disparities are large even in some countries that are relatively poor as ranked by income per capita – an internal disparity that would be far more dramatic if we could visually depict, say, the top 1% or 0.1% of income earners in each country – the commanding heights of the worldwide income distribution are occupied by rich people in rich countries. "In 2005 [when the original version of this graph was published] the top one-tenth of US citizens [received]

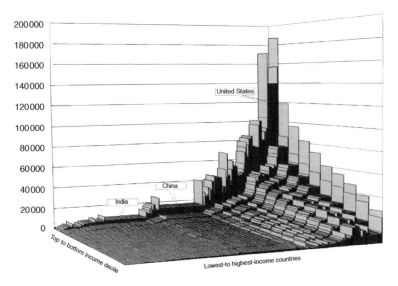

Figure 2.5 Global income distribution: the world is *not* flat. Annual income (adjusted for purchasing power parity) by income decile, 140 countries, 2008.
Source: Graph generated by Bob Sutcliffe © 2009. Used with permission.

a total income equal to that of the poorest 2 200 000 000 citizens in the world" (Sutcliffe, 2005, p. 12). Wealth is more concentrated than income, within countries and globally (Davies *et al.*, 2008), and as noted the tendency of global markets is to increase the concentration of both; this tendency is not beyond the ability of national policies to reverse, although efforts to do so often confront formidable domestic opposition.

Birdsall's second dynamic is illustrated by the development of a multilateral trade regime with intellectual property provisions driven by the interests of major US pharmaceutical and information technology corporations (Sell, 2003), and the rise in bilateral "strong-arming" negotiations to increase access to developing country markets given the slow pace of negotiations in multilateral trade talks (where developing countries have more combined bargaining power). More generally, and as noted in other chapters in this volume, globalization as it has emerged over the past few decades was actively promoted by the governments of major G7 powers, acting on their own and through multilateral institutions like the World Bank and the International Monetary Fund (IMF); by transnational corporations that now routinely reorganize production across multiple national borders; and by owners of financial assets who can now shift them across national borders in search of higher returns and lower risks, often destabilizing national economies and plunging millions into poverty as a result.[6] In many cases, notably the structural adjustment programs demanded by the World Bank and IMF as the condition for loans that would enable governments to maintain their ability to borrow on international markets, the results included increased economic inequality and a decline in the ability of governments to meet basic health-related needs. Such measures generated social and economic conditions that may have contributed to the spread of HIV infection in Africa (De Vogli & Birbeck, 2005). Similar economic "shock therapy," applied to the former Soviet Union, contributed to economic decline that reduced male life expectancy, in particular, as GDP shrank by roughly 50% with drastic increases in poverty and economic inequality (Field *et al.*, 2000). If health was considered at all in such macroeconomic prescriptions, it

was on the basis described by a team of World Bank economists writing about the former Soviet Union and its Eastern European satellites: that "In the long run, the transition towards a market economy and adoption of democratic forms of government should ultimately lead to improvements in health status ... In the short run, however, one could expect that health status would deteriorate" (Adeyi *et al.*, 1997, p. 133). As in other cases, the anticipation of long-term gains is better understood as an expression of faith than as an evidence-based assessment.

As an empirical test of the performance of globalization in delivering health benefits over the first two decades (1980–2000) of intensified economic integration, Cornia and colleagues (2008) carried out an innovative econometric exercise based on data from 136 countries in which they first identified five main influences on mortality: (i) material deprivation; (ii) psychological stress; (iii) unhealthy lifestyles; (iv) inequality and lack of social cohesion; and (v) medical progress: the variable identified by Preston and Deaton as the primary influence on worldwide life expectancy during an earlier period. They then described a range of variables that affect these influences, classifying them as either (a) related to policy choices made in the context of globalization (e.g. income inequality, immunization rates); (b) endogenous, and therefore unrelated to globalization for purposes of the analysis (medical progress); or (c), describable as "shocks" (e.g. wars and natural disasters, HIV/AIDS). The final stage of their analysis consisted of a simulation that compared trends in LEB over the period 1980–2000 with those that would be predicted based on a counterfactual set of assumptions in which trends in all the relevant variables did not follow the actual 1980–2000 pattern, but rather remained at the 1980 value or continued the trend they followed over the pre-1980 period. Thus, it was assumed in the counterfactual (for instance) not only that income distribution within countries, one of the globalization-related variables, did not change over the period 1980–2000, but also that there was no progress in medical technology and that HIV incidence remained at its 1980 level.

This simulation indicated that, on a worldwide basis over the period 1980–2000, (a) globalization cancelled out most of the progress toward better health (as measured by LEB) attributable to the diffusion of medical progress, and (b) the effects of shocks (wars, natural disasters and AIDS) combined with globalization resulted in a slight worldwide decline in LEB as

[6] Due to space limitations, we are unable to provide citations to the extensive social science literature on the global marketplace. Readers are referred to our earlier published work, in particular Labonté & Schrecker, (2007) and Labonté *et al.* (2009).

compared with the counterfactual. Globalization's most conspicuous effects on LEB occurred in the transition economies and the former Soviet Union (where globalization accounted for essentially the entire decline) and sub-Saharan Africa (where globalization contributed almost as much as the AIDS epidemic). Although data limitations mean that "the establishment of a causal nexus between globalization policies and health cannot be but tentative" (Cornia *et al.*, 2008, p. 1), the study nonetheless represents a remarkable rebuttal of claims about globalization's health benefits to date, notably including the performance of the "growth superstars," India and China (Cornia *et al.*, 2008, p. 31). Its authors emphasize that "the negative association noted between liberalization-globalization policies, poor economic performance and unsatisfactory health trends … seems to be quite robust" (Cornia *et al.*, 2008, p. 36).

Long-term benefits?

It can always be argued that the longer-term benefits of integration into the global marketplace have simply yet to materialize; growth should eventually generate resources to improve health for all. But against the background of lost development progress that followed the financial crisis of 2008 (World Bank & International Monetary Fund, 2009, chapter 1), this might be called the *Waiting for Godot* approach to population health. Even before the crisis, the issue identified in passing by Deaton was an urgent one from an ethical point of view: how long should the majority of the world's people be asked to wait for the presumed benefits of globalization to reach them? As Thomas Pogge has pointed out in his important work on poverty and global justice, it is not difficult to envision alternative sets of economic and political institutions that would not involve long periods of pain in anticipation of health gains at some indeterminate point in the future (Pogge, 2002, 2007). A focus on the institutions of the global marketplace is also necessary because – although the point cannot be pursued further here – globalization has probably created major obstacles to countries wishing today to emphasize widely shared improvements in human welfare and the redistributive policies that bring these about. Foreign investors and the purchasers at the top of global commodity chains for manufactured products demand cost containment and "flexible" labor regimes; a liberalized financial marketplace facilitates capital flight in anticipation of higher taxation; and trade policies limit countries' ability to favor domestic producers

while enforcing intellectual property protections, few of which existed when the high-income countries were starting their path to riches.

Prospects for the future: money matters

Despite the uncertainties created by globalization, some efforts to improve the health status of people outside the metaphorical castle walls have succeeded in recent years. Improvements in vaccination coverage have reduced measles deaths from more than 700 000 in 2000 to an estimated 164 000 in 2008 (Dabbagh *et al.*, 2009). At the end of 2008, 4 million people were receiving antiretroviral therapy for AIDS in low- and middle-income countries, a tenfold increase over 7 years, although still a long way from WHO's stated goal of universal coverage (World Health Organization, UNAIDS & UNICEF, 2009). Conversely, despite abundant evidence on the effectiveness and cost of the relevant interventions, only limited progress has been made in reducing maternal mortality – within the limits of available data, none in sub-Saharan Africa, where it is highest (United Nations, 2009) – and progress in reducing child mortality remains far inferior to what could have been achieved based on available evidence (Bryce *et al.*, 2005a). An extensive list exists of demonstrably effective interventions to improve maternal and child health (Bryce *et al.*, 2005b; Bhutta *et al.*, 2008). Meeting the challenge of improving the availability of these interventions will require strengthening the public-sector health systems that are essential to deliver them. This is a formidable task, particularly since it often entails not only addressing the "brain drain" of health professionals from LICs but also, more generally, repairing damage done by long periods of underfunding that were driven in part by the imperatives of globalization.

Although detailed analysis is beyond the scope of this chapter, the success stories cited in the preceding paragraph depended on effective and sustained mobilization of financial and other resources, both domestically and internationally. Apprehensions are being expressed about the availability of resources to continue these initiatives in the future (Dabbagh *et al.*, 2009), with one US commentator referring to antiretroviral therapy as a "ballooning entitlement burden" (Over, 2008). According to recent estimates, the value of all public development assistance for health increased from $4.15 billion in 1990 to $14.08 billion in 2007

(Ravishankar *et al.*, 2009). By contrast, one assessment of the need for such assistance is based on estimates by the World Health Organization's Commission on Macroeconomics and Health of the cost of financing basic health care and preventive interventions in all LICs: $40/person/year, in 2007 dollars (Sachs, 2007a). *Even if* all the world's low-income countries were to commit 15% of their general government expenditures to health – and many governments' spending on health is well below that figure – annual spending of $28–36 billion by the high-income countries would be necessary to provide a "global social health protection floor" (Ooms, 2009). Factually, this approach recognizes the implausibility of insisting that health systems in LICs can be financed primarily from domestic revenues in the near future (Sachs, 2007b). Normatively, this approach is a direct challenge to the "entitlement burden" view of financing health protection outside the high-income countries. This figure, however, represents only part of the resources needed to support widely shared improvements in population health – for example, by investing in the provision of safe drinking water, sanitation, and slum upgrading. Still less would such a commitment satisfy the critical need, identified by the Commission on Social Determinants of Health (2008, see generally chapters 3, 11 and 15), for "changes in the functioning of the global economy" that would redress the unequal distribution of power and resources that it identified as a fundamental cause of ill health.

Rather, the figure is cited here to make two points by way of conclusion. First, money matters, and global health ethics must start from the position that rhetoric is no substitute for commitments of resources to protect health on a much larger scale than at present. This can serve as a point of agreement even among researchers and practitioners who disagree about the relative value of improving social determinants of health and those who emphasize the "upstream" social determinants of health, usually with a focus on poverty and economic inequality, and those who dismiss interventions to address these factors as "romantic but impracticable notions" (Jha *et al.*, 2005), arguing instead for a focus on biomedical innovations and scaling up health systems. In fact, all of these are necessary, with the relative importance depending on context: no amount of investment in health systems will undo the damage caused by indoor air pollution from cooking smoke; no investment in social determinants of health will substitute for the skilled birth attendance that is essential to

reducing maternal mortality; and neither problem can be addressed without real resources.

Second, in today's global environment a preoccupation with setting priorities in "resource-constrained" contexts is a diversion (Schrecker, 2008). In addition to providing a harsh demonstration of the vulnerabilities created by globalization, the financial crisis that swept across the world in 2008 emphasized a point that Jeffrey Sachs has been making for years: "in a world of trillions of dollars of income every year," the resources needed to address emergencies of the kind described in our introductory paragraph *are available* (Sachs, 2003). Pogge has often made a similar point in the context of global poverty. The fact that resource scarcities condemn millions every year to premature and avoidable deaths, and millions more to shorter and less healthy lives than most readers of this volume take for granted, must be understood as policy-generated, resulting from choices that could have been made differently and institutions that can function differently.

Acknowledgment

Research for this chapter was partially supported by Canadian Institutes of Health Research Grant # 79153.

References

Adeyi, O., Chellaraj, G., Goldstein, E., Preker, A. S. & Ringold, D. (1997). Health status during the transition in Central and Eastern Europe: development in reverse? *Health Policy and Planning* **12**, 132–145.

Bates, I., Fenton, C., Gruber, J. *et al.* (2004). Vulnerability to malaria, tuberculosis, and HIV/AIDS infection and disease. Part I: determinants operating at individual and household level. *Lancet Infectious Diseases* **4**, 267–277.

Bhutta, Z., Ali, S., Cousens, S. *et al.* (2008). Alma-Ata: Rebirth and Revision 6 – Interventions to address maternal, newborn, and child survival: what difference can integrated primary health care strategies make? *Lancet* **372**, 972–989.

Birdsall, N. (2006). *The World is Not Flat: Inequality and Injustice in our Global Economy*. WIDER Annual Lectures. Helsinki: World Institute for Development Economics Research. www.wider.unu.edu/publications/annual-lectures/en_GB/AL9/_files/78121127186268214/default/annual-lecture-2005.pdf.

Birn, A.-E., Pillay, L. & Holtz, T. H. (2009). *Textbook of International Health*. (3rd edn.) Oxford: Oxford University Press.

Braveman, P. & Egerter, S. (2008). *Overcoming Obstacles to Health: Report from the Robert Wood Johnson Foundation* to the Commission to Build a Healthier America. Princeton, NJ: Robert Wood Johnson Foundation. www.rwjf.org/files/research/obstaclestohealth.pdf.

Bryce, J., Black, R. E., Walker, N. *et al.* (2005a). Can the world afford to save the lives of 6 million children each year? *Lancet* **365**, 2193–2200.

Bryce, J., Boschi-Pinto, C., Shibuya, K. & Black, R. E. (2005b). WHO estimates of the causes of death in children. *Lancet* **365**, 1147–1152.

Chen, S. & Ravallion, M. (2008). *The Developing World Is Poorer Than We Thought, But No Less Successful in the Fight against Poverty.* Policy Research Working Papers No. 4703. Washington, DC: World Bank. www-wds.worldbank.org/external/default/WDSContentServer/IW3P/IB/2008/08/26/000158349_20080826113239/Rendered/PDF/WPS4703.pdf.

Coker, R. J. (2004). Review: Multidrug-resistant tuberculosis: public health challenges. *Tropical Medicine & International Health* **9**, 25–40.

Commission on Social Determinants of Health (2008). *Closing the Gap in a Generation: Health equity through action on the social determinants of health (final report).* Geneva: World Health Organization. http://whqlibdoc.who.int/publications/2008/9789241563703_eng.pdf.

Cornia, G. A., Rosignoli, S. & Tiberti, L. (2008). *Globalization and Health: Impact Pathways and Recent Evidence.* WIDER Research Papers No. 2008–74. Helsinki: World Institute for Development Economics Research. www.wider.unu.edu/publications/working-papers/research-papers/2008/en_GB/rp2008–74/.

Dabbagh, A., Gacic-Dobo, M., Simons, E. *et al.* (2009). Global measles mortality, 2000–2008. *Morbidity and Mortality Weekly Reports*, **58**, 1321–1326.

Davies, J. B., Sandström, S., Shorrocks, A. & Wolff, E. N. (2008). *The World Distribution of Household Wealth.* WIDER Discussion Papers No. 2008/03. Helsinki: World Institute for Development Economics Research. www.wider.unu.edu/publications/working-papers/discussion-papers/2008/en_GB/dp2008–03/_files/78918010772127840/default/dp2008–03.pdf.

De Vogli, R. & Birbeck, G. L. (2005). Potential impact of adjustment policies on vulnerability of women and children to HIV/AIDS in Sub-Saharan Africa. *Journal of Health Population and Nutrition* **23**, 105–120.

Deaton, A. (2003). Health, inequality, and economic development. *Journal of Economic Literature* **41**, 113–158.

Deaton, A. (2004). Health in an age of globalization. *Brookings Trade Forum* 2004, 83–130.

Deaton, A. (2006). Global patterns of income and health. *WIDER Angle* **2**, 1–3.

Eyoh, D. & Sandbrook, R. (2003). Pragmatic neo-liberalism and just development in Africa. In A. Kohli, C. Moon & G. Sørensen (Eds.), *States, Markets, and Just Growth: Development in the Twenty-first Century* (pp. 227–257). Tokyo: United Nations University Press.

Ezzati, M. & Kammen, D. M. (2002). Household energy, indoor air pollution, and health in developing countries: knowledge base for effective interventions. *Annual Review of Energy and Environment* **27**, 233–270.

Ezzati, M., Vander Hoorn, S., Lawes, C. M. *et al.* (2005). Rethinking the 'diseases of affluence' paradigm: Global patterns of nutritional risks in relation to economic development. *PLoS Medicine* **2**, 404–412.

Field, M. G., Kotz, D. M. & Bukhman, G. (2000). Neoliberal economic policy, "state desertion," and the Russian health crisis. In J. Y. Kim, J. V. Millen, A. Irwin & J. Gershman (Eds.), *Dying for Growth: Global Inequality and the Health of the Poor* (pp. 155–173). Monroe, ME: Common Courage Press.

Garau, P., Sclar, E. D. & Carolini, G. Y. (2005). *A Home in the City: UN Millennium Project Task Force on Improving the Lives of Slum Dwellers.* London: Earthscan.

Gwatkin, D. R., Rutstein, S., Johnson, K. *et al.* (2007). *Socio-Economic Differences in Health, Nutrition and Population within Developing Countries: An Overview.* Washington, DC: World Bank. http://go.worldbank.org/XJK7WKSE40.

Halstead, S. B., Walsh, J. A. & Warren, K. S., Eds. (1985). *Good Health at Low Cost.* New York: Rockefeller Foundation.

Hawkes, C. (2005). The role of foreign direct investment in the nutrition transition. *Public Health Nutrition* **8**, 357–365.

Hawkes, C., Chopra, M. & Friel, S. (2009). Globalization, trade, and the nutrition transition. In R. Labonté, T. Schrecker, C. Packer & V. Runnels (Eds.), *Globalization and Health: Pathways, Evidence and Policy* (pp. 235–262). New York, NY: Routledge.

Jha, P., Brown, D., Nagelkerke, N., Slutsky, A. S. & Jamison, D. T. (2005). Global IDEA: Five members of the Global IDEA Scientific Advisory Committee respond to Dr. Moore and Colleagues. *Canadian Medical Association Journal* **172**, 1538–1539.

Labonté, R. & Schrecker, T. (2007). Globalization and social determinants of health: the role of the global marketplace (part 2 of 3). *Globalization and Health* **3**(6), 1–17.

Labonté, R., Schrecker, T., Packer, C. & Runnels, V., Eds. (2009). *Globalization and Health: Pathways, Evidence and Policy.* New York, NY: Routledge.

Lister, J. & Labonté, R. (2009). Globalization and health systems change. In R. Labonté, T. Schrecker, C. Packer & V. Runnels (Eds.), *Globalization and Health: Pathways, Evidence and Policy* (pp. 181–212). New York, NY: Routledge.

Marmot, M. (2005). Social determinants of health inequalities. *Lancet* **365**, 1099–1104.

Mathers, C. (2010). Global burden of disease among women, children, and adolescents. In J. Ehiri (Ed.), *Maternal and Child Health: Global Challenges, Programs, and Policies* (pp. 19–42). New York, NY: Springer.

McCord, C. & Freeman, H. P. (1990). Excess mortality in Harlem. *New England Journal of Medicine,* **322**, 173–177.

Mendez, M. & Popkin, B. (2004). Globalization, urbanization and nutritional change in the developing world. In *Globalization of Food Systems in Developing Countries: Impact on Food Security and Nutrition (FAO Food and Nutrition Paper 83)* (pp. 55–80). Rome: Food and Agriculture Organization of the United Nations. ftp://ftp.fao.org/docrep/fao/007/y5736e/y5736e00.pdf.

Monteiro, C. A., Conde, W. L. & Popkin, B. M. (2004). The burden of disease from undernutrition and overnutrition in countries undergoing rapid nutrition transition: a view from Brazil. *American Journal of Public Health* **94**, 433–434.

Monteiro, C. A., Conde, W. L. & Popkin, B. M. (2007). Income-specific trends in obesity in Brazil: 1975–2003. *American Journal of Public Health* **97**, 1808–1812.

Moser, K., Shkolnikov, V. & Leon, D. (2007). World Mortality 1950–2000: Divergence replaces convergence from the late 1980s. In M. Caraël & J. R. Glynn (Eds.), *HIV, Resurgent Infections and Population Change in Africa* (pp. 11–25). Dordrecht: Springer.

Murray, C. J. L., Kulkarni, S. C., Michaud, C. *et al.* (2006). Eight Americas: Investigating mortality disparities across races, counties, and race-counties in the United States. *PLoS Medicine* **3**, e260.

Omran, A. R. (1971). The epidemiologic transition: a theory of the epidemiology of population change. *Milbank Memorial Fund Quarterly* **49**, 509–538.

Ooms, G. (2009). *From the Global AIDS Response towards Global Health?* Brussels: Hélène de Beir Foundation. www.internationalhealthpartnership. net//CMS_files/documents/ global_health_discussion_paper_b_EN.pdf.

Over, M. (2008). *Prevention Failure: The Ballooning Entitlement Burden of U.S. Global AIDS Treatment Spending and What to Do About It.* Working Paper No. 144. Washington, DC: Center for Global Development. www.cgdev.org/files/15973_file_Presidential_AIDS_ Policy_FINAL.pdf.

Pogge, T. (2002). *World Poverty and Human Rights.* Cambridge: Polity.

Pogge, T. (2007). Severe poverty as a human rights violation. In T. Pogge (Ed.), *Freedom from Poverty as a Human Right: Who Owes What to the Very Poor?* (pp. 11–53). Oxford: Oxford University Press.

Popkin, B. M. (2002). The shift in stages of the nutrition transition in the developing world differs from past experiences! *Public Health Nutrition* **5**, 205–214.

Popkin, B. M. (2006). Technology, transport, globalization and the nutrition transition food policy. *Food Policy* **31**, 554–569.

Popkin, B. M. (2008). Will China's nutrition transition overwhelm its health care system and slow economic growth? *Health Affairs,* **27**, 1064–1076.

Popkin, B. M. (2009). Global changes in diet and activity patterns as drivers of the nutrition transition. In S. C. Calhan, A. M. Prentice & C. S. Yagnik (Eds.), *Emerging Societies – Coexistence of Childhood Malnutrition and Obesity* (pp. 1–14). Basel: Karger.

Preston, S. H. (2007). The changing relation between mortality and level of economic development. *International Journal of Epidemiology* **36**, 484–490 (original publication 1975).

Prüss-Üstun, A., Bos, R., Gore, F. & Bartram, J. (2008). *Safer Water, Better Health.* Geneva: World Health Organization. www.who.int/quantifying_ehimpacts/ publications/saferwater/en/index.html.

Ravishankar, N., Gubbins, P., Cooley, R. J. *et al.* (2009). Financing of global health: tracking development assistance for health from 1990 to 2007. *Lancet* **373**, 2113–2124.

Riley, J. C. (2005). Estimates of regional and global life expectancy, 1800–2001. *Population and Development Review* **31**, 537–543.

Riley, J. C. (2008). *Low Income, Social Growth and Good Health: A History of Twelve Countries.* Berkeley, CA: University of California Press.

Sachs, J. (2003). *Achieving the Millennium Development Goals: Health in the Developing World.* Speech at the Second Global Consultation of the Commission on Macroeconomics and Health. Geneva: World Health Organization. www.earthinstitute.columbia.edu/about/ director/pubs/CMHSpeech102903.pdf.

Sachs, J. (2007a). The basic economics of scaling up health care in low-income settings. In Working Party on Biotechnology (Ed.), *Horizontal Project on Policy Coherence: Availability of Medicines for Emerging and Infected Neglected Diseases. DSTI/STP/BIO(2007)6* (pp. 7–23). Paris: OECD.

Sachs, J. (2007b). Beware false tradeoffs. *Foreign Affairs* [On-line]. www.foreignaffairs.org/special/global_health/ sachs

Say, L., Inoue, M., Mills, S. & Suzuki, E. (2007). *Maternal Mortality in 2005: Estimates developed by WHO, UNICEF, UNFPA, and the World Bank.* Geneva: Department of Reproductive Health and Research, World Health Organization. www.unfpa.org/publications/detail. cfm?ID=343.

Schrecker, T. (2008). Denaturalizing scarcity: a strategy of inquiry for public health ethics. *Bulletin of the World Health Organization* **86**, 600–605.

Sell, S. K. (2003). *Private Power, Public Law: The Globalization of Intellectual Property Rights*. Cambridge: Cambridge University Press.

Stillwaggon, E. (2006). *AIDS and the Ecology of Poverty*. Oxford: Oxford University Press.

Sutcliffe, B. (2005). *A Converging or Diverging World?* DESA Working Paper Series No. ST/ESA/2005/DWP/2. New York, NY: United Nations Department of Economic and Social Affairs. www.un.org/esa/desa/papers/2005/wp2_2005.pdf.

Taub, S. (2008). Best-paid hedge fund managers. Alpha Magazine [On-line]. www.alphamagazine.com/Article.aspx?ArticleID=1914753

The Coca-Cola Company (2009). Per capita consumption of company beverage products. The Coca-Cola Company [On-line]. www.thecoca-colacompany.com/ourcompany/ar/pdf/perCapitaConsumption2008.pdf.

UNAIDS (2009). *AIDS Epidemic Update 2009*. Geneva: UNAIDS. http://data.unaids.org/pub/Report/2009/2009_epidemic_update_en.pdf.

Unger, A. & Riley, L. W. (2007). Slum health: from understanding to action. *PLoS Medicine* **4**, e295.

UNICEF (2008a). *Progress for Children: A Report Card on Maternal Mortality (No. 7)*. New York, NY: UNICEF. www.unicef.org/publications/index_45454.html.

UNICEF (2008b). *The State of the World's Children 2008*. New York, NY: UNICEF. www.unicef.org/sowc08/.

United Nations (2009). *The Millennium Development Goals Report 2009*. New York, NY: United Nations. www.un.org/millenniumgoals/pdf/MDG_Report_2009_ENG.pdf.

United Nations Development Program (2006). *Human Development Report 2006: Beyond Scarcity – Power, Poverty and the Global Water Crisis*. New York, NY: Palgrave Macmillan. http://hdr.undp.org/hdr2006/statistics/indicators/124.html.

United Nations Food and Agriculture Organization (2009). *More People than ever are Victims of Hunger*. Rome: UNFAO. www.fao.org/fileadmin/user_upload/newsroom/docs/Press%20release%20june-en.pdf.

van Doorslaer, E., O'Donnell, O., Rannan-Eliya, R. P. et al. (2006). Effect of payments for health care on poverty estimates in 11 countries in Asia: an analysis of household survey data. *Lancet* **368**, 1357–1364.

Wang, Y. (1998). *Life Expectancy in Chicago*. Chicago: Epidemiology Program, Chicago Department of Public Health.

World Bank (2009). World Development Indicators 2009. World Bank [On-line]. http://ddp-ext.worldbank.org/ext/DDPQQ/member.do?method=getMembers&userid=1&queryId=135

World Bank & International Monetary Fund (2009). *Global Monitoring Report 2009: A Development Emergency*. Washington, DC: World Bank. http://siteresources.worldbank.org/INTGLOMONREP2009/Resources/5924349-1239742507025/GMR09_book.pdf.

World Health Organization (2009a). *Global Health Risks: Mortality and Burden of Disease Attributable to Selected Major Risks*. Geneva: World Health Organization. www.who.int/healthinfo/global_burden_disease/GlobalHealthRisks_report_full.pdf.

World Health Organization (2009b). *Global Status Report on Road Safety: Time for Action*. Geneva: World Health Organization. http://whqlibdoc.who.int/publications/2009/9789241563840_eng.pdf.

World Health Organization, UNAIDS & UNICEF (2009). *Towards Universal Access – Scaling up Priority HIV/AIDS Interventions in the Health Sector: Progress Report 2009*. Geneva: World Health Organization. www.who.int/entity/hiv/pub/tuapr_2009_en.pdf.

Xu, K., Evans, D. B., Carrin, G., Aguilar-Rivera, A. M., Musgrove, P. & Evans, T. (2007). Protecting households from catastrophic health spending. *Health Affairs* **26**, 972–983.

Zhang, H. & Cai, B. (2003). The impact of tobacco on lung health in China. *Respirology* **8**, 17–21.

Chapter

3

Addressing the societal determinants of health: the key global health ethics imperative of our times

Anne-Emanuelle Birn

> If the rich could hire others to die for them, we, the poor, would all make a nice living.
>
> – *Mordcha, the innkeeper,* Fiddler on the Roof

In 2006, Costa Ricans and Cubans had a life expectancy of 78, identical to that of the USA. Yet the US per capita GDP was almost five times that of Costa Rica and almost ten times Cuba's. Moreover, the US outstripped total health spending in Costa Rica and Cuba by a factor of 9 and 19, respectively (WHOSIS, 2009). Even more striking, in 2000, inhabitants of the southern Indian state of Kerala, earning, on average, less than US$3000 per year, had a life expectancy of 74.6 (Government of Kerala, 2005), while Washington, DC residents, with almost $30 000 per capita annual income, had a life expectancy of 72.6 years (Phillips & Beasley, 2005; US Government, 2005). Why are Costa Ricans, Cubans and Keralites so healthy, and why does US wealth not enable greater longevity? The answer to this question has far less to do with the nature of the people living in these settings or of their disease and epidemiological profile than with the structure of their societies.

A political economy approach to health (see Figure 3.1 and Gill and Bakker, Chapter 19, this volume) examines the role of the distribution of power and of political, economic and social resources in shaping the health of populations, showing that factors such as genetic endowment, human behavior and medical care explain only a small fraction of health and disease and of patterns of inequalities in health. Here we discuss these patterns in terms of a broad range of factors – societal determinants – that shape health at personal, household, community, national and global levels.

What makes the underlying determinants of health societal as opposed to individual?

Most of us experience ill health as individuals. Yet virtually every bout of ill health or injury can be understood in societal terms. For example, picture a construction worker who takes a 10-story fall from scaffolding and dies. On one level, he may have been inattentive and insufficiently conscious of safety. But if we look to the societal context in which this worker lives, we learn that he was exhausted due to his long commute to work – he can only afford to reside in a distant slum – and his inability to get a good night's sleep, because the thin walls of his dwelling fail to block out night-time noise. At an intermediary level, we learn that his low earnings derive from poor enforcement (and inadequacy) of minimum wages and his precarious status as an undocumented worker. Lack of government oversight and poor regulation also contribute to the meager safety training he received from his employer and the poor quality materials the company purchased to build the scaffolding. At the highest level, we may understand the fall to be linked to a free market economic system where profits come before worker safety and working class efforts to organize and ensure social security and occupational protections are constrained by threats of job loss and repression. In sum, the construction worker's fall may be construed as a personal accident, but when viewed through a lens of societal determinants can be clearly understood as the product of interlocking social, economic, and political factors.

At a population level, patterns of premature death and disability can also be examined in societal terms.

Global Health and Global Health Ethics, ed. Solomon Benatar and Gillian Brock. Published by Cambridge University Press.
© Cambridge University Press 2011.

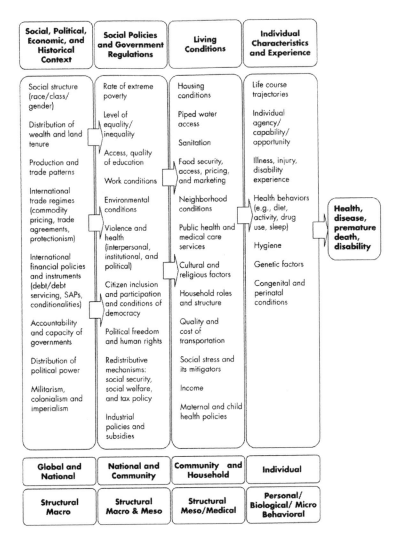

Social, Political, Economic, and Historical Context	Social Policies and Government Regulations	Living Conditions	Individual Characteristics and Experience
Social structure (race/class/gender)	Rate of extreme poverty	Housing conditions	Life course trajectories
Distribution of wealth and land tenure	Level of equality/inequality	Piped water access	Individual agency/capability/opportunity
Production and trade patterns	Access, quality of education	Sanitation	Illness, injury, disability experience
International trade regimes (commodity pricing, trade agreements, protectionism)	Work conditions	Food security, access, pricing, and marketing	Health behaviors (e.g., diet, activity, drug use, sleep)
	Environmental conditions	Neighborhood conditions	
International financial policies and instruments (debt/debt servicing, SAPs, conditionalities)	Violence and health (interpersonal, institutional, and political)	Public health and medical care services	Hygiene
		Cultural and religious factors	Genetic factors
Accountability and capacity of governments	Citizen inclusion and participation and conditions of democracy	Household roles and structure	Congenital and perinatal conditions
Distribution of political power	Political freedom and human rights	Quality and cost of transportation	
Militarism, colonialism and imperialism	Redistributive mechanisms: social security, social welfare, and tax policy	Social stress and its mitigators	
		Income	
	Industrial policies and subsidies	Maternal and child health policies	

Health, disease, premature death, disability

Global and National	National and Community	Community and Household	Individual
Structural Macro	Structural Macro & Meso	Structural Meso/Medical	Personal/Biological/Micro Behavioral

Figure 3.1 Political economy of international health – societal determinants of health framework. *Source:* Courtesy of Anne-Emanuelle Birn, Yogan Pillay & Timothy H. Holtz, *Textbook of International Health: Global Health in a Dynamic World* (3rd edn.). New York: Oxford University Press, 2009, Figure 4–2, p. 138. Adapted with permission from Stephen Gloyd, "Child Survival and Resource Scarcity." *World Congress of Public Health Associations.* Mexico City, March 1987.

Population health is linked to and explained by a range of societal factors and conditions, from neighborhood conditions to the work environment, availability of and access to social services, such as education and health, to the overall class and political structure (see Figure 3.1). These determinants function on multiple levels simultaneously. If the social determinants of health are the "causes of the causes" (Marmot, 2005), the societal determinants of health are the "causes of the causes of the causes" of health and disease.[1]

A political economy of health approach, then, considers the political, social, cultural, and economic contexts in which disease and illness arise and examines the ways in which societal structures interact with the

and structural forces underpinning health and health inequalities. The social determinants of health generally refer to interactions among people and communities, whereby public policies and private sector actions shape hierarchies of exposure to factors that determine health. Societal determinants of health, by contrast, refer to the political-economic order and structures of power, in which health inequities derive from elite groups wielding power against oppressed groups. As such, addressing the societal determinants of health requires fundamentally rectifying unequal political power (Birn, 2009).

---

[1] Although the term *social determinants of health* is widely employed, a growing contingent prefers *societal determinants of health* to make explicit the political

particular conditions or factors that lead to good or ill health. This approach contrasts sharply with behavioral and biomedical models, which largely attribute ill health to personal features and actions and ascribe its resolution to individual and medical measures (see Box 3.1).

Box 3.1. Models for understanding health and disease

The *biomedical model* views health and illness at the individual level, with the body conceptualized as a machine with constituent parts (i.e. genes, organs, etc.) that can be manipulated or repaired. While the biomedical approach is largely curative, it also includes a preventive armamentarium (such as vaccines, screening and genetic testing) and considers the role of behavioral determinants of health. Much of the appeal of the biomedical approach stems from the dramatic technological advances in medical treatment over the last century, in pharmacotherapy, surgery and other areas.

The *behavioral model* views health and illness primarily as a consequence of individual actions and beliefs. Poor health status is characterized as the outcome of poor lifestyle choices, such as unsafe sexual behavior, smoking, alcohol and drug consumption, poor diet, excessive stress and insufficient exercise. This approach focuses primarily on the regulation or modification of personal conduct and cultural attitudes through education, counseling and incentives. Although the behavioral approach sometimes addresses social and structural issues, it mainly views the individual (and sometimes the household or community) as responsible for health.

The *political economy approach* considers the political, social, cultural and economic contexts in which disease and illness arise, and examines the ways in which societal structures interact with particular health conditions. This approach views health as a function and reflection of linked determinants that operate at multiple levels: individual, household, community, workplace, social class, nation and the global political and economic context. These determinants are addressed through, for example, public policy aimed at improving transportation and housing conditions. These efforts include, but are not reduced to, biomedical technologies and behavior/lifestyle strategies.

While there is no doubt that individual actions have a bearing on health outcomes (i.e. reckless driving can lead to automobile fatalities), behaviors are mediated by political, economic, cultural and other societal determinants of health. For example, notwithstanding the well-known correlation between smoking and lung cancer, the associated mortality is considerably higher among working-class smokers than upper-class smokers. As well, smoking cessation and education efforts have been far more successful among privileged populations who are better able to relieve stress or cope with the challenges of quitting smoking. Indeed, other than major genetic conditions passed down through Mendelian inheritance patterns, every occurrence of disease, death or disability includes varying degrees of societal influence. Moreover, even the health outcomes of genetic conditions are socially mediated. Congenital and perinatal conditions, for example, are affected by prenatal care and maternal well-being, which are in turn influenced by nutrition, household resources, employment, housing, social security measures and health policies.

What is wrong with the individual perspective? Is it not important to live a healthy life? Of course it is, but this approach covers only one small component of multiple influences on health. It assumes that people are perfect decision makers with day-to-day control over work and neighborhood conditions, not to mention production, pollution control, trade and marketing patterns, ignoring the clear evidence that life chances are structurally constrained. Further, in placing the blame on individuals for poor health, this approach removes responsibility for change from government, private business and other actors. With this in mind, we turn to the influence of living conditions on health.

Living conditions (community and household levels)

Numerous ailments result from poor living conditions, in particular cardiovascular, respiratory, gastrointestinal, endocrine, nutritional and metabolic diseases, injuries, and violence. Living conditions refer to housing and neighborhood characteristics, availability of potable water and adequate sanitation, food quality and security, maternal and child health facilities and policies, household roles and income, social services such as public health and transportation, and social stress and its mitigators, including support from friends and leisure activities. Cultural and religious practices are also intertwined with and affect health at the community and household level.

Water and sanitation

Water is fundamental to life, yet over one-sixth of the world's population lives without an adequate supply of safe water. Approximately one-third of the world's population lives on land with moderate to severe water stress. Competition for water also precipitates conflict, as evidenced in the Middle East and elsewhere over thousands of years. Almost half the world's population (2.6 billion people, mostly in rural areas) lacks access (either unpaid or paid) to even the most basic sanitation and must resort to using pit latrines, fields and ditches. This leads to water and soil contamination and increased rates of communicable diseases, especially diarrhea. Water and sanitation-related illnesses kill some 3 million people each year and are among the leading causes of preventable mortality and morbidity. Diarrhea alone causes 2 million annual deaths, mostly among children (UNICEF, 2007).

The connection between water/sanitation and health is complicated. For instance, the World Health Organization (WHO) argues that hand washing can reduce diarrheal diseases by close to 50% (WHO, 2004b). However, this is not simply a matter of personal habits, but rests on access to clean water (and soap). Paradoxically, poorer populations tend to pay more for water use than richer ones, who typically live closer to utility systems. Women, girls and refugees are particularly affected by poor water supply. They typically bear responsibility for collecting water, often over great distances, making them vulnerable to assault and to sustaining injuries from carrying heavy loads, as well as jeopardizing school attendance and other activities.

Nutrition and food security

Feeding children is a foremost family and societal responsibility. A healthy diet is essential to child development and growth, and to human flourishing. Over 50% of child deaths are the result of poor nutrition or undernutrition (Sanchez et al., 2005), and it is estimated that hunger and malnutrition kill more people per year than do AIDS, malaria and tuberculosis (TB) combined (WHO, 2002a).

For approximately one-seventh of the world's population, hunger is a severe problem. Although global food production far exceeds the nutrient and caloric needs of the world's population, over 850 million people go hungry every day. Personal, household and community food insecurity are heavily determined by structural factors. World food production and trade are big business, and power is concentrated in a few large corporations: 30 retailers control one-third of global grocery sales, and 90% of world grain trade is controlled by just five companies (Eagleton, 2005). This affects the existence of local, sustainable farming practices – and in turn food stability – especially since over 50% of the population in developing countries works in agriculture.

For billions of other people, poor nutrition is the main problem. In the past, malnutrition was a matter of insufficient calorie intake (in terms of protein, fresh fruits and vegetables). Today, malnutrition is increasingly associated with consumption of so-called empty calories – chemically processed foods with high sugar and fat content – that are cheap, widely available and heavily marketed in almost every society. Not only does this food have little nutritional value, its consumption can lead to obesity, cardiovascular disease, certain cancers, dental caries, low birth weight babies, diabetes and vitamin deficiencies. Throughout the world, 2 million people suffer from nutrient shortages, even when their daily caloric needs are met or exceeded (Sanchez et al., 2005).

While medical authorities often attribute poor diet to bad individual choices and lack of education, these issues are rooted in the mass production and marketing of food. For example, marbled (fatty) meat is a result of an industrial meat processing system that overfeeds livestock, uses growth hormones and limits animals' exercise in order to accelerate production and increase profits. Although tradition, culture and household resources play an important role, dietary patterns are profoundly influenced by the industrialization of food production, which has made processed food cheaper per calorie than fresh produce and basic foodstuffs, despite use of multiple ingredients and elaborate production methods, marketing costs and distribution chains. For households with restricted food storage and cooking facilities, and/or in which household members work long hours or non-coinciding shifts, "fast food" is indeed convenient.

Food production and consumption affect health in other ways. Pesticide residues, industrial chemical run-off in soil and waterways, and other contaminants in food cause a variety of cancers and infertility. In addition, food-borne illnesses due to contamination in the production and distribution process affect millions of people each year. Moreover, agricultural irrigation is the biggest single use of water worldwide, accounting for two-thirds of water consumption, affecting water access for millions of people.

Housing conditions

Along with food and water, shelter is a basic human need that (ideally) provides safety, stability, a place for rest and leisure and fosters physical and mental health. Poor housing conditions, however, can cause or exacerbate a range of health problems. For example, housing that is cold, damp, and/or moldy can lead to upper- and lower-respiratory tract diseases, meningococcal infections and asthma. Furthermore, housing in which open stoves are used for heating or cooking have high rates of fire accidents and lung disease. Overcrowding and inadequate ventilation and sanitation facilitate the spread of air-borne, water-borne, and skin ailments, including TB, diarrhea, lice and scabies. Beds shared by many increases the spread of disease and the possibility of the molestation of minors and other vulnerable persons. Flimsy structures provide little or no protection from storms, fires and earthquakes, and the use of recycled industrial materials and lead paint in housing can cause fatal poisonings and severe neurological and cognitive problems. All of these aspects of poor housing also affect psychological well-being.

In areas with endemic malaria, dengue and other vector-borne diseases, bed nets and door and window screens protect against mosquito bites, but they are usually prohibitively expensive. If there is no indoor plumbing (or regular refuse collection), water storage containers often serve as mosquito breeding sites. In areas where Chagas disease is endemic, low-cost thatched roofs can pose a problem because insects that are vector hosts of *Trypanosoma cruzi* spend daylight hours hidden in them, only to descend and bite at night.

The most extreme housing problem is homelessness. Estimates of global homelessness range from 100 million to 1 billion people. In high-income European countries, 2 million people depend on homelessness services. More than 7 million US residents have experienced homelessness at some point in their lives, with over 600 000 people homeless every night. Homelessness estimates in developing nations range from 1.5 million people in South Africa to 18.5 million in India (Kellett & Moore, 2003).

The death rate among homeless people is two to ten times higher than that of the non-homeless. This differential is partially mitigated by social services, but even societies with extensive services for the homeless – including free health care, accessible shelters, food banks and employment training programs – cannot compensate for the health effects of not having a permanent home. In many locales, homeless people may be jailed or abused by the police. Children who live on the streets in cities across Latin America and other regions are subject to violence by shopkeepers, gangs or political authorities. The desperate conditions of homelessness can also lead to drug use, sex work and deterioration of mental health.

Neighborhood conditions

Neighborhood conditions affect the quality of housing, water, and sanitation, food availability and other determinants of health. Neighborhood infrastructure and institutions, including schools, health and social services, parks, stores, transport and recreation and community spaces affect health along with other less tangible neighborhood features, such as unemployment rates; crime and stress levels; community solidarity and organization; social, racial and cultural tolerance; political empowerment; and civic engagement.

Across the world, nearly 1 billion people (32% of the world's urban population, and 43% of the developing world's urban population) live in "slums" characterized by open sewers, stagnant water, rotting garbage, toxic dumpsites, an unstable land base, shoddy housing, abandoned lots and buildings, unpaved roads, overcrowding, gang violence, high eviction rates, few legal protections and inadequate electricity, sanitation, schools, clinics and other infrastructure (Rice & Steinkopf Rice, 2009). Because factories and waste facilities located near slums often evade regulations, air and soil pollution in slums is often extensive. All of these factors generate high infant, child and maternal mortality rates among slum dwellers (higher even than among the rural poor). These conditions also generate poor health from infectious diseases such as TB, HIV and diarrhea, as well as cancer, trauma and stress-related cardiovascular disease. Other ailments that particularly affect slum dwellers include salmonella, plague and other diseases that have rodent vectors. Although not all slum dwellers are poor, they include large numbers of destitute migrants from rural areas (many of whom are socially marginalized), and chronically unemployed and exploited long-time urban residents.

Public health and health-care services

A range of community-level public health activities are important determinants of health. These include food safety inspection and standards; epidemic and chronic disease surveillance, control and clinics; collection and disposal of refuse; road safety; monitoring of environmental health, sanitation and water quality; school health services and lunches; maternal and child health programs; housing regulations and inspection; and workplace safety and inspection. These activities influence other determinants of health and can have a significant role in reducing mortality.

Health-care services, particularly primary care, constitute another key determinant of health: approximately 10% of premature deaths are preventable through medical care. Indeed, the provision of primary health care in countries such as Cuba and Costa Rica partially explains why health indicators are high even when economic indicators are not. Costa Rica's 1970s health system reform, for example, emphasized primary care for underserved areas together with nutritional and educational improvements. In the 15 years following the reform, infant mortality rates dropped from 60/1000 to 19/1000, and life expectancy increased dramatically (Starfield *et al.*, 2005).

Finally, the health system itself can also promote or jeopardize health depending on how equitably it is financed (the presence or absence of user fees and national health insurance), its accessibility and quality (especially to rural populations and slum dwellers), and the extent to which it prioritizes preventive services and public health over curative services.

Culture

Culture refers to socially transmitted frameworks of meaning. These form the basis through which people interpret and engage with the world, including ways in which health and illness are defined and understood. Culture influences what actions may be taken to prevent or treat illness, and which healing authorities to consult. Although the International Classification of Diseases has been in use for more than a century, most people view health through cultural filters other than the biomedical lens (which is itself an assemblage of cultural values, symbols, preferences, rituals, practices and traditions). For example, in some cultures, pregnancy is medicalized and treated as though it were a disease; in others it is understood in more spiritual or kinship terms.

Identifying cultural influences on health is fraught with issues of relativism. What one cultural group determines is a disease or to be harmful to health is unlikely to be universally accepted. For example, fatigue-inducing anemia accompanying chronic malnutrition may not be understood as a disease by subsistence farmers, but rather as an inevitable part of their lives.

Cultural influences on health can be over-emphasized, particularly when the illness and/or treatments are sensationalized. For example, most HIV/AIDS prevention work in sub-Saharan Africa focuses primarily on sexual practices, to the neglect of larger structural issues such as poor nutrition and housing and extremely limited access to safe employment and social services.

Transport

Transport influences health through a variety of mechanisms: car use results in road injuries and fatalities as well as poor air quality, whereas public transportation may improve air quality and increases human interaction, interpersonal security and overall quality of urban life. Inadequate or unaffordable transport can affect other determinants, such as school attendance and access to employment and (preventive) health-care services. Most directly, road traffic accidents are the second leading cause of death for children between 5 and 14 years of age. Traffic fatality and injury rates vary by class, income and education levels, with poor and working classes disproportionately affected. In high-income countries, most casualties are among drivers and passengers, whereas in low- and middle-income countries pedestrians, cyclists and public transport passengers account for 90% of deaths. In Haiti, the word for local transport is *molue* ("moving morgue") and in southern Nigeria it is the *danfo* ("flying coffins") (Nantulya & Reich, 2003).

Social policies and government regulations (national and community levels)

A range of social, political and economic policies at the national and sub-national levels influence health. These include education, health, taxation, labor, social welfare, human rights and environmental policies and regulations.

Income and poverty

Each year, 18 million deaths (more than one-third of all deaths worldwide) are directly attributable to the conditions of poverty (Pogge, 2005), with women, children and indigenous populations disproportionately affected. These numbers say nothing of the untold millions of deaths *indirectly* linked to poverty. Living on less than US$1/day is the indicator of extreme poverty used by international agencies such as the United Nations and the World Bank. Extreme poverty is characterized by very low income and lack of access to the basic necessities of health and life – food, shelter, water and other living requirements. However, absolute poverty alone does not explain global mortality patterns; relative poverty is also a determinant of health. Indeed, although per capita income and health are roughly correlated up to a level of approximately US$5000, above this level the correlation is far hazier and is affected more by inequality in power and resources than by per capita (average) income levels (see Labonté and Schrecker, Chapter 2, this volume).

Education

Education has long been associated with health status through two primary means: it increases the likelihood of finding a well-paid, safe job with benefits and room for advancement, and it influences the ability to take, or advocate for, protective health measures. Compared with those with little schooling, people who are more educated have a wider range of employment possibilities and selection of neighborhoods, engage more in the political process, and have a better understanding of, and ability to avoid or respond to, a variety of impediments to health. Moreover, early childhood development and education can help ameliorate some of the negative effects of social disadvantage throughout the life span. In general, people who are better educated have lower levels of infectious diseases, hypertension, emphysema, diabetes, anxiety and depression; improved physical and mental functioning; and healthier behaviors (e.g. lower rates of smoking, heavy drinking and drug use; higher rates of exercise; and better management of stress and chronic health conditions).

Access to and quality of education are both important. In growing numbers of underdeveloped countries, students must pay user fees (and fees for books, uniforms and supplies) in order to attend school, excluding millions of children from formal education. Girls' ability to attend school is particularly jeopardized when families favor having girls contribute to household work over paying for their school fees, and boys are perceived as benefiting more from education. In many countries, deregulation and reductions in social sector spending have led to a marked deterioration in the quality of education. In some settings, the ranks of educators have been decimated in recent decades by high rates of migration to developed countries, civil conflict and HIV/AIDS. Neighborhood conditions (safety, existence of schools, transport) and the household environment (a quiet space, light to study by, and few economic and family care-giving responsibilities) also affect school attendance.

Work conditions/employment status

Globally, there are 250 million occupational injuries, 1.6 million occupationally related deaths, and 350 000 injury-related deaths (on the job or job-related) every year (Driscoll *et al.*, 2005). Typically, those who are employed in many of the most dangerous employment sectors (forestry, fishing, agriculture, construction, commercial sex work and transport) are not covered by workers' compensation for any injury. Altogether, only 10% of workers in developing countries are covered by occupational health and safety laws (LaDou, 2003). In turn, ill health and disability affect employment status. Those who are ill may be more likely to lose a job, be unable to keep a steady job, and become sicker as a result of stress and anxiety, inability to pay for care and so on. In many societies, persons with disabilities are unable to find steady employment due to discrimination.

In work environments where there is low or no worker control and inadequate rewards, psychosocial stress is exacerbated. Seasonal employment, including construction and agricultural migrant work, also generates high levels of stress because employment from year to year is not guaranteed, and seasonal workers usually lack benefits, workplace protections, or recourse against abuse, such as lack of payment and physical violence.

Employment can have major negative health effects, but unemployment is even more deleterious. Precarious or no employment increases stress, anxiety and mental health problems, leading to excess ill health and mortality, particularly following job loss. Developing countries have unemployment rates of approximately 30% compared with 4–12% in developed countries (Benach *et al.*, 2007), with concomitant health effects. Unemployment soars to much higher rates during economic recessions.

Finally, income from employment is a key determinant of health but employment is also important in providing social protections such as health benefits and pensions (in some societies), and in offering education and training, social networks, opportunities for labor organizing and a sense of solidarity.

Environmental conditions

Environmental conditions are one of the major determinants of health. Environmental problems and their health consequences derive from two key processes: depletion and contamination. Depletion of water, forests, the earth's protective ozone layer, soil, and flora and fauna generally affect human health by limiting the availability of, and access to, basic necessities such as arable land, thereby impeding livelihoods. Contamination, which occurs largely through industrial production and consumption processes, leads to human exposure to a variety of chemical, biological and physical agents, with endocrinological, physiological, genetic and other effects. As well, greenhouse gas emissions have led to global warming, which decreases land productivity, water availability and biodiversity, and threatens climate disasters, all of which have profound effects on human health.

Violence

Violence is an important determinant of health due to the deaths and disability it causes but also because it generates fear and destruction and restricts day-to-day activities and dreams for the future. The *World Report on Violence and Health* (WHO, 2002b) categorizes violence as: (a) self-directed, including suicide and self-mutilation; (b) collective, which may be socially, economically or politically motivated; and (c) interpersonal, including partner or family violence and violence in settings outside the home. Of the 5 million deaths from injuries in 2000, approximately 1.6 million were the result of violence, with 49% from suicides, 18% due to war and 31% from homicides (WHO, 2004a).

Currently rates of violent death are two to three times higher in low- or middle-income countries than in high-income countries due to high poverty rates, political and economic inequality, rapid urbanization, competition for resources, military conflict and repressive political regimes. During the twentieth century, almost 200 million people lost their lives directly or indirectly as a result of wars, with civilians constituting over half of those killed (WHO, 2002b). Weapon use can cause acute physical trauma and long-term disability. Men, particularly those between the ages of 15 and 29, are disproportionately killed in violent conflict. Sexual violence – both within families during conflict and as a weapon of war – especially affects women.

Human rights

A society's recognition and enforcement of human rights – including civil and political rights *and* economic, social, and cultural rights – is a key determinant of health and is associated with many other determinants relating to political, economic, living and employment conditions. The breach of rights, through conscious policies, programs and practices, or through neglect, has an enormous negative impact on collective health and is manifested through an array of household, community and national level determinants of health.

Although the actions of the private sector and civil society have great bearing on human health, it is governments that are responsible for enabling their populations to achieve "health as a human right." This government obligation is met through respecting, protecting and fulfilling rights (i.e. not violating rights, preventing rights violations and creating policies, structures and resources that promote and enforce rights), including tackling societal determinants of health such as adequate education, housing, and food, and favorable working conditions (Gruskin & Tarantola, 2005).

The right to health is a central component of the World Health Organization's constitution. Key international human rights treaties, such as the Convention on the Rights of the Child and the International Covenant on Economic, Social and Cultural Rights, protect the right to societal determinants of health including education, food and nutrition, an adequate standard of living, social security, civil participation and protection from violence and discrimination.

Redistributive mechanisms

Redistributive mechanisms including social security, social well-being programs, and progressive tax policy, based on both broad and targeted social protections, are the scaffolding of welfare states. The welfare state has been recognized as a crucial determinant of population health due to its central functions of ensuring income redistribution; protecting against immiseration, unemployment and ill health; providing universal public health care and education; and enforcing occupational health and safety standards.

The main welfare state policies positively correlated with health are those that ensure high rates of female employment, high levels of unemployment compensation, universal access to health care and adequate subsidies to single mothers and divorced women (Chung & Muntaner, 2007). Other factors include having strong unionized labor movements and socialist political parties, high corporate taxes, progressive income taxes, high expenditures on social security and health care and high levels of employment, particularly in the public sector.

The relationship between welfare states and health is complex (Beckfield & Krieger, 2009) and may unfold over many years. When evaluated according to the impact of particular social policies, strong welfare states are associated with positive health outcomes, but whether this is due to politics or policies is debated (Lundberg, 2008; Muntaner et al., 2009). In addition, little attention has been paid to the long-term effects of both welfare state policies and politics. It may be that the very political activism that builds welfare states has other beneficial outcomes, including the positive health characteristics of bona fide political participation.

Ultimately the more egalitarian a country is on political, economic and social grounds, the fewer inequalities are found in health. Though there is limited systematic research on the relationship between redistributive mechanisms and health outside high-income countries, the experiences of Cuba, Costa Rica and Kerala demonstrate that there is a strong relationship between social and economic redistribution and health outcomes, including life expectancy and infant mortality, in low-income countries as well.

Social, political, economic, and historical context (global and national levels)

At the broadest level, the societal determinants of health can be understood in relation to social, political, economic and historical forces as played out in national and global arenas. At the national level, these forces include forms of stratification such as patriarchy, racism and class structure, the nature of land tenure and the structure of the political system. At the international level, these forces include trade agreements and international financial instruments. Many

other societal forces operate at both national and global levels, including militarism, colonialism and imperialism. In the following section, we detail how these forces affect population health. Although here they are identified one by one, they are highly interrelated (Waitzkin, 2007).

Wealth distribution

Half the world's population controls just 1% of global wealth, living on less than US$730 per person per year. To put it more starkly, there is a 10 000 to 1 difference between the wealthiest 10% of Americans and the poorest 10% of Ethiopians (Birdsall, 2005). Wealth inequalities have been increasing over the last four decades within countries as well.[2] Four-fifths of the world's population lives in countries that have seen large increases in income inequality, including Colombia, Indonesia, Zambia, Poland, China, South Africa, India and the United States. In Brazil, the poorest 10% of the population earns just 0.7% of national income, while the wealthiest 10% amasses 47% (UNDP, 2005).

Stepwise differences in health indicators by wealth quintile have been found in certain developing countries. For instance, in Peru, child mortality is almost five times higher for children of the lowest wealth quintile than those of the highest wealth quintile. But Tanzania, which is a less unequal society, has far smaller differences by wealth quintile (although higher infant mortality rates overall) (Gwatkin et al., 2007). Some point to income inequality as key to understanding population health patterns, arguing that for high-income countries, relative income inequality is more important than GDP/capita in determining shorter life expectancy. An accompanying assertion is that the mortality effects of inequality, while most deeply felt by the poorest, are also experienced among the well-off due to the psychosocial impact of inequality and of low levels of social cohesion (including among elites seeking to protect their status) (Wilkinson & Pickett, 2009).

But the relationship between income inequality and health outcomes is not as direct as these findings suggest (Lynch et al., 2004). With the exception of the USA, income inequality is not a major determinant of population health differences within or between

---

[2] Measurements of wealth (as opposed to income) take into account property, stock, interest and other non-income assets.

countries and is only one feature of the distribution of wealth and power. In fact, though raising the incomes of the poorest would help to lift people out of absolute poverty and reduce health inequalities, the maldistribution of political influence and power associated with income and wealth inequalities would likely persist. As such, a range of universal and redistributive social policies – that are themselves both the result and the makings of greater equality in political power – are likely to have a far greater impact on health than income redistribution per se (Starfield & Birn, 2007).

Land tenure

While property ownership is a key feature of assets and wealth in most societies, land tenure is particularly salient where small-scale agriculture and subsistence farming is practiced because holding and farming the land is often the sole source of livelihood which provides access to food, income, decent living conditions and other determinants of health. In some countries, land redistribution has been a key feature of political movements and revolutions and has served as a means of raising the living conditions of millions of small-scale farmers.

As agricultural production has become industrialized over the past two centuries, however, big business interests and free trade policies have squeezed out small rural landholders through a variety of mechanisms. In nineteenth-century Britain, for example, collective landholdings were forcibly split after reform of official inheritance laws, making small plots no longer sustainable. At the same time, guaranteed crop prices were abandoned by the state (with repeal of the Corn Laws), driving small farmers off the land and forcing them into factories. More recently, large agribusinesses have used technologies and unfair competitive practices to drive down prices, similarly squeezing out small landholders. In Brazil, for example, recent corporate takeovers by Nestlé and Parmalat caused 50 000 small dairy farmers to lose their livelihoods. In various countries, governments have nationalized large swaths of land – forcing local farmers or nomadic hunters and pastoralists onto unproductive land – only to resell the property to private interests. Millions of landless farmers in South Asia, Latin America and elsewhere have been forced to migrate to urban settings. Though they have begun to organize politically (e.g. through Brazil's Landless Workers' Movement), they continue to be among the most marginalized of the world's population.

As environmental scientist-activist Vandana Shiva has poignantly demonstrated in her examination of agriculture in India, the rise of agribusiness, free trade agreements, and the marketing of genetically modified (GM) seeds has had devastating effects. Unlike local varieties, GM seeds are patented and expensive to purchase; many farmers lured into GM seed dependence soon become indebted. Millions of small farmers have lost their livelihoods, unable to survive against large competitors. Since 1997 more than 200 000 farmers in India have committed suicide (Shiva, 2009).

Social structure

The political, social and economic context into which we are born and live significantly influences health. This context, in turn, is shaped by the class, gender, and racial organization of society, that is, how power is structured. Understanding extant inequalities in structural, spatial and social position terms is central to rectifying social inequalities in health.

Class

Social class, theorized by Karl Marx to define people's relationship to the production process – in a capitalist system, whether one is an owner or a worker – is among the most powerful determinants of health (Navarro, 2001). According to the political economy of health approach, the structures, institutions and relations of the capitalist economic system generate, and are reflected in, social inequality. In classical Marxism, the foremost inequality is between owners and workers. More recently, neo-Marxist thinkers have elaborated on class structure theory to analyze contradictory class location – for example, people who are simultaneously owners and workers (such as factory employees with pension plans tied to company profits) or neither owners nor workers (managers, administrators, professors etc.). Critical gender and race theorists further show that class location, race, and gender are intertwined (see ahead).

How does class affect health? To begin, the material conditions of life, as discussed throughout this chapter, have an enormous bearing on health. These conditions, whether referring to neighborhoods, assets and possessions, or workplace environment, indicate material advantage or disadvantage over the life-span (Shaw *et al.*, 2002). Material conditions are associated with physical (infections, malnutrition, chronic disease and injuries), developmental (delayed or impaired cognitive, personality and social development), educational (learning disabilities, poor learning, early school leaving) and social (socialization, preparation for work and family life) problems. Income affects these conditions in terms of consumption of health care and private transportation, for example, but cannot explain why highly paid industrial workers have far worse health than lower-paid teachers; occupational exposures, control over work processes, workplace social policies and decision making all have to do with structures of class power in the polis and in the workplace, regardless of income.

Where there are more inequalities in political structures and institutions (disadvantaging the working class), there is less redistribution of material resources, fewer social services, reduced economic and social security, and lower democratic decision-making capacity, reflected in inequalities in virtually every other determinant of health. In the workplace, class struggle and class inequality have enormous health effects. The lower one is in a workplace hierarchy, the less decision latitude and employment security is enjoyed, and the more one is subject to oversight, repetitive activities and deprivation, all leading to higher stress levels, with the health consequences described above.

Where workers have less political power (i.e. where unions are limited or illegal), stress is compounded by precarious work conditions, with higher exposure to workplace hazards, fewer protections against dangers and job loss, and more repression. While social democratic societies with universal and comprehensive social security systems and strong unions, such as Sweden, experience less inequality than less redistributive societies, class-based inequalities remain and redressing them is a prime societal concern.

Gender

Gender, referring to social conceptions and roles rather than biological differences, is a key determinant of health (Sen & Östlin, 2009). In other words, health differences due to sex-based differences in biology are not gendered per se, whereas health differences between women and men (whether heterosexual, transsexual, gay, lesbian, bisexual or of ambiguous sexuality) due to their differing household responsibilities, decision-making powers, occupational roles or legal rights are gendered. Even health issues that are largely biological may be inextricably linked to gender. For example, the health of women during pregnancy and delivery is affected by their lifelong nutritional status, level of social support, as well as access to health care – factors which are all influenced by gender roles.

Gender-based differences in health status vary over time and place, just as gender roles vary according to era and context. That said, in most societies, women, together with sexual minorities, bear the brunt of gender oppression and prejudice. In most high- and middle-income countries today, women experience lower levels of mortality and longer life expectancy (though higher morbidity) than men do, in large part due to reductions in childbirth-related deaths over the past century. Yet in certain developing countries, maternal mortality remains extremely high, shortening women's life expectancy.

Gendered roles by no means consistently favor men. In the former USSR, men have disproportionately higher mortality rates as well as higher rates of smoking, alcohol consumption and obesity. Men are also more likely to be involved in road traffic accidents. Globally, violence is a gendered phenomenon, with women experiencing much higher rates of domestic and sexual violence and men experiencing higher rates of homicide.

The sexual division of labor leads to differential health outcomes, with men more likely to undertake dangerous or high-stress employment outside of the home, while women – especially in developing countries – are exposed to dangerous household-related activities such as indoor cooking and water collection. But this is changing with women's greater integration into the paid labor force. Moreover, a significant number of women are engaged in some of the most hazardous occupations, including farming and sex work. Although women generally benefit from higher levels of social support through friends and kin, this support can be a demand as well as a resource, potentially increasing stress levels.

Gender interacts with class, race and other categories of difference in determining access to education, employment, health and social services. Poverty increases morbidity and mortality for both men and women, but women typically have less control over the material and social conditions of life that foster good health. In settings such as Kerala, where there have been investments in education for girls and an emphasis on increasing women's participation in civil and political life, there have been improvements not only in gender equity but also in population health in general.

Race and racism

Race, like gender, is a social construction that is used to classify groups into categories based on arbitrary, usually visible, characteristics (e.g. skin color, shape of eyes, etc.). Historically, racial distinctions have been created by dominant societal groups in order to establish or maintain power and privilege at the expense of "the other" (Krieger, 2003). Racism is the enactment of structural and systematic forms of oppression and discrimination against particular racial groups by individuals and/or institutions, with racial definitions themselves arising from oppressive systems of race relations. Racial or "ethnic" inequities are observed in numerous health outcomes. In the USA, for example, the infant mortality rate among African–Americans is more than twice that of the population of European descent, and the death rate from heart disease, as well as lung and colorectal cancer, is higher among African–Americans than in the population as a whole (Kington & Nickens, 2001).

Racial inequalities in health are often theorized to reflect biological differences in susceptibility to disease. But this approach disregards the overwhelmingly social rather than biological basis of race, and may in itself reinforce racial discrimination. Moreover, because of the genetic heterogeneity within socially designated racial/ethnic groups, it is implausible that innate genetics alone can explain patterns and trends in racial/ethnic health inequities.

If, as current research suggests, the basis of racial/ethnic health inequities is not genes, however, then what is? Certainly, the rate of poverty is higher among African–Americans than among most other ethnic/racial groups in the USA. But higher poverty rates do not explain everything: death rates among African–Americans are higher than among Euro-Americans in every social class. Rather, these inequities are the result of the legacy of slavery and oppression, and the continued and pervasive effects of institutional and everyday racism. Indeed, a small but rapidly growing body of research documents the impact of racial discrimination on somatic health, mental health, and health behaviors, including self-rated health, blood pressure, pre-term delivery, obesity and tobacco and other substance use. In South Africa, the legacy of the racist apartheid system continues to manifest itself in unequal health conditions, with a three- to fourfold difference in infant mortality rates between blacks and whites.

Across the world there are also marked discrepancies in the health status of indigenous versus non-indigenous populations. In virtually every society (Russia, throughout Latin America, China, North America, Iceland, Australasia and elsewhere), aboriginal populations experience greater oppression and worse health. Colonization and continued discrimination against indigenous peoples – including forcible removal from ancestral lands, denial of heritage, loss of livelihood, government neglect and absence of social protections – has had many negative health effects. In Australia and Canada, thousands of indigenous children were forced from their families and communities into residential schools over almost a century, where they faced violence, overcrowding, poor nutrition and forced labor. Almost one-fourth of students in residential schools died of TB in early twentieth-century Canada.

The continued marginalization of indigenous populations is reflected in disproportionate poverty rates, limited access to potable water, poor quality housing and high exposure to environmental toxins. In Canada, indigenous groups have twice the poverty rate of non-indigenous populations; in Mexico, almost 90% of indigenous communities live in extreme poverty (Castro et al., 2007); and in El Salvador, 95% of water sources that are used by indigenous populations are contaminated (PAHO, 2002). The poor health status of many indigenous populations is compounded by lack of access to health care. All told, aboriginal children have death rates four times higher than non-aboriginal counterparts in Canada, Australia, New Zealand and the USA. Throughout the Americas, 40% of indigenous groups do not receive health services for geographic and economic reasons, and often there are large cultural, linguistic and social barriers to care (Montenegro & Stephans, 2006).

Global data reveal a consistent pattern across societies: groups subjected to racial discrimination – whether through conquest, slavery, segregation or subjugation – typically are the poorest and have the worst health status. It is important to note, however, that not all people of racialized origins are poor and not all poor people are of these origins. Most importantly, there is nothing inherent (genetically or culturally) that correlates racial/ethnic background with poverty. Rather, it is racism and its social application in everyday life that explains the poverty and poor health status of racialized groups around the world. In sum, worse health status among historically oppressed and marginalized groups is a reflection of *both* poverty and racism and must be analyzed as such.

Militarism, colonialism and imperialism

The legacies of colonialism, militarism and imperialism have shaped the historical trajectories of many, if not all, societal determinants of health in the domains of political self-determination, resource control, social policy, law and order and so on. Although few colonies remain, the current global political structure reflects geopolitical relations that have been in place for centuries. Systems of trade and commodity pricing, debt and global finance regimes, and international organizations for the most part maintain the historical power imbalances between colonizer (read high-income, developed, industrialized) and colonized (low-income, underdeveloped) countries.

Militarism escalates all forms of violence within and between countries, with extremely damaging consequences to soldiers and civilians alike. Militaristic societies often have excessively harsh judicial systems. For example, the USA has the highest number of people (2.3 million) and proportion of the population (1%) in prison in the world. Those incarcerated are disproportionately poor, young African–American and Latino men. Military spending also channels resources away from social and infrastructural endeavors, such as building parks, schools and quality housing, investing in safe employment and so on. The diamond business provides one example of the combined damage that militarism and imperialism can wreak on global health. Recent civil wars in Angola, the Democratic Republic of Congo and Sierra Leone – where over 5 million people have died – were largely fueled and financed by trade in "conflict diamonds."

Neo-liberal globalization, international trade regimes, financial instruments and policies

The neo-liberal paradigm, on which the current system of global trade is premised, purports that economic growth through integration into global markets – and deregulation, privatization and a reduced role for the state – are tools for poverty alleviation and reduction in national and international disparities, including health disparities. However, economic integration has had the opposite effect, with inequality increasing over the past three decades. Where economic growth has led to poverty reduction, most notably in China, vulnerability and insecurity have typically increased alongside dangerous work and environmental conditions (such as in mining and agriculture), lack of regulation, and deterioration of health and social infrastructure (Reddy, 2008).

Indeed, the global trade system damages health by creating and maintaining unequal power relations. In many developing countries, primary materials and labor-intensive goods are extracted and produced at far lower cost than in higher-income countries thanks to low wages, lax environmental and occupational standards and few, if any, taxes, all of which have negative health repercussions. Producer countries receive few gains (although corrupt politicians often benefit enormously), as they have little control over commodity pricing. Moreover, in many countries, a combination of subsistence living and political repression makes it difficult for workers to unionize and form effective political movements to lobby for more protective (health) measures.

Free trade agreements, a cornerstone of the global trade system, undermine worker rights and environmental protection policies, while promoting privatization of public sectors, such as water, health care and education. Reductions in tariffs and taxes also lower state income that could be spent on social services (Gershman et al., 2003). Similarly, the economic instruments and policies of international financial agencies, commercial banks and dominant corporate interests, namely structural adjustment programs and poverty reduction strategies, have affected health by influencing national policies and environments regarding work, production and economic patterns, and social welfare. More specifically:

(1) Agriculture and mining sector reforms have undermined the viability of small producers, weakened food security and damaged the natural environment.

(2) Privatization and civil and labor sector reforms have increased rates of unemployment and precarious employment, weakened worker protections and decreased wages.

(3) Deregulation has increased environmental contamination, occupational exposures and hazards in the home and community.

(4) Privatization, user fees and social spending cuts have decreased access to essential services, including education, health care, and housing.

(5) The emergence of large multinational companies has devastated local industries, especially small and medium enterprises.

The burden of these policies and reforms has been borne disproportionately by the poorest and most vulnerable populations (children, women, indigenous groups and small-scale farmers), while the benefits have been disproportionately enjoyed by local and international elites, large private sector enterprises and transnational corporations.

Conclusion

As we have seen, the societal determinants of health are both distinguishable from one another *and* inter-related at progressive levels (Starfield, 2007; Krieger, 2008). Poverty, for example, is both the outcome of local, national and global activities and is accompanied by material deprivation leading to, among other things, inadequate access to nutritious food, clean water, housing, safe neighborhoods and so on (Marmot, 2005). These factors, in turn, increase exposure and susceptibility to, and reduce resistance and recovery from, disease and disability. Ultimately, patterns of unequal political power and resource distribution drive the societal determinants of health, which synergistically interact with biological processes, leading to inequalities in health within and across population groups. There is no natural or inherent reason for these health inequalities: they are societally produced.

Many of the deleterious health effects of the societal determinants explored in this chapter have been known for hundreds of years. As early as the seventeenth century, Bernardino Ramazzini uncovered the damaging effects of environmental and occupational chemicals on the health of workers. As soon as French cities began collecting statistics, laissez-faire advocate Louis-René Villermé found that untoward housing conditions and poverty were associated with ill health. And before the germ theory was elaborated in the late nineteenth century, medico-social observers such as Friedrich Engels and Rudolf Virchow recognized the capitalist system of production and lack of political representation as underlying determinants of health in industrializing Europe, which, they argued, had to be addressed by redistributing power via revolution and democracy.

More recently, the clearest articulation of the need to address the political and social (i.e. societal) determinants of health was made in 1978 by the *Alma Ata Declaration on Primary Health Care*, signed by 175 countries. It called for a new international economic order, emancipatory development of decolonized countries, and a commitment to addressing the roots of leading health problems, including food insecurity, poor sanitation and social and economic inequality, from a community-based, primary-care approach. Though the *Alma Ata Declaration* generated enormous discursive currency, in practice it was quickly fragmented and criticized for being overtly political (Banerji, 2003).

> The existing gross inequality in the health status of the people particularly between developed and developing countries as well as within countries is politically, socially, and economically unacceptable and is, therefore, of common concern to all countries. Alma Ata Declaration (WHO, 1978 p. 1)

In the last several years, the WHO has returned to these concerns. In 2008, a special commission issued the report *Closing the Gap in a Generation: Health Equity Through Action on the Social Determinants of Health*. Bold enough to show the global dimensions of social inequalities in health and calling on them to be monitored and addressed, the report nonetheless refrained from "making it political," that is, it failed to spell out what the "causes of the causes of the causes" are, viz. why inequalities exist in the first place (ALAMES, 2008; Birn, 2009; Navarro, 2009). As Alison Katz passionately puts it, genuinely employing a societal determinants approach to reducing health inequalities "will not be possible unless the multiple crises that we are confronting today – in energy, water, food, finance, the environment, science, information, and democracy – are recognized as capitalist crises and addressed in these terms. In short, the invisible hand of the market must be replaced by the visible hand of social justice" (Katz, 2009, p. 568). This is, undoubtedly, the global health ethics imperative of our times.

Acknowledgments

I am grateful to Oxford University Press for allowing me to adapt this material from Birn, A. E., Pillay, Y. & Holtz, T. H. (2009). *Textbook of International Health: Global Health in a Dynamic World*, 3rd edn. New York: Oxford University Press. I also thank Danielle Schirmer for editing assistance.

References

ALAMES (Latin American Social Medicine Association) (2008). Taller Latinoamericano sobre Determinantes Sociales. Mexico City, Mexico. www.alames.org/documentos/ponencias.pdf (Accessed September 15, 2009).

Banerji, D. (2003). Reflections on the twenty-fifth anniversary of the Alma-Ata Declaration. *International Journal of Health Services* **33**, 813–818.

Beckfield, J. & Krieger, N. (2009). Epi + demos + cracy: a critical review of empirical research linking political systems and priorities to the magnitude of health inequities. *Epidemiologic Reviews* **31**, 1–26.

Benach, J., Muntaner, C. & Santana, V. (2007). *Employment Conditions and Health Inequalities: Final Report to the WHO Commission on Social Determinants of Health*. Geneva: Employment Conditions Knowledge Network (EMCONET).

Birdsall, N. (2005). Rising inequality in the new global economy. In *WIDER Annual Lecture*: United Nations University.

Birn, A.-E. (2009). Making it politic(al): closing the gap in a generation: health equity through action on the social determinants of health. *Social Medicine* **5**, 166–182.

Castro, R., Erviti, J. & Leyva, R. (2007). Globalización y enfermedades infecciosas en las poblaciones indígenas de México. *Cadernos de Saúde Pública* **23**, S41–S50.

Chung, H. & Muntaner, C. (2007). Welfare state matters: a typological multilevel analysis of wealthy countries. *Health Policy* **80**, 328–339.

Driscoll, T., Takala, J., Steenland, K., Corvalan, C. & Fingerhut, M. (2005). Review of estimates of the global burden of injury and illness due to occupational exposure. *American Journal of Industrial Medicine* **48**, 491–502.

Eagleton, D. (2005). *Power Hungry: Six Reasons to Regulate Global Food Corporations*. Johannesburg: ActionAid International.

Gershman, J., Irwin, A. & Shakow, A. (2003). Getting a grip on the global economy: Health outcomes and the decoding of the development discourse. In R. Hofrichter, (Ed.), *Health and Social Justice: Politics, Ideology, and Inequity in the Distribution of Disease*. San Francisco, CA: Jossey-Bass.

Gruskin, S. & Tarantola, D. (2005). Health and human rights. In S. Gruskin, M. Grodin, G. Annas & S. Marks (Eds.), *Perspectives on Health and Human Rights*. New York, NY: Routledge.

Gwatkin, D. R., Rutstein, S., Johnson, K. *et al.* (2007). *Socio-Economic Differences in Health, Nutrition and Population within Developing Countries: An Overview*. Washington, DC: World Bank. http://go.worldbank.org/XJK7WKSE40.

Katz, A. R. (2009). Prospects for a genuine revival of primary health care – through the visible hand of social justice rather than the invisible hand of the market: part I. *International Journal of Health Services* **39**, 567–585.

Kellett, P. & Moore, J. (2003). Routes to home: homelessness and home-making in contrasting societies. *Habitat International* **27**, 123–141.

Kington, R. S. & Nickens, H. W. (2001). Racial and ethnic differences in health: recent trends, current patterns, future directions. In N. Smelser, W. Wilson & F. Mitchell (Eds.), *America Becoming: Racial Trends and Their Consequences*. Washington, DC: National Academy Press.

Krieger, N. (2003). Does racism harm health? Did child abuse exist before 1962? On explicit questions, critical science and current controversies: an ecosocial perspective. *American Journal of Public Health* **93**, 194–99.

Krieger, N. (2008). Proximal, distal, and the politics of causation: what's level got to do with it? *American Journal of Public Health* **98**, 221–230.

LaDou, J. (2003). International occupational health. *International Journal of Hygiene and Environmental Health* **206**, 303–313.

Lundberg, O., Åberg Yngwe, M., Kölegård Stjärne, M. *et al.* (2008). The role of welfare state principles and generosity in social policy programmes for public health: an international comparative study. *Lancet*, **372**, 1633–1640.

Lynch, J., Davey Smith, G., Harper, S. *et al.* (2004). Is income inequality a determinant of population health? Part 1. A systematic review. *The Milbank Quarterly* **82**, 5–99.

Marmot, M. (2005). The social determinants of health inequalities. *Lancet* **365**, 1099–1104.

Montenegro, R. & Stephans, C. (2006). Indigenous health in Latin America and the Caribbean. *Lancet* **367**, 1859–1869.

Muntaner, C., Borrell, C., Espelt, A. *et al.* (2009). Politics or policies vs politics and policies: a comment on Lundberg. *International Journal of Epidemiology*, doi:10.1093/ije/dyp220.

Nantulya, V. M. & Reich, M. R. (2003). Equity dimensions of road traffic injuries in low- and middle-income countries. *Injury Control and Safety Prevention* **10**, 13–20.

Navarro, V., Ed. (2001). *The Political Economy of Social Inequalities*. Amityville, NY: Baywood Publishing Company.

Navarro, V. (2009). What we mean by social determinants of health. *Global Health Promotion* **16**, 5–16.

PAHO 2002. Health of indigenous people: a challenge for public health. www.paho.org/english/DPI/100/100feature32.htm (Accessed November 17, 2009).

Phillips, J. & Beasley, R. (2005). *Income and Poverty in the District of Columbia: 1990–2004*. Washington, DC: State Data Centre, D.C. Office of Planning.

Pogge, T. (2005). World poverty and human rights. *Ethics and International Affairs* **19**, 1–7.

Reddy, S. G. (2008). Death in China: Market reforms and health. *International Journal of Health Services* **38**, 125–141.

Rice, J. & Steinkopf Rice, J. (2009). The concentration of disadvantage and the rise of an urban penalty: urban slum prevalence and the social production of health inequalities in the developing countries. *International Journal of Health Services* **39**, 749–770.

Sanchez, P., Swaminathan, M. S., Dobie, P. & Yuksel, N. (2005). *Halving Hunger: It Can Be Done*. New York, NY: UN Millennium Project.

Sen, G. & Östlin, P., Eds. (2009). *Gender Equity in Health: The Shifting Frontiers of Evidence and Action*. New York, NY: Routledge.

Shaw, M., Dorling, D. & Mitchell, R. (2002). *Health, Place and Society*. Harlow, UK: Prentice Hall.

Shiva, V. (2009) Why Are Indian Farmers Committing Suicide and How Can We Stop This Tragedy? May 23, 2009. voltairenet.org Non Aligned Press Network. www.voltairenet.org/article159305.html (Accessed July 27, 2009).

Starfield, B. (2007). Pathways of influence on equity in health. *Social Science and Medicine* **64**, 1355–1362.

Starfield, B. & Birn, A-E. (2007). Income redistribution is not enough: income inequality, social welfare programs, and achieving equity in health. *Journal of Epidemiology and Community Health* **61**, 1038–1104.

Starfield, B., Shi, L. & Macinko, J. (2005). Contribution of primary care to health systems and health. *Milbank Quarterly* **83**, 457–502.

UNDP (2005). *Human Development Report 2005: International Development at a Crossroads: Aid, Trade and Security in an Unequal World*. New York, NY: UNDP.

UNICEF (2007). *Facts on Children: Water and Sanitation*. New York, NY: UNICEF.

US Government (2005). Average life expectancy at birth by state for 2000 and ratio of estimates and projections of deaths: 2001 to 2003. www.census.gov/population/projections/MethTab2.xls (Accessed November 17, 2009).

Waitzkin H. (2007). Political economic systems and the health of populations: historical thought and current directions. In S. Galea (Ed.), *Macrosocial Determinants of Population Health*. New York, NY: Springer.

WHOSIS (2009). WHO Statistical Information System. www.who.int/whosis/en/ (Accessed November 12, 2009).

Wilkinson, R. & Pickett, K. (2009). *The Spirit Level: Why More Equal Societies Almost Always Do Better*. London: Allen Lane.

World Health Organization (WHO) (1978). *Declaration of Alma Ata*. International Conference on Primary Health Care. Alma Ata, USSR.

World Health Organization (WHO) (2002a). *World Health Report*. Geneva: World Health Organization.

World Health Organization (WHO) (2002b). *World Report on Violence and Health*. Geneva: World Health Organization.

World Health Organization (WHO) (2004a). *Handbook for the Documentation of Interpersonal Violence Prevention Programs*. Geneva: World Health Organization.

World Health Organization (WHO) (2004b). *Water, Sanitation and Hygiene Links to Health*. Geneva: World Health Organization.

Chapter

4

Gender and global health: inequality and differences

Lesley Doyal and Sarah Payne

Introduction

Gender equity and gender equality appear increasingly often in the health policies and mission statements of national governments and international organizations. These concepts are found not only in the more obvious locations such as the World Health Organization (WHO), United Nations Development Program (UNDP) or the United Nations Population Fund (UNFPA) but also in settings as apparently unlikely as the World Bank. But do we really know what these terms mean and how they could be achieved? Indeed would we recognize them if we saw them?

This chapter will explore these issues from a number of different perspectives. First it will spell out the differences between male and female patterns of health and illness. Second it will offer the conceptual tools necessary for understanding them. This will involve a clarification of the distinction between biological sex and social gender as well as an exploration of their inter-relationships. Given this background we can then explore the differences between equity and equality in the context of gender and health policy.

Men and women: patterns of health and illness

Any attempt to compare the health and well-being of women and men is faced with considerable challenges. All the available data have limitations in terms of what is counted, and how accurately and inclusive these statistics are. These limitations are greatest in the poorest parts of the world. Despite these problems such data offer a useful indication of various health inequalities, including those between men and women.

Measurements of mortality

The most reliable data on differences between males and females are those relating to deaths. Overall they suggest that women can expect to live longer than their male counterparts in virtually every country in the world. In 2006, for example, male life expectancy at birth was higher than that of females in only two out of the 193 member countries of the World Health Organization (WHO, 2009b). There were three countries where men and women had the same life expectancy. But in all of the other 188 countries women could expect to live longer than men.

However, the gap between women and men varies. The narrowest differences in life expectancy are found in those settings in which life expectancy is low overall. In most cases these are the poorest countries in the world, notably those in the sub-Saharan region of Africa where there has been a reversal in both male and female life expectancy in recent years as a result of the increasing burden of HIV/AIDS together with persistent poverty (WHO, 2004).

The widest gap in life expectancy between males and females, 19 years, is found in Iraq (WHO, 2009b). However, men are also much more likely to die before women in Eastern Europe, particularly in those countries which were formerly part of the Soviet Union. In the Russian Federation, for example, women might expect to live up to 13 years longer than men (WHO, 2009b). This gap reflects a reduction in male life expectancy towards the end of the twentieth century, following the rapid growth in poverty in the post-communist era, with high levels of male unemployment and changing patterns of alcohol and substance abuse.

The ways in which the gap between women and men varies across different cultures, time periods, locations and levels of development suggests that the

Global Health and Global Health Ethics, ed. Solomon Benatar and Gillian Brock. Published by Cambridge University Press.
© Cambridge University Press 2011.

underlying reasons for these differences do not reflect a single cause but need to be explained in each setting by a range of more complex influences involving both biological and social factors.

When we look at what men and women die from, male and female causes of death are very similar. Around one-third of both men and women die from communicable diseases such as respiratory infections, tuberculosis (TB) or HIV/AIDS (WHO, 2004). Similarly, around 60% of both men and women die from non-communicable diseases, including cardiovascular disease and cancer. However, there are two important differences in male and female mortality patterns that are useful to highlight here. The first draws attention to social factors while the second focuses on biological ones that are mediated by social inequalities.

First, men are much more likely than women to die from both intentional and non-intentional injuries with over 1 million male deaths each year from such causes (WHO, 2004). In the Russian Federation, for example, four times as many men as women die from such injuries (WHO, 2009a). Around the world, more men than women die each year as a result of homicide, especially among younger age groups. Men are also much more likely than women to die or be injured as a result of conflict.

On the other hand many women still have to face the hazards of reproduction which can result in maternal mortality. Overall more than half a million women die each year from complications following pregnancy and childbirth, including those arising from miscarriage and terminations (WHO, 2005). Although these account for less than 2% of all female deaths worldwide, most are relatively easy to prevent. In 2005 for example, the maternal mortality rate in Sierra Leone was 2100 per 100 000 live births compared with only 8 per 100 000 in the UK (WHO, 2009b). This reflects gendered aspects of poverty as well as the fact that about three-fifths of births in Sierra Leone are unattended.

Figures for deaths are useful for making broad comparisons between women and men but they also have major limitations. Most importantly, they do not accurately capture health experience across the life course. An alternative measure of health is morbidity, which refers to illness, both short-term acute periods of ill-health and also longer term or chronic illness. This can be measured in a number of different ways, each of which may throw a different light on comparisons between women and men. Three of these measures will be illustrated here.

Self-reported health

It has long been assumed that women experience poorer health during their lives in comparison with men: that "women get sicker but men die quicker" (Lorber, 1997). But the true picture of the gap between women and men is more complex and varied.

In most countries women report their overall health to be worse than that of men. This is especially true in poorer communities. In the World Health Organization's *World Health Surveys*, for example, figures from China, India, Malawi, the Russian Federation and Pakistan (among others) all revealed that more women than men reported their health as either bad or very bad, while more men than women reported their health as either good or very good (WHO, 2009c).

However, women do not always report poorer health than men. In Australia, for example, national survey data for 2004–5 show that women are slightly more likely than men to say their health is either very good or excellent (ABS, 2006). In the UK, similar numbers of men and women report their health as bad (ONS, 2006) while in the USA more men than women report good health, although the gap is again narrow (Schiller & Bernadel, 2004).

These differences are difficult to interpret. They might reflect variations in wording and cultural perceptions of survey questions and may also be influenced by whether or not the data are age-standardized. They might reflect class or income differences, as poorer health is reported by those in lower income groups, which in some countries may include a greater proportion of women.

Composite health indicators

We can also assess the health gap between women and men through composite indicators of health at population level. One of the best known of these is the estimate of healthy life expectancy (HALE) produced by the World Health Organization. HALE is a measure which starts from life expectancy at birth and is then adjusted downwards to reflect an estimate of time spent during the life course in poor health (WHO, 2004). This estimate is carried out for each of WHO's member countries, using a range of survey statistics and other measures to calculate the adjustment separately for men and women.

HALE figures for 2002 revealed that in 14 out of 192 countries males had either the same or a better healthy life expectancy than females. In the remaining

178 countries women could expect to live a longer time in full health. As with mortality and life expectancy, the extent of female advantage varies – in the Russian Federation, for example, female healthy life expectancy was over 11 years greater than male HALE. Yet as we have seen, fewer Russian women than men describe themselves as being in good health.

If we look not at years spent in healthy life but instead at the proportion of overall life expectancy that is lost due to poor health, women appear to do rather less well. For the same 192 countries, there were only four countries in 2002 where men lost a greater proportion of their life expectancy to illness and disability. In the remaining countries the proportion of life expectancy lost was higher for women (WHO, 2004).

An alternative measure of health, using disability adjusted life years (DALYs), highlights the distribution of the burden of disease. DALYs are based on calculations of the value of years of disability-free life which are lost as a result of either premature death or the onset of disability (Lopez *et al.*, 2006). DALYs can be used in relation to specific conditions as well as overall health and may also be used to indicate the value of particular interventions which reduce mortality or disability.

Overall, there is only a narrow gap between women and men in their experience of morbidity using this measure: men comprise 52% of total DALYs lost per annum and women comprise the remaining 48% (WHO, 2004). But men are much more likely than women to suffer illness or disability as a consequence of accidental and non-accidental injury, as well as from heart disease, alcohol use disorders and some cancers. Males also have higher risks of perinatal disabilities. Healthy years lost by women are especially likely to result from pregnancy and childbirth, depression, sensory disorders including cataracts and sexually transmitted infections.

However DALYs have been criticized for their focus on economic rather than social costs of disease and poor health – the loss of income or the costs of care, for example, rather than suffering, stigma and individual well-being (Sen & Bonita, 2000). In addition some have argued that DALYs fail to measure the full consequences of some health conditions. This is because the severity of their impact was estimated by experts in the field rather than individuals with experience of a condition.

This means that calculations of what has been lost tend to underestimate the burden of illness that has wider individual and social costs (Dejong, 2006).

Very often this will vary between women and men. For example, obstetric fistulae are debilitating conditions which arise as a result of prolonged or obstructed labor, often in women who have undergone female genital mutilation (FGM). Various health consequences may follow including infection, ulcers and incontinence. Fistulae are also highly stigmatizing and create enormous social problems for the women involved. But this stigma and the consequences are not counted as part of the burden of DALYs, leaving the social and functional disabilities facing many women uncounted (Dejong, 2006).

Use of health services

Finally health differences between women and men can be measured through data on consultations with health professionals. But again these figures are likely to be influenced by a range of factors that may be different in women and men. For example, in some settings men are reluctant to seek care for fear of appearing "weak" and are more likely to soldier on when faced with symptoms of poor health (Robertson, 2007). Men also may experience difficulty taking time off from paid employment to use health care (Wilkins *et al.*, 2008). Women on the other hand can face other material obstacles in accessing services.

For example, they are more often responsible for the care of children and vulnerable dependents and this can limit their ability to seek help. Women are also less likely to have control over the resources needed to pay for health consultations in many countries. In some cultural settings women also need to be accompanied when using services and are therefore dependent on someone being available to take them (Baghadi, 2005).

Though few data are available to confirm this, it seems likely that these limitations have a greater impact on women's use of health care in resource-poor settings. In more developed countries such as the UK on the other hand, women consult more often than men throughout the health-care system and also take more prescribed medication (GHS, 2004). Similar gendered patterns of consultation are also found in the USA and Australia (Payne, 2006).

There are further differences between women and men in terms of what they are treated for. For example, in general practice in the UK, more women than men are treated for hypertension, depression and anxiety while men are more often treated for coronary heart disease and diabetes (Wilkins *et al.*, 2008). The difference in treatment for depression is particularly large with women being more than twice as likely to receive such a diagnosis in general practice (Wilkins *et al.*, 2008).

Taken together, the various ways of measuring morbidity or ill-health among women and men suggest that the situation is a complex one. On the whole, women report poorer health, use services more, particularly where health care is relatively accessible, and experience more chronic problems, especially those associated with reproduction. Men experience higher levels of illness and disability from those conditions which also contribute to their higher mortality rates, as well as apparently under-using health care.

Sex and gender influences on health are central to explanations of these differences. The next section will therefore explore the ways in which each (and both together) might affect health and health outcomes.

Sex, gender and health

There is now a growing literature on both sex and gender influences on health. But this has not always led to a clearer understanding of the issues. Two problems need our attention here. The first is the continuing confusion between the terms "biological sex" and "social gender" (Krieger, 2003). The second is the tendency to discuss gender issues only in the context of women. Men too are "gendered" and this has huge significance for their narratives of health and illness.

Those working within the paradigm of biomedicine have traditionally talked of "sex differences" between women and men, defined mainly in relation to their reproductive systems. However, the last decade has seen an extension of this concept to "sex-related biology" which includes a broader range of hormonal and metabolic variations between women and men (Wizeman & Pardue, 2001). There has also been increasing recognition of the differences between males and females in the way they experience diseases that affect both sexes.

The term "gender" came into use during the 1960s to describe the ways in which maleness and femaleness are socially constructed. Feminist writers and activists of the period were concerned to challenge the essentialism so often inherent in the use of the term "sex." Their main aim was to show that many of the supposedly "natural" differences between women and men were in fact the result of the ways in which societies were organized. Moreover, they demonstrated that many of these differences were inequalities which

were potentially damaging to women's health in various ways (Doyal, 1995; Payne, 2006).

These literatures on biological sex and social gender have developed separately but there continues to be confusion between them. In the biomedical arena in particular, the terms sex and gender are often used both interchangeably and inappropriately. Too often, researchers ascribe differences in results between women and men to either sex or gender influences without any supporting argument for their choice of term. Indeed it seems that the use of "gender" often derives from an erroneous belief that this is the more "politically correct" option. As a result the interconnected but different domains of biological and social causality become confused and research findings may be hard to interpret (Krieger, 2003).

These problems are confounded by the fact that sex and gender differences need to be understood both separately and also in combination. In the case of HIV, for example, aspects of women's biology interact with gender inequalities to heighten their vulnerability to infection and also to shape their experience of the illness. Hence we need to be very clear about the impact of both sex and gender as well as their complex interactions in order to fully understand the different patterns of health between men and women in different settings. As Nancy Krieger has pointed out:

> The relevance of gender relations and sex-linked biology to a given health outcome is an empirical question, not a philosophical principle; depending on the health outcome under study, *both*, *neither*, *one*, or the *other* may be relevant – as sole, independent, or synergistic determinants. (Krieger, 2003, p. 656, emphasis in the original)

Krieger & Zierler (1995) describe such interactions in terms of *the biologic expression of gender* and the *gendered expression of biology*. The biologic expression of gender refers to the ways in which gender becomes embodied. For example, in many societies gender is constructed to mean that women see themselves, and are seen by others, as weaker than men. This in turn may result in women taking less exercise, or choosing less strenuous forms of activity, which in turn affect the female body.

The gendered expression of biology on the other hand, refers to the ways in which biological understandings of women and men lead to gendered differentiations, which often take the form of discrimination. Women's reproductive capacity, for example, is used to justify their exclusion from some forms of paid work on the basis that it is unsafe. Similarly their exclusion from medical research is said to be justified on the basis that it may cause harm to an unborn child. This exclusion in turn strengthens social constructions of gender in which women are seen as less able to undertake some forms of paid work, or are less likely to have some symptoms recognized by health-care professionals because of stereotypes about "candidacy" for certain conditions, such as heart disease.

We turn now to explore these influences – sex, gender and the interaction between the two – in more detail.

Sex and health

Biological influences on health include not only differences between women and men based on their reproductive systems, but also those reflecting genetic and hormonal factors. The most obvious of these differences is the greater vulnerability of males throughout the life course (Waldron, 1983). Even studies of fetal mortality – deaths in the womb at any gestational age – reveal higher rates of mortality among males than females.

Female sex hormones appear to protect women against a range of conditions including, for example, ischemic heart disease (Waldron, 1985). One explanation for this advantage is that estrogen increases the flexibility of the female circulatory system, and that high blood pressure is less damaging for premenopausal women (Bird & Rieker, 1999). Similarly, estrogen increases high-density lipoprotein (HDL) cholesterol levels and decreases low-density lipoprotein (LDL) cholesterol, improving the functioning of the heart (Wizeman & Pardue, 2001).

There are also differences in male and female immune systems which in turn reflect reproductive factors, particularly the capacity of women to conceive and carry a child. These differences mean that women are more at risk than men from auto-immune disorders (Bird & Rieker, 1999). During pregnancy women are also at higher risk of some communicable diseases ranging from measles to malaria (Wizeman & Pardue, 2001).

However, we must be wary of attributing too much to biology. Wizeman & Pardue (2001) also point out the limitations in this area of knowledge. Despite many years of research on the ways in which biology impacts on health, conclusive evidence and clear understanding of the pathways concerned remain scarce. There are various reasons for this, including often the failure to disaggregate research results for men and women. There is also evidence that negative findings which

show no differences between women and men are often not published despite the fact that they too could advance our understanding of overall sex differences (Emslie et al., 1999).

What remains clear, however, is that biological or sex-linked factors shape the health of both women and men through their interaction with a wide range of environmental factors, including socially constructed gender differences in particular.

Gender and health

Gender affects the health of both men and women in a number of interlocking ways. First, gender mediates the effect of physical and psychological risks encountered in daily life. Men and women will often be affected in different ways by both their unwaged work and their employment, for example. Second, gender roles and expectations are closely associated with individual behavior which in turn may impact on the health of women and men.

Thus far these issues have been explored mainly through a female lens. This concentration on women is not surprising given the structural disadvantage so many face in accessing the resources needed to optimize their health. But as we shall see the focus is now beginning to open up as the links between "maleness" and health are increasingly explored (Courtenay, 2000; Robertson, 2007).

There is an extensive literature on the links between women's health problems and their relative poverty, their heavy burden of both waged and domestic labor, their low social status and their vulnerability to gendered violence and other forms of abuse (Doyal, 1995; Payne, 2006). In many parts of the world women are more likely than men to be poor. This is due to lower wages, reduced access to paid work as a result of caring responsibilities and in some countries cultural restrictions, and inequalities in the allocation of household resources. Poverty is often especially severe among older women whose health is already frail (Arber & Cooper, 1999).

Paid employment also exerts significant and gendered effects on health. There are a range of hazards associated with particular jobs, including exposure to unsafe chemicals, hazardous work environments and dangers inherent in the nature of the work itself (Ostlin, 2000). The gender division of labor which sees men more often employed in certain sectors and in certain occupations creates a gendered division of occupational risk (Payne, 2006). Men typically work in industries and in jobs with a higher mortality risk – including construction, transport and the emergency services, for example.

However, in recent years the occupational injury gap between women and men has narrowed, following the rise in the numbers of women in the labor force with corresponding increases in some forms of injury-related mortality (Waldron *et al.*, 2005). Some hazards which increase the risk of poor health – repetitive strain injury (RSI), for example, from keyboard work and some production processes in manufacturing – are more common among women partly as a result of the jobs in which they are placed and partly because the design of workstations is often based on male rather than female physiology (de Zwart *et al.*, 2001; Lacerda *et al.*, 2005).

Exposure to violence creates further risks including poor mental health, post-traumatic stress disorders and physical injuries. Violence is one of the most important causes of death for younger age groups (WHO, 2002c) but there are marked gender differences not only in the level of risk from violence but also in the source. Although both women and men are at risk from interpersonal violence, violence against men is more common in the public domain, and they are more at risk from strangers (Payne, 2006).

Women on the other hand are more likely to be exposed to violence in the home – from partners and members of their family (WHO, 2002c). Women are at particular risk from sexual violence, and the consequences for their health can include pregnancy and sexually transmitted infections as well as mental health problems. Although sexual violence against men is less common, it may be especially damaging for mental health due to feelings of stigma and shame (Ganju *et al.*, 2004).

Taken together, these varied aspects of daily life can create particular health stresses which are often different for men and women. To these health risks, we can add those associated with "doing gender" – the ways in which men and women adopt certain behaviors as a result of social constructions of masculinity and femininity, which in turn impact on health risk (Connell, 2005).

There are still important differences between women and men in behaviors such as smoking, alcohol and substance use, physical activity, diet, risk-taking behavior, and use of health-care services including preventive care and screening. The nature of these differences will vary across communities but taken together they are a key part of the explanation for men's higher

mortality. Indeed a number of writers in this area have highlighted the extent to which masculinity itself increases risks to men's health across a range of cultural settings (Courtenay, 2000; Robertson, 2007).

One of the most damaging behaviors – smoking and tobacco use – has a strongly gendered history. More men than women die each year from smoking-related diseases: lung cancer, for example, killed twice as many men as women worldwide in 2002 (WHO, 2004). This reflects the gender ratio in smokers: throughout the world more men smoke than women and in countries where the epidemic is relatively new, the great majority of those using tobacco are male (WHO, 2002b).

However, more developed countries have seen increasing numbers of female smokers: in Norway and Sweden for example, women now smoke in roughly similar numbers to men (WHO, 2002b). In the USA around 23% of men and 18% of women smoke, while in the UK the comparable figures are 27% of men and 24% of women (GHS, 2004; CDC, 2009). In younger age groups in the UK, female smokers now outnumber males and there are also more women smokers than men in some minority ethnic groups in the UK, particularly those described as "mixed race" (GHS, 2004).

Patterns of nutrition also reflect gender differences. The diets of men are often less healthy than those of women, particularly in more developed countries where they are more likely to consume inadequate amounts of vegetables and fruit, and high levels of red meat (Courtenay, 2000; Payne, 2006). However, in many less-developed countries where there is an increased risk of food insecurity, women and girls are less likely than men to be eating adequate levels of important nutrients. In some countries, there are also cultural differences in the distribution of food within households, in expectations about what men and women will eat, and also in what will be given to male and female children (Sayers, 2002).

Overall, then, gender differences in roles, expectations and behavior combine to increase the likelihood of premature mortality for men and women's vulnerability to chronic health problems. Masculinity, in so far as it involves risk-taking and unhealthy behaviors, increases the chance of accidental and non-accidental injury, and non-communicable diseases associated with smoking, alcohol and substance use. Masculine practices also increase some health risks for women, particularly the risks associated with male violence, sexually transmitted communicable diseases and poor reproductive health.

Female gender roles and expectations, on the other hand, may lead to reduced risks of some conditions, due to lower rates of smoking, alcohol and substance use, better diets and less risk-taking. But these have to be offset against the physical and psychological damage often wrought by wider gender inequalities.

We can illustrate some of these complex associations between sex and gender in the context of a specific case study using the example of cardiovascular disease.

How biological sex and social gender shape cardiovascular diseases

Cardiovascular diseases are a category of illness including coronary heart disease (CHD) and stroke. Taken together they account for around one-tenth of the global burden of disease, with more men than women affected (WHO, 2004). Coronary heart disease is the major contributor to this burden, particularly among men, while strokes account for similar proportions of illness among men and women. These conditions are also important in overall mortality: more men than women die as a result of CHD but women are more likely to die from a stroke (WHO, 2004).

One of the key differences between women and men in these illnesses is the age at which risk increases: men are more likely than women to die prematurely from coronary heart disease and the male to female ratio is greatest in mid-life. Women die on average 10 years later than men (Wizeman & Pardue, 2001). Although trends in CHD have changed over time, the greater risk men experience of premature death and illness associated with this condition is found throughout the world (Khaw, 2006; Payne, 2006).

Why do men have higher risks than women for CHD at an early stage in the life course? In the etiology of CHD, raised blood pressure and blood cholesterol are significant risk factors, and behavioral factors associated with these risks – particularly poor diet and smoking – are more common among males and are important underlying explanations. While women gain protection from heart disease due to female hormones, men increase their risks with poorer health behaviors. However, there also appear to be differences in the impact of different risks. Low levels of HDL cholesterol, for example, are predictive of CHD risk but the risk associated with low HDL cholesterol is greater for women than for men (Fodor & Tzerovska, 2004).

The later age at which women appear to be at risk of CHD has led to speculation that until the menopause, female hormones might offer women some degree of protection. However, most recent research has failed to support this suggestion. For example, women's CHD risk does not increase immediately following the menopause but some years later, suggesting that other factors may be important instead of, or alongside, female hormones. In addition hormone replacement therapy does not appear to offer women protection from CHD (Khaw, 2006).

There are also debates concerning possible differences between women and men in the recognition and treatment of CHD. Women themselves may be less likely to seek help because they assume that heart disease is a "male" problem (Moser et al., 2005). Based on the same presumption, health workers may also be less likely to diagnose their illness quickly or to offer appropriate treatment. There is now considerable evidence that in some settings women with heart disease are less likely than men to receive particular interventions (Wilkins et al., 2008). However the reasons for this remain unclear and it is uncertain whether it represents an under-treatment of women or an over-treatment of men (Raine et al., 2002).

It should now be clear that there are marked differences in the health needs of women and men and that these are both biological and social in origin. It is also evident that these differences are not reflected appropriately in health services or in wider public policy. Though "equality" and "equity" are frequently cited as policy goals there is little clarity about what this means in practice.

Gender equality and gender equity in health policy

One of the most significant debates about gender justice in public policy occurred at the 1994 Cairo Conference on Population and Development (ICPD). The initial aims of the meeting were broadly drawn to include the promotion of gender equality as well as gender equity. However, the meanings of these terms were strongly contested among participants (Petchesky, 2003).

It was argued by faith-based organizations in particular that women were "natural" homemakers and hence did not need equal rights at work. Similarly the domestic relations between women and men were said to be divinely ordained, making the notion of female sexual rights inappropriate. Hence "gender equity" required that the two groups should be treated differently because of what were seen as "natural" and unchangeable differences between them. But for many of the other participants this meant "freezing" women into their current state of socially constructed inequality which was perceived to be unfair and inappropriate (Barton, 2004).

Given the nature of these debates, the UN adopted "gender equality" in preference to "gender equity" in developing the objectives for the Beijing Platform for Action the following year. Cairo had shown that the term "gender equity" could be predicated on perceptions of "difference" and concepts of social justice which were not in themselves value-free or objective. Hence the notion of gender equality was deemed to be preferable in order to avoid perpetuating what could be seen as gender-based discrimination (UN, 2001).

This continues to be the preferred term for the majority of organizations and institutions charged with reducing the inequalities between men and women. Within the United Nations, for example, responsibility for gender mainstreaming is held by the Office of the Special Advisor on Gender Issues and the Advancement of Women (OSAGI). Their aim is to achieve "gender equality" between women and men which is defined as follows:

> the equal rights, responsibilities and opportunities of women and men and girls and boys. Equality does not mean that women and men will become the same but that women's and men's rights, responsibilities and opportunities will not depend on whether they are born male or female. (OSAGI, 2001, p. 1)

Similarly the World Bank and the International Monetary Fund both use the concept of gender equality in defining their approach to development work and funding, and in the working of their own internal organizations (World Bank, 2007). In the European Union discourses around gender also use the concept of equality rather than equity, and the UK and Norway have both recently passed legislation which requires the public sector actively to promote "gender equality" throughout all their activities.

But despite this growing preference for the term "gender equality," some organizations specifically concerned with health are continuing to use the notion of "gender equity." The clearest argument for the importance of both "gender equality" and "gender equity" in discourse concerning health can be found in documents from WHO (WHO, 2002a; 2008). The differences in the meaning and implications of the two concepts are described as follows:

> Gender equality means the absence of discrimination on the basis of a person's sex in opportunities, allocation of resources or benefits, and access to services.

while

> Gender equity means fairness and justice in the distribution of benefits, power, resources and responsibilities between women and men. The concept recognizes that women and men have different needs, power and access to resources, and that these differences should be identified and addressed in a manner that rectifies the imbalance between the sexes. (WHO, 2002a, p. 3)

So why are these issues of terminology different in the context of health? Why should "equity" be a central concept alongside "equality" when this option has been rejected in other policy arenas? The key reason for this lies in the distinction between gender inequalities and gender differences and in the sex differences in biology between women and men.

In the context of education or employment, for example, it is social obstacles which prevent gender equality in outcomes. In order for girls and boys to achieve their potential, a range of gendered obstacles need to be removed. It is then theoretically possible to imagine equality of outcomes between women and men.

However, the same argument cannot be applied in the context of health. Of course the many inequalities experienced by women will need attention if their health and health care are to be optimized. These will be especially important for the poorest women where appropriate and effective reproductive health services are essential as well as gender-sensitive strategies for poverty alleviation and for the promotion of physical security.

For men too, the removal of social obstacles to health will be important. However, it is important to recognize the fact that these stem not from gender inequalities per se but from the shaping of masculinities in different cultural settings. And policies will need to take this crucial difference into account.

But even complex strategies of this kind will not be sufficient. As we have seen, biology itself is also a major determinant of health and failure to recognize this can promote further inequalities between women and men. Though biological characteristics can rarely be changed, some potentially harmful effects can be mitigated through social policies which take them properly into account. However these biological factors will make it impossible to ever achieve "equal" health for women and men.

Thus the only realizable goal will be to ensure that both men and women are able to optimize their potential for health *within the constraints of their biological sex* (Anand & Sen, 1995). And it is here that strategies for gender equity will need to come into play alongside those of gender equality to meet the inherently different needs of women and men. To take just one example, it may never be possible to give men and women equal life expectancy. But equitable policies will ensure that both are able to reach their potential for a long and healthy life.

Strategies for enabling women and men to reach their health potential will need to begin with a commitment to both equality and equity in the delivery of services. This in turn will require the development of health care which is based on an improved knowledge base of both sex and gender differences in health needs and their implications for appropriate interventions. This will be a challenging task. But the promotion of gender equality in health itself will be even harder.

The differences between the social constructions of "maleness" and "femaleness" are deeply embedded in all aspects of the individual psyche and in the wider social order. Any shift towards "healthier" models of gender will be a complex and difficult process and will involve changes far beyond the health sector. These issues have been at the heart of many feminist debates over the years and are beginning to emerge in the literature on men's health (Robertson, 2007). However, there are no easy solutions.

The goal of gender justice is even more challenging. As we have seen, gender inequalities are often more pervasive and more damaging to women than they are to men, while men may have more to gain from the status quo. If this unfairness is to be tackled it will require a radical transformation of gender relations. A major restructuring will be needed in the divisions of labor, of resources and of status between women and men across a range of social and economic settings.

These changes would be complex and difficult to achieve and as we have seen, they are likely to be resisted at both individual and institutional levels. It is always difficult to persuade those (mainly men) with status and power to relinquish them. But without such changes, neither women (nor men) will be able to fully realize their biological potential for health.

References

ABS (2006). *National Health Survey 2004–05*. Australian Bureau of Statistics: Canberra.

Anand, S. & Sen, A. (1995). *Gender Inequality in Human Development: Theories and Measurement*. Occasional Paper 19. Washington, DC: UNDP.

Arber, S. & Cooper, H. (1999). Gender differences in health in later life: the new paradox? *Social Science and Medicine* **48**, 61–76.

Baghadi, G. (2005). Gender and medicines: an international public health perspective. *Journal of Women's Health* **14**, 82–86.

Barton, C. (2004). Global women's movements at a crossroads: Seeking definition, new alliances and greater impact. *Socialism and Democracy* **18**, 151–184.

Bird, C.E. & Rieker, P.P. (1999). Gender matters: an integrated model for understanding men's and women's health. *Social Science and Medicine* **48**, 745–755.

Centers for Disease Control and Prevention (CDC) (2009). Cigarette smoking among adults and trends in smoking cessation – United States, 2008. *MMWR* **58**, 1227–1232. www.cdc.gov/mmwr/PDF/wk/mm5844.pdf (Accessed November 2009).

Connell, R. (2005). *Masculinities*. Berkeley, CA: University of California Press.

Courtenay, W. (2000). Constructions of masculinity and their influence on men's well-being: a theory of gender and health. *Social Science and Medicine* **50**, 1385–1401.

De Zwart B., Frings-Dressen, M. & Kilbom, A. (2001). Gender differences in upper extremity musculoskeletal complaints in the working population. *International Archives of Occupational and Environmental Health* **74**, 21–30.

Dejong, J. (2006). Capabilities, reproductive health and well-being. *Journal of Development Studies* **42**, 1158–1179.

Doyal, L. (1995). *What Makes Women Sick: Gender and the Political Economy of Health*. London: Macmillan.

Emslie, C., Hunt, K. & MacIntyre, S. (1999). Problematizing gender, work and health: the relationship between gender, occupational grade, working conditions and minor morbidity in full-time bank employees. *Social Science and Medicine* **4**, 33–48.

Fodor, J. & Tzerovska, R. (2004). Coronary heart disease: is gender important? *Journal of Men's Health and Gender* **1**, 32–37.

Ganju, D., Jejeebhoy, S., Nidadavoluand V. *et al.* (2004). *Sexual Coercion: Young Men's Experiences as Victims and Perpetrators*. New Delhi: Population Council.

GHS (2004). *Living in Britain: Results from the 2002 General Household Survey*. London: The Stationery Office.

Khaw, K-T. (2006). Epidemiology of coronary heart disease in women. *Heart* **92**, 2–4.

Krieger, N. (2003). Genders, sexes and health: what are the connections – and why does it matter? *International Journal of Epidemiology* **32**, 652–657.

Krieger, N. & Zierler, S. H. (1995). Accounting for the health of women. *Current Issues in Public Health* **1**, 251–256.

Lacerda, E., Nacul, L., da S., Augusto, L. *et al.* (2005). Prevalence and associations of symptoms of upper extremities, repetitive strain injuries (RSI) and 'RSI-like condition': a cross sectional study of bank workers in Northeast Brazil. *BMC Public Health* **5**, 107.

Lopez, A. D., Mathers, C. D., Ezzati, M., Jamison, D. T. & Murray, C. J. H. (2006). Measuring the global burden of disease and risk factors, 1990–2001. In A. D. Lopez, C. D. Mathers, M. Ezzati, D. T. Jamison & C. J. H. Murray (Eds.), *Global Burden of Disease and Risk Factors*. Oxford: The World Bank and Oxford University Press.

Lorber, J. (1997). *Gender and the Social Construction of Illness*. London: Sage.

Moser, D., McKinley, S., Dracup, K. & Chung, M. L. (2005). Gender differences in reasons patients delay in seeking treatment for acute myocardial infarction. *Patient Education and Counseling* **56**, 45–54.

Office for National Statistics (ONS) (2006). 2001 Census Data: Focus on Health. www.statistics.gov.uk/cci/nugget.asp?id=1325 (Accessed July 2009).

OSAGI – Office of the Special Advisor on Gender Issues and the Advancement of Women (2001). *Gender Mainstreaming: Strategy for Promoting Gender Equality*. Washington: OSAGI, United Nations.

Ostlin, P. (2000). *Gender Inequalities in Occupational Health*. Cambridge, MA: Harvard Center for Population and Development.

Payne, S. (2006). *The Health of Men and Women*. Cambridge: Polity.

Petchesky, R. (2003). *Global Prescriptions: Gendering Health and Human Rights*. London: Zed Books.

Robertson, S. (2007). *Understanding Men and Health: Masculinities, Identity and Well-being*. Maidenhead: Open University Press.

Raine, R., Black, N. A., Towker, T. J. & Wood, D. A. (2002). Gender differences in the management and outcome of patients with acute coronary heart disease. *Journal of Epidemiology and Community Health* **56**, 791–797.

Sayers, J. (2002). Feeding the body. In M. Evans & E. Lee (Eds.), *Real Bodies: A Sociological Introduction*. Basingstoke: Palgrave Macmillan.

Schiller, J. S. & Bernadel, L. (2004). *Summary Health Statistics for the US Population: National Health Interview Survey*. Vital Health Stat Series 10 Number 220. Washington, DC: National Centre for Health Statistics.

Sen, K. & Bonita, R. (2000). Global health status: two steps forward, one step back. *Lancet* **356**, 577–582.

United Nations (2001). *Important Concepts Underlying Gender Mainstreaming*. New York, NY: United Nations, UN Office of the Special Adviser on Gender Issues and the Advancement of Women.

Waldron, I. (1983). Sex differences in human mortality: the role of genetic factors. *Social Science and Medicine* **17**, 321–333.

Waldron, I. (1985). What do we know about the causes of sex differences in mortality? *Population Bulletin of United Nations* **18**, 59–76.

Waldron, I., McCloskey, C. & Earle, I (2005). Trends in gender differences in accidents mortality. *Demographic Research* **13**, 415–454.

Wilkins, D., Payne, S., Granville, G. & Branney, P. (2008). *Gender and Access to Health Services*. London: Department of Health www.dh.gov.uk/prod_consum_dh/groups/dh_digitalassets/@dh/@en/documents/digitalasset/dh_092041.pdf (Accessed November 2009).

Wizeman, T. & Pardue, M. (2001). *Exploring the Biological Contributions to Human Health: Does Sex Matter?* Washington, DC: National Academy Press.

World Bank (2007). *Global Monitoring Report 2007: Confronting the Challenges of Gender Equality and Fragile States*. New York, NY: World Bank.

World Health Organization (WHO) (2002a). *Mainstreaming Gender Equity in Health: The Need to Move Forward – Madrid Statement*. Geneva: World Health Organization.

World Health Organization (WHO) (2002b). *Tobacco Atlas*. Geneva: World Health Organization.

World Health Organization (WHO) (2002c). *World Report on Violence and Health*. Geneva: World Health Organization.

World Health Organization (WHO) (2004). *World Health Report 2004: Changing History*. Geneva: World Health Organization.

World Health Organization (WHO) (2005). *World Health Report 2005: Make every Mother and Child Count*. Geneva: World Health Organization.

World Health Organization (WHO) (2008). *Strategy for Integrating Gender Analysis and Actions into the Work of WHO*. Geneva: World Health Organization.

World Health Organization (WHO) (2009a). European health for all database (HFA-DB). World Health Organization Regional Office for Europe http://data.euro.who.int/hfadb/ (Accessed October 2009).

World Health Organization (WHO) (2009b). WHO Statistical Information System (WHOSIS). www.who.int/whosis (Accessed October 2009).

World Health Organization (WHO) (2009c). World Health Survey Results. www.who.int/healthinfo/survey/whsresults/en/index.html (Accessed October 2009).

Chapter

5

Health systems and health

Martin McKee

What are health systems for?

It is easy to forget that one of the primary purposes of a health system should be to improve health (McKee, 1999). For decades, debates on health systems have been dominated by discussions of how much they cost to run (typically questioning whether they are affordable, as if there was an alternative in a civilized society) or how many resources they require (typically expressed in an arbitrary fashion as people, usually doctors and nurses but not managers or physiotherapists, or facilities and items of furniture, usually hospitals but not primary-care clinics or beds, but not examination couches). The nature of this discourse has meant that health systems have tended to be regarded as a cost to society from which there is little return, instead of as an investment whereby appropriately directed expenditure leads to better health. Indeed, some studies even suggested that more resources were associated with higher mortality, possibly as a consequence of higher rates of discretionary surgery (Cochrane *et al.*, 1978), a finding supported by the observation that death rates fell when doctors went on strike (Roemer, 1981).

This chapter is based on a very different vision, in which health, health systems and economic growth can exist together, in a mutually supportive virtuous circle. Drawing on work undertaken for a ministerial conference organized by the European Region of the World Health Organization in Tallinn, Estonia, in 2008, it builds on what is now a substantial body of research on these three sets of mutual inter-relationships (Figure 5.1). First, health care delivered appropriately and equitably has achieved substantial gains in population health while the promotion of better health reduces future demands for health care. Second, while, in general, wealthy countries have better health than poor ones, better population health leads to faster economic growth, as it enables

individuals to make a greater contribution to the labor market and to be more productive. Finally, while economic growth makes more resources available for health care, the health-care system can, if harnessed in support of regional development and innovation, contribute to economic growth. These mutually beneficial relationships will not, however, emerge spontaneously. Rather, they require collective action by governments and others to create health systems that address the health needs of their populations and respond to them with equitable and effective policies and practices.

There is a longstanding debate about whether social and economic rights should be considered, like political rights, as fundamental human rights. While respecting the different perspectives, the available evidence shows how appropriate and equitable investment in health systems is an important means of conferring on individuals the right to life.

This chapter begins by examining the much misunderstood contribution of health care to population health.

Some controversies about the contributions of medicine

Although by the 1970s some were making impressive claims for the achievements of modern health care, many demographers subscribed to a contrary view. These were exemplified by the work of Thomas McKeown, a British professor of public health who argued that over the preceding century and a half, therapeutic interventions had added little if anything to gains in life expectancy which instead were driven by improvements in living standards and, especially, nutrition (McKeown, 1979). At the same time Ivan Illich, in his book *Medical Nemesis*, argued that modern health care was actually harmful (Illich, 1977). Coining

Global Health and Global Health Ethics, ed. Solomon Benatar and Gillian Brock. Published by Cambridge University Press.
© Cambridge University Press 2011.

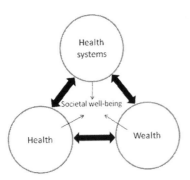

Figure 5.1 Health systems, health and wealth.
Source: World Health Organization (adapted with permission).

the term iatrogenesis, or doctor created, he described its clinical form in which the growth of diagnostic technology was being used to label variants on normality as illness, leading in turn to unnecessary treatment and adverse side effects. He also described a social and cultural form, whereby the increasing medicalization of life encouraged a growing number of essentially normal people to feel that they had something wrong and thus become dependent on doctors. This created a vicious circle whereby the health system expanded yet the population felt worse. A consequence was that medicine increasingly took on a role of social control, defining who was normal and who was not. Similar views were being expressed by others working in the field of mental health, where the role of medicine as a form of social control was especially apparent. Laing, for example, saw what was labeled as mental illness as a rational reaction to an abnormal society (Laing, 1965). Szasz argued that to qualify as an illness an entity must be capable of being assessed or measured in a scientific way and be demonstrable at the cellular or molecular level. Many so-called "mental illnesses" were, in his view, false illnesses, representing a judgment by society about what is or is not acceptable. Hence "If you talk to God, you are praying; If God talks to you, you have schizophrenia. If the dead talk to you, you are a spiritualist; If you talk to the dead, you are a schizophrenic" (Szasz, 1974). From this perspective, psychiatry is a means of controlling those seen to be deviant, with those deemed to be mentally ill assuming the role previously occupied by witches and certain religious minorities.

All these arguments have some truth. Although McKeown's attribution of much of the improvement in life expectancy in nineteenth century England to nutrition has been challenged by subsequent, more detailed analyses (Colgrove, 2002), it is true that, at least until the 1950s, health care could do little to address the common causes of premature death. And while Illich may have overestimated the harmful effects of health care, his term iatrogenesis has become established within mainstream medicine. He was writing at a time when the thalidomide scandal was unfolding, in which a sedative given to pregnant women was found, despite initial denials by its manufacturers, to cause serious birth defects (Rosen, 1979). However, in 2000, a report by the US Institute of Medicine estimated that as many as 44 000 deaths each year could be attributed to medical errors (Institute of Medicine, 2000), findings since replicated elsewhere (Thomson, 2007). These findings have influenced the development of what is now a global alliance of health professionals seeking to improve patient safety. Similarly, the once firmly opposed camps represented by psychiatry and anti-psychiatry have moved closer together, at least in the developed world, as the treatment of people with mental illness is increasingly underpinned by commitments to patients' rights. Yet what health care could deliver in the 1960s and 1970s, when McKeown and Illich were writing, has changed almost beyond recognition.

The changing nature of health care

The antibiotic era

Perhaps the most spectacular example of how health care has changed is the discovery of antibiotics. The early sulphonamides, such as Salvarsan, developed by Domagk, for which he won the 1939 Nobel Prize for Medicine, did work against some common bacteria but they were of limited effectiveness in severe cases and they had important side effects. Penicillin, discovered by Fleming and subsequently mass produced following work by Florey and Chain, achievements for which all three shared the 1945 Nobel Prize in Medicine, was much safer and more effective. It now became possible to cure many common but previously often fatal bacterial infections. In time these compounds were supplemented by new classes of drugs, each with their own mode of action, range of activity against different organisms and side effects. Thus, the advent of aminoglycosides made it possible to treat serious infections with gram-negative bacilli that often followed major abdominal surgery albeit at a risk of side effects from some of the more effective drugs in this class, such as deafness or kidney damage. The results were especially dramatic with tuberculosis, until then a not uncommon cause of death of young people. McKeown had used the example of tuberculosis to argue against the contribution of medicine to declining mortality, showing how the death rate had already fallen substantially even before Koch had identified the tubercle bacillus as the cause of the disease and longer before either immunization, with the BCG vaccine, or treatment with drugs became available. However, an examination of age-specific death rates in England and Wales shows a striking year-on-year decline in mortality in young people between 1947, when streptomycin began to be available, and 1954 when it was in widespread use (Nolte & McKee, 2004). This remarkable achievement was repeated 40 years later when the introduction of antiretrovirals transformed infection with HIV from a rapidly fatal illness into one that its victims were as likely to die with as from (Atun *et al.*, 2009).

Unlike some of the other successes of medicine, however, the development of antibiotics has not been without its setbacks. Within a decade of the widespread introduction of antibiotics it was already becoming clear that humans and micro-organisms were engaged in a massive evolutionary struggle, as the process of natural selection allowed those few bacteria in which a mutation had conferred resistance to an antibiotic to survive and multiply, a process facilitated in some cases by the transfer of tiny fragments of DNA called plasmids. The emergence of resistance was detected early in cases of tuberculosis, leading physicians to employ multiple therapy regimes, on the basis that it was extremely unlikely that sufficient organisms would develop resistance against three or more drugs acting on different mechanisms. However, tuberculosis was seen as a special case because of the long duration of treatment, at that time often two years or more, which offered many opportunities for resistance to develop.

Multiple therapy was not seen as an option for more easily cured infections. However, within a few decades, humans had created the conditions that allowed resistance to many common antibiotics to flourish. One factor was the almost ubiquitous use of antibiotics as a growth promoter in the rapidly expanding industrial agricultural plants, in which tens of thousands of chickens and pigs were kept in appalling conditions where they were at constant risk of growth-retarding infections. Another was the inappropriate use of antibiotics for often self-limiting infections, a practice encouraged by widespread over-the-counter sales in many countries. This is exemplified by tuberculosis. Problems arose

once anti-tuberculous drugs became widely available in countries with fragile health systems that had weak systems of governance. These were initially in Latin America and the countries emerging from the Soviet Union but now include many parts of the developing world. The absence of an effective laboratory infrastructure means that patients are treated without knowledge of the drugs to which their infections are sensitive. Patients whose infections are already resistant to two of the usual combination of three drugs are at great risk of developing resistance to the third, a risk that could be countered by giving them one or more second-line drugs to which their infections are still sensitive. The resultant multidrug-resistant tuberculosis (MDR-TB) and, initially in South Africa, extensively resistant tuberculosis (XDR-TB) were the inevitable consequences.

Tuberculosis is, however, only one of many examples. *Staphylococcus aureus*, a common bacterium often found on the skin, was initially killed rapidly by penicillin. For many years it was possible to keep one step ahead by the development of new antibiotics until finally a strain resistant to methicillin emerged. This is now widespread in hospitals in some countries and is extremely difficult to eradicate. It can therefore be concluded that, in the case of antibiotics, while health systems have achieved a great deal, the final chapter has yet to be written.

Advances in the treatment of chronic diseases

The situation is rather more encouraging with regard to drugs for chronic diseases. The discovery of insulin in the early 1920s by Banting and Best transformed the management of type 1 diabetes. Children who, until then, had been dying slowly over a period of about 18 months after diagnosis could be treated, enabling them to achieve an almost normal life expectancy (at least after subsequent developments allowed prevention or treatment of many of the long-term complications of this disease). This was the first time ever that a disease was treated by a drug that the patient would remain on for the rest of their lives. The introduction of progressively purified thyroid hormones in the 1930s followed for patients with myxedema, but in both cases the numbers of people in the population affected by these disorders were relatively small. By the 1950s, however, the first drugs that were both effective and well-tolerated in treating hypertension were becoming available. The subsequent discovery of safe and effective bronchodilators for people with asthma and chronic obstructive airways disease, major tranquillizers for those with mental disorders, and anti-inflammatory drugs for those with arthritis, led to a situation whereby a substantial share of the middle-aged population would be commenced on medication they would take for the rest of their lives. Progress was gradual. For example, treatment of hypertension was initially prescribed only for those whose blood pressure was extremely high and who were clearly suffering adverse consequences, manifest as cerebrovascular, ocular and renal dysfunction. In the early 1960s, research showed how the treatment of asymptomatic hypertension could reduce the subsequent incidence of stroke (Hamilton *et al.*, 1964). The new drugs, thiazide diuretics and later beta-blockers, were initially prescribed predominantly for younger men with substantially elevated blood pressure, reflecting both the widespread tendency to under-treat cardiovascular disease in women and an erroneous view that the observed increase in blood pressure with age was both natural and of little danger. In time, the population offered treatment expanded and the threshold for treatment fell, accompanied by a steady decline in mortality from stroke in developed countries that continues to this day.

Advances in surgery

Progress was also seen in the outcome of surgery. The development of anesthesia and asepsis in the nineteenth century made it possible to operate inside the abdominal and thoracic cavities. Over the subsequent century surgical, anesthetic and post-operative techniques progressively developed. Over the past three or four decades rates of peri-operative mortality associated with many procedures have fallen markedly. A major factor has been the ability to recognize and treat complications, as is apparent from studies using a measure of "failure to rescue," which assess mortality in those suffering complications (Silber *et al.*, 2007). At the same time, advances in surgical technique have reduced the trauma associated with surgery, in particular through the use of minimally invasive techniques. Although there is little evidence that these methods are, overall, safer than open procedures, they do increase the number of otherwise unfit patients who can benefit from surgery. A related development is the introduction of medical alternatives to surgery, most notably the introduction of H2 blockers for peptic ulcers, followed later by the use of drugs to eradicate *Helicobacter* infection, now known to be the cause of most ulcers.

Cancer therapy

Although less successful overall, there have also been achievements in the struggle against cancer. Within a decade of the discovery of X-rays by Röntgen in 1895 electromagnetic radiation was being used to treat cancers. However, its use was limited to tumors that were radiosensitive, such as lymphomas and germ cell tumors rather than those developing from epithelial cells, and to those that were localized to one part of the body. By the 1940s a number of chemotherapeutic agents were being used, initially derived from chemical weapons such as mustard gas. The combination of chemo- and radiotherapy transformed the management of some cancers, such as Hodgkin's disease and testicular cancer, but for many others the only option was surgical removal. This was only successful where resection was complete and before metastases had developed. From the 1980s, advances in understanding of cell biology and, in particular, the role of hormones and the complex relationship between tumors and their blood supply, have progressively extended the pharmacologic armamentarium, with drugs such as tamoxifen transforming the survival of patients with that form of breast cancer that is estrogen-receptor positive. Deaths from some cancers have also been reduced by the development of screening programs that have enabled tumors or pre-malignant lesions to be detected and treated at an early stage, exemplified by breast and cervical cancer screening programs. However, as the experience with screening for prostate cancer shows, the decision to implement screening requires careful consideration as it may simply detect many lesions that are slow growing and which may never cause problems, while the resulting diagnosis may provoke considerable anxiety and treatment may give rise to unnecessary complications, while conferring no survival benefit.

Technological advances in diagnosis and treatment

There have also been a number of technological developments that have impacted substantially on the ability to improve health or prevent premature death more generally. These include a wide range of diagnostic methods, such as improved imaging that facilitates the targeting of radiotherapy. In other cases the benefits have been unexpected. For example, the widespread use of new forms of abdominal imaging may have detected many early cancers of the kidney that would have been missed using barium enemas. In other cases, technology has provided a new form of treatment, with dialysis enabling those with renal failure to remain alive, ideally until they can receive a transplant.

The influence of evidence on medical practice

Finally, it is necessary to consider the massive expansion of evidence-based medicine. The expansion of randomized controlled trials into areas such as surgery or organizational interventions (such as the evaluation of stroke units) has generated a vastly increased body of knowledge on the effectiveness of health care. This, in turn, has been taken advantage of by those engaged in the synthesis of evidence, most notably by the Cochrane Collaboration. Its use of meta-analysis to combine the results of multiple studies has made it possible to identify effective treatments where single trials have been inconclusive and to reject treatments previously thought to be effective, while also delineating areas where more primary research is required. These activities are not, however, limited to synthesizing knowledge. There is increasing emphasis on the translation of evidence into practice, encouraged in some countries by the creation of specialized agencies such as the British National Institute for Health and Clinical Evidence (NICE) or the German Institut für Qualität und Wirtschaflichkeit im Gesundheitswesen (IQWiG), both generating guidelines tailored to the needs of practicing clinicians. This is supported by a growing body of research on how to influence clinical practice. The consequences can be seen in a study of the outcome of major trauma in British hospitals, where steadily improving outcomes could not be attributed to a single intervention but rather to the increased seniority and skills of the doctors involved, coupled with greater use of evidence-based guidelines (Lecky et al., 2000). Together, these illustrate the importance of strong institutions committed to the generation, synthesis and transmission of evidence in modern health systems (Moon et al., 2010).

The dream and the reality

The potential value of health systems

Modern health care holds out enormous promise, but only if it can be delivered effectively to those in need

through well-organized health-care systems. However, these do not emerge spontaneously. As Frenk has noted, health systems have received far too little attention by policy makers, regarded as a "black box" whose contents are too complex to understand, a "black hole," which absorb unlimited amounts of resources to little effect or a "laundry list," whereby it is sufficient to put all the components, such as facilities, people and technologies, in place and hope that something useful will emerge (Frenk, 2010). Rejecting these concepts, he calls for a greater emphasis on four essential elements for health system success, coining the mnemonic LIST: leadership, institutions, systems design and technologies.

So what do health systems achieve at a population level? This can be assessed using the concept of avoidable mortality that Rutstein and colleagues developed over three decades ago (Rutstein et al., 1976). They identified a number of conditions from which premature death should not occur in the presence of timely and effective care. Such deaths were termed "avoidable." The initial list included many infectious diseases, common surgical conditions, such as acute appendicitis or cholecystitis, and some chronic conditions for which life-sustaining medication was available, such as diabetes or hypertension. They were writing at a time when the scope of medical practice had changed beyond all recognition.

This concept has been refined and updated taking account of factors such as the increase in life expectancy (Rutstein considered only those deaths before 65 years of age as avoidable whereas life expectancy at birth now exceeds 80 years in many industrialized countries) and the greater scope of medicine to prevent premature death, as discussed above (Nolte & McKee, 2004). Taking a historical perspective, the consequences at a population level can be seen from a comparison of the experiences of two countries, one of which had access to both modern health care and to the evidence underpinning it and one that had neither (McKee, 2007). Death rates from avoidable mortality were very similar in England and Wales and in Russia in 1965, at a time when these medications were just becoming available (Andreev et al., 2003). However, the trends then diverged, remaining high in Russia but falling away progressively in England and Wales.

Subsequent work has examined trends in avoidable mortality in many countries, usually showing how, since the 1970s, deaths from these causes have fallen at a faster rate than deaths where health care plays little role (Charlton & Velez, 1986). However, this work has also focused attention on the differences in performance of health systems and develops what is perhaps the best known attempt to compare health systems, the 2000 World Health Report (WHO, 2000).

A global ranking of health systems

The 2000 World Health Report identified three measures of a health system's performance: health attainment, responsiveness, and fairness of financing. Both health attainment and fairness of financing were assessed in terms of both the level achieved and their distribution within the population. The resulting five measures were then combined using weights obtained from a survey of public health experts in 100 countries. It was recognized that what countries could achieve was constrained by their economic and human resources so they were assessed against a predicted frontier derived from each country's economic performance and level of education.

Health attainment was measured in terms of Disability-Adjusted Life Expectancy at birth, a synthetic measure combining data on population structure, mortality rates at different ages, and the prevalence and severity of disability. A year lived with disability was given a lower value than one in perfect health, with the reduction calculated according to the severity of disability. The distribution of health attainment was calculated using data on child survival.

The approach taken was constrained by the need to rank all 192 of the World Health Organization's member states. Data on adult mortality were only available from about 60 countries so, in most, life expectancy was estimated by applying standard life tables to data from child mortality obtained from surveys, in particular the Demographic and Health Survey series. Disability levels were then modeled using the mortality data, taking account of other characteristics of each country.

The resulting rankings have been welcomed by some, especially in those countries such as France which came first overall, but criticized in others, typically those that fared less well, such as the USA and Brazil. Beyond these headline criticisms, there are a substantial number of technical issues that have attracted controversy and debate, including the weightings applied when combining each dimension of performance and the values underpinning the measures chosen (Almeida *et al.*, 2001). However, those who constructed the rankings recognize the many limitations but see them as a means of getting health system performance on to the political agenda, thus acting as a stimulus to obtain better data in the future.

In the present context, however, the greatest problem is that so few countries have cause-specific mortality data. The 2000 World Health Report partially circumvented this problem by defining the health system as "all organizations, people and actions whose primary intent is to promote, restore or maintain health," thereby justifying the use of a measure of health attainment that included death and disability from all causes. However, this also captures efforts undertaken in many other sectors, such as education, transport and employment. Hence, more recent work in industrialized countries has employed measures more specifically to health care, such as rates of deaths that should not occur in the presence of timely and effective care, or avoidable mortality, as described above.

One recent example was a comparison of trends in avoidable mortality in industrialized countries between 1997/8 and 2002/3 (Nolte & McKee, 2008). This study has attracted considerable political attention, especially in the USA where it has been cited extensively and accurately by those favoring President Obama's proposals for health-care reform but has attracted criticism in equal measure from those opposed to reform, who have attacked it, invariably on the basis of a misreading, deliberate or otherwise, of its findings. Its key finding was that the average decline in avoidable mortality in all the countries studied was 17% during this period. The one exception was the USA, where the decline was only 4%. It was estimated that, had the USA achieved the levels of avoidable mortality seen in the three best performing countries, it would have experienced over 100 000 fewer deaths at ages under 75 each year. It is, however, important to note that there are substantial differences within the USA with some states, such as Minnesota achieving a level comparable to that in the best performing European countries (63.9/100 000 in 2007), while in others the death rate is more than twice as high (e.g. Mississippi, at 142/100 000) (McCarthy *et al.*, 2009). For completeness, it is however necessary to recognize that there is one area where the USA does perform better than many European countries. While cancer survival rates at young ages are broadly comparable on both sides of the Atlantic, after account is taken of the unrepresentativeness of American cancer registry data and biases introduced by widespread use of ineffective screening activities, such as those for prostate cancer that provide earlier diagnosis but do not affect prognosis, the USA does manage to achieve substantially better outcomes for those aged over 65 (Gatta *et al.*, 2000). This is unsurprising as this group is covered by Medicare, which spends substantially more per capita than European health systems. Paradoxically, the inference is that the USA would achieve better outcomes with a strong, well-funded public insurer, precisely the opposite conclusion of those who draw attention to America's better cancer survival (Preston & Ho, 2009).

Those advocating the use of avoidable mortality in comparative research have consistently argued that this measure should only be used as an indicator that may suggest underlying problems. Hence, it is necessary to look beyond the aggregate figures to ascertain why this difference occurs. A more detailed analysis of broad categories of avoidable deaths showed that deaths from ischemic heart disease had increased in the USA but fallen elsewhere. However, some of the largest relative differences, where there has been least progress in the USA, are those common chronic diseases requiring long-term coordinated care, such as diabetes. Death rates from diabetes among young people are several times higher in the USA than in any western European country and while it can be argued that the epidemic of obesity in the USA means that there are more people at risk, it is difficult to accept that, in the twenty-first century, anyone should die from diabetes under the age of 50.

Diabetes as a lens to view the health system

This suggests that the experience of those suffering from diabetes may offer a useful lens through which to view the health system. Diabetes is an entirely treatable disorder. It has a number of advantages, in that it is common, those with diabetes (at least those using insulin) can easily be identified to participate in research, and mortality is demonstrably sensitive to health-system performance (Nolte *et al.*, 2006). This is illustrated by the experience of countries emerging from the turmoil accompanying the collapse of the Soviet Union in the late 1980s. The Soviet health system, despite its many weaknesses, did manage to keep many people with diabetes alive, albeit often with a poor quality of life. As health systems broke down following independence, death rates increased rapidly, only beginning to recover in the mid 1990s.

Diabetes is also of interest because its effective treatment requires the coordinated application of a range of different resources, which if inadequate have implications for many other disorders. First, it requires human resources, in the form of trained staff, from different professions but working collaboratively, and empowered patients who can employ self-care. Second, it requires physical resources, such as adequate and affordable supplies of insulin and drugs required for the complications of diabetes, as well as treatment facilities and testing equipment that make it possible to monitor the disorder. Third, it requires knowledge resources, such as evidence-based guidelines for treatment (appropriate to the needs of patients and professionals). Finally, there is a need for social resources, such as mechanisms to enable those with diabetes to lead lives that are as normal as possible, and systems of communication that ensure seamless referrals and transfer of information across the various layers of the health system.

This framework, and ones that are similar to it, have been employed in studies in several countries. A recent example is from Georgia, in the former Soviet Union (Balabanova *et al.*, 2009). The essential inputs needed to provide diabetes care were in place, including free insulin and training for primary-care physicians but constraints within the system hampered the delivery of accessible and affordable care. There were no evidence-based guidelines for diabetes management and no mechanisms to ensure quality of care. Primary care practitioners confined their activities to basic provision of care and saw diabetes as something that should be managed in specialist hospitals. In practice, access to insulin was problematic in rural areas and even in cities it was often difficult to obtain syringes, hypoglycemic drugs, and self-monitoring equipment and related consumables. Preventable complications were frequent and, when they occurred, involved hospital admission, often incurring prohibitive out-of-pocket payments. Referral pathways were complex, inhibiting the provision of seamless care, and follow-up was ineffective, with no monitoring of outcomes. Patients were disempowered, being viewed as invalids, and there was little effort to promote self-care, adherence to drug regimens, or appropriate lifestyles. These findings were very similar to those from an earlier study in Kyrgyzstan (Hopkinson *et al.*, 2004).

The situation is much worse in many developing countries. Beran and colleagues have developed the RAPIA instrument as a means of assessing the quality of care for people with diabetes, with an emphasis on access to insulin (Beran *et al.*, 2006). So far studies have been undertaken in Mali, Mozambique, Nicaragua, Vietnam, and Zambia. In each case, the analyses identified major weaknesses in the systems that have implications well beyond the management of diabetes. In Mali, for example, there was no standardized means of collecting information on patients. Insulin was available but supplies in the public system were often disrupted. Private pharmacists did have supplies but these were expensive due to high profit margins along the supply chain. Syringes were unavailable in the public sector and attracted 5% Value Added Tax. There were no guidelines or treatment protocols and care was uncoordinated, with long waiting times for referral. Frontline health-care workers had little understanding of diabetes and traditional healers played an important role in provision of care.

These examples illustrate the complexity involved in assessing health systems. While it is clearly necessary to have sufficient levels of inputs, such as hospitals, physicians, and essential drugs, knowledge of their numbers says nothing about how they are used and, especially, whether they form part of an integrated managed system rather than a chaotic and disorganized mix. This highlights once again the importance of ensuring that there are functioning systems of governance in place to ensure that health systems actually work as systems, and not as a disorganized and disconnected set of activities that lack any clear purpose or direction, as is unfortunately the case in many countries.

The contribution of health to health systems

So far this chapter has focused on the evidence that health care can contribute to population health. However there is a potential reciprocal relationship, whereby the level of health impacts on health systems. This is intuitively important; if everyone were to live to 100 years without significant illness and then die suddenly there would be no need for organized health care. However, the implication of the possibility that efforts to improve the health of a population may save future costs of health care has attracted surprisingly little attention. In fact, some have argued quite the contrary. In a now notorious example, consultants acting on behalf of a major tobacco company sought to persuade the Czech government not to implement anti-smoking measures on the grounds that the resulting increase in

people surviving into old age would increase the cost to the taxpayer.

The Wanless Report, prepared for the UK Treasury, was a seminal document in this respect (Wanless, 2001). Asked to assess future options for funding the National Health Service, Wanless, a banking executive, developed a series of scenarios of future expenditure on health care varying according to the nature and extent of adoption of policies to promote health and ensure timely and effective care. He concluded that the difference in expenditure between slow progress on these policies compared to what was described as "full engagement" would be £30 billion by 2022/3, representing approximately 40% of the total National Health Service budget in 2002. This evidence was seen as compelling by the Treasury, contributing to a substantial increase in health-care funding in the UK, a necessary measure given the need to make up for the long-term effects of under-spending over several decades.

There are others who are more pessimistic, arguing that an aging population will inevitably render health care unaffordable. This argument is based, in large part, on the evidence that older people incur greater health-care costs. However, initial research on the costs of aging was cross-sectional. Longitudinal studies have since confirmed that it is proximity to death that drives costs, with those dying at older ages actually being less expensive as they are treated less intensively (McGrail *et al.*, 2000). Furthermore, as a recent review has shown, there is much that can be done to encourage healthy aging and thus mitigate the economic consequences (Doyle *et al.*, 2009). This suggests that it may be possible to create a mutually beneficial situation whereby investments in health reduce future costs of health care while effective health care, especially where it prevents the onset or progression of disease and avoids the emergence of complications, may be mutually reinforcing.

Bring the economy into the equation: health systems and wealth

This concept, whereby health and health systems are mutually beneficial, has recently been extended to links with the wider economy. Self-evidently, there is a relationship between economic development and the ability to provide health care, although this is complicated by the fact that some inputs to health care have local prices, such as salaries (although even here there is to some degree a global market, depending on the ease with which health workers can migrate), while others, such as technology and pharmaceuticals, have international prices. A key question is how much to spend. This cannot be answered easily and, to some extent, the answer will depend on the political priorities of each government, especially because health care spending is fundamentally redistributive, not only from healthy to ill but, because the latter are typically concentrated among the most deprived, from rich to poor.

Once again there is a reciprocal relationship. Paying for health care, especially when serious illness strikes, is a major burden in many developing countries. Consequently, health systems are increasingly seen as playing a role in macroeconomic policy by lifting the fear of catastrophic expenditure (Anand & Ravaillon, 1993). Provision of funds for health care will not only benefit the poor directly, but will also give them the security to invest their meager resources in wealth creation rather than hoarding it to protect their families from possible disaster. This is also becoming a concern in the USA, the only industrialized country (at the time of writing) unwilling to pay for health care for all its citizens, where medical expenses are the leading cause of personal insolvency. The provision of health infrastructure is also being recognized increasingly as one component of a comprehensive approach to regional development, especially where procurement systems are established that provide a level playing field for local suppliers, for example by breaking up large tenders into smaller packages that enable small and medium enterprises to bid. Health infrastructure can also support regional development through tie-ups with the health industry, for example through academic medical centers linked to biotechnology start-ups.

Health and wealth

There is a considerable body of evidence, reviewed recently in the report of the Commission on Social Determinants of Health, that greater wealth is, all else being equal, associated with better health (Commission on Social Determinants of Health, 2008). Those with greater command over resources are better able to make healthy choices, enabling them to live healthier lifestyles and to access timely and effective health care.

The key question is, however, whether better health leads to greater wealth. This has already been answered in developing countries by the Commission on Macroeconomics and Health, which assembled an impressive body of evidence that poor health is

an important constraint on economic growth. It also showed that the return on investment from many basic health interventions is considerable (Commission on Macroeconomics and Health, 2001). However, it was by no means clear that the Commission's conclusions could be applied to high-income settings. One reason is that the nature of work differs. In poor countries much work involves physical activity, in agriculture, extractive industries or non-mechanized manufacturing, while in rich countries much work is sedentary. Another is that in poor countries substantial health gains can be achieved by scaling up basic interventions, such as immunization and treated bed nets, whereas in rich countries the burden of disease is dominated by chronic disorders so that the interventions needed are complex, multifaceted and often expensive.

Subsequent work has, however, examined the situation in both high-income and transition countries in Europe (Suhrcke et al. 2005, 2007). This work explores several pathways by which better health can increase economic growth. First, healthy people are more likely to be employed and are less likely to take sickness absence or to retire early. Second, they are more productive at work. It has been suggested that, as people realize that they are likely to live longer, they invest more time and money in their education, itself a driver of economic growth, and although the available evidence is limited, what does exist supports this pathway. Finally, in poor countries, people expecting to live longer are likely to save more for retirement, providing greater resources for capital investment. Here the evidence from rich countries remains inconclusive. Contemporary research is consistent with historical studies that have shown how a substantial share of the economic wealth in rich countries today can be linked to gains in health and nutrition in the past two centuries (Fogel, 1994; Arora, 2001), with several cross-country growth studies documenting a significant effect of better health on economic growth (Sala-I-Martin X, 2004).

This work has been complemented by research on the economic losses attributable to health inequalities in Europe, both in terms of the additional cost of health care and the wider impact on productivity (Mackenbach et al., 2007). It estimated that, if European Union governments could raise levels of good health among the least well educated to those of the best educated, they could achieve a 22% reduction in hospitalizations and gain €141 billion in productivity (equivalent to 1.4% of Gross Domestic Product) each year.

Summary

Too often health systems have been seen as a safety net, dealing with the immediate effects of illness but not actually enhancing health or contributing to economic growth. This chapter sets out a vision in which health, health systems, and economic growth can exist together, in a mutually supportive virtuous circle.

The importance of well-functioning health systems has been accepted by the global community of nations when they established the health-related Millennium Development Goals. It has also been accepted by governments of the European Union when they decided to invest in the health of their citizens as a key element of their Lisbon Strategy that seeks to make Europe the most competitive economy in the world (European Commission, 2008), by the World Bank's approach to investing in health in transition countries (World Bank, 2005), and by the governments of the World Health Organization's European Region, meeting in Tallinn in 2008 (McKee et al., 2009).

This chapter has described the enormous strides that have been made over recent decades by medical science. Yet these advances can only be dreamt of by the majority of the world's populations and, even in the USA, one of the richest countries in the world, those striving to provide universal health coverage face an enormous struggle against powerful vested interests. Governments and international agencies now need to deliver on the commitments that have been made, developing coordinated policies to structure effective health systems that meet the needs of their populations while establishing systems to monitor whether they are achieving what they promise.

References

Almeida, C., Braveman, P., Gold, M. R. et al. (2001). Methodological concerns and recommendations on policy consequences of the World Health Report 2000. Lancet 357(9269), 1692–1697.

Anand, S. & Ravaillon, M. (1993). Human development in poor countries: on the role of private incomes and public services. Journal of Economic Perspectives 7, 133–150.

Andreev, E. M., Nolte, E., Shkolnikov, V. M. et al. (2003). The evolving pattern of avoidable mortality in Russia. International Journal of Epidemiology 32, 437–446.

Arora, S. (2001). Health, human productivity, and long-term economic growth. Journal of Economic History 61, 699–749.

Atun, R. A., Gurol-Urganci, I. & McKee, M. (2009). Health systems and increased longevity in people with HIV and AIDS. British Medical Journal 338, b2165.

Balabanova, D., McKee, M., Koroleva, N. et al. (2009). Navigating the health system: diabetes care in Georgia. Health Policy and Planning 24, 46–54.

Beran, D., Yudkin, J. S. & De Courten, M. (2006). Assessing health systems for type 1 diabetes in sub-Saharan Africa: developing a "Rapid Assessment Protocol for Insulin Access". British Medical Council Health Service Research 6, 17.

Charlton, J. R. & Velez, R. (1986). Some international comparisons of mortality amenable to medical intervention. British Medical Journal (Clinical Research Edition) 292(6516), 295–301.

Cochrane, A. L., St Leger, A. S. & Moore, F. (1978). Health service "input" and mortality "output" in developed countries. Journal of Epidemiology and Community Health 32, 200–205.

Colgrove, J. (2002). The McKeown thesis: a historical controversy and its enduring influence. American Journal of Public Health 92, 725–729.

Commission on Macroeconomics and Health (2001). Macroeconomics and Health: Investing in Health for Economic Development. Geneva: World Health Organization.

Commission on Social Determinants of Health (2008). Closing the Gap in a Generation: Health Equity through Action on the Social Determinants of Health. Geneva: World Health Organization.

Doyle, Y., McKee, M., Rechel, B. & Grundy, E. (2009). Meeting the challenge of population ageing. British Medical Journal 339, b3926.

European Commission (2008). Lisbon Strategy. http://europa.eu/scadplus/glossary/lisbon_strategy_en.htm (Accessed October 11, 2009).

Fogel, R. W. (1994). Economic growth, population theory, and physiology: the bearing of long-term process on the making of economic policy. American Economic Review 84, 369–395.

Frenk, J. (2010). The global health system: strengthening national health systems as the next step for global progress. PLoS Med 7(1): e1000089. doi:10.1371/journal.pmed.1000089.

Gatta, G., Capocaccia, R., Coleman, M. P. et al. (2000). Toward a comparison of survival in American and European cancer patients. Cancer 89(4), 893–900.

Hamilton, M., Thompson, E. M. & Wizniewski, T. K. (1964). The role of blood-pressure control in preventing complications of hypertension. Lancet 1(7327), 235–238.

Hopkinson, B., Balabanova, D., McKee, M. & Kutzin, J. (2004). The human perspective on health care reform: coping with diabetes in Kyrgyzstan. International Journal of Health Planning and Management 19(1), 43–61.

Illich, I. (1977). Limits to Medicine. Medical Nemesis: the Expropriation of Health. Harmondsworth, UK: Penguin.

Institute of Medicine (2000). *To Err is Human: Building a Safer Health System*. Washington, DC: National Academy Press.

Laing, R. D. (1965). *The Divided Self: An Existential Study in Sanity and Madness*. London: Penguin.

Lecky, F., Woodford, M. & Yates, D. W. (2000). Trends in trauma care in England and Wales 1989–97. UK Trauma Audit and Research Network. *Lancet* **355**(9217), 1771–1775.

Mackenbach, J. P., Meerding, W. J. & Kunst, A. E. (2007). *Economic Implications of Socio-economic Inequalities in Health in the European Union*. Luxembourg: European Commission.

McCarthy, D., How, M. B. A., Sabrina K. H. *et al.* (2009). *Aiming Higher: Results from a State Scorecard on Health System Performance, 2009*. New York, NY: Commonwealth Fund.

McGrail, K., Green, B., Barer, M. L. *et al.* (2000). Age, costs of acute and long-term care and proximity to death: evidence for 1987–88 and 1994–95 in British Columbia. *Age and Ageing* **29**, 249–253.

McKee, M. (1999). For debate – Does health care save lives? *Croat Medical Journal* **40**, 123–128.

McKee, M. (2007). Cochrane on Communism: the influence of ideology on the search for evidence. *International Journal of Epidemiology* **36**, 269–273.

McKee, M., Suhrcke, M., Nolte, E. *et al.* (2009). Health systems, health, and wealth: a European perspective. *Lancet* **373**(9660), 349–351.

McKeown, T. (1979). *The Role Of Medicine: Drama, Mirage or Nemesis?* Oxford: Blackwell.

Moon, S., Szlezák, N. A., Michaud, C. M. *et al.* (2010) The global health system: lessons for a stronger institutional framework. *PLoS Medicine* **7**(1), e1000193. doi:10.1371/journal.pmed.1000193

Nolte, E., Bain, C. & McKee, M. (2006). Diabetes as a tracer condition in international benchmarking of health systems. *Diabetes Care* **29**(5), 1007–1011.

Nolte, E. & McKee, C. M. (2008). Measuring the health of nations: updating an earlier analysis. *Health Affairs (Millwood)* **27**, 58–71.

Nolte, E. & McKee, M. (2004). *Does Health Care Save Lives? Avoidable Mortality Revisited*. London: Nuffield Trust.

Preston, S. H. & Ho, J. Y. (2009). *Low Life Expectancy in the United States: Is the Health Care System at Fault?* PSC Working Paper Series. Philadelphia, PA: Population Studies Center, University of Pennsylvania.

Roemer, M. I. (1981). More data on post-surgical deaths related to the 1976 Los Angeles doctor slowdown. *Social Science and Medicine C* **15**(3), 161–163.

Rosen, M. (1979). *The Sunday Times Thalidomide Case: Contempt of Court and the Freedom of the Press*. London: Writers and Scholars Educational Trust.

Rutstein, D. D., Berenberg, W., Chalmers, T. C. *et al.* (1976). Measuring the quality of medical care. A clinical method. *New England Journal of Medicine* **294**(11), 582–588.

Sala-I-Martin X, D. G. & Miller, R. I. (2004). Determinants of long-term growth: a Bayesian averaging of classical estimates (BACE) approach. *American Economic Review* **94**, 813–835.

Silber, J. H., Romano, P. S., Rosen, A. K. *et al.* (2007). Failure-to-rescue: comparing definitions to measure quality of care. *Medical Care* **45**, 918–925.

Suhrcke, M., McKee, M., Sauto Arce, R., Tsolova, S. & Mortensen, J. (2005). *The Contribution of Health to the Economy in the European Union*. Brussels: European Commission.

Suhrcke, M., Rocco, L. & McKee, M. (2007). *Health: a Vital Investment for Economic Development in Eastern Europe and Central Asia*. Copenhagen: WHO Regional Office for Europe on behalf of the European Observatory on Health Systems and Policies.

Szasz, T. S. (1974). *The Second Sin*. London: Routledge and Kegan Paul.

Thomson, R. P. (2007). *Safer Care for the Acutely Ill Patient: Learning from Serious Incidents*. London: National Patient Safety Agency.

World Health Organization (WHO) (2000). *Health Systems: Improving Performance*. World Health Report. Geneva: World Health Organization.

Wanless, D. (2001). *Securing our Future Health: Taking a Long-Term View; Interim Report*. London: Her Majesty's Treasury.

World Bank (2005). *Dying too Young*. Washington, DC: World Bank.

Global health ethics, responsibilities and justice: some central issues

Chapter

6

Is there a need for global health ethics? For and against

David Hunter and Angus J. Dawson

Introduction

To provide an answer to the question of whether we need global health ethics we set ourselves three goals in this chapter. First, we explore a number of different ways that we might understand the term "global health ethics." Second, we consider the arguments that could be used either to support or dismiss what we call "substantive accounts" of global health ethics. Finally, we make some suggestions in relation to what (if any) "global" obligations may bind us. Our discussions will use public health as an example throughout to illustrate our points. The reason for this focus is that, in our view, we ought to think of public health as providing systematic structural support for population health, with the key aim of fulfilling the basic requirements to protect health and prevent illness. This is not to suggest that other forms of health care are unimportant, just that public health will fulfill a primary role in any attempt to address questions of global justice in relation to existing health inequalities.

Global health ethics is an important topic. We do not need to accept the view that health is of special consideration in a range of possible aims or outcomes, to accept that it is, nevertheless, a key constitutive part of how well our lives go (Daniels, 1985, 2007; Segall, 2007; Wilson, 2009). Health may not be the only or the primary good to be promoted, but it is important for both prudential and ethical reasons. One reason to explore global health ethics is that it is a striking feature of many health-care issues, particularly in the field of public health, that they fail to respect national boundaries. For example if we look at the ethical issues in infectious disease control, given that epidemics often spread between countries, policies adopted in one country have cross-border effects. Likewise, issues in resource allocation for individual countries can

exacerbate or ameliorate health outcomes depending on what their neighbors do. Similarly, issues about the control and regulation of new medical technologies can be affected by cross-border considerations (Hunter & Oultram, 2008). Global and cross-border considerations, therefore, have clear implications for individual and population health. If we assume this is true, what does this mean for thinking about the ethics of health and health care? The place to start is with trying to become clearer about what we mean by "global health ethics."

What is "global health ethics"?

Despite its clear importance, there is surprisingly little literature directly on this topic. The key question, in particular, namely "what is global health ethics?" appears to have been neglected. In this section of the chapter we will consider three possible interpretations of the phrase: first as a purely geographical account, second as an account focused on content and, finally, as a normative account.

A geographical account of global health ethics

When thinking about how we might define "global health ethics" we might focus on the *global* aspects of the phrase to give a purely descriptive definition. On this view, global health ethics is defined spatially. It is about ethical issues related to health at the global level. This, in turn, may be filled out by specifying that such issues might be global in two senses: issues that spatially *affect* the world (e.g. climate change or global pandemics etc.) or issues that can perhaps only be *solved* by worldwide activity and collaboration (e.g. infectious disease control, global tobacco control etc.).

Global Health and Global Health Ethics, ed. Solomon Benatar and Gillian Brock. Published by Cambridge University Press.
© Cambridge University Press 2011.

On this view, then, global health ethics would be an area of study within the broader field of health-care ethics: one with a particular focus on ethical issues that span or sit outside of national boundaries or require global solutions.

The main strength of this approach is that it is relatively uncontroversial. It requires people discussing global health ethics to make few normative assumptions or commitments, and relies on a clear and generally accepted definition of "global." It might, arguably, also help to refocus attention on issues that are neglected in mainstream medical ethics, where there is often a tendency to focus on micro-level interactions between patients and health-care practitioners with minimal concern for more macro-level considerations (Hunter, 2007; Dawson, 2010).

However, this definition applies, uncontroversially, only to a limited set of issues. This may leave the field of global health ethics as relatively small and unimportant, possibly reinforcing its neglect. Furthermore, there is a risk here of creating a silo of thought that is then difficult to integrate into our thinking about health-care ethics in other contexts. Given that there will be issues that impact both on the global and the local scale, we must ensure that we have an integrated approach.

Finally it is difficult to see how one could be either for or against global health ethics on this definition since it is largely descriptive and assumes that we can agree that such global problems and solutions exist. It may seem trivially true to state that they are important and need to be addressed.

A content account of global health ethics

Rather than defining global health ethics in terms of geography we might instead define it in terms of the issues it addresses. In other words we could consider global health ethics to be specified by discussion of a set of important issues that might include: global justice, health inequalities, infectious diseases, resource allocation, international research and so on. On this view global health ethics would be a field of study or area of activity with a range of different topics and focal areas within it. The relevant content would be specified by convention, in the sense that whichever topics were the focus of those involved in the discussions, would count as *being* global health ethics. This would mean that such issues might well change over time. For example, smallpox may once have counted as a relevant issue, but since its elimination, it does no longer.

This content approach contrasts with the descriptive focus of the geographical account we gave previously, and provides for an arguably richer approach that allows for greater normativity to be built in, as including something in the range of topics, immediately calls attention to it.

This view has the advantage of focusing on specific issues and allows for considerable flexibility in the approaches taken to each issue. In principle, since its concerns are not just limited to the global sphere, but also address issues that cut across the global sphere and into the realms of individual countries, it is less likely to encourage silos of thought than the previous approach.

However, this focus on specific issues could be accused of being vague, and lacking both coherence and unity in its approach. This objection is seen most clearly when we consider which issues might be held to be the core issues of global health ethics. Without a coherent account of why something would count as a global health ethics issue it seems difficult to appropriately limit the scope of the field. Indeed, on this view, global health ethics might be seen not as a part of medical ethics/bioethics but instead as a competitor: an entirely new field of study which encompasses the concerns of conventional health-care ethics as well as other concerns, topics and issues.

As with the first account the conventional nature of the account seems to make a nonsense of the question of whether global health ethics is something we ought to be either for or against. As a field of study, as long as we agree the topics within it are worthy of consideration there seems little to say in regard to whether we ought to be for it or against it. All interesting debate switches to arguments about which items ought to be on the list and what we ought to do in relation to each particular topic.

A normative account of global health ethics

The third alternative way to approach the definition is to see "global health ethics" as being, explicitly, a normative project. On this view, to be working on global health ethics is to be committed and engaged in identifying global wrongs related to health, and seeking to have them redressed. For example, we might take global health ethics to be an approach requiring us to address global injustice in regard to health, motivated by existing and historical wrongs characteristic of global trade, structural global inequalities, inequalities in global power etc.

This approach has the strong advantage of being a clearly defined project, with key aims, rather than merely being a field of study. However, this strength comes with a parallel weakness in that this account of global health ethics requires substantive normative commitments, and these commitments are not merely conclusions to arguments, but serve as premises, often taking it as given, for example, that global injustice has occurred, and that such a fact provides us with good (even, overriding) reasons to act. There is a significant danger here of an unjustified drift into mere ideology, where writers in the field of global health ethics move from addressing arguments and evidence into prioritizing their role as activists.

Nonetheless in terms of an account of global health ethics, here is something one could be either for or against. This account seems to be the most plausible candidate for being a distinctive account of global health ethics, but it is also the most contentious. If this is what global health ethics is (and ought to be) then we need some strong arguments in favor of such views. Let us call such a view: substantive global health ethics.

Arguments in favor of substantive global health ethics

To be successful an argument for substantive global health ethics needs to provide compelling normative reasons for being concerned about global inequalities in health outcomes. The starting point for such a view may be establishing plausible empirical claims about the existence of inequalities in global health outcomes. Fortunately (at least for the argument) there is considerable evidence of significant disparities in global health outcomes.

For example, children have dramatically different life expectancies depending on where they are born. In Japan or Sweden they can expect to live more than 80 years; India, 63 years; and in several African countries, fewer than 50 years (CSDH, 2008). The infant mortality rate is just 2 in every 1000 babies born in Iceland, but it is over 120 in every 1000 babies born in Mozambique. And it is no better for mothers in developing nations, the lifetime risk of maternal death is 1 in 8 in Afghanistan; it is 1 in 17 400 in Sweden (WHO *et al.*, 2007).

If we switch from children to adults we see that low- and middle-income nations fare no better here. It was estimated that 17.5 million people died from cardiovascular diseases in 2005, representing 30% of all global deaths. Over 80% of these deaths occurred in developing countries (WHO, 2010a). Of people with diabetes, a disease which is making a rapidly increasing contribution to the global disease burden and mortality rate, 80% live in developing countries (WHO, 2010b). These are only a few examples of the evidence available outlining the significant inequalities in the global disease burden, but it serves to illustrate the key point in relation to the reality of the inequalities that currently exist.

Merely demonstrating the existence of global inequalities in health outcomes does not provide us with the normative grounding necessary for the substantive claim we are interested in. It would need to be shown that there was something ethically problematic about such inequalities, either in and of themselves or because of the nature of their causes. There are several arguments that can be given to show that we ought to take the existence of global inequalities in health outcomes as being ethically troubling, and we will canvas some of the more compelling arguments here to assess whether they show that we ought to be committed to substantive global health ethics. We will consider: beneficence, harm and certain accounts of justice as plausible a priori grounds for such a substantive view.

Beneficence

There are a number of ethical positions that consider global inequalities in health outcomes as morally objectionable in and of themselves because they hold that differences in outcomes need to be morally justified, and that there does not seem to be a justification in this case (Unger, 1996). These views might focus on our claims relating to common humanity, needs, capabilities or disadvantages. However, we focus here on a beneficence claim deriving from a particular form of consequentialism as an example of this kind of approach to ethics. We discuss Peter Singer's account of the obligation of the developed world to those in dramatic need in the developing world. Singer argues in an influential paper called "Famine, affluence and morality" that those in the developed world have direct responsibilities to aid those in the developing world (Singer, 1972). While Singer was not directly discussing health-care needs, his account straightforwardly applies to these as well as other forms of aid. What makes such accounts relevant for supporting substantive global health ethics is their impartiality towards individuals. On this view, given that the possession of a given property entails moral relevance or value, we are provided with a reason to support an account of our obligations that responds to cross-border and global issues where global health inequalities exist.

Singer's argument is relatively simple, yet compelling. He suggests we ought to accept one of two versions of a principle of comparable moral importance. The weaker version of this principle, which Singer argues should be broadly acceptable to someone from any moral perspective, holds that:

> If it is in our power to do or prevent something bad from happening, without thereby sacrificing anything of moral importance, we ought, morally, to do it. (Singer, 1972)

Singer himself holds a stronger version of this principle:

> If it is in our power to do or prevent something bad from happening, without thereby sacrificing anything of comparable moral importance, we ought, morally, to do it. (Singer, 1972)

It is this stronger version that is most discussed in the literature, and we will focus on this version.

From here the argument for redistributing from those in the developed world towards those in the developing world is relatively simple:

(1) Suffering and death from lack of food, shelter, and medical care are bad.

(2) "If it is in our power to do or prevent something bad from happening, without thereby sacrificing anything of comparable moral importance, we ought, morally, to do it."

(3) It is within our power to prevent such suffering.

Conclusion: Therefore, we ought to prevent such suffering.

The first premise seems, in light of the evidence we have already given, uncontroversial. Such suffering and death clearly does occur and can only be counted as bad. Likewise the third premise is empirical in nature, and while we do not want to address it in detail here, it seems plausible. Even if it is the case that a significant amount of suffering cannot be prevented, nonetheless a significant amount could be. For these reasons, discussion of Singer's argument usually focuses on the second premise, either by debating whether it holds true, or alternatively whether Singer is right to claim that nothing of comparable moral worth would be sacrificed in this case.

To justify this premise Singer offered a thought experiment to help guide our intuitions:

> If I am walking past a shallow pond and see a child drowning in it, I ought to wade in and pull the child out. This will mean getting my clothes muddy, but this is insignificant, while the death of the child would presumably be a very bad thing. (Singer, 1972)

He notes that saving the child in this case would be supported and explained by the principle of comparable moral importance. We will not focus on criticisms of Singer's view here, though we will address some of these later in the chapter. Instead we will simply conclude that Singer's beneficence-based argument is likely to give us a prima facie reason to accept substantive global health ethics.

Justice and harm

Thomas Pogge agrees with Singer that we have demanding obligations to respond to those in need in the developing world. However, contrary to Singer he argues that our duties to aid do not derive from our positive obligations to *benefit* others, but rather from claims of justice and our negative duties to both not harm others, and to provide restitution when we have harmed them (Pogge, 2008). This is potentially a very powerful argument because some theorists argue (as we will see in the following section) that negative duties (e.g. do not harm) bind strictly (they must always be followed), whereas whilst individuals are bound by positive duties (e.g. give to charity), they have latitude to decide when they ought to act from them.

There are two primary strands to Pogge's argument, an appeal to historic injustices, and an appeal to present injustices, although these two strands are conceptually linked.

It seems unarguable that the present global world order rests in part on the back of significant and systemic historic injustices stemming from a shared global history. Many developing nations were colonized by developed nations, and their resources and people exploited for economic gain by the developed nations. Pogge argues that this creates obligations that bind those countries that were involved in exploitation to aid those which were historically exploited. However, in response it can be argued that there are significant epistemic difficulties both with tracing the causal pathway of past harms and in assigning the degree of responsibility of restoration, given that the present members of the "relevant" group are distinct from the past members of that "same" group.

However, if we choose to focus on the impact of past injustice in the present we can sidestep these epistemic concerns to some degree.

First, it is clear that whoever is present in a developed nation is likely to have benefited from the effects of historic injustice. This fact, in turn, generates some obligations to aid those who are likely to have been harmed by such injustice. Furthermore, as Jeremy Waldron argues, unjust transactions are particularly pernicious because they impact upon all the other transactions in a market (Waldron, 1992). To see this point, consider the market for car stereos. Given that a significant number of probably stolen car stereos are available secondhand through such outlets as ebay, someone who wants to sell a legitimate secondhand car stereo will have to price their stereo at a lower price point to be able to compete with the stolen car stereos on the market. Hence the availability of some unjust transactions in a market has an effect on all prices in a market.

Second, the relative power relationships that have developed (based on economies bolstered by historical unjust acts) have allowed the negotiation of a world order that heavily favors the powerful, and disadvantages the weak. Pogge argues this is a systemic problem and notes, for example, that the way we have decided to recognize people as having the right to alienate the resources of a country if they have effective military control, creates strong incentives for dictators to seize control of developing countries, financing their revolution on the basis of future profits from selling off the country's resources to the highest bidder.

As Pogge puts it:

> It is hardly obvious that the basic institutions we participate in are just or nearly just. In any case, a somewhat unobvious but massive threat to the moral quality of our lives is the danger that we will have lived as advantaged participants in unjust institutions, collaborating in their perpetuation and benefiting from their injustice. (Pogge, 1989)

To give an example of this in the context of health care Pogge, in his paper, "Human rights and global health: a research program," argues that the present medical-patenting system formed by the *trade-related aspects of intellectual property rights* (TRIPs) agreement is patently unjust because of the avoidable mortality and morbidity it produces (Pogge, 2005). At present, medical research is overwhelmingly focused on the needs of those in relatively affluent nations, since there is little incentive for innovation if there is no market that can afford to purchase that innovation. For example, statistics from the Global Forum for Health Reform show that only 0.31% of all public and private funds devoted to health research is spent on research into medication for malaria, pneumonia, diarrhea and tuberculosis, which together account for 21% of the global burden of disease (GFHR, 2004). But this means that much of new medical research makes little impact on the global disease burden since this burden is disproportionately borne by those in relatively poor nations (Pogge, 2008). This has led to what is often referred to as the 90/10 gap, 90% of medical research funding is spent on conditions affecting only the top 10% of people in terms of wealth. As Pogge notes in his paper, the TRIPs agreement developed out of the Western pharmaceutical industry's concerns that companies in the developing world failed to respect patents and produced considerably cheaper versions of their drugs for local markets.

While Pogge, like Singer, has critics, some of whom we will discuss later in this chapter, it nonetheless appears that considering harms and justice, likewise, can provide a *prima facie* reason for accepting a substantive global health ethics.

Cosmopolitan justice

Cosmopolitanism is a term that applies to a broad range of views perhaps best summed up by the quote from the fourth century BC cynic Diogenes who, when asked where he came from, replied "I am a citizen of the world" (Kleingeld & Brown, 2009). The essence of cosmopolitanism can be found in either the denial or reduction of the importance of nations and nationality (Scheffler, 1999). For our purposes this range of views can be divided into moral cosmopolitanism and political cosmopolitanism.

Moral cosmopolitanism focuses on moral judgments and obligations as being universal and impartial in nature. Singer's account of our obligations counts as a version of moral cosmopolitanism, so we will not discuss moral cosmopolitanism further here.

Political cosmopolitanism, on the other hand, generally focuses on institutions and argues for no or a weakened role for the state in politics (although not all political cosmopolitans argue for this, see Brock (2009) for example). This is then replaced either with a world government, or global institutions such as the United Nations or the International Court of Justice. Such global institutions mitigate and limit the power of individual nation states (both in terms of interfering with their neighboring states, but also in regard to states acting upon their own citizens). Because political cosmopolitanism downplays the importance of individual nation states, and focuses instead on fair world governance, it might, indirectly, provide a possible grounding for a substantive global health ethics. This is because injustices in health outcomes that may exist across the globe are to be assessed in terms of comparisons across the world, and are therefore a concern for all.

A variety of different arguments can be offered for political cosmopolitanism. In his book, *Realizing Rawls*, Thomas Pogge develops a strong case for political cosmopolitanism, arguing, ironically, that Rawls himself is mistaken about the implications of his views in the international context (Pogge, 1989). Pogge suggests that precisely the same arguments that Rawls makes for the (potentially radical) reformation of the nation state likewise apply in the global context. The argument can be established through an intuitive appeal to a revised version of the Veil of Ignorance example, wherein the participants don't know which society they will end up in (Rawls, 1971). This results in the establishment of principles of international governance similar to the principles that Rawls derives for the internal governance of nation states. Or it can be established on the basis of the moral argument offered by Rawls in *A Theory of Justice* for a certain model of a just state, abstracted to the worldwide level. In either case this would lead to a global system which protected basic liberties, and critically in terms of supporting substantive global health ethics, would call for a redistribution of global resources on the basis of the difference principle: namely, that the distribution of resources ought to be such that the person in the worst off position is as well off as possible.

Another possible ground for the establishment of political cosmopolitanism is luck egalitarianism (Caney, 2005). Luck egalitarianism is (broadly) the view that the distribution of resources ought to be such that it is insensitive to matters of brute luck (Dworkin, 2000). As Ronald Dworkin puts it, the distribution of resources ought to be ambition sensitive, but insensitive to natural endowments (Dworkin, 2000). When this view is applied to questions of global justice it appears to straightforwardly lead to cosmopolitan conclusions (at least in relation to the, presumably, quite extensive elements of global health injustice related to brute luck).

As Simon Caney puts it:

Underpinning our commitment to equality of opportunity is the deep conviction that it is unfair if someone enjoys worse chances in life because of class or social status or ethnicity. This deep conviction implies, however, that we should also object if some people have worse opportunities because of their nationality or civic identity. The core intuition, then, maintains that persons should not face worse opportunities because of the community or communities they come from. This point can be expressed negatively: people should not be penalized because of the vagaries of happenstance, and their fortunes should not be set by factors like nationality or citizenship. Or it can be expressed positively: People are entitled to the same opportunities as others. If, then, we object to an aristocratic or medieval scheme that distributes unequal opportunities according to one's social standing, or to a racist scheme that distributes unequal opportunities according to one's race, we should, I am arguing, also object to an international order that distributes unequal opportunities according to one's nationality. In short, then, the rationale for accepting equality of opportunity within the state entails that we should accept global equality of opportunity. (Caney, 2001)

Alternatively, a Republican justification could be offered for political cosmopolitanism. This view is centered on the claim that the common understanding of political freedom as a claim about non-interference is a mistake (Pettit, 1997). Instead, we should consider true political freedom to be what Phillip Pettit dubs freedom as non-domination. Pettit argues that the usual characterization of liberty as either positive or negative leaves out an important alternative, namely freedom from the ability of others being able to arbitrarily interfere with us – freedom from domination. Since the state is an important potential source of domination, Republicans argue that we need to have a state which has a significant division of powers, to ensure that checks and balances are in place. In the international arena strong global institutions provide a reassuring limitation on governments for Republicans, and since those who are unhealthy are often vulnerable to domination, this provides a ground for a concern about global health inequalities.

Whichever of these grounds we accept for political cosmopolitanism may provide, once again, a *prima facie* ground for substantive global health ethics.

So, in this section, we have shown that there are several arguments that might be offered for a substantive global health ethics. However, there are also several arguments that are often offered against any substantive view of global health ethics. These either aim to show that the arguments we have thus far given are mistaken, or that there is some independent reason for denying the legitimacy of the obligations that supposedly derive from substantive global health ethics.

Arguments against substantive global health ethics

Obligations of charity are imperfect duties

One argument that might be offered against substantive global health ethics is that, as has already been mentioned, on some views of morality, a positive duty to assist others is of a different nature to a negative duty not to cause harm.

One way of putting this position forward is in regards to Kant's distinction between what he calls perfect and imperfect duties. A perfect duty is one that you can fulfill all the time, simply by refraining from doing something. Not lying is a good example of such a duty. Whereas, an imperfect duty is one that you have latitude over when you can choose to fulfill it. Benefiting others through charitable activity might be a good example of such an imperfect duty. Such a duty is binding upon you, but you cannot be expected to always be acting charitably.

Given the imperfect nature of the obligation of charity, some have argued that it is a matter of choice how and where we ought to carry it out. Whilst we may choose to give charity to developing nations, there would be nothing wrong in choosing to fulfill our obligation of charity in other ways, such as donating money to allow a local child to travel overseas to receive potentially life-saving, but expensive, treatment.

If this truly is the nature of our obligation to give, then it undermines arguments such as that offered by Singer. Even if he is able to establish that we have a duty to give to those in need, it might be argued that the obligation is not of the nature he suggests, and so we are not necessarily obliged to give to anything like the extent he suggests. However, in the face of massive global inequalities in health outcomes, it is worth considering how compelling this argument might be. Is it really the case that what matters is the mere fact *that* we act charitably rather than *how* and *when* we act charitably? For this objection to be entirely telling it would have to be the case that it didn't matter what the subject of our charity was, only that we engaged in some charitable act or other. However, even if it

is the case that our duty to give charitably is weaker than that which Singer defends, it is surely the case that the nature of our charitable actions will still matter morally. Is it really the case that we ought to just give to someone on some occasion, rather than focusing on potentially life-threatening health inequalities? Perhaps what has convinced some people of this argument is a misunderstanding about the differences between praiseworthy actions and right actions. It seems that whilst the giving of large but inefficient donations to individuals may be praiseworthy, we may not see it as being the right action, given what else that money could do. Even if we think the positive/negative duties distinction is morally relevant, we have a choice about priorities when it comes to our actions, and it is hard to imagine a more pressing priority than at least some of the inequalities in relation to global health care.

Furthermore this objection is not telling against all of the arguments for substantive global health ethics since some, such as Pogge's position, focus on negative rather than positive duties. Nonetheless, this objection may cause some doubt about an argument for a substantive global health ethics. At the very least, we are pushed into the necessity of grappling with deep and contested normative theory, and it certainly looks as though there is no easy intuitive support for the radical conclusions that some supporters of global health ethics wish for.

We have no obligations to the distant needy

Some theorists have argued, contra Peter Singer, that the distance we are from those in need does make a moral difference. Our duties to aid decrease as the needy become further away from us (Kamm, 2000).

This might be based on the ease of aiding those who are closer, or in determining their need. Kamm puts forward an argument to claim that distance does make a moral difference in her paper "Does distance matter morally to the duty to rescue?" (Kamm, 2000) where she criticizes Singer for relying on single cases to try and show that distance does not matter (since single cases only show that distance does not matter in that case, not all cases). She suggests that we have to carefully construct cases to test our intuitions and that the following example is a better test of our intuitions in regard to the role of distance:

Near Alone Case: I am walking past a pond in a foreign country that I am visiting. I alone see many children drowning in it and I alone can save one of them. To save the one, I must put the $500 I have in my pocket into a machine that then triggers (via electric current) rescue machinery that will certainly scoop him out.

Far Alone Case: I alone know that in a distant part of a foreign country that I am visiting, many children are drowning, and I alone can save one of them. To save the one, all I must do is put the $500 I carry in my pocket into a machine that then triggers (via electric current) rescue machinery that will certainly scoop him out. (Kamm, 2000)

Kamm concludes that it is intuitive to recognize a difference in our moral obligations between these two cases. Singer, however, defends the idea that distance is irrelevant. This underlies his argument that we outlined earlier. He insists that if you accept "any principle of impartiality, universalizability, equality, or whatever" then you ought to hold distance as morally irrelevant (Singer, 1972). He suggests that to hold otherwise is to be guilty of a form of discrimination. He allows that *psychologically* it might make a difference whether an individual is starving to death in front of your eyes or in a far-away country, but that it makes no *moral* difference.

As with the previous objection at best this argument undermines only some of the arguments for substantive global health ethics – namely those founded on beneficence and other such positive obligations.

Property rights as trumps

Perhaps a more powerful argument against substantive global health ethics is a libertarian argument, based around the ideal of freedom and the notion of the ownership of property. On this view, we only can have positive duties if we ourselves have caused harm. Whilst the suffering of others is unfortunate, it is not unfair. On this view, it would be good of us to intervene, but it is not, and cannot be compulsory to give, for that would violate our property ownership rights. If this position can be defended then this is a problem for champions of substantive global health ethics because it would block the significant redistribution that substantive global health ethics requires.

Typically, such a response is based on Nozick's account of Lockean property rights (Locke, 1690 [1960]) (Nozick, 1974). Such a view starts from an account of the fair initial acquisition of property, and then holds that as long as procedurally fair transactions led us, from that initial distribution of resources to the current distribution of resources, then the current distribution is just and fair, and interference with it would be illegitimate. The account of initial acquisition relies on the idea that prior to anyone owning anything it is reasonable to believe that we all have a right to everything. In other words everything is owned in common. This generates a puzzle though, since to be able to use something we usually need to alienate it: to make it ours and ours alone. While in a small group we could simply ask if anyone minded; but when everything is owned in common, we would need to ask everyone. Locke thought that no one could object to the alienation of some bit of property provided two conditions were met. First, that you left enough for others and that what was left was as good for them, and that, second, you didn't just waste the common stock.

Similarly to the last objection, if this argument holds, then this would seem to undermine some of the arguments put forward for substantive global health ethics. However, there seem to be three main objections that could be raised to it.

The first objection is to point out, as Pogge does, that there is *in fact* a systemic history of the violent and unjust acquisition of resources (Pogge, 2008). In the face of this undeniable fact it seems difficult to justify resisting redistribution.

The second objection challenges the first condition of initial acquisition – that enough and as good has been left. Given that all or most resources have been acquired is it really possible to leave enough and as good? The typical libertarian response to this is to point to the benefits for all of economic development which is dependent on the alienation of the means of production and the notion that people who have worked hard deserve a reward for their work. However this seems based on the notion of first come – first served, and it is hard to see why late comers would automatically accept that this is a fair way to determine who owns resources, especially if there are no limits on the control of those resources.

The final objection is that the appeal to desert leaves libertarians open to a desert-based challenge. This challenge is commonly made by egalitarians, who point out that some of the income we earn does not seem to be deserved since it is just a matter of luck. This is the part of our income that is derived from the exercise of our natural talents. Which talents we have, and which talents are valued, is a matter of brute luck; and if a distribution should reflect deservingness, then natural talents and differences ought not make a difference to who gets what. So while we might not be in a position to tax people and remove all of their income, we might still be able to justly redistribute (at least) some of it.

As with the last argument, at best, this is only telling against some of the positive arguments for substantive global health ethics. Nonetheless, in so far as it is compelling, it does provide reasons to question the acceptance of a substantive global health ethics.

We have a duty to prioritize our compatriots

There seem to be two main versions of this objection, the first of which argues we have more significant duties to our compatriots than to others. The second version argues that we have duties not to interfere directly in the governance of other societies. This is a different sort of objection to the first three because if it works it is a global objection to substantive global health ethics.

Broadly, the first version of the objection might be called nationalism, and might seem to run directly counter to the claims made by cosmopolitans that we discussed earlier. On this view there is something central and important about the nation state. To maintain and develop our nations we are required to prioritize the needs of our citizens first, even if others are in greater need (Miller, 1995).

A variety of arguments might be offered for this claim, for example we might claim that there is something important about the shared cultural and moral understandings that flourish in a common culture. Alternatively, we might argue that to properly flourish, individuals need a cultural context that they are comfortable within, and that the nation state is an essential part of this. Or we might simply claim that nationality is an important constitutive part of our personal identity, and if we allow our nation to be undermined, then, in a sense we are undermining our own identity. On each of these claims there is the underlying notion that the nation is important psychologically to underwrite our behavior, moral or otherwise. While this position does seem to weaken the strength of substantive global health ethics it does not seem to negate it entirely. Even if we must prioritize our compatriots, given, as we pointed out earlier, the scale of health inequalities between nations, even a nationalist might admit there are significant opportunities to aid others without undermining our own nation.

The second version of these arguments, if compelling, would be more telling against substantive global health ethics since it would establish that there is no obligation to aid those individuals outside of our nation, or even a positive obligation to not interfere in others' ways of life. These arguments tend to be based on social contract theory that sees both political and moral obligations as based on an unspoken agreement as the basis for society. Hobbes, one of the early social contract theorists, held that moral obligations were only possible within the context of a society, but modern social contract theorists often see our obligations to our compatriots as being far stronger than our obligations to those in other countries (Hobbes, 1651 [1992]). We focus on John Rawls as the exemplar of this sort of position.

Rawls has been a very influential writer on justice within liberal societies and his position on justice inside liberal societies had, as we outlined earlier, been applied to the global context. However, Rawls felt that these approaches misconstrued an appropriate approach to global considerations, because they applied his theory, which was targeted at individuals within a particular context, in a parallel way to countries within the global context.

As Rawls says:

> Two main ideas motivate the Law of Peoples. One is that the great evils of human history – unjust war and oppression, religious persecution and the denial of liberty of conscience, starvation and poverty, not to mention genocide and mass murder – follow from political injustice, with its own cruelties and callousness ... The other main idea, obviously connected with the first, is that, once the gravest forms of political injustice are eliminated by following just (or at least decent) social policies and establishing just (or at least decent) basic institutions, these great evils will eventually disappear. (Rawls, 1999)

On the basis of this Rawls put forward eight principles for ordering the international basic structure:

(1) Peoples are free and independent, and their freedom and independence are to be respected by other peoples.

(2) Peoples are to observe treaties and undertakings.

(3) Peoples are equal and are parties to the agreements that bind them.

(4) Peoples are to observe the duty of non-intervention (except to address grave violations of human rights).

(5) Peoples have a right of self-defense, but no right to instigate war for reasons other than self-defense.

(6) Peoples are to honor human rights.

(7) Peoples are to observe certain specified restrictions in the conduct of war.

(8) Peoples have a duty to assist other peoples living under unfavorable conditions that prevent their having a just or decent political and social regime. (Rawls, 1999)

Many theorists, who held that the difference principle ought to be applied globally, were surprised by Rawls' rejection of this idea, and his insistence instead on a much more limited set of obligations. The aim of aid was not to achieve global equality but to ensure instead that nations could achieve and maintain liberal or decent political institutions.

As we mentioned earlier, Rawls' views have been criticized by Pogge pointing out that while starvation and poverty are related to internal political injustice, they are not solely derived from this – unjust international institutions and a lack of natural resources also have an impact. And it seems that the points that Simon Caney makes in favor of global equality of opportunity above still hold. It seems unfair that an arbitrary factor such as where one is born ought to have a significant role to play in determining how well one's life goes. Nonetheless, while Rawls' position might weaken support for a substantive global health ethics it need not remove it, since Rawls does recognize that there is a duty to assist those who are living in conditions which prevent them living in a just or decent political and social regime, which, arguably, is the case in countries with the severest needs.

Practical – what obligations bind us here?

So what can we now say about substantive global health ethics? At best the arguments for substantive global health ethics could not be described as uncontroversial, and while we have expressed doubt about whether the arguments against are decisive, the case for, likewise, does not seem entirely compelling. Given this, it seems inappropriate, at the very least, to take substantive and controversial normative conclusions as our starting point and to approach issues in global health ethics from there.

However it might be asked, do we have to accept substantive global health ethics to achieve many of the goods it aims to achieve? It seems to us that the answer to this question is clearly no.

As we saw in our discussion of the arguments for substantive global health ethics there are powerful ethical arguments for being concerned with global issues. Even if these do not carry us as far as someone committed to substantive global health ethics would like us to go, nonetheless any reasonable theory/view is going to accept that global ethical and political concerns need to be addressed, if only because when they are not, there is a tendency for this to end up in our own backyard, as can happen for example in regard to infectious diseases and other public health issues. Drug-resistant tuberculosis or increasingly ineffective antibiotics ought to be a concern to us all. Given that health-care issues rarely respect borders, even the staunchest nationalist will have to sometimes consider taking action on health-care issues while they are still "someone else's problem."

Indeed, taking a purely prudential approach might lead even the purely self-interested to address significant global ethical and political concerns. It has been argued that this might arise out of consideration of global public goods.

Public goods are classically defined as being:

(a) *non-rival* (my enjoyment of clean air has no consequences for your enjoyment of the same thing)

(b) *non-excludable* (it is not possible to exclude others from enjoying the benefits of clean air).

Global public goods are public goods that benefit a substantial region of the world, or the whole world. Suggested candidates include: climatic and environmental stability, financial stability, infectious disease control, human rights etc. If we accept these as global public goods then it is in *each individual state's interests* to create and maintain such goods. Whatever the merits of such an approach, discussion of global public goods is one way to motivate self-interested nation states to act to improve (at least some) global health inequalities.

So, we conclude that it seems there is something to be said for the aims of substantive global health ethics. However, even if we choose to interpret the phrase "global health ethics" in either the geographical or content sense, we might end up with significant overlap with a more substantive account, when it comes to justifying many actions.

It is also worth noting how a focus on the wider issue of global inequalities can, helpfully, stress the problems for more narrow approaches, such as the autonomy-obsessed state of present medical ethics. So even if we adopt one of the less substantive approaches to global health ethics that we have outlined, there are still things to be said in favor of giving a higher priority to justice in relation to health outcomes. Such an approach focused on considering issues broadly within the field of global health ethics, might give us new ideas and approaches that can then be used to critique and develop traditional medical ethics (Dawson, 2010).

This chapter has focused on the moral/political case for being concerned about inequalities and justice in health across the world (particularly in relation to public health).

We can call this global health ethics if we wish, but it is the issues that require action. Labels are far less important. We have argued we are obligated to respond to global inequalities (whatever you think of the idea of global health ethics).

References

Brock, G. (2009). *Global Justice: A Cosmopolitan Account*. Oxford: Oxford University Press.

Caney, S. (2001). Cosmopolitan justice and equalizing opportunities. *Metaphilosophy* **32**, 113–134.

Caney, S. (2005). *Justice Beyond Borders: A Global Political Theory*. Oxford: Oxford University Press.

Commission on Social Determinants of Health (CSDH) (2008). *Closing the Gap in a Generation: Health Equity through Action on the Social Determinants of Health. Final Report of the Commission on Social Determinants of Health*. Geneva: World Health Organization.

Daniels, N. (1985). *Just Health Care*. Cambridge: Cambridge University Press.

Daniels, N. (2007). *Just Health: Meeting Health Needs Fairly*. New York: Cambridge University Press.

Dawson, A. (2010). The future of bioethics: three dogmas and a cup of hemlock. *Bioethics* **24**, 218–225.

GFHR (2004) *The 10/90 Report on Health Research 2003–2004*. www.globalforumhealth.org/filesupld/1090_report_03_04/109004_chap_5.pdf (Accessed March 11, 2010).

Dworkin, R. (2000). *Sovereign Virtue*. Cambridge, MA: Harvard University Press.

Hobbes, T. (1651). *Leviathan*. E. Curley (trans. 1992). London: Hackett.

Hunter, D. (2007). Am I my brother's gatekeeper? Professional ethics and the prioritisation of healthcare. *Journal of Medical Ethics* **33**, 522–526.

Hunter, D. & Oultram, S. (2008). The challenge of "sperm ships": the need for the global regulation of medical technology. *Journal of Medical Ethics* **34**, 552–556.

Inge, K., Conceicao, P., Le Goulven, K. & Mendoza, R. (2003). *Providing Global Public Goods: Managing Globalization*. New York, NY: Oxford University Press.

Kamm, F. M. (2000). Does distance matter morally to the duty to rescue? *Law and Philosophy* **19**, 655–681.

Kleingeld, P. & Brown, E. (2009). Cosmopolitanism. In E. N. Zalta (Ed.), *The Stanford Encyclopedia of Philosophy* (Summer 2009 edn). http://plato.stanford.edu/archives/sum2009/entries/cosmopolitanism/ (Accessed March 11, 2010).

Locke, J. (1690 [1960]). *Two Treatises of Government*, P. Laslett (Ed.). New York, NY: Cambridge University Press.

Miller, D. (1995). *On Nationality*. Oxford: Oxford University Press.

Nozick, R. (1974). *Anarchy, State, and Utopia*. New York, NY: Basic Books.

Pettit, P. (1997). *Republicanism: A Theory of Freedom and Government*. Oxford: Clarendon Press.

Pogge, T. (1989). *Realizing Rawls*. Ithaca, NY: Cornell University Press.

Pogge, T. (2005). Human rights and global health: a research program. *Metaphilosophy* **36**, 182–209.

Pogge, T. (2008). *World Poverty and Human Rights: Cosmopolitan Responsibilities and Reforms*. (2nd edn.) Cambridge: Polity Press.

Rawls, J. (1971). *A Theory of Justice*. Cambridge, MA: Harvard University Press.

Rawls, J. (1999). *The Law of Peoples*. Cambridge, MA: Harvard University Press.

Scheffler, S. (1999). Conceptions of cosmopolitanism. *Utilitas* **11**, 255–276.

Segall, S. (2007). Is health care (still) special? *Journal of Political Philosophy* **15**, 342–361.

Singer, P. (1972). Famine, affluence, and morality. *Philosophy and Public Affairs* **1**, 229–243.

Unger, P. (1996). *Living High and Letting Die*. Oxford: Oxford University Press.

Waldron, J. (1992). Superseding historic injustice. *Ethics* **103**, 4–28.

Wilson, J. (2009). Not so special after all? Daniels and the social determinants of health. *Journal of Medical Ethics* **35**, 3–6.

World Health Organization (WHO) *et al.* (2007). *Maternal Mortality in 2005: Estimates Developed by WHO, UNICEF, UNFPA and the World Bank*. Geneva: World

Health Organization. www.who/reproductive-health/
publications/maternalmortality2005/mme2005.pdf
(Accessed March 11, 2010).

World Health Organization (WHO) (2010a). *Cardiovascular
Diseases: What are Cardiovascular Diseases?*
Geneva: World Health Organization. www.who.int/
mediacentre/factsheets/fs317/en/index.html (Accessed
March 11, 2010).

World Health Organization (WHO) (2010b). *Quick
Diabetes Facts*. Geneva: World Health Organization.
www.who.int/diabetes/en/ (Accessed March 11,
2010).

Justice, infectious diseases and globalization

Michael J. Selgelid

The ethical importance of infectious diseases

The ethical importance of infectious diseases partly relates to the fact that their consequences are almost unrivalled. Historically they have caused more morbidity and mortality than any other cause, including war (Price-Smith, 2001). The Black Death eliminated one-third of the European population in just a few years during the mid-fourteenth century (Ziegler, 1969); the 1918 flu epidemic killed between 20 and 100 million people (Crosby, 2003); tuberculosis (TB) killed a billion people during the past two centuries (Ryan, 1992); and smallpox killed between 300 and 500 million people during the twentieth century alone – i.e. three times more than were killed by all the wars of that period (Oldstone, 1998).

Second, because the public health measures used to control them sometimes involve infringement of widely accepted individual rights and liberties, infectious diseases raise difficult philosophical questions about how to strike a balance between the goal to protect the greater good of public health and the goal to protect individual rights and liberties. Quarantine and travel restrictions, for example, violate the right to freedom of movement. Other public health measures – such as contact tracing, the notification of third parties, and the reporting of the health status of individuals to authorities – can interfere with the right to privacy. Mandatory treatment and vaccination, finally, conflicts with the right to informed consent. Though measures such as these may sometimes be necessary to avert public health disasters, how great must a public health threat be for such measures to be justified? Most would deny that either the goal to promote the greater good of society in the way of public health or the goal to protect individual rights and liberties should always take priority over the other.

Third, because infectious diseases primarily affect the poor and disempowered,[1] the topic of infectious disease is closely connected to the topic of justice (Selgelid, 2005). Malnutrition, dirty water, crowded living conditions, bad working conditions, poor education, lack of sanitation and hygiene, and lack of decent health-care provision all increase chances that those who suffer from poverty will also suffer from infectious disease. Malnutrition weakens immune systems, for example, and this increases chances of infection. Dirty water harbors infectious pathogens. Crowded living and working conditions facilitate the spread of disease from person to person. Those who are poorly educated fail to take sufficient disease-avoidance measures. And poor communities often lack adequate resources to improve sanitation and hygiene. Finally, when the poor do become infected they suffer worse consequences than would otherwise be the case because health-care systems are weak in poor countries and because impoverished individuals cannot afford to pay for the medicines they need. Factors like these explain why the bulk of infectious disease morbidity and mortality occurs in developing countries.

Infectious diseases raise additional issues of global ethics because they fail to respect national borders. An epidemic in one country or region can quickly spread to others. The international spread of infectious diseases is facilitated by the dramatic increase in trade and travel associated with globalization. The mobility of infectious diseases is illustrated by the spread of AIDS from Africa to the rest of the world during the 1980s, and by the rapid spread of SARS from Asia to

---

[1] Which is not to say that infectious diseases cannot, or do not, also severely affect the affluent.

An earlier versions of this work has appeared: Selgelid M. J. (2009). Infectious diseases. In *A Companion Bioethics* (Second Edition), edited by Helga Kuhse and Peter Singer (pp. 430–440). Malden, MA: Wiley-Blackwell.

Canada in 2003. For many years experts have worried that avian influenza (H5N1) might become transmissible between humans and lead to a global pandemic rivaling that of 1918. In the meanwhile, a pandemic of H1N1 swine influenza (originating in Mexico) was declared by WHO in June 2009. At the time of this writing (in January 2010), however, the death toll of H1N1 swine influenza does not appear to be greater than that of seasonal influenza. The danger that H1N1, H5N1 or other strains of influenza might mutate into more dangerous forms nonetheless remains.

One implication of infectious disease mobility is that the poverty and poor health-care conditions in developing countries have negative implications for health in rich countries. In order to protect their own populations, rich countries should thus take greater interest in both poverty reduction and health-care improvement in poor countries.

The global infectious disease status quo: AIDS and TB

Infectious diseases cause approximately 15 million deaths worldwide yearly, and they cause almost one in two deaths in developing countries. AIDS, TB and malaria are the biggest killers. Together they account for approximately 5 million deaths each year. Approximately 30–36 million people are presently living with HIV worldwide. During 2007, 2.7 million people became newly infected with HIV and there were 2 million HIV-related deaths (UNAIDS, 2008); 67% of cases and 75% of AIDS deaths occur in sub-Saharan Africa, where adult HIV prevalence rates commonly reach (and sometimes exceed) 30%. Ninety-five percent of AIDS deaths occur in developing countries. Although prices for antiretroviral medications have dropped considerably (to as low as US$100 for a year of treatment), they are still relatively expensive and thus unaffordable to the very poor. At the beginning of the twenty-first century, only 5% of those in need received antiretroviral medication. Though coverage improved as a result of the WHO/UNAIDS "3 by 5" program that aimed to provide treatment to 3 (i.e. half) of the 6 million people who needed it by the end of 2005, only 24% of those in need were receiving treatment at the end of 2006. AIDS has killed over 25 million people since the disease was first recognized in 1981.

Tuberculosis kills 1.7 million people each year. Though considered eradicable during the 1950s, TB "is now more prevalent than in any previous period

in human history" (Gandy & Zumla, 2002, p. 385). One-third of the human population is infected with the latent form of the disease, and a tenth of these are expected to develop active illness. The WHO declared TB a global health emergency in 1993, and in 2002 the WHO estimated "that between [then] and 2020, approximately 1000 million people will be newly infected, over 150 million people will get sick, and 36 million will die of TB – if control is not further strengthened" (WHO, 2002). Ninety-five percent of TB cases and 98% of TB deaths occur in developing countries (WHO, 2007).

There are numerous reasons why it is especially tragic that TB kills nearly as many people as AIDS each year. Curative TB drugs have existed for over 50 years, and they are much less expensive than AIDS medications (which are not themselves curative). A standard course of TB medication costs only US$10 to US$20. From an economic standpoint, therefore, the morbidity and mortality resulting from TB is more easily preventable. Another reason for concern is that TB, being airborne, is contractible via casual contact and is much more contagious than AIDS. While behavior modification (with respect to intravenous drug use and sexual practice) can essentially eliminate the risk of infection with AIDS, TB can be passed from one individual to another via coughing, sneezing and even talking. In some ways, then, the threat to "innocent individuals" – and public health in general – is greater in the case of TB.

Though the consequences of TB rival those of AIDS – and though TB is especially problematic for reasons mentioned immediately above – it is worth noting that bioethics discussion of AIDS has, to date, dwarfed that of TB. The comparative lack of attention to ethical issues associated with TB is revealed via searches on the internet. A *Pubmed* search of titles and abstracts (conducted in October 2007) for the terms "ethics" and "AIDS" yielded 2998 entries; while a similar search for the terms "ethics" and "tuberculosis" yielded only 179.

AIDS and TB are, in any case, mutually reinforcing. Those with AIDS are more likely to contract TB, and TB is the leading cause of death in AIDS patients.

Infectious diseases like these are driven by poverty (for the reasons noted above); but such diseases themselves in turn promote poverty. A vicious cycle exists between poverty and infectious disease. AIDS and TB have brought numerous communities in sub-Saharan Africa to the verge of economic collapse. Economies suffer when those who are sick or die cannot work, when employers need to hire and train new personnel, when consumers shift spending away from durable things goods to necessities like funerals and health care, and for numerous other complex reasons.

Poverty alleviation would be one way to reduce disease; and disease reduction would be one way to alleviate poverty. There are numerous implications from the standpoint of justice. If international justice requires poverty reduction – and thus provision of means for poverty reduction – then international justice requires reduction of major infectious diseases like TB and AIDS.

Many of the social, political and economic conditions (including poverty) that promote infectious diseases like AIDS and TB are themselves products of past injustices and human rights abuses. Examination of the social, political and economic causes of AIDS and TB reveal that current prevalence rates in southern Africa are partly a legacy of slavery, colonialism, cold war manipulation (by superpowers), racist oppression and (in the case of South Africa) apartheid (Barnett & Whiteside, 2002). Rather than being a product of mere bad luck, the health-care status quo in southern Africa is rooted in historical injustice (Benatar, 1998). Some would argue that reparations are therefore called for. If this is correct, then rich countries that have caused or been complicit in the exploitation of African countries have obligations to help improve the situation (Pogge, 2002; Singer, 2002).

Drug resistance

The increase in drug-resistant disease is a paramount growing global concern. A recent WHO report claimed that:

> Drug resistance is the most telling sign that we have failed to take the threat of infectious diseases seriously. It suggests that we have mishandled our precious arsenal of disease-fighting drugs, both by overusing them in developed nations and, paradoxically, both misusing and underusing them in developing nations. In all cases, half-hearted use of powerful antibiotics now will eventually result in less effective drugs later … [O]nce life-saving medicines are increasingly having as little effect as a sugar pill. Microbial resistance to treatment could bring the world back to a pre-antibiotic age … The potential of drug resistance to catapult us all back into a world of premature death and chronic illness is all too real. (WHO, 2000)

The WHO considers drug resistance to be one of the three most important issues in global health. The personal opinion of Karl Ekdahl, Strategic Advisor to the Director of the European Centre for Disease Prevention and Control (ECDC), is that "drug resistance is the greatest threat to health over the next 25 years;" and he agrees that "the antibiotic era may soon be a thing of the past" (Ekdahl, 2006).[2]

A major cause of drug resistance is that patients do not always complete a full course of therapy. When a patient starts but fails to complete a course of antimicrobial therapy, this selects for drug-resistant strains of disease: bacteria most vulnerable to the drugs are killed, allowing mutant resistant strains (that might have been killed if therapy had been completed) to thrive in the absence of microbial competitors in the environment of the patient's body.

Though "non-compliant" patients are often blamed for the problem of drug resistance, it is often impossible for patients in poor countries to complete a course of medication when drug supplies run out at local clinics due to a lack of resources and the general weakness of local health-care infrastructure. Poor patients are also often unable to complete treatment because they cannot afford to continue to pay for medications they have started, or because they cannot afford (often difficult) transportation to (often faraway) medical facilities (Farmer, 1999).

When a drug-resistant strain of disease emerges in one person's body, this has implications for others because drug-resistant diseases, like infectious diseases in general, are usually contagious. There are also implications for global health because contagious drug-resistant diseases, like contagious infectious diseases in general, show no respect for international borders. Lack of access to medicine in poor countries thus has adverse affects on health in rich countries.

One way of addressing the problem of drug resistance would be to make medicines more accessible to poor populations in developing countries, as this would help stall the emergence of drug resistance. In the meantime, however, new antibiotics (and other antimicrobials) are desperately needed, because the power of our existing supply has increasingly declined. Vaccine development is also important, because vaccination prevents infection to begin with. There has been a dearth of vaccine and antibiotic drug development for decades, however. Almost no new classes of antibiotics have been developed since 1970. Lack of antimicrobial research and development reflects the fact that these

---

[2] For earlier warnings regarding drug resistance, see Garrett (1994) and Benatar (1995).

have been unattractive areas of investment for the profit-driven pharmaceutical industry.[3] Because infectious diseases primarily affect the poor, the potential for recouping antimicrobial drug development costs is low. This explains "the 10/90 divide," a phenomenon whereby less than 10% of medical research resources are spent on diseases accounting for 90% of the global burden of disease. Rather than addressing the world's most important health-care needs, a majority of funds are spent on research aimed at meeting the wants and needs of a minority of the world's population – those who are relatively wealthy. This unjust distribution of research resources may come back to haunt us all, rich and poor alike, if we do in fact return to a situation analogous to the pre-antibiotic era (Selgelid, 2007).

The reality of the threat is well illustrated by the case of TB, for which there was "a 40 year standstill in … drug development" (WHO, 2004) – and for which no new drugs can realistically be expected before 2015. Multidrug-resistant TB (MDR-TB) is defined as TB resistant to at least two of the four "first-line" TB medications. While ordinary TB can be cured with an inexpensive six-month course of treatment, MDR-TB takes two years to treat, and treatment can be 100 times more expensive. The "second-line" medications used to treat MDR-TB are, furthermore, both more toxic and less effective than "first-line" drugs.

More alarming still is the emergence and spread of virtually untreatable "extreme" or "extensively" drug resistant TB (XDR-TB), as announced by the US Centers for Disease Control and Prevention (CDC) and the WHO in 2006 (CDC, 2006; WHO, 2006). XDR-TB is defined as TB resistant not only to first-line but also to several second-line medications (CDC, 2006; WHO, 2006). The most dramatic epidemic of XDR-TB is currently underway in South Africa, where a recent study showed that 41% of suspected patients were infected with MDR-TB and that 24% of these had XDR-TB. Of the 53 patients with the latter, 52 died within 25 days (Médecins Sans Frontières, 2006). Implications of XDR-TB for the international community are starkly revealed by the CDC's statement that XDR-TB "has emerged worldwide as a threat to public health and

TB control, raising concerns of a future epidemic of virtually untreatable TB" (CDC, 2006). In the meantime, a suspected case of XDR-TB in 2007 already led to the first imposition of Federal isolation/quarantine restrictions in the USA since 1963 (Selgelid, 2008a).

Limiting liberty in contexts of contagion

Isolation and quarantine were also imposed in Asia and Canada during the SARS crisis of 2003 – and, in many countries, in response to H1N1 swine flu. As noted above, however, coercive social distancing measures conflict with the right to freedom of movement. Quarantine can also violate the right to life. If an airplane carrying a passenger infected with a deadly strain of flu is quarantined, for example, then other previously uninfected passengers held in close confinement may become infected and die as a result. Does this mean that the coercive imposition of quarantine would be unethical or wrong? Not necessarily. Individual rights and liberties matter and we should not run roughshod over individuals in the name of public health, but the goal of promoting utility in the way of public health matters greatly too.

If a disastrous epidemic would result from the maximal protection of individual rights and liberties, then individual rights and liberties must be compromised. Even arch-libertarian Robert Nozick hints that we might need to violate "side-constraints" (i.e. human rights as he perceives them) when this is necessary to avoid "catastrophic moral horror" (Nozick, 1974, p. 30n). Though it should be considered an extreme or exceptional measure, there is no reason in principle to rule out quarantine altogether, even if it sometimes ends up killing innocent people, just as there is no ethical reason to rule out participation in just wars which also inevitably involve compromise of innocent individuals' rights, including the right to life.

Ethical principles regarding coercive isolation and quarantine should arguably include the following. First, extreme measures such as these should not be employed unless there are compelling reasons to believe that they would provide effective means of controlling disease in the circumstances under consideration. While authors such as George Annas deny that quarantine actually works (Annas, 2005), this is of course an empirical question. We should avoid making and/or accepting sweeping empirical claims in the absence of empirical evidence. There are historical cases – such as

---

[3] As the problem of drug resistance grows (and increasingly affects patients in relatively affluent countries), however, the financial incentives of the pharmaceutical industry to develop more new antimicrobial treatments will hopefully increase. Fears regarding liability, meanwhile, have been a persistent disincentive regarding vaccine development.

that of American Samoa during the 1918–19 flu pandemic – where long-term coercive social distancing measures appear to have been highly effective (Crosby, 2003). This important case reveals that we should, in addition to rejecting the sweeping claims of Annas, perhaps be skeptical about Gostin's (2006) claim that measures like quarantine would only play an early and minor role in the event of a major flu pandemic. That might be true for most places on large continents, but demographic context matters here – and islands, at least, may be a different story.

The evidence for or against the effectiveness of quarantine warrants further study. Given the difficulty of conducting controlled studies in the context of quarantine, however, it will not be easy to conclusively demonstrate whether or not quarantine would be effective in any given circumstance, and greater uncertainty will arise in the case of unknown novel pathogens. There is an ethical imperative, in any case, that researchers with relevant expertise further examine this issue as best they can; relevant data are required for solving ethical/policy questions as well as questions more purely concerned with public health science.

Second, mandatory isolation and quarantine should not be employed unless they are actually required. If alternative, less restrictive means are available to achieve the same ends regarding public health protection, then these should be employed instead (Upshur, 2002). If voluntary quarantine, for example, would likely be just as effective as mandatory quarantine, then the latter should not be imposed. Mandatory quarantine should only be used as a last resort (Gostin, 2006).

Third, extreme measures such as these should not be imposed unless the consequences would otherwise be severe. It would be wrong to think that rights violations and the imposition of harms on individuals are justified whenever this would lead to a net payoff for society as a whole. The maximal promotion of public health should not be the sole goal of ethical public health policy. The stakes would need to be high in order for liberty-infringing measures to be permissible.

Fourth, for isolation and quarantine to be ethically acceptable, they must be implemented in an equitable manner. It would be unjust, that is, if quarantine were used (as it often has been in the past) in a discriminatory fashion against those who are already socially marginalized or disempowered. One could argue that the grounds for imposing isolation or quarantine must be strongest when, other things being equal,

those being considered for confinement are members of the worst-off groups in society. Just as research ethics guidelines give special protection to those who are vulnerable, isolation/quarantine guidelines should arguably do the same. If justice requires improving the situation of the worst-off groups of society (Rawls, 1971), then we should be especially reluctant to infringe upon the rights and liberties of – or impose harms upon – such groups' members.

Fifth, isolation and quarantine, if implemented, should be made as minimally burdensome as possible. Those confined should be provided with basic necessities such as food, water, comfort and health care. A sixth, and related, point is that those who endure confinement for the benefit of society should be compensated in return. If there are limited amounts of medicine and vaccine available, for example, then those who have been confined deserve special priority when allocation decisions about medical resources are made. If the overall benefits of confinement outweigh the costs – as would have to be the case for confinement to be justified in the first place – then a net social dividend results from liberty infringement. Part of this should be returned to the victims of coercion. It would be wrong if confined individuals are expected to shoulder the burdens required for the protection of society, and then receive nothing in return. The burdens associated with epidemic disease are shared more fairly if those who make sacrifices by succumbing to confinement are provided with compensation for doing so. This is a matter of reciprocity (University of Toronto Joint Centre for Bioethics, 2005). A final benefit of putting a compensation/reward scheme into place is that this would likely enhance trust in – and thus cooperation with – public health systems (Ly *et al.*, 2007). It is well known that trust is important for public health systems to succeed.

Improving global health

The section above presents a conflict between social values: the aim to promote utility in the way of public health conflicts with the aim to protect individual rights and liberties in situations where coercive social distancing measures or other intrusive public health-care measures are called for. We then ask what balance to strike between these goals. In a way, however, this is a false dilemma. If global health were better, the conflict (requiring sacrifice of either utility or human rights/liberties) would arise less often. Infectious diseases, recall, primarily affect the poor; and infectious disease contributes to the poverty of the poor. If the health of those who are now poor were better to begin with, then the global infectious disease threat would diminish; and we would not so often be forced to choose between promoting utility in the way of public health, on the one hand, and protecting human rights and liberties, on the other. Improvement of global health (and thus poverty reduction) would promote multiple important social goals: equality, human rights/liberty and utility.

From a global perspective, one of the most important questions is whether or not – or why – wealthy developed nations should be motivated to do more to help improve the health-care situation in developing countries (given that the latter lack sufficient resources to adequately do so on their own). In what follows, we see that cumulative ethical and self-interested reasons justify wealthy world funding of disease reduction in poor countries (Selgelid, 2008b).

There are numerous ways in which health-care improvement in developing countries would promote equality. One of the best developed arguments for treating health care as a special kind of good is that provided by Norman Daniels in *Just Health Care* (1985). Disease interferes with species-typical functioning and thus detracts from equality of opportunity – and equality of opportunity is a requirement of justice. We should thus, according to Daniels, guarantee equal access to a basic minimum package of health care for all members of society. Daniels appeals to Rawls' theory of justice for domestic society, however; and Rawls resists application of domestic principles of justice to the global scene. Several have persuasively argued, on the other hand, that Rawls' weaker requirements for international justice are inconsistent with what he says elsewhere (Moellendorf, 2002; Pogge, 2002). Theory aside, Daniels' argument that health is crucial to equality of opportunity holds; and the idea that equality of opportunity matters in other countries, just as it matters in our own, will be accepted by many as a common sense precept.

Another egalitarian reason for improving the health of the poor is that this would make the worst-off better off. The sick and poor in southern Africa are, by any measure, clearly among the worst-off members of global society; and increased provision of health care is one of the things most needed to improve their situation. Improvement of health in developing countries would also reduce *undeserved inequalities* in well-being. Despite the fact that some suffer from AIDS as a result of their own (informed) careless sexual or drug-injecting behavior, most who suffer from AIDS, TB and other infectious diseases in developing countries are in no way responsible for, nor do they deserve, the illnesses from which they suffer.

It can also be argued that many of those who suffer from these diseases are, directly or indirectly, victims of injustice. In so far as rich countries have (benefitted from) and contributed to the exploitation of developing countries – while this in turn has promoted poverty and disease in the latter – rich countries should recognize obligations to amend unjust inequalities that they are partly responsible for.

In addition to promoting equality in these ways, health improvement in poor countries would promote human rights. It is commonly believed that human beings have rights to have their most basic needs (for things like shelter, clothing, housing, food and clean water) met. The idea that there is a human right to health care is reflected by the existence of universal health-care systems in every industrialized nation except the USA. Such rights are, furthermore, enshrined by authoritative international documents such as the Universal Declaration of Human Rights, which claims in Article 25 that "Everyone has the right to a standard of living adequate for the health and well-being of himself and his family, including food, clothing, and medical care … [and that] every individual and every organ of society … shall strive … by progressive measures, national and international, to secure [its] universal and effective recognition" (United Nations, 1999). Because human rights are supposedly taken seriously in other contexts of foreign policy making – as grounds for waging war to prevent their violation, for example[4] – it is inconsistent to ignore their violation in the context of health care.

Utilitarian reasons strengthen the case for health-care improvement in developing countries. Given that a $20 course of TB medication or even a $100 yearly course of AIDS medication can each make all the difference between life and death – and enable

---

4 One might object that those who appeal to rights violations to justify waging war usually refer to negative rights violations as opposed to a failure to promote "more aspirational" positive rights of people to have basic necessities met. Whether or not this is true – or always the case – is an empirical question that warrants further study. In any case the (rights-based) justification for providing aid presumably need not be so stringent (as that required for waging war).

prevention of enormous suffering – these are among the very best uses that can be made of such sums of money in terms of positive impact on human lives, especially when compared with the frivolous way such sums are routinely spent in wealthy countries. Promotion of the greater good in terms of human well-being provides *a* reason for taking one action rather than another, even if other potentially over-riding legitimate social aims must also be taken into consideration. One need not subscribe to utilitarianism to think that the greater good of humanity is (one of the things that is) morally important and should thus be taken into consideration by policy makers in rich countries. Only a minor sacrifice by wealthy developed nations would be required to achieve tremendous benefits in terms of reduced suffering and saved lives in poor countries. According to Jeffrey Sachs:

> The [Commissission on Macroeconomics and Health] concluded that donor aid [to invest in global health] ought to rise from around [US]$6 billion per year [in 2001] to $27 billion per year (by 2007). With combined GNP of the donor countries equal to around $25 trillion dollars as of 2001, the commission was advocating an annual investment of around one thousandth of rich-world income. The commission showed, on the best epidemiological evidence, that such an investment could avert eight million deaths per year. (Sachs, 2005)

Improvement of health care in developing countries is thus justified on numerous ethical grounds. This would promote equality, restorative justice, the human right to health care, and utility – and only a minor sacrifice would be required for wealthy developed nations to achieve enormous benefits. As noted above, it would also help protect liberty, because the reduction of infectious diseases in poor countries would diminish their prevalence worldwide, and so the need for liberty restricting public health-care measures would arise less often (in rich and poor countries alike). (The aim to avoid liberty restrictions within their own borders might be considered both an ethical and a self-interested reason why wealthy nations should do more to improve health care in developing countries.)

Additional straightforward self-interested reasons should motivate wealthy nations to do more to improve health care in developing countries (Benatar, 1998). When infectious diseases thrive in poor countries, this has negative implications for health in rich countries. One implication of poverty and the lack of health care in poor countries is that everyone everywhere is subject to greater risk of infection than would otherwise be the case. This was well illustrated in the above discussion of drug resistance. When the poor lack adequate health care, drug-resistant strains of disease emerge and threaten global health. The idea that we might soon return to a situation analogous to the pre-antibiotic era – and the *fact* that we already again live in a world with untreatable TB – should not be taken lightly.

Acknowledgment

An earlier version of this paper was published as "Infectious Diseases" in *A Companion to Bioethics*, Second Edition, edited by Helga Kuhse and Peter Singer. Malden, MA: Wiley-Blackwell, 2009, pp. 430–440. I thank Wiley-Blackwell for permission to reprint this material here. I am grateful to Solomon Benatar and Gillian Brock for numerous suggestions which led to improvement of the paper. Work on this paper was partly supported by an Australian Research Council Discovery Grant for a project on Infectious Diseases, Security and Ethics.

References

Annas, G. J. (2005). *American Bioethics: Crossing Human Rights and Health Law Boundaries*. New York, NY: Oxford University Press.

Barnett, T. & Whiteside, A. (2002). *AIDS in the Twenty-First Century: Disease and Globalisation*. New York, NY: W.W. Norton.

Benatar, S. R. (1995). Prospects for global health: lessons from tuberculosis. *Thorax* 50, 489–491.

Benatar, S. R. (1998). Global disparities in health and human rights: a critical commentary. *American Journal of Public Health* 88, 295–300.

Centers for Disease Control and Prevention (CDC) (2006). Emergence of *Mycobacterium tuberculosis* with extensive resistance to second-line drugs – worldwide, 2000–2004. *Morbidity and Mortality Weekly Report* 55, 301–305.

Crosby, A. W. (2003). *America's Forgotten Pandemic: The Influenza of 1918*. (2nd edn.) Cambridge: Cambridge University Press.

Daniels, N. (1985). *Just Health Care*. New York, NY: Cambridge University Press.

Ekdahl, K. (2006). Ethical issues from the ECDC perspective. Paper presented at the Bioethical Implications of Globalisation Processes (BIG) Workshop on Globalisation and New Epidemics: Ethics, Security and Policy Making, Brussels.

Farmer, P. (1999). *Infections and Inequalities*. Berkeley, CA: University of California Press.

Gandy, M. & Zumla, A. (2002). The resurgence of disease: social and historical perspectives on the "new" tuberculosis. *Social Science and Medicine* **55**, 385–396.

Garrett, L. (1994). *The Coming Plague: Newly Emerging Diseases in a World Out of Balance*. New York, NY: Penguin.

Gostin, L. O. (2006). Public health strategies for pandemic influenza. *Journal of the American Medical Association* **295**, 1700–1704.

Ly, T., Selgelid, M. J. & Kerridge, I. (2007). Pandemic and public health controls: toward an equitable compensation system. *Journal of Law and Medicine* **15**, 318–324.

Médecins Sans Frontières (2006). Extensive drug resistant tuberculosis (XDR-TB). www.accessmed-msf.org (Accessed February 15, 2007).

Moellendorf, D. (2002). *Cosmopolitan Justice*. New York, NY: Westview Press.

Nozick, R. (1974). *Anarchy, State, and Utopia*. New York, NY: Basic Books.

Oldstone, M. B. A. (1998). *Viruses, Plagues, and History*. New York, NY: Oxford University Press.

Pogge, T. W. (2002). *World Poverty and Human Rights*. Cambridge, MA: Polity Press.

Price-Smith, A. T. (2001). *The Health of Nations: Infectious Disease, Environmental Change, and their Effects on National Security and Development*. Cambridge, MA: MIT Press.

Rawls, J. (1971). *A Theory of Justice*. Cambridge, MA: Harvard University Press.

Ryan, F. (1992). *The Forgotten Plague: How the Battle Against Tuberculosis was Won – and Lost*. Boston, MA: Bay Back Books.

Sachs, J. (2005). *The End of Poverty*. London: Penguin.

Selgelid, M. J. (2005). Ethics and infectious disease. *Bioethics* **19**, 272–289.

Selgelid, M. J. (2007). Ethics and drug resistance. *Bioethics* **21**, 218–229.

Selgelid, M. J. (2008a). Ethics, tuberculosis and globalization. *Public Health Ethics* **1**, 10–20.

Selgelid, M. J. (2008b). Improving global health: counting reasons why. *Developing World Bioethics* **8**, 115–125.

Singer, P. (2002). *One World: The Ethics of Globalization*. Melbourne: The Text Publishing Company.

UNAIDS (2008). Report on the global AIDS epidemic. http://www.unaids.org/en/KnowledgeCentre/HIVData/GlobalReport/2008/2008_Global_report.asp (Accessed January 12, 2010).

United Nations (UN) (1999). *Universal Declaration of Human Rights*. www.un.org/Overview/rights.html (Accessed February 8, 2006).

University of Toronto Joint Centre for Bioethics, Pandemic Influenza Working Group (2005). Stand on guard for thee: ethical considerations in preparedness planning for pandemic influenza. www.utoronto.ca/jcb/home/documents/pandemic.pdf (Accessed January 6, 2006).

Upshur, R. (2002). Principles for the justification of public health intervention. *Canadian Journal of Public Health* **93**, 101–103.

World Health Organization (WHO) (2000). Report on infectious diseases 2000 – overcoming antimicrobial resistance. www.who.int/infectious-disease-report/2000/ (Accessed August 30, 2006).

World Health Organization (WHO) (2002). Fact sheet no 104. Tuberculosis. www.who.int/mediacentre/factsheets/fs104/en/print.html (Accessed June 2004).

World Health Organization (WHO) (2004). Drug resistant tuberculosis ten times higher in Eastern Europe and Central Asia. www.who.int/mediacentre/releases/2004/pr17/en/print.thml (Accessed March 7, 2004).

World Health Organization (WHO) (2006). *Weekly Epidemiological Record*, September 2006. www.who.int/wer (Accessed February 2007).

World Health Organization (WHO) (2007). *Global Tuberculosis Control: Surveillance, Planning, Financing*. Geneva: World Health Organization. WHO/HTM/TB/2007.376.

Ziegler, P. (1969). *The Black Death*. London: Penguin.

Chapter

International health inequalities and global justice: toward a middle ground

Norman Daniels

Disturbing international inequalities in health abound. Life expectancy in Swaziland is half that in Japan.[1] A child unfortunate enough to be born in Angola has 73 times as great a chance of dying before age 5 as a child born in Norway.[2] A mother giving birth in southern sub-Saharan Africa has 100 times as great a chance of dying from her labor as one birthing in an industrialized country.[3] For every mile one travels outward toward the Maryland suburbs from downtown Washington, DC on its underground rail system, life expectancy rises by a year – reflecting the race and class inequities in American health.[4] Are the glaring, even larger, international health inequalities also unjust?

All of us no doubt think they are grossly unfortunate. Many of us think they are unfair or unjust. Why should some people be at such a health disadvantage through no fault of their own, losers in a natural and social lottery assigning them birth in an unhealthy place? Others of us are troubled by the absence of the kinds of human relationships that ordinarily give rise to the claims of egalitarian justice that we make on each other – for example, being fellow citizens or even interacting in a cooperative scheme. Who has obligations of justice to reduce these international inequalities? And do those obligations hold regardless of how the inequalities came about? What institutions are accountable for addressing them?

My account of just health (Daniels, 2008), alas, gives us no simple or straightforward answers to these important questions about global justice. Some will see that as a serious shortcoming, perhaps insisting that an adequate account of justice and health must apply uniformly to all citizens of the globe or even the cosmos. Others are less troubled by the silence of my account because they reject the idea that justice can apply to people regardless of the relationships they stand in to each other. For them justice is fundamentally relational – indeed it depends on the relationship of being fellow citizens in a state – and not cosmopolitan.

My task here is to point, in a very preliminary way, to a relatively unexplored middle ground where I hope it is possible to clarify what kinds of international obligations of justice exist.

When are international inequalities in health unjust?

Health inequalities between social groups count as unjust or unfair when they result from an unjust distribution of the socially controllable factors that affect population health and its distribution. To illustrate what such a just distribution of these factors might be, consider Rawls' principles of justice as fairness. They assure equal basic liberties and the worth of political participation rights, assure fair equality of opportunity through public education, early childhood supports, and appropriate public health and medical services, and constrain socio-economic inequalities in ways that make the worst off groups as well off as possible. Together, this distribution of the key determinants of population health would significantly flatten the socio-economic gradient of health and would minimize various inequities in health, including race and gender inequities.

Judged from this ideal perspective, we see that there are indeed many health inequities – by race and ethnicity,

[1] 40 vs 80+ years. www.os-connect.com/pop/p1.asp?which page=10&pagesize=20&sort=Country (Accessed August 23, 2005).
[2] The State of the World's Children, www.unicef.org/sowc00/stat2.htm (Accessed August 23, 2005).
[3] See WHO/UNICEF/UNFPA (2005). *Maternal Mortality in 2004 – Estimates Developed by WHO, UNICEF, and UNFPA.* www.childinfo.org/Areas/maternalmortality (Accessed August 23, 2005).
[4] Michael Marmot, presentation at Harvard School of Public Health, 2006.

An earlier version of this work has appeared: Daniels, N. (2008). *Just Health: Meeting Health Needs Fairly.* Chapter 13: International health inequalities and global justice. Cambridge University Press.

by class and caste, and by gender – in many countries around the world, both developed and developing. At the same time, not all health inequalities between social groups count as inequities. For example, the health inequality that results when a religious or ethnic group achieves better health outcomes than other demographic groups because of special dietary or restrictive sexual practices would not count as an inequity if appropriate health education were available to the other groups.

This account tells us when health inequalities between groups in a given society are unjust, not when inequalities between different societies are. It tells us what we as fellow citizens owe each other regarding the promotion and protection of health, but not what other societies owe, if anything, by way of improving the health of the population in less healthy societies. The account, for example, fails to address this issue: suppose countries A and B each do the best they can to distribute the socially controllable factors affecting health fairly, and, as a result, there are no sub-group inequities within them. Nevertheless, health outcomes are unequal between A and B because A has more resources to devote to population health than B. Is the resulting international inequality in health a matter of justice? Suppose we vary the case: Now B, whether or not it has resources comparable to A, fails to protect its population health as best it can, leading again to population health worse than A's. Is the resulting health inequality a matter of international justice? Our account of just health informs us about intra-societal obligations to eliminate health inequities, but it is silent about important questions of international justice.[5]

Those who claim the gross health inequalities are unjust have quite different, incompatible ways of justifying that view. For example, those who believe that any disadvantage that people suffer through no fault or choice of their own is unjust would assert that the disadvantage facing the Angolan child is therefore unjust. The underlying principle of justice is applied to individuals wherever they are in the cosmos and regardless of what specific relationships they stand in to others (roughly, the cosmopolitan perspective) – contrary to

the Rawls–Nagel account, which applies principles of justice to the basic structure of a shared society (the statist view). The disadvantage of the Angolan child might also be thought unjust by those who, like statists, think principles of justice are "relational" and apply only to a basic social structure that people share, but who believe we already live in a world where international agencies and rule-making bodies constitute a robust global basic structure that is appropriately seen as the subject of international justice developed perhaps through a social contract involving representatives of relevant groups globally (Beitz, 1979, 2000). Fair terms of cooperation involving that structure would, some argue, reject arrangements that failed to make children in low-income countries as well off as they could be. Clearly, there may be more agreement about some specific judgments of injustice than there is on the justification for those judgments or on broader theoretical issues.

I shall briefly examine two ways of trying to break the stalemate between statist and cosmopolitan perspectives. One approach aims for a minimalist (albeit cosmopolitan) strategy that focuses on an international obligation of justice to avoid "harming" people by causing "deficits" in the satisfaction of their human rights (Pogge, 2002, 2005b). It is a minimalist view in the sense that people may agree on negative duties not to harm even if they disagree about positive duties to aid. This approach handles some international health issues better than others, and to identify its limitations more clearly, I shall distinguish various sources of international health inequalities, some of which are not addressed by negative duties. A more promising (relational justice) approach, which I can only briefly illustrate, requires that we work out a more intermediary conception of justice appropriate to evolving international institutions and rule making bodies, leaving it open just how central issues of equality would be in such a context (Cohen & Sable, 2006). Properly developed, such an approach may address more of the sources of international health inequalities.

Harms to health: a minimalist strategy

If wealthy countries engage in a practice or policy – or impose an institutional order – that foreseeably makes the health of those in poorer countries worse than it would otherwise be, specifically, making it harder than it would otherwise be to realize a human right to health

---

[5] Nor does the appeal to the international law framework for a right to health answer the question about which inequalities are unjust. The primary obligations for promoting health fall to states, even if there are international obligations to assist states, and the progressive realizability of such rights mean that significant health inequalities will persist despite international and national efforts.

or health care, then, Pogge (2005b) argues, it is harming that population by creating this "deficit" in human rights. Since this harm is defined relative to an internationally recognized standard of justice, the protection of human rights, Pogge concludes that imposing the harm is unjust. Moreover, if there is a foreseeable alternative institutional order that would reasonably avoid the deficit in human rights, there is an international obligation of justice to produce the rights-promoting alternative.

There remains some lack of clarity about how the baseline against which harm is measured is specified. When is there a "deficit" in a human right to health? Whenever a country fails to meet the levels of health provided, say, by Japan, which has the highest life expectancy? Or is there some other, unspecified standard? Consider two examples.

The brain drain of health personnel

The brain drain of health personnel from low-income to OECD countries may exemplify Pogge's concerns. Rich countries have harmed health in poorer ones by solving their own labor shortages of trained health-care personnel by actively and passively attracting immigrants from poorer countries. In developed countries such as New Zealand, the UK, USA, Australia, and Canada, 23–34% of physicians are foreign-trained.

The situation that results in developing countries is dire. For instance, over 60% of doctors' trained in Ghana in the 1980s emigrated overseas (WHO, 2004). In 2002 in Ghana 47% of doctors posts were unfilled and 57% of registered nursing positions were unfilled. Whereas there are 188 physicians per 100 000 population in the USA, there are only 1 or 2 per 100 000 in large parts of Africa. The brain drain does not cause the whole of the inequality in health workers, but it significantly contributes to it.

International efforts to reduce poverty, lower mortality rates, and treat HIV/AIDS patients – the Millennium Development Goals (MDG) agreed upon in 2000 – are all threatened by the loss of health personnel in sub-Saharan Africa. An editorial in the *Bulletin of the World Health Organization* points out that the MDG goals of reducing mortality rates for infants, mothers, and children under five cannot be achieved without a million additional skilled health workers in the region (Chen & Hanvoravongchai, 2005).

What about causes? There is both a "push" from poor working conditions and opportunities in low-income countries and a "pull" from more attractive

conditions elsewhere. Is this simply "the market" at work, backed by a "right to migrate"?

Pogge's argument about an international institutional order has more specific grip than the vague appeal to a market. When economic conditions worsened in various developing countries in the 1980s, international lenders, such as the World Bank and International Monetary Fund (IMF) insisted that countries severely cut back publicly funded health systems as well as take other steps to reduce deficit spending. In Cameroon, for example, in the 1990s, measures included a suspension of health-worker recruitment, mandatory retirement at 50 or 55 years, suspension of promotions and reduction of benefits. The health sector budget shrank from 4.8% in 1993 to 2.4% in 1999, even while the private health sector grew (Liese *et al.*, 2004). As a result, public sector health workers migrated to the private sector and others joined the international brain drain. Cost cutting imposed on the country led to cuts in the training of health workers, increasing the shortage. Another consequence of salary cuts was an increase in "under the table" payments to secure domestic treatment and an increase in "shadow providers" who collected public salaries but practiced privately during public sector hours. The international institutional order thus increased the push and at the same time harmed the health system in various ways.

The "pull" attracting health workers to OECD countries is also not just diffuse economic demand. Targeted recruiting by developed countries is so intensive that it has stripped whole nursing classes away from some universities in the South. In 2000, the Labour Government in the UK set a target of adding 20 000 nurses to the NHS by 2004. It achieved the goal by 2002. The UK absorbed 13 000 foreign nurses and 4000 doctors in 2002 alone. Recruitment from EU countries was flat (many of these countries also face shortages in the face of aging populations), but immigration from developing countries continued, despite an effort to frame a policy of ethical recruitment (Deeming, 2004). Arguably, even if there were a diffuse economic "pull," in the absence of active recruiting the harm would be much less.

The remedy for this harm is not a prohibition on migration, which is protected by various human rights. The UK has recently announced a tougher code to restrict recruitment from 150 developing countries. In addition it has initiated a US$100m contribution to the Malawi health system aimed at creating better conditions for retaining health personnel there. The UK has thus taken two steps that are intended to reduce both the push and the pull behind the brain drain. Other countries have not followed suit.

International property rights and access to drugs

The minimalist strategy becomes harder to apply in a clear way to other international health issues, such as access to drugs. Major pharmaceutical companies have long been criticized for a research and development bias against drugs needed in developing country markets and for opposition to relaxing their monopoly control over such drugs as antiretroviral cocktails for treating HIV/AIDS.[6] Indeed, they have responded to existing incentives by concentrating on "blockbuster" drugs for wealthier markets, including many "me too" drugs that marginally improve effectiveness or reduce side effects slightly. Funding the research needed to develop a vaccine against malaria, for example, has fallen to private foundations.

Do intellectual property rights and the incentive structures they support create a foreseeable deficit in the right to health that can be reasonably avoided? Pogge (2005b) argues that they do. Nevertheless, many drugs developed by major pharmaceutical companies under existing property right protections have filtered into widespread use as generics on "essential drug" formularies in developing countries. Health outcomes in those countries are much better than they would be absent such drugs. Since many of these drugs would not have been produced in the absence of some form of property right protections, people are not worse off than they would be in a completely free market with no temporary monopolies on products.

Arguably, however, different incentive schemes would make people in these poor countries with poor markets better off than they currently are. Which schemes ought we to select? Pogge (2005a) proposes that we revise incentives for drug development by establishing a tax-based fund in developed countries that would reward drug companies in proportion to the impact of their products on the global burden of disease.[7] The program could be limited to "essential drugs" leaving existing incentives in place for other drug products. How do we pick which alternative level of tax and thus incentives to use as a baseline against which a "deficit" in the right to health is specified? Pogge does not tell us.

Leaving aside the problem of vagueness, Pogge's proposal cannot be justified by appealing to the "no harm" principle alone. The proposed incentive fund would better help to realize human rights to health, as Pogge argues, but "not optimally helping" is not the same as "harming" and so the justification has shifted. There may well be good reasons for an account of international justice to consider the interests of those affected by current property right protections more carefully than those agreements now do – but that takes us into more contested terrain than the minimalist strategy.

International harming is complex in several ways. The harms are often not deliberately imposed, and sometimes benefits were arguably intended. The harms are often mixed with benefits. In any case, great care must be taken to describe the baseline against which harm is measured. Such a complex story about motivations, intentions, and effects might seem to weaken the straightforward appeal of the minimalist strategy, but the complexity does not undermine the view that we have obligations of justice to avoid harming health.

Where do international health inequalities come from?

Pogge (2005a) emphasizes the fact that 18 million premature, preventable deaths are associated with global poverty. It is tempting, then, to infer that country wealth determines population health and that if rich countries help to keep poor countries poor, they thus harm the health of those populations. If this inference is sound, it gives the minimalist strategy considerable power in addressing international health inequalities. Unfortunately, the inference is not sound, since the relationship between country wealth and country health is more complex than the inference presupposes. We need to examine the sources of international health inequalities more systematically.

---

[6] Patent holders on antiretroviral drugs led a fight, until recently, to restrict access to generic versions of their drugs. The consequence was a direct harm to those who might have benefited from antiretrovirals and died instead. Still, the emergence of these generics that do save other lives would not have happened had there not been the incentives created by the existing patent system – or so the dominant view about intellectual property maintains.

[7] Unfortunately, measuring this impact is exceedingly difficult since many factors besides a drug may be at work.

We can divide the sources of international health inequalities[8] into three categories:

(1) Those that result from domestic injustice in the distribution of the socially controllable factors determining population health and its distribution. Included here would be inequalities by race, caste, ethnicity, religion, or gender, or geography in the distribution of the determinants of health. Also included are failure to fund adequately (relative to capacity) the health sector, including intersectoral public health measures, immunizations and comprehensive community based primary care; misallocation of resources, for example, diverting funds from public health and primary care to hospital care serving best-off groups in response to their demand and greater political power.

(2) Those that result from international inequalities in other conditions that affect health. These include inequalities in natural conditions, such as poor natural resources, including arable land, or susceptibility to droughts and floods, or disease vectors, such as mosquitoes carrying malaria or dengue. They also include socially produced inequalities, such as significant inequalities in capital, in human capital and in political culture.

(3) Those that result from international practices – institutions, rule-making bodies, treaties – that harm the health of some countries. The harms can be direct, as in the case of the brain drain of health workers, or more indirect, as in failures to build worker health and safety protections into international trade agreements, or through international loans or other means that may perpetuate poverty.

These sources of inequality are not exclusive. Some international practices (category 3) may help create the social inequalities in the second category that in turn increase health inequalities; they may also make it more difficult for states to distribute the determinants of health in a just way (category 1). Some of the inequalities in the second category may also contribute to the

injustices of the first. The minimalist strategy would have great scope if category 3 sources dominated categories 1 and 2, but this seems unlikely. Only more robust accounts of international justice can address the broader sources of inequality.

To see why the kinds of inequalities referred to in the second category cannot exhaust the problem of international inequalities in health, consider how much health inequality across countries is simply the result of wealth inequalities. The wealth of a country has an effect on aggregate measures of health, at least up to some fairly moderate level of aggregate wealth, say $6–8000 gross domestic product per capita (GDPPC). Above that level, there is little influence of aggregate wealth on aggregate health. This may be some evidence that international inequalities in wealth have some contribution to international health inequalities, and to the extent that wealthy countries cause or sustain that inequality, the minimalist strategy obtains a grip on the problem.

But even more striking than the fact that great wealth is not needed to secure high levels of population health is the amount of variation in life expectancy both above and below that middle-income figure. Some poor countries, with GDP per capita less than $3000, such as Cuba, or the even poorer state of Kerala in southern India (which has lower income per capita than the average in India), have health outcomes rivaling those achieved in wealthy ones. Among the wealthiest countries, there are also significant differences in life expectancy.

I draw the conclusion from these facts that policy matters greatly: what is done with national resources explains much of the wide variation across countries that are equally rich or equally poor. Cuba invests great effort in public health, including ecologically sound environmental policies, as well as in basic education. It invests heavily in training health personnel (its doctor per population ratio is comparable to the USA), and it sends doctors abroad to worse off countries. Indeed, it does so despite US economic and travel sanctions intended to undermine its government by inflicting economic harm.

Cuba's success in health outcomes despite the harms imposed by the USA does not show that other international practices play no causal role in producing poor health outcomes elsewhere. But the Cuban example shows how hard it is to specify the baseline against which harm is to be measured. The minimalist strategy supposes that international practices that

---

[8] Not all international health inequalities plausibly raise questions about injustice, just as not all domestic inequalities between groups raise those questions. For example, religious or ethnic differences in lifestyle (diet, sex, social cohesiveness) might give rise domestically and internationally to health inequalities that we would not consider unjust.

make a country poorer than it would otherwise have been would thereby make it less healthy than it would otherwise be. But international practices may make a country poorer than it would otherwise be, but determined public policy may nevertheless result in much better health outcomes than is typical for countries with those levels of poverty. The harm to health can be specified only by assuming that no good health policy is put in place – but why that assumption holds when it does may have nothing to do with the economic harm.

Kerala, like Cuba, also invests heavily in basic education, securing high literacy rates even for poor women, as well as in public health and primary care. The positive treatment of women stands out as a contrast with practices in many other areas of India and South Asia in general. In the case of Kerala, it is popularly believed that the lack of gender bias in education and in reproductive and marriage rights is the result of a left-wing state government, but the story is more complex. Kerala, in contrast to the rest of India, had a history of matrilineal property transmission for two thousand years. As a result, women could not be discounted as in many other states of India. Its cultural tradition was a base on which a more egalitarian social policy could take root. Given a culture in which women retain significant autonomy and power, both within and outside the home, more egalitarian education and control over reproduction are realistic social goals, and both contribute significantly to population health. Though Kerala, unlike Cuba, was not the victim of focused antagonism, its superior health outcomes were achieved despite a long period of slow economic growth. To the extent that the slow growth resulted from a lack of foreign investment prompted by fears of its left-wing government, we have an even stronger counter-example to the assumption that externally caused economic harm produces lower health outcomes.

In short, good health policy in even poor countries can yield excellent population health. This suggests that primary responsibility for meeting rights to health and health care in a population should rest with each state. The fact that some poor states can and do produce excellent population health makes this point dramatically.[9]

Even if primary responsibility for population health rests with each state, that does not mean the state has sole responsibility. Where we can explain why states cannot do as well as others because of being harmed by international practices, the minimalist strategy applies. Where other international inequalities are important, but they cannot be attributed to international practices, there may still be room for other considerations of global justice.

The new terrain of global justice: where the action is

Global justice is a hotly disputed area of philosophical work in part because it is so new. Not only are the complex economic and social forces underlying globalization themselves fairly recent developments, but the international agreements, institutions, and rule-making bodies that regulate those forces are just emerging and evolving, forming a moving target for our understanding. Their powers and effects are newly grasped and felt, and moral understanding of their consequences and their potential is in its infancy. The content of a theory of global justice and the justification for it can only emerge from the work of a generation of thinkers and doers grappling with the problem. The process will involve working back and forth between judgments, based on arguments and evidence, about what is just in particular practices or decisions of the operation of international agencies or rule-makers and more theoretical considerations. We need time for reflective equilibrium to do its work.

Accordingly, my modest goal here is not to provide a theory of international justice and global health inequalities, but to suggest where I think the most promising area of inquiry lies. Specifically, inquiry should focus on a middle ground between strongly "statist" claims that egalitarian requirements of social justice are solely the domain of the nation-state and its well-defined basic structure (Rawls, 1999; Nagel,

---

compatible with well-ordered societies producing justice for their populations. He argues that if two well-ordered societies make different decisions about population policy, with the result that one becomes wealthier than the other over time, then the wealthier one should not then have to make transfers to the other in accordance with some international Difference Principle aimed at making the worst off as well off as possible. Arguably, an analogous point holds for health policy and health inequalities.

---

[9] In *The Law of Peoples*, Rawls (1999) makes the claim that international inequality in wealth or income is quite

2005), and strong cosmopolitan claims that principles of justice apply to individuals globally, regardless of the relations in which they stand or the institutional structures through which they interact.[10] This intermediary ground consists of relatively recently formed and evolving international agencies, institutions, and rule-making bodies. Even if this intermediary ground is not equivalent in all its morally relevant features or functions to the basic structure of a state, some of its functions may have morally important similarities to such a basic structure. These similarities may justify seeking fair terms of cooperation for them, perhaps intermediary in content between strongly egalitarian concerns appropriate within a state and the skeptical rejection of international justice that strongly statist views make (Cohen & Sabel, 2006). Working out what international justice means for these international institutions, including what it means for global health, is the crucial task facing political philosophy and international politics in the next generation.

To motivate exploring this intermediary ground, we need good reason to resist the pulls of both the cosmopolitan views and the strongly statist views that form the poles of the current debate. We also need some illustrations of what it would mean for these intermediary institutions to make decisions or implement practices that address gross international health inequalities as matters of justice. What results is not a roadmap of how to get to an account of international justice, let alone a blueprint of one, but at best a satellite map revealing some key features of the new terrain.

Resisting the pull of the cosmopolitan intuition

Earlier, I invoked the powerful intuition that the vast gulf in life prospects between the Angolan child and the Norwegian one is not just unfortunate but unfair. Many people think such dramatic health inequalities are unjust when they occur between the rich and the poor or between ethnic or racial groups within a country because morally arbitrary contingencies,

such as the luck of being born into one group rather than another, should not determine life prospects in such a fundamental way. The same contingency, however, applies to being born Angolan rather than Norwegian, and it seems no less morally arbitrary and troubling. By abstracting from all relations that might hold among people, including the institutions through which they interact and can make claims on each other, the intuition seems to support egalitarian forms of cosmopolitanism.

The support the egalitarian intuition appears to give to cosmopolitanism derives in part from theoretical considerations that carry weight in many ethical theories, including non-egalitarian ones. A feature of many ethical theories is that persons or moral agents deserve equal respect or concern regardless of certain contingent differences between them. Whatever the differences in the content of equal respect among theories, there is considerable theoretical agreement on what counts as the contingent or morally arbitrary differences that equal respect must ignore: mere physical distance, the color of skin, religion, gender and ethnicity. Nationality seems to be part of the same family. The egalitarian intuition about the Angolan and Norwegian children thus draws power from the broader theoretical agreement about what generally counts as a mere contingency and therefore a morally arbitrary difference between moral agents.

The agreement about what counts as contingency and morally arbitrary difference, however, slides past a significant point of controversy, and that is the importance of nationality. If we think of nationality as a set of relationships in which one stands to others, and if we think that being in certain political relationships with others, including interacting through certain kinds of institutions, has moral import, then being a member of one nation rather than another may be a less morally arbitrary fact than it first seemed, though this requires argument.

One of the strengths of a relational view such as Rawls' is that an account of the requirements of justice will have to include an explanation of how institutions that are just can remain stable and sustain commitment to them over time. Justice must be in this sense feasible. Indeed, principles of justice are not acceptable as such if conformance with them in a society's basic structure does not over time lead to a stable or feasible social arrangement. Strains of commitment, for example, must be tolerable, that is, less demanding than for alternatives.

---

[10] Beitz (1979) holds a relational view, though it is global in scope, since he has argued that the emerging international institutions constitute a global basic structure, even if not a global state, that demands fair terms of cooperation. This view is distinct from the cosmopolitan individualism that is being contrasted with statism.

By abstracting justice from any account of the institutions that can deliver just outcomes in a sustainable way, the cosmopolitan view risks falling into hand wringing. It can lament injustice, but it has failed to set itself the task of showing that justice is a stable product of institutions structured in certain ways. Making justice a set of outcomes among individuals, abstracted from the institutional structure through which individuals cooperate, is utopian in a strong sense: we have no real description of what can produce or sustain it.[11]

Resisting strongly statist versions of relational justice

An important obstacle to exploring this international space comes from one version of a relational theory of justice, a strongly statist alternative to cosmopolitanism. Nagel (2005), stimulated by Rawls' (1999) articulation of what a liberal state's foreign policy ought to include, argues that socio-economic justice, with its concerns about equality of opportunity and economic inequality, requires that people stand in the specific relationship to each other defined by a nation-state. Within such a state, socio-economic justice has application because the terms of fair cooperation must be justifiable, that is acceptable, to all, since all citizens are at once subject to coercion and are parties to laws made in their name. Outside the state, there is a moral order, but it is limited to more fundamental humanitarian obligations to assist those facing grave risks and having urgent needs; it must also not violate some fundamental human rights, and we must keep our agreements. We do not, however, have obligations of justice to distribute health fairly, or to protect equality of opportunity, or to assist other societies to become as well off as they can be with regard to the satisfaction of rights to health or education or political participation.

Why is it only within a state that we are obliged to mitigate or eliminate morally arbitrary inequalities and pursue social and economic justice? As subjects of a state, individuals are exposed to coercively imposed rules, in contrast to the constraints imposed by voluntary cooperative enterprises for mutual advantage. The coercively imposed rules are imposed in the name of all citizens, who are putatively the authors of the rules. Consequently, they must take responsibility as authors

and insist on the justifiability of the rules to all involved. In this context the concern for arbitrary inequalities becomes a matter for all to address.

In contrast, Nagel argues, international institutions and rule-making bodies, such as the World Trade Organization (WTO), the World Health Organization (WHO), the World Bank (WB), or the International Monetary Fund (IMF), do not directly coerce individuals, as states do, nor do they make rules directly in the name of individuals. Where international rules or agreements are made, as in establishing the North American Free Trade Agreement (NAFTA), they are the result of voluntary agreements or bargains made by states and are not made in the name of citizens of those states. Since these two features are missing, Nagel concludes, the kind of engagement of the will that holds for citizens of states is missing from international institutions. Consequently, the condition that necessitates a justification of inequalities and a mitigation of morally arbitrary inequalities is missing. More specifically, whereas (to use his examples) Nagel's relation to the New Yorker who irons his shirts is a contract mediated by a complex configuration of laws defining contracts and property rights that forms a system of social justice, trade agreements within the Americas that establish his relations with the Brazilian who grows his coffee constitute much "thinner" agreements or "pure" contracts that pursue mutual self-interest at the state level. They contain no assurance that background conditions of justice are met and give rise to no obligations to make such assurances.

We should resist Nagel's strong statism for two reasons. First, some international institutions impose conditions in a manner that is coercive and that arguably involves the wills of those in the participant states. Second, some obligations of justice may arise in institutions that are not coercive. Cohen & Sable (2006, p. 29) address the first reason by noting that when the WTO sets certain standards, there is no way for citizens of a country to opt out of their application. In effect, there is coercive application of rules, albeit by agencies not directly elected by the various citizenries. This mediated agency, however, is common within complex states and still involves rules made in the name of the citizens.

We may also resist Nagel's strong statist position because obligations of justice can arise in international institutions even if they are not coercive and do not engage the will of citizens as subjects and authors in the way Nagel says is necessary. Cohen & Sable (2006)

---

[11] The cosmopolitan can attribute instrumental importance to institutions, as a way to achieve what can be independently specified as what justice requires.

argue that considerations about inclusion, falling short of fully equal concern or egalitarianism but still within the domain of justice, arise within a range of international institutions. Concerns about inclusion have implications for governance. If worker organizations were suddenly excluded from participation in the International Labour Organization, that would be seen to violate important concerns about inclusion (Cohen & Sabel, 2006). Similarly, if a policy enables better off groups or states to advance their interests and leaves worst off groups with little or no benefits, and if significantly better benefits could be gained by the worst off groups at little sacrifice by others, then there has been inadequate inclusion of the interests of all in the deliberations of the institution (Cohen & Sabel, 2006). Nagel is then wrong to insist that only humanitarian concerns apply internationally.

Illustrations of obligations of justice in international organizations

Cohen & Sabel (2006, p. 153) sketch three types of international relationships that might give rise to obligations of justice going beyond humanitarian concerns, international agencies charged with distributing a specific good, cooperative schemes and some kinds of interdependency. Each may give rise to obligations of justice, such as concerns about inclusion. These may range from an obligation to give more weight to the interests of those who are worse off if it can be done at little cost to others, to obligations of equal concern, perhaps yielding far more egalitarian obligations. I shall illustrate each of these relationships and the obligations they give rise to with examples focused on key issues of global health.

The World Health Organization plausibly illustrates the idea that institutions charged with distributing a particular, important good, such as public health expertise and technology, must show equal concern in the distribution of that good. The organization would be charged with being unfair if it ignored the health of some and attended more to the health of others. For instance, the WHO is constrained by its mission of improving world health to consider equity in distribution in all contexts in which it works – within and across countries.

Concerns about equity show up in the WHO's programmatic discussions as well. The WHO paid attention to equity in the distribution of antiretroviral treatments (ARTs) for HIV/AIDS. The WHO also

sponsors a Commission on the Social Determinants of Health that has a strong focus on equity in health. Both of these examples illustrate behavior compatible with and required by the institutional charge to the WHO. Either this is a misguided focus of energy for the WHO, as seems to be implied by Nagel's strong statist view, or it is an implication of the obligation of justice to show equal concern that arises within institutions charged with delivering an important good – whether they operate within states or across them.

Consider now the international bodies that establish rules governing intellectual property rights, including those that are key to creating temporary monopolies over new drugs. Such a scheme is "consequential" in that it increases the level of cooperation among affected parties in the production of an important collective good, research and development of drugs, and it does so in a way that has normatively relevant consequences (Cohen & Sabel, 2006, p. 153, n. 12). Suppose we conclude that this mutually cooperative scheme generates considerations of equal concern, or at least that it must be governed by a principle of inclusion.

We might then view quite favorably Pogge's (2005a) suggestion about structuring drug development incentives so that they better address the global burden of disease. Earlier, I said Pogge's proposal could not be defended on the minimalist grounds that it avoided doing harm because of the problem of specifying the relevant human rights baseline. Now, however, we have a new basis on which to defend the justice of Pogge-style incentives. Such an incentive scheme arguably would greatly enhance the benefits to those who are largely excluded from new drug benefits for a significant period of time, and it would do so at only modest cost to those profiting from the endeavor. Minimally, it illustrates what a more inclusive policy should include; one can build into it even stronger egalitarian considerations, if the cooperative scheme gives rise to concerns about equality and not simply inclusion. Exactly what form the policy would take, or the justification for it deriving from the form of cooperative scheme involved, remains a task for further work. With these issues worked out, we might then support Pogge's incentive schemes as a way of moving some countries closer to satisfaction of a right to health, connecting the effort to human rights goals as he does.

Consider again the example of the brain drain of health personnel from low- and middle-income countries to wealthier ones. Nagel (2005, p. 130) notes that nations generally have "immunity from the need to justify to outsiders the limits on access to its territory," though this immunity is not absolute, since the human rights of asylum seekers act as a constraint. Still, the decisions different countries make about training of health personnel and about access to their territories have great mutual impact on them. There is an important interdependency affecting their well-being, specifically, the health of the populations contributing and receiving health personnel. The British decision in 2000 to recruit 30 000 new nurses from developing countries rather than try to train more greatly affected the fate of people being served by health systems in southern Africa.

Arguably, this relation of interdependence brings into play obligations of inclusion, perhaps those of equal concern, going beyond in any event humanitarian considerations. In addition to Pogge's "no harm" or minimalist approach, we thus have available obligations of inclusion requiring us to consider the interests of all those in the interdependent relationship. These obligations can be translated into various policy options that address the brain drain: it may be necessary to restrict the terms of employment in receiving countries of health workers from vulnerable countries; it may be necessary to seek compensation for lost training costs of these workers; it may be important to contribute aid to contributing countries aimed at reducing the push factors; it may be necessary to prohibit active recruitment from vulnerable countries.

We might combine these relationships of interdependence with the relationships and obligations that arise from cooperative schemes. The International Organization for Migration, established in 1951 to help resettle displaced persons from World War II, now has 112 member states and 23 observer states. It "manages" various aspects of migration, providing information and technical advice, and arguably goes beyond its initial humanitarian mission. Suppose it took on the task of developing a policy that helped to coordinate or manage the frightening health personnel brain drain.

Minimally, it might seek internationally acceptable standards for managing the flow – standards on recruitment, on compensation, on terms of work. More ambitiously, it might seek actual treaties that balanced rights to migrate with costs to the contributing countries, countering at least some of the pull factors and even providing funds that might alleviate some of the push factors underlying the brain drain. In seeking these, it might work together with the ILO, with the WTO, with the WHO and with the UN. Such a cooperative endeavor would reflect the common interest in all countries of having adequate health personnel – and thus being able to assure citizens a right to health and health care – as well as the common interest in protecting human rights to dignified migration.

The way forward

There is a fertile area of emerging international institutions where the task of working out considerations of international justice lies. This is where the action is. We must move beyond a minimalist strategy that justifies only avoiding and correcting harms. How far we go toward robust egalitarian considerations is a matter to be worked out. In any case, how far we can go will depend specifically on the nature of the international relationships in which we stand. It will depend on the institutional structures that are still developing. This work in progress has barely started, but it must break out of the framing of the problem posed by the poles of statism and cosmopolitan individualism.

Earlier I posed the question, When are international inequalities in health unjust? This discussion falls short of providing an answer because we remain unclear just what kinds of obligations states and international institutions and rule-making bodies have regarding health inequalities across countries. We characterized domestic health inequalities as unjust when they arise from an unjust distribution of the socially controllable factors that determine population health and its distribution – and we illustrated what was meant by a just distribution by reference to conformance to Rawls' principles of justice as fairness. Internationally, we must carry out the task of explaining the substance of international obligations for the various kinds of cooperative schemes, international agencies and international rule-making bodies in order to specify when the internationally socially controllable factors affecting health are justly distributed and regulated. My account of just health remains, then, a work in progress.

Acknowledgments

This paper is based on the more detailed discussion in chapter 13 of my book *Just Health: Meeting Health Needs Fairly* (Cambridge University Press, 2008), and is published with permission from Cambridge University Press. I thank Gillian Brock for editorial suggestions about shortening the original.

References

Beitz, C. R. (1979). *Political Theory and International Relations*. Princeton, NJ: Princeton University Press.

Beitz, C. R. (2000). Rawls's law of peoples. *Ethics* **110**, 669–696.

Chen, L. & Hanvoravongchai, P. (2005). HIV/AIDS and human resources. *Bulletin of the World Health Organiztion* **83**, 143–144.

Cohen, J. & Sabel, C. (2006). Extra rempublicam nulla justitia. *Philosophy and Public Affairs* **34**, 147–175.

Daniels, N. (2008). *Just Health: Meeting Health Needs Fairly*. Cambridge: Cambridge University Press.

Deeming, C. (2004). Policy targets and ethical tensions: UK nurse recruitment. *Social Policy and Administration* **38** (7), 227–292.

Liese, B., Blanchet N. & Dussault, G. (2004). The human resource crisis in health services in Sub-Saharan Africa. *Background Paper: World Development Report 2004, Making Services Work for Poor People*. Washington, DC: The World Bank.

Nagel, T. (2005). The problem of global justice. *Philosophy and Public Affairs* **33**, 113–147.

Pogge, T. W. (2002). *World Poverty and Human Rights: Cosmopolitan Responsibilities and Reforms*. Oxford: Blackwell.

Pogge, T. W. (2005a). Human rights and global health: A research program. *Metaphilosophy* **36**, 182–209.

Pogge, T. W. (2005b). Severe poverty as a violation of negative duties. *Ethics and International Affairs* **19**, 55–83.

Rawls, J. (1999). *The Laws of Peoples*. Cambridge, MA: Harvard University Press.

UNICEF (2000). *The State of the World's Children*. www.unicef.org/sowcoo/stat2.htm (Accessed August 23, 2005).

World Health Organization (WHO) (2004). *Recruitment of Health Workers from the Developing World*. Geneva: World Health Organization.

World Health Organization/UNICEF/UNFPA (2005). *Maternal Mortality in 2004 – Estimates Developed by WHO, UNICEF, and UNFPA*. www.childinfo.org/Areas/maternalmortality (Accessed August 23, 2005).

Chapter

9

The human right to health

Jonathan Wolff

Introduction: The global health duty

It is hardly news that the health and life expectancy of many of the peoples of the developing world is truly shocking. For example, according to one source, in 2009 life expectancy at birth was over 82 for those born in Japan, but, astonishingly, around 32 for those born in Swaziland (Central Intelligence Agency (CIA), 2009). If this figure is to be believed then it may well be that adult male life expectancy in Swaziland is as low as it has ever been, or at least not far above.[1]

The crisis in global health is staggering (Garrett, 1995). Within political philosophy this crisis intersects with the topic of global justice, which has seen a surge in interest in recent years (Rawls, 1999; Pogge, 2002; Caney, 2005; Brock, 2009a). However in the mainstream of political philosophy the health agenda remains relatively undeveloped, typically focusing on a small number of issues, such as redistributive transfers (Sreenivasan, 2002), the health brain drain (Brock, 2009b) and access to medicine and drug discovery (Pogge, 2005), although a broader agenda is also beginning to emerge (O'Neill, 2002; Childress, 2002; Benatar *et al.*, 2003, 2009; Daniels, 2006).

Philosophical debates need to absorb a wave of critical examination of existing policies both from development commentators (Easterley, 2006; Collier, 2007; Moyo, 2009) and the health activist literature (Global Health Watch, 2008) which suggest that traditional forms of assistance are far less effective than their proponents hope or believe. For example, it is said that the research effort has been driven by the agenda of funders and researchers, looking for glamorous, headline-grabbing, potentially prize-winning outcomes, and concentrating on a "technological fix," when community and health system strengthening may be more effective.

These criticisms of development aid should not stop political philosophers arguing that there is a duty for wealthy nations and their citizens to take steps to attempt to remedy the global health crisis. Moreover, we should acknowledge that while finding solutions will be complex, these should not exclude seeking imaginative ways of improving financial flows, changing drug discovery and migration incentives and funding health interventions. Nevertheless there remains work to be done to bring political philosophy into contact with the concerns of development and global health specialists.

Possible foundations of the global health duty

Yet, before deciding which global health programs to support there is a prior question. Why should peoples of the developed world take an interest in the health of those in the developing world? To put the point bluntly, what business is it of ours? Possible answers can be divided into three types (which are not exclusive of each other) (Wolff, forthcoming). First, taking on this duty may be in our own interests – either as nations, or as particular individuals. For example, perhaps the best protection against global pandemics is to strengthen public health in the developing world. Or for an individual, it may be that attending to the health needs of others is highly fulfilling.

This individualized self-interest argument shades into another; that there is a humanitarian duty of assistance to people in the developing world. Such a moral duty could be grounded in moral arguments such as Peter Singer's claim that if we can save a life without sacrificing anything of significant moral importance, we have a duty to do so (Singer, 1972). Many international

---

[1] I have used the example of an adult male to abstract from the benefits of improved infant and maternal survival.

Global Health and Global Health Ethics, ed. Solomon Benatar and Gillian Brock. Published by Cambridge University Press.
© Cambridge University Press 2011.

charities implicitly appeal to such considerations, especially in times of emergencies. Third, there are arguments from justice, which go beyond humanitarian arguments by positing not only a duty to act, but a right of those in the developing world to receive assistance.

Three forms of the justice arguments are particularly salient. First, "cosmopolitans" argue that there is no moral significance to distinctions between countries, and each person has duties of justice to all others regardless of where they live (Steiner, 2005). Second, it is argued that many of the problems of the developing world are either the legacy of shamefully brutal colonization, or the consequence of unfair contemporary international trade policies, for which justice requires reparation (Pogge, 2002; Benatar *et al.*, 2003). Finally, it is also increasingly argued that each person on earth has a set of human rights, and these rights include the human right to health. It is the responsibility of the global community to advance and protect the human rights of all. Therefore we each have a justice-based responsibility to act in accordance with the human right to health (Clapham & Robinson, 2009). The claim that there is a human right to health will be the focus of the remaining discussion here.

Why do foundations matter?

Each of the arguments set out in the previous section appeals to plausible considerations. However, given the apparent convergence on the result that we have a duty to help it may be asked why it is worth pursuing the philosophical debate. How can it matter? It seems indulgent to spend time and energy on obtuse philosophical questions when our duties are so clear and so pressing.

I have a great deal of sympathy for this objection (Wolff & de-Shalit, 2007). Indeed, I will make a version of this argument later here. However, in the present case, in the words of health activist James Orbinski, "language matters" (Orbinski, 2008, p. 341). It matters not only because it can be important to get the philosophical details right, but because different ways of understanding the basis of the duty have different consequences.

Consider the question of agency: who has a duty to act? Cosmopolitan justice arguments put the duty on everyone, whereas reparative justice arguments assign it to those who have caused, or have benefited from, previous injustice, while humanitarian arguments place the duty on those who are best able to help. (Human rights arguments raise more complex issues

of agency, to which we will return.) Another issue is one of enforcement. Human rights, and in some cases, reparative justice, arguments have international institutions associated with them, and so offer some hope, however small, of judicial remedy, whereas none of the others do (Wolff, forthcoming). Indeed, the pragmatic advantages of using the idea of a human right to health are clear, potentially at least: human rights are an internationally respected currency, backed by 60 years of institution building, an enforcement mechanism and ever-growing in influence.

Human rights conventions

Various declarations and conventions have attempted to establish the human right to health. Perhaps the boldest statement is to be found in the Constitution of the World Health Organization (WHO):

> The enjoyment of the highest attainable standard of health is one of the fundamental rights of every human being without distinction of race, religion, political belief, economic or social condition. (WHO, 1946/2006)

The same year that the WHO Constitution came into effect, 1948, saw also the Universal Declaration of Human Rights (UDHR), article 25(1) of which reads:

> Everyone has the right to a standard of living adequate for the health and well-being of himself and of his family, including food, clothing, housing and medical care and necessary social services, and the right to security in the event of unemployment, sickness, disability, widowhood, old age or other lack of livelihood in circumstances beyond his control. (United Nations, 1948)

The Universal Declaration, therefore, while recognizing the right to medical care as a determinant of well-being, falls short of the expansive right to health set out by the WHO. However in 1966, The International Covenant on Economic, Social and Cultural Rights (ICESCR) was adopted, coming into force in 1976 when ratified by the required 30 countries. Here, in Article 12, we see the most elaborate statement of the Human Right to Health:

(1) The States Parties to the present Covenant recognize the right of everyone to the enjoyment of the highest attainable standard of physical and mental health.

(2) The steps to be taken by the States Parties to the present Covenant to achieve the full realization of this right shall include those necessary for:

(a) The provision for the reduction of the stillbirth-rate and of infant mortality and for the healthy development of the child;

(b) The improvement of all aspects of environmental and industrial hygiene;

(c) The prevention, treatment and control of epidemic, endemic, occupational and other diseases;

(d) The creation of conditions which would assure to all medical service and medical attention in the event of sickness. (United Nations, 1966)

Furthermore, at least for children the WHO right was recognized in the UN Convention on The Rights of the Child that came into force in 1990. Article 24(1) reads:

> States Parties recognize the right of the child to the enjoyment of the highest attainable standard of health and to facilities for the treatment of illness and rehabilitation of health. States Parties shall strive to ensure that no child is deprived of his or her right of access to such health care services. (United Nations, 1989)

Although ICESCR is far from universally adopted, the position is more encouraging for the Convention on the Rights of the Child. According to UNICEF, it has been ratified by all countries of the world, except Somalia, with no effective government, and the USA, which is always very slow to ratify human rights conventions (UNICEF, 2006). In consequence, virtually all countries in the world have accepted the right to the highest attainable standard of health for children, and many have accepted it for all their citizens.

Yet looking at the terms in which these treatises are stated, one may be filled with a sense of hopelessness. What could it mean to guarantee to all the people of the world "the right to the highest attainable standard of health"? Does everyone in the world have the right to the health and life expectancy of the Japanese? How could that be achieved? Without a huge increase in budgets, which is not in prospect, attempting to provide everyone with the right to health could drain resources from other vital areas, such as education and housing. Many will view such conventions as no more than fine words and sentiments.

In response the ICESRC adopts the notion of "progressive realization" rather than "full immediate realization" of the rights (Article 2(1)) (United Nations, 1966) (see also Hessler & Buchanan, 2002). In 2000 this was further clarified when the Committee on Economic, Social and Cultural Rights issued "General Comment 14" to explain how the human right to health can be approached in practice. The Committee understood the difficulties of the task, writing, in Article 5:

The Committee is aware that, for millions of people throughout the world, the full enjoyment of the right to health still remains a distant goal. Moreover, in many cases, especially for those living in poverty, this goal is becoming increasingly remote. The Committee recognizes the formidable structural and other obstacles resulting from international and other factors beyond the control of States that impede the full realization of article 12 [of the ICESCR] in many States parties. (United Nations, 2000)

Accordingly General Comment 14 clarifies that the right to health is not the right to be healthy (Article 8). Nevertheless, the right to health is not merely the right to medical care, which is merely one of the many determinants of health. Healthy living and working conditions, for example, are just as vital (Article 11).

Furthermore, resource constraints provide a legitimate reason why a state may not be able fully to realize the right to health. Nevertheless General Comment 14 insists that:

> 30. ... States parties have immediate obligations in relation to the right to health, such as the guarantee that the right will be exercised without discrimination of any kind (art. 2.2) and the obligation to take steps (art. 2.1) towards the full realization of article 12 [of the ICESCR]. Such steps must be deliberate, concrete and targeted towards the full realization of the right to health.

Finally, in the earlier General Comment 3, the notion of a state's "minimum core obligations" is clarified, which instructs that States must use whatever resources they have to supply essential primary health care (United Nations, 1990). To help promote, protect and advocate for the human right to health, in 2002 Professor Paul Hunt was appointed "Special Rapporteur" on the right to health, with the obligation to undertake country-based missions and to produce reports.

Skepticism about the human right to health

The Covenants are full of fine words. General Comment 14 attempts to translate those words into action. Yet given that over the decades the global health crisis has, if anything, increased, it appears that the various conventions on human rights have not been effective (Benatar, 2002). Of course, such claims are hard to assess, yet one must concede that progress has not been encouraging. Some argue that this is a consequence of an irreparably flawed conceptual structure. For example, it has even been suggested that philosophers do themselves no credit by associating themselves with the human right to health (Baumrin, 2002). In response it will be suggested here that while there are problems these are in the process of being addressed, and although far from perfect the human rights approach is arguably one of our best hopes for improving global health.

Many arguments against the human right to health are parasitic on a more general argument against the notion of human rights: that the notion of human rights is confused, empty, useless or damaging. Some of these arguments go back several centuries (Bentham, 1796[1987]; Marx, 1843[1975]), though here we will concentrate on more recent arguments, such as that once we accept a wide range of human rights, and also that states do not have an obligation to realize them all fully, then we have devalued the currency of human rights. This is the criticism of "rights inflation;" that once rights such as the right to health are accepted, then rights against arbitrary arrest, even rights against torture, will be taken even less seriously and abused (for discussion see Nickell, 2009). To guard against this, it is said, human rights must be limited to a relatively small set of absolutely indispensable rights that should always be fully, rather than progressively, realized.

It is unclear whether there is evidence that rights inflation has devalued the currency, but to guard against it, rights-based claims and actions must be made sparingly. And still it is not obvious that a minor weakening of civil and political rights is too high a price to pay for the establishment of the right to health, and other social and economic rights. This is controversial, but there are costs and benefits on both sides. However, it is important to use rights claims sparingly for a different reason: that a quick recourse to rights will encourage an unattractive and unproductive legalistic culture in which people encounter each other as opponents, rather than as fellow citizens who need to negotiate their way out of a collective difficulty (O'Neill, 2005). Human rights are something close to a last resort, for when all else has failed, rather than the first moral weapon to hand. It would be a better world if we never had to mention human rights. But unfortunately that is not the world we are in.

Proliferation of rights makes conflicts more probable (Freeman, 2002, p. 5). So, for example, the right for people to choose to spend their resources their own way may lead to wealthy people looking to the private sector for health care, leaving the public sector in a state of political and economic neglect. Hence one right may undermine another. Once more, we must accept that this may happen. But it is not clear that the solution is to restrict the list of human rights in advance. For even if that does have the virtue of ruling out conflict by privileging one set of values, avoidance of conflict is not the highest good, if it comes at a high price.

It has also been argued that it is incoherent to claim that a person has a right unless it is possible to identify a duty holder in respect of that right, and in the case of the claimed human right to health it is not obvious who the duty holder will be (this returns us to the vexed question of "agency" raised above) (Baumrin, 2002; O'Neill, 2005; see also Benatar, 2002). However, it is possible to deny that it is always necessary to identify a particular duty holder. Or more concessively, it could be said that the duty holder is the government of the state in which the person resides. Now, this can be problematic. Some people are stateless, or are refugees across borders, and this is where some of the greatest human rights challenges are to be found. Furthermore some states are unwilling or unable to act, while others that may be willing are hobbled by the power of globalizing forces that inhibit their release from sustained poverty. Nevertheless, we can still say that in the first instance the duty falls on the state of which the person is a citizen; if that is problematic then the country of residence; and as a last resort the international community.

Other critics have focused on the individualism of human rights discourse, suggesting, instead, that it can be a grave obstacle to achievement of global health (Benatar *et al.*, 2003). First, a focus on individual rights inevitably tends to bring issues of access to health care into sharper focus than public health, which, from the point of view of global health is far more important. Second, access to human rights courts is likely to be the exclusive recourse of those who are wealthy or have powerful connections. Hence, it appears, a human right to health agenda threatens to reduce health to health care and to reinforce health inequalities. These are serious problems. The question is whether they are intrinsic to the human rights approach. It may be possible to refocus the human rights agenda to include the rights of groups of individuals, and, to some degree, this is already in process, as we will see below. Furthermore, although court action is the ultimate sanction for human rights abuse, in reality it is rare, while policies of "naming and shaming" are more common and effective (Birn, 2008), and may be pursued in respect to the poor and vulnerable. Consider, for example, the study of "excess deaths" in the aftermath of the invasion of

Iraq, which although was not explicitly part of a human rights agenda is highly appropriate for that purpose (Burnham *et al.*, 2006).

Naturally following on from this observation, however, is a quite different argument based on the political sociology of human rights, and in particular rights advocacy and empowerment. Human rights organizations, such as Amnesty International and Human Rights Watch campaign, lobby and take action on behalf of those whose rights have been violated. This, it is said, while often highly beneficial and effective, nevertheless has the effect of continuing to marginalize disadvantaged people. Human rights activists will tend to be relatively privileged people from the developed world acting on behalf of others, who are passive beneficiaries of their activities. Once more we must admit that this is a danger. For this reason some of the most encouraging developments in human rights activism are those facilitating disadvantaged people's self-advocacy. The role for NGOs is to provide training and support, and to help form a radicalized and empowered community, able to fight its own battles. It is important for NGOs to focus not only on the goals of their campaigns, but the means by which those goals are obtained. Every NGO should consider whether making itself redundant should be part of its mission statement.

However, a recent, and very urgent, criticism, made by William Easterley, is that advocacy for the human right to health has done more harm than good by distorting health priority setting, diverting resources, effectively, to those who shout the loudest and are most effective in their advocacy, to the detriment of general health promotion (Easterley, 2009). Easterley claims that societies – developed and developing – would be better off with cost-effective health-maximizing strategies.

Single-issue advocacy can be damaging to health systems. For example in some areas of sub-Saharan Africa as ever more money is spent on HIV/AIDS programs, the proportion of attended births goes down (Haacker, 2010; see also WHO, 2009). Health workers are drawn to the well-funded campaign areas, away from general practice which is left depleted. This is a very serious problem. It is unclear, though, that it is somehow intimately connected with the right to health. Human right to health advocacy is as likely to be addressed to health system strengthening as to single-issue projects, and as we will see later, there is no evidence from case law that the human right to health has led to judicial decisions overturning cost-effective

state decisions about health services. However, it may be possible that it has distorted spending priorities to pre-empt legal challenges, although it is hard to find evidence. But the lesson from Easterley's challenge is important. We should never complacently assume that attempts to do good can do no harm. This is as true for rights advocacy as it is for anything else.

Philosophical foundations of human rights

Skepticism about human rights, we saw, takes many forms. Philosophers, whose training instructs them to take nothing for granted, have often led the skeptical charge. Yet this is puzzling. For it is possible to see the Declaration of Human Rights as a philosophical triumph. After two and a half thousand years of dispute about the fundamental terms on which human beings should live together, a series of international discussions, meetings and debates arrived at a detailed consensus statement of the fundamental rights of human beings.

Yet until very recently philosophers have tended to treat the UDHR as if it had very little to do with philosophy. If one looks at some of the most important works of twentieth century political philosophy, such as John Rawls' *A Theory of Justice* (Rawls, 1971) and Robert Nozick's *Anarchy State and Utopia* (Nozick, 1974) almost nothing is said about human rights. The general attitude among philosophers seems to have been that there is something problematic either about the idea of human rights or in the catalog of rights included. This can be seen, for example, even in the title of James Griffin's paper "Discrepancies between the best philosophical account of human rights and the international law of human rights" (Griffin, 2001).

Griffin argues that when one properly understands the foundations of human rights not all of the rights in the standard list can be justified. Griffin believes that human rights must be seen as "protections of our normative agency" (Griffin, 2008, p. 2) and, for example, pours scorn on the "human right" to "periodic holidays with pay" as stated in Article 24. But much more importantly, Griffin acutely observes that the convention documents provide the *names* of rights, but, typically, say very little about their *content*, and so, it appears, philosophical and ethical reflection is needed to complete the account of human rights, as well as to refine it (Griffin, 2008, p. 5). In the case of the right to health, Griffin argues, its contours must be determined by what is necessary to preserve agency: a decent life span, and protection of the capacities that promote agency. This will have consequences, for example, for the right to health care at the end of life, when agency cannot be restored in any meaningful way (Griffin, 2008, pp. 98–99). This is important, for if it was thought that the correct ethical foundation for the human right to health was that of need, then there is no special reason to give priority to those interventions that would protect or promote individual agency.

It may seem, therefore, that strengthening the philosophical foundations of the rights is necessary to provide a concrete account of the rights. Yet the matter is problematic. There is no ultimate agreement on the foundation of human rights. Is it normative agency? Human dignity? Vital human interests? Each of these may provide subtly different accounts of the precise contours of human rights, and how are such disputes to be settled?

However, this repeats a debate that took place in the context of drafting the Universal Declaration. For what is as true now as 60 years ago is that there is much greater agreement on the list of human rights than there is on their moral foundations. Of course, there are disagreements about content, but the convergence on doctrine is remarkable, given the divergence on foundations.

Jacques Maritain, who helped provide background material for the convention at which the Universal Declaration was drafted, commented:

> During one of the meetings of the French National Commission of UNESCO at which the Rights of Man were being discussed, someone was astonished that certain proponents of violently opposed ideologies had agreed on the draft of a list of rights. Yes, they replied, we agree on these rights, *provided we are not asked why*. (Maritain, 1951, p. 77, emphasis in original)

Indeed, Maritain names the section heading in which this discussion is contained "Men mutually opposed in their theoretical conceptions can come to a merely practical agreement regarding a list of human rights" (Maritain, 1951, p. 76). Unfortunately, the point is rather spoilt by the inclusion of the words "merely practical." To use Rawlsian terminology we might argue that the Universal Declaration of Human Rights is a superb example of an overlapping consensus, in which each person can endorse a political doctrine for his or her own moral reasons (Rawls, 1993/1996, pp. 135–172). While they share the political doctrine, and can justify it on the basis of their own moral reasons, none of the moral perspectives has a privileged place as providing the core foundation for the doctrine. Different people

will find their own justifications. In sum, then, on this view human rights have moral foundations, but no particular moral foundation. This, perhaps, explains the appeal of human rights doctrine within a broadly liberal framework.

But what do we do about residual differences in interpretation? Arguably, however, the right response at this point is simply to acknowledge the limits of philosophical argument, and allow the resulting disputes to be resolved through the development of democratic politics and legal doctrine (Hessler & Buchanan, 2002). Such a proposal fits well with the account of human rights provided by Joseph Raz (Raz, 2010; see also Beitz, 2009). In summary, Raz believes that human rights should now be seen as a branch of international law, and, luckily, a branch of law in reasonably good order. This is essential, Raz argues, if the discussions of philosophers are to engage with the concerns of human rights practice. Seeing matters this way allows us to draw an analogy with other branches of law such as family law or property law. In such cases the broad contours of the law can be seen as having a philosophical foundation, setting limits to what can reasonably be part of the law. So, for example, no doubt any reasonable view would wish to give parents duties of care towards their children. Yet it would be unrealistic to think that precise details of maintenance payments for children in case of divorce can be given a philosophical foundation. Such issues will be worked out in the practical context of politics and legal casework. The same is possible for the details of human rights. While the overall framework can be justified from a range of philosophical positions, it is not necessary to think that each particular human right needs a single philosophical justification, or even that the details of its determinate content need to be acceptable from all points of view.

Of course this does not settle all disputes. For example, the USA has complained that General Comment 14 has expanded the human right to health beyond its initial basis in an arbitrary and unaccountable fashion (United States Government, n.d.).[2] But it is unrealistic to think that all disputes about doctrine can be settled. Sometimes we have to accept that doctrine is living: contested and permanently developing, rather than entirely static and stable.

Still, this understanding of the doctrine of human rights raises the question of what human rights are

---

[2] I owe this reference to Douglas Reeve.

for: why, exactly, do we have this branch of international law? Raz takes his cue, initially, from John Rawls' account (Rawls, 1999, pp. 80–81) that the point of human rights law is to legitimate one state's interest, and possible interventions, in the affairs of another. Such interventions can, of course, take a variety of forms, from sending a note expressing concern to the ambassador, through public criticism and sanctions, to full-scale invasion (Raz, 2010). Beitz points out the importance of mechanisms such as reporting requirements and trade incentives (Beitz, 2009, pp. 31–47). Of course many aspects of a state's internal arrangements are simply not the business of other states. For example, the particular pension regime one country has may seem unacceptable from the point of view of another country, but still, attempts to influence it may seem an illegitimate interference with a sovereign state's internal affairs. No such defense may be available if a country tortures prisoners, or, arguably, fails to take steps progressively to realize universal access to health care.

This international law understanding of human rights allows both outsiders and insiders to criticize a regime for failing to meet the human rights of its citizens, and to exert pressure. On this understanding a human right is claimed against a particular government, which has the duty to meet the right. The international community is not directly expected to meet the claim itself, but has the second-order duty to help enforce the duty of the national government. It is this second-order character, placing duties of enforcement on the international community that, arguably, marks the distinction between a *human right* to health and a *right* to health.

Case law

The human right to health has to be seen from two perspectives. From a philosophical point of view, it is a right that, in outline, can be justified from a variety of perspectives, as an overlapping consensus. However, in trying to go further to specify the right, and to connect it with human rights practice, philosophy runs out, and the second perspective needs to be engaged, that of the development of legal doctrine. Accordingly, to explore the detailed contours of the human right to health it is necessary to look at case law, in addition to the conventions, declarations and general comments outlined above.

It has to be admitted that case law is, at present, rather limited in extent, and that the human right to health is at a relatively early stage of development. On the whole courts have not been keen to engage with the human right to health. For example, in the important British case of Rogers v Swindon NHS Primary Care Trust ([2006] EWCA civ392 Case No: C1/2006/0312), an action was brought under the European Convention of Human Rights, against the decision not to prescribe the claimant the breast cancer drug herceptin on the National Health Service. The court, however, felt able to decide the case in the claimant's favor, ordering a review of the decision, without entering discussion of the human rights issues. Hence the issue of human rights was simply left untouched in the judgment.

Some more instructive cases come from South Africa, where the right to health is included in Article 27 of the South African Constitution, which took effect in 1997, and includes "the right to have access to health care services, including reproductive health care" and the right to "emergency medical treatment" (Republic of South Africa, 1996).

One case, Soobramoney v Minister of Health, was brought very soon after the adoption of the new constitution, in 1997 ((KwaZulu Natal) CCT32/97 (1997) ZACC 17: 1998 (1) SA 765 (CC)). The claimant, Thiagraj Soobramoney, who was just 41, was unemployed and suffering from many health problems. In 1996 his kidneys failed and his life was in danger. He sought access to dialysis treatment, at public expense, in hospital in Durban, but dialysis machines, which are very expensive, were in short supply. The hospital had set up tight guidelines for access, but sadly he fell outside the criteria. He had managed to pay for private dialysis to keep him alive, but was running out of money. Accordingly he brought a legal action under Article 27 and in particular to the right not to be denied emergency medical treatment, as well as Article 11 which states, bluntly enough, that: "Everyone has the right to life."

The court emphasized, however, that the even the right to life has to be understood in the context of resource constraints, and followed other precedents that it simply is not the right authority to make resource allocation decisions. Consequently the judges concentrated on the question of whether the rules applied by the hospital for access to scarce dialysis machines could be justified, and here they found no objection. Hence the case did not succeed.

Given the courts' reasonable reluctance to make decisions concerning resource allocation, one might wonder whether there will be anything to be gained by pursuing a human right to health action. However, the position is not entirely bleak. In the Soobramoney case the judges referred to the Indian case of *Paschim Banga Khet Mazdoor Samity and others v State of West Bengal and another*, where it was argued that the right to medical treatment falls under the constitutionally protected right to life. In this case a patient with severe head injuries was turned away from a number of state-funded hospitals and had to seek treatment at a private hospital. But at least some of these hospitals did in fact have available facilities, and denied him access on arbitrary grounds. Hence the court felt it could determine the case in the claimant's favor without distorting health resource allocation decisions.

Another important and well-known case in which the court found in favor of the claimant also comes from South Africa, and is part of a series of activities led by TAC – the Treatment Action Campaign – which has taken up the vital issue of HIV/AIDS in South Africa. It was founded in late 1998 to demand right of access to treatment for HIV/AIDS, believing this to be supported by the South African constitution article 27(a) providing "access to health care services including reproductive health" which was especially important for mothers affected by HIV.

In 1999 TAC pressed for the government to make Nevirapine – the leading antiretroviral drug – available to HIV-infected pregnant women. The manufacturers had, in fact, offered the drug to the government free of charge for a period, so the resource implications were very limited. The treatment is very simple: the administration of a single dose to the mother and a few drops to the baby. However, even after treatment there remains a risk of passing on infection through breastfeeding. Therefore a comprehensive package of treatment involves replacing breastfeeding with bottle feeding, which is not a trivial matter, especially given the strong cultural attachment to breastfeeding, advocacy of breast feeding by the World Health Organization, the cost of formula milk and the difficulty of obtaining safe water in some parts of the country. There would also be the need for infrastructural change and staff training. Citing concerns about safety and efficacy, as well as the need to assess management issues, the government allowed only small-scale pilot studies, which it was very slow to implement. The Constitutional Court accepted that there were good public health reasons for having a pilot program, but was dismayed that the infants of mothers without access to private health care were suffering while the government dragged its feet. They did not accept the government's contention that

providing less than the more comprehensive package would be ineffective or harmful. Accordingly, the court ordered the government to make Nevirapine available where it was clinically indicated to prevent transmission to infants (Heywood, 2009).

There are a number of important differences between Soobramoney and the TAC case. First of all, Soobramoney was an individual with a specific, fatal condition, which the health service chose not to treat, even though they could have done. However, to have chosen to treat Soobramoney would have left another person facing the same plight as him, and so it was declared appropriate for the health authorities to make these decisions, as long as they did so on defensible and rational grounds. In the TAC case the government's stand is much harder to understand. Although the government appealed to the importance of providing a more comprehensive package of care, which was unaffordable as well as having other difficulties, the court was persuaded by the evidence that drug treatment, alongside testing and counseling, would save the lives of thousands, and would have minimal cost implications. Indeed, it was argued, there would eventually be cost savings, compared with the burden on the health system of caring for thousands of HIV-positive infants. Some commentators have attempted to explain the government's position as being linked to Mbeki's "AIDS denialism" or even the ANC's hope to be able to provide its own, lucrative, therapy for AIDS, although such issues were not discussed in the judgment (Heywood, 2009).

Legally, then, the difference appears to be that in the Soobramoney case the authorities acted reasonably in difficult circumstances while in the TAC case no such defence was available. A further difference is that TAC is, after all, a campaign, building up a groundswell of support among people who themselves were suffering from adverse government policy. TAC was able to ride on the support of a people's movement. There was no equivalent support for Soobramoney, even though no doubt there was great public sympathy.

It should be made clear too that TAC is not the only human right to health success story. For example, Brazil extended many lives by manufacturing generic antiretroviral drugs, defending its action in international fora against accusations of patent violation in terms of protecting the human rights of its citizens. Here, too, a constitutional right to health, and human right case law, has strengthened human rights campaigns (Galvao, 2005).

Realizing the right to health

While philosophers may continue to puzzle over the foundation, even the existence, of human rights, and philosophers and lawyers wrangle over their content, activists are most concerned about their realization (Clapham & Robinson, 2009). The current state is patchy, to say the least (Backman *et al.*, 2008). Nevertheless, the TAC example is in some respects very encouraging. It was, after all, a successful human rights case, saving many lives. Yet it is also limited. The South African context was very unusual and the government stance appeared quite unreasonable. In legal terms, the situation appears unlikely to reoccur, and the case will rarely, if ever, be used as a precedent.

On the other hand, the organization of TAC provides a model for activism, in which legal action could be a useful threat, even if it is rarely taken forward. At its foundation TAC was originally concerned about the high price of HIV/AIDS related pharmaceuticals. Later it broadened out as it became clear that realizing human rights requires governments to act over a much wider range of areas. In contrast to other NGO campaigns, which often work through elites, academics, professionals, press and communications, TAC aimed to set up a situation in which "poor people become their own advocates" (Heywood, 2009, p. 17) and build a political movement for health, with an understanding both of health and governance. A rights approach, backed by a popular movement can have considerable power and influence. Yet the right to health is still at a relatively early stage; realization is at present a struggle.

Nevertheless, it is worth reminding ourselves of some of the criticisms explored above. Used the wrong way a human right to health approach can prioritize the claims of the powerful, vocal, troublesome and well-organized, leaving the most vulnerable unprotected. Health system strengthening, rather than single-issue campaigning, would surely be far more generally beneficial, but there is, no doubt, great difficulty of organizing campaigns and popular movements in such a way.

Conclusions

Whatever philosophical, or practical, doubts one may have about human rights in general, or the human right to health in particular, there can be no doubt that they exist at least in the sense of being objects of international agreement, with some mechanisms of enforcement. This gives the human rights approach a powerful advantage over other philosophical arguments aimed at improving the health status of the poor and vulnerable. The general point has been made with great force by health activist Gorik Ooms:

> [We are] trying to achieve a goal: to describe a bad situation, to explain why it is as bad as it is, and to convince decision-makers to change their decisions. So the very pragmatic question for me is: which are the arguments most likely to convince these decision-makers? One line of arguments could be: "what goes around comes around, if you continue to abandon a huge part of humanity in its present misery, it will come back to you". Another line of arguments could be: "this is really extremely unfair". Or it could be: "the way you (leaders of high-income countries) are organising the global economy, refusing to share your or our wealth, and using your powers in the World Bank and the IMF to make countries invest less in social expenditure, is in fact a permanent and deliberate violation of human rights, for which you should be put on trial". Perhaps that would help? (Ooms, private communication)[3]

Of course, Ooms and other activists would not wish to suggest that human rights abuses are a consequence purely of the negligence or corruption of public officials. Much more important is creating resilient and supportive national and international health and governance structures and systems. Yet even the reform of structures has to be initiated, in the first instance, through the action of individuals with the power – individually, or collectively – to bring about those reforms.

References

Backman, G., Hunt, P., Khosla, R. *et al.* (2008). Health systems and the right to health: an assessment of 194 countries. *Lancet* **372**, 2047–2085.

Baumrin, B. (2002). Why there is no right to health care. In R. Rhodes, M. Pabst Battin & A. Silvers (Eds.), *Medicine and Social Justice: Essays on the Distribution of Health Care*. Oxford: Oxford University Press.

Beitz, C. (2009). *The Idea of Human Rights*. Oxford: Oxford University Press.

Benatar, S. R. (2002). Human rights in the biotechnology era 1. *BMC International Health and Human Rights* **2**, 3.

Benatar, S., Daar, A. & Singer P.A. (2003). Global health: the rationale for mutual caring. *International Affairs* **79**, 107–138.

---

3 I am extremely grateful to Gillian Brock, Solomon Benatar, Douglas Reeve and Gorik Ooms for their comments on an earlier draft.

Benatar, S., Gill, S. & Bakker, I. (2009). Making progress in global health: the need for new paradigms. *International Affairs* **85**, 347–371.

Bentham, J. (1796 [1987]) "Anarchical Fallacies" and "Supply Without Burden". In J. Waldron (Ed.), *Nonsense Upon Stilts*. London: Methuen.

Birn, A.-E. (2008). Health and human rights: historical perspectives and political challenges. *Journal of Public Health Policy* **29**, 32–41.

Brock, G. (2009a). *Global Justice*. Oxford: Oxford University Press.

Brock, G. (2009b). Health in developing countries and our global responsibilities. In A. Dawson (Ed.), *The Philosophy of Public Health* (pp. 73–83). Farnham: Ashgate.

Burnham, G., Lafta, R., Doocy, S. & Roberts, L. (2006). Mortality after the 2003 invasion of Iraq: a cross-sectional cluster sample survey. *Lancet* **368**, 1421–1428.

Caney, S. (2005). *Justice Beyond Borders*. Oxford: Oxford University Press.

Childress, J. F., Faden, R. R., Gaare, R. D. *et al.* (2002). Public health ethics: mapping the terrain. *Journal of Law, Medicine & Ethics* **30**, 170–178.

Central Intelligence Agency (CIA) (2009). *The World Factbook: Life Expectancy at Birth*. www.cia.gov/library/publications/the-world-factbook/rankorder/2102rank.html (Accessed November 25, 2009).

Clapham, A. & Robinson, M. (Eds.) (2009). *Realizing the Right to Health*. Zurich: Rüffer & Rub.

Collier, P. (2007). *The Bottom Billion*. Oxford: Oxford University Press.

Daniels, N. (2006). Equity and population health: toward a broader bioethics agenda. *Hastings Center Report* **36**, 22–23.

Easterley, W. (2006). *The White Man's Burden*. Oxford: Oxford University Press.

Easterley, W. (2009). Human Rights Are the Wrong Basis for Health Care. *Financial Times* October 12, 2009. www.ft.com/cms/s/0/89bbbda2-b763–11de-9812–00144feab49a.html (Accessed November 25, 2009).

Freeman, M. (2002). *Human Rights*. Cambridge: Polity.

Galvao, J. (2005). Brazil and access to HIV/AIDS drugs: a question of human rights and public health. *American Journal of Public Health* **95**, 1110–1116.

Garrett, L. (1995). *The Coming Plague*. London: Virago.

Global Health Watch (2008). *Alternative World Health Report 2*. London: Zed Books.

Griffin, J. (2001). Discrepancies between the best philosophical account of human rights and the International Law Of Human Rights. *Proceedings of the Aristotelian Society* **101**, 28.

Griffin, J. (2008). *On Human Rights*. Oxford: Oxford University Press.

Haacker, M. (2010). The Macroeconomics of HIV/AIDS. In M. Hannam & J. Wolff (Eds.), *Southern Africa: 2020 Vision*. London: e9 Publishing.

Heywood, M. (2009). South Africa's treatment action campaign: combining law and social mobilization to realize the right to health. *Journal of Human Rights Practice* **1**, 14–36.

Hessler, K. & Buchanan, A. (2002). Specifying the content of the human right to health care. In R. Rhodes, M. Pabst Battin & A. Silvers (Eds.), *Medicine and Social Justice: Essays on the Distribution of Health Care*. Oxford: Oxford University Press.

Maritain, J. (1951). *Man and the State*. Chicago: University of Chicago Press.

Marx, K. (1843 [1975]) On The Jewish Question. In L. Colletti (Ed.), *Early Writings*. Harmondsworth: Penguin.

Moyo, D. (2009). *Dead Aid*. London: Allen Lane.

Nickel, J. (2009). Human Rights. In E. N. Zalta (Ed.), *The Stanford Encyclopedia of Philosophy*. http://plato.stanford.edu/archives/spr2009/entries/rights-human/

Nozick, R. (1974) *Anarchy, State, and Utopia*. Oxford: Blackwell.

O'Neill, O. (2002). Public health or clinical ethics: thinking beyond borders. *Ethics & International Affairs* **16**, 35–45.

O'Neill, O. (2005). The Dark Side of Human Rights. *International Affairs* **81**, 427–439.

Orbinski, J. (2008). *An Imperfect Offering*. London: Rider.

Pogge, T. (2002). *World Poverty and Human Rights*. Cambridge, MA: Cambridge University Press.

Pogge, T. (2005). Human rights and global health: a research programme. *Metaphilosophy* **36**, 182–209.

Rawls, J. (1971). *A Theory of Justice*. Oxford: Oxford University Press.

Rawls, J. (1993/1996). *Political Liberalism*. New York, NY: Columbia University Press.

Rawls, J. (1999). *The Law of Peoples*. Cambridge, MA: Harvard University Press.

Raz, J. (2010). Human rights without foundations. In J. Tasioulas & S. Besson (Eds.), *The Philosophy of International Law*. Oxford: Oxford University Press.

Republic of South Africa (1996). *Constitution*. www.info.gov.za/documents/constitution/1996/96cons2.htm (Accessed November 26, 2009).

Singer, P. (1972). Famine, affluence and morality. *Philosophy and Public Affairs* **1**, 229–243.

Sreenivasan, G. (2002). International justice and health: a proposal. *Ethics and International Affairs* **16**, 81–90.

Steiner, H. (2005), Territorial justice and global redistribution. In G. Brock & H. Brighouse (Eds.), *The Political Philosophy of Cosmopolitanism* (pp. 28–38). Cambridge: Cambridge University Press.

UNICEF (2006). *Convention on the Rights of the Child: Frequently Asked Questions.* www.unicef.org/crc/index_30229.html (Accessed November 26, 2009).

United Nations (1948). *Universal Declaration of Human Rights.* www.un.org/en/documents/udhr/ (Accessed November 26, 2009).

United Nations (1966). *International Covenant on Economic, Social and Cultural Rights.* www2.ohchr.org/english/law/cescr.htm (Accessed November 26, 2009).

United Nations (1989). *Convention on the Rights of the Child.* www2.ohchr.org/english/law/crc.htm (Accessed November 26, 2009).

United Nations (1990). General Comment 3. www.unhchr.ch/tbs/doc.nsf/(symbol)/E.C.12.2000.4.En (Accessed November 26, 2009).

United Nations (2000). *General Comment 14.* www.unhchr.ch/tbs/doc.nsf/(symbol)/E.C.12.2000.4.En (Accessed November 26, 2009).

United States Government (ND) *Response to Request.* www.globalgovernancewatch.org/docLib/20080213_US_Hunt_Response.pdf (Accessed November 26, 2009).

Wolff, J. (forthcoming). Global justice and health: the basis of the global health duty. In E. Emanuel & J. Millum (Eds.), *Global Justice and Bioethics.* Oxford: Oxford University Press.

Wolff, J. & de-Shalit, A. (2007). *Disadvantage.* Oxford: Oxford University Press.

World Health Organization (WHO) (1946/2006). *Constitution.* www.who.int/governance/eb/who_constitution_en.pdf (Accessed November 26, 2009).

World Health Organization (WHO) (2009). *Positive Synergies.* www.who.int/healthsystems/GHIsynergies/en/index.html (Accessed December 6, 2009).

Chapter

10

Responsibility for global health

Allen Buchanan and Matthew DeCamp

Introduction

Growing concern about global health

"Global health" is becoming a fashionable term among scholars, human rights activists, state officials, leaders of international and transnational organizations and others.[1] Until recently, health as a matter of collective concern largely implied national health. When the health problems of people in other countries became a public issue, it was usually within the confines of the notion of disaster relief, short-term responses to acute health crises caused by natural disasters or wars. Global health is a relatively new category of moral concern, empirical investigation and institutional action.

There are several reasons for the current prominence of global health issues. First, there is a widening recognition that some major risks to health are global in three senses: Their adverse impact on health is potentially worldwide, the conditions for their occurrence include various transnational dependencies that are lumped together under the rubric of globalization and an effective response to them requires cooperation on a global scale. Examples of global health risks that are global in each of these three senses include emerging infections, pollution of the oceans, depletion of the ozone layer, global warming, nuclear terrorism and bioterrorism. Second, due to the revolution in information technologies and the emergence of transnational epistemic communities equipped with powerful empirical methodologies for measuring and

explaining health and disease, we now know more about the health problems of people in other countries than ever before. We also now have greater institutional resources, both within wealthier states and through international and transnational organizations, for applying this new knowledge to ameliorate global health problems. Finally, human rights discourse and, more generally, the articulation of a cosmopolitan ethical perspective, provide a normative basis for taking global health seriously as a moral issue.[2]

An inadequate response: Duty Dumping

Having reliable information about the nature and causes of global health problems, the capacity to ameliorate them, and a cosmopolitan ethical perspective that regards the need to ameliorate them as urgent is not sufficient, however. It is also necessary to move from the judgment that these problems must be addressed to concrete conclusions about who should do what to solve them. Call this the Problem of Concrete Responsibilities.

One response to the Problem of Concrete Responsibilities is what might be called Duty Dumping. To "dump" a duty in global health means to ascribe obligations to individuals or institutions, holding them accountable for the adverse health effects of their policies, without offering adequate justification for why

---

[1] "International organization" here means an organization in which states are the primary participants. "Transnational organization" refers to an organization that encompasses individuals or groups across state borders and in which states may not be the primary participants.

[2] A cosmopolitan ethical perspective is one that takes individual human beings – regardless of where they happen to reside and independently of what national or ethnic group they are members of – as the fundamental objects of moral concern. Of course, the cosmopolitan perspective may not be the only possible normative basis for taking global health to be an important moral issue. On its most plausible reconstruction, however, the contemporary conception of human rights is a cosmopolitan conception.

An earlier version of this work has appeared: Buchanan, A. & Decamp, M. (2006). Responsibility for global health. *Theoretical Medicine and Bioethics* 27(1), 95–114.

particular obligations should be imposed on particular individuals or institutions. The mistake might be that the putative obligation is too onerous or that it has been assigned to the wrong entity. In either case, Duty Dumping occurs when critics assign duties or obligations without good – or sometimes, without any – reason. However, we do not use Duty Dumping to signify *only* a mistake in assigning duties; in the complex area of global health, such errors might be expected. Instead, we reserve the term for errors of a particularly egregious sort that would be easily rejected in other contexts. Duty Dumping is both morally unjustified and potentially counterproductive for the overall goal of improving global health.

A prominent example of Duty Dumping is the claim that pharmaceutical companies that produce antiretroviral HIV/AIDS drugs have a duty to supply these drugs to all of those who could benefit from them at prices they can afford. The claim here is not just that it would be a good thing for drug companies to do this, nor simply that they have a moral obligation to do *something* to make their medicines more affordable to the worst off. Instead, those who criticize these private corporations often imply something much stronger: that the companies are acting wrongly if they do not do *whatever* it takes to make the drugs affordable to all who need them. In this case, the assigned obligation seems too demanding. Analogously, two decades ago in the USA, it was often said that for-profit hospitals ought to provide free care for the medically indigent and that, if they did not do so, they were guilty of acting unjustly (Gray, 1986).[3] Duty Dumping seems to proceed on something like a "can implies ought" principle or a principle to the effect that the producers of health-care goods or services have a determinate obligation to provide them to those who cannot pay. But such a principle cannot withstand scrutiny. There is no more reason to believe that drug companies are responsible for providing drugs to all who need them or that for-profit hospitals are to provide care to all that need it, than there is to believe that grocers have an obligation to ensure that no one goes without sufficient food.

Duty Dumping may be an effective political strategy, but it is unprincipled, evasive and in the end most likely counterproductive. It may well be true that drug companies ought to do something to make their drugs more affordable. In the language of traditional moral theory, perhaps they have an imperfect duty of beneficence – a moral obligation to do something to help some of the needy. Whether they should do this by lowering their drug prices or by engaging in some other form of beneficence (say, funding scholarships to train people from poor countries to become doctors or scientists) is another matter.

Duty Dumping is not only morally unjustifiable; it also is a powerful mechanism for the evasion of responsibility. The analogy with the problem of securing access to care for the indigent in the USA is illuminating: The obligation to make basic health care affordable in the USA is a societal obligation; therefore, the lack of affordable basic health care is a moral failing of the citizens of the USA. To pretend that for-profit hospitals are the villains conveniently diverts attention from our failure to fulfill our obligations. Similarly, to focus exclusively or even primarily on the supposed obligations of drug companies is to divert attention from a whole range of responsibilities for responding to the HIV/AIDS crisis. From a cosmopolitan moral standpoint, all of us, as individuals, whether we happen to be leaders of corporations or not, have a moral obligation to help ensure that all persons have access to institutions that protect their basic human rights (Buchanan, 2003, chapters 1, 2 and 3). From the perspective of the principle of humanity or benevolence, we also have an obligation to relieve the sufferings of others. From either of these vantage points, we might all have moral obligations for responding to the HIV/AIDS crisis. This includes the major multinational pharmaceutical companies, but it is substantially different because it recognizes our collective obligation, rather than dumping this obligation solely on these companies (as if only they were responsible for the HIV/AIDS crisis). It is one thing to say that an appropriate collective effort to ensure that HIV/AIDS medications are affordable will include specific obligations on the part of drug companies; it is quite another to pretend that such specific obligations already exist.

Because of their own lack of resources and inability to participate effectively in political processes, however, many individuals are not in a position to do much to act on this obligation. Those of us who are fortunate enough to have resources beyond what we need for a decent and fulfilling life, and who have the freedom to organize with others to influence political processes, have many opportunities to fulfill our obligations regarding human rights and benevolence. Perhaps

---

[3] For a further account of why for-profit health-care organizations do not have determinate obligations to provide access to the indigent, see Brock & Buchanan (1986).

most important, we have the capacity – if we can muster the will – to work together to create an effective specification of responsibilities.

Duty Dumping is also a short-sighted and inherently conservative response to global health problems. The problem is not simply that it leaves the root causes of both illness and lack of access to health care untouched, though that is bad enough. In addition, by focusing arbitrarily on unpopular private organizations (such as big drug companies), it gives political cover to institutions that do have determinate responsibilities for health and which are failing to fulfill them. Chief among these, we shall argue, are states.[4]

A satisfactory account of determinate responsibilities for ameliorating the most serious global health problems will have to do three things. First, it should correctly identify whatever reasonably determinate responsibilities for health already exist in our world (rather than simply foisting imagined determinate responsibilities on whatever resource-rich agents are conveniently at hand – Duty Dumping). Second, it should recognize "responsibility gaps;" that is, it should acknowledge that, in many cases, determinate responsibilities will have to be *created* through the development of new institutions or through modifying existing institutions. Third, it must make clear that the responsibility for holding powerful agents accountable for the determinate responsibilities they already have, and for creating institutions that assign new determinate responsibilities, lies with all of us – but especially with those who have surplus personal resources and political clout.

We have noted that from a cosmopolitan standpoint there are two sources of moral concern about global health: the obligation to help ensure that every person has access to institutions that protect their basic human rights (including the human right to health, and other rights, such as rights against discrimination, which have implications for health), and the so-called imperfect obligation of humanity, or benevolence. Both of these moral obligations are indeterminate – taken by themselves, they provide insufficient guidance for ameliorating the complex problems of

global health. Taking them seriously requires a commitment to collective action to construct a moral division of labor that is both fair and effective. In most cases, successful collective action requires institutions.

Consider first the imperfect obligation of humanity or benevolence. Because of the impact of health status on human well-being, those who act from the duty of humanity will naturally be concerned about improving health, whether by efforts to help ensure that the sick receive medical care or through the amelioration of social and economic conditions that adversely affect health. However, if they act alone, individuals cannot do much to alleviate large-scale health problems. Instead of continuing to act independently and inefficiently, they can and should create institutions for health-care research and for the provision of services, thereby coordinating their efforts and achieving great efficiencies of scale, as well as the benefits of the division of labor. Such institutions will assign various determinate duties to a range of individuals occupying various institutional roles; they will create determinate duties, not simply identify pre-existing determinate duties.

How is this different from Duty Dumping? Consider again the case of HIV/AIDS medications. We have already noted that it is a mistake to assume that drug companies already have determinate obligations to ensure that such medicines are available to all who could benefit from them. It might be possible, however, to create determinate obligations on the part of drug companies. For example, one way might be to modify existing intellectual property rules. As a condition of receiving drug patents – a form of intellectual property right of particular import to the pharmaceutical industry – drug companies might be required to contribute a certain percentage of future sales to a global fund for subsidizing purchases of medications by the health services of poor countries. This hypothetical example is not offered as a policy proposal, but rather as an illustration of the difference between the unprincipled attribution of determinate responsibilities (Duty Dumping) and a collective effort – in this case, new legislation regarding intellectual property rules to create determinate obligations.

Acting conscientiously on the obligation to help ensure that all have access to just institutions also requires collective *institutional* action, for at least two reasons. First, in some cases institutions are needed to give determinate shape to abstract principles of justice, through legitimate processes for selecting particular "justice-regimes" from among a range of feasible

---

[4] Onora O'Neill argues against states as the primary agents of global justice; her view is at least partly based on the failure of states to accomplish justice beyond their borders in the past. This does not necessarily mean that states do not have, or are ill suited to carry out, at least some of the determinate responsibilities we describe. See O'Neill (2004).

alternatives. For example, even if it is true that justice requires some form of private property, there are many alternative private property rights regimes. Yet to reap the benefits a property rights regime can produce, a society must have some way of settling on one particular arrangement, and the process of choosing a particular arrangement must itself accord with principles of justice. Within the constraints of a constitution, democratic institutions are needed to specify a particular property rights regime as one important element of the establishment of justice.

Second, institutions are needed to create or collect resources need for the provision of justice and for ensuring that the costs of providing justice are distributed fairly (Buchanan, 1984). For example, if a particular society, through its institutional processes, recognizes that all its members have a right to a "decent minimum" or "adequate level" of health care, it will also need institutions for raising the revenues needed to secure this right for all and for ensuring that the costs of doing so are distributed fairly. Finally, institutions are often needed to enforce the fulfillment of the duties that institutions create.

Once these various roles of institutions are understood, it becomes clear that whenever human needs are not fulfilled this need not be the result of someone's failure to fulfill a determinate duty; it could be primarily a failure of collective action. To revert to an earlier example, the fact that millions of people are dying whose lives could be prolonged by antiretroviral drugs does not necessarily show that any particular party has failed to perform a determinate duty. Instead, it may indicate a deeper failure of many people to undertake collective action to establish the sorts of institutions that make the ascription of determinate duties both morally justifiable and efficacious.

In the next section, we begin the task of identifying the most important existing determinate responsibilities regarding global health by outlining some of the main responsibilities of states. On our view, it is important to begin with the responsibilities of states both because state behavior plays a larger role in the burden of disease than is usually recognized and because at present, states are the primary agents of distributive justice. Then, in the following section, we consider, also in a preliminary way, the responsibilities of some of the most important non-state actors, including global corporations and certain types of global governance institutions, such as the World Trade Organization (WTO) and the World Bank.

Our inquiry will focus on responsibilities for ameliorating the most serious health problems of the world's worst off people. Apart from the fact that this is literally a life and death matter, and for that reason morally urgent, there is another reason to concentrate on the most serious health problems of those who have the least resource for addressing them. This commitment can be seen as the focus of an "overlapping consensus" among quite disparate views of justice, ranging from strict egalitarianism to an extreme prioritarianism, according to which only the well-being or resources of the worst off count from the perspective of distributive justice. This is a signal advantage because it allows us to make some progress on the Problem of Concrete Responsibilities without having first to determine which of a number of competing conceptions of justice is correct (Sreenivasan, 2002).

The responsibilities of states

The recognition that some health problems occur globally and may require supranational responses should not blind us to the fact that, in our world, states are not only the primary agents of justice, but also the institutions that have the greatest impact on the health of individuals.

Even if it were true, as libertarian political theorists argue, that there are no positive general moral rights, states would still have significant responsibilities for ameliorating those health problems that are caused by the injustices they commit or support – responsibilities that they are not now fulfilling.

The responsibilities of states: justice and membership in the state system

The first responsibility of states regarding global health is to avoid committing acts of injustice that have health-harming effects. This general obligation implies more determinate obligations. Among the most important of these are the obligation to refrain from fighting unjust wars abroad and using violence for oppression at home. In addition, states have a moral obligation to put an end to the common practice – especially among some of the wealthiest countries – of equipping and training the military forces of states that are likely to use this power unjustly, whether against their own people or others.

Another important source of rather determinate obligations of states is their participation in the state system. A key aspect of participation in the state system is the practice of recognizing the legitimacy of other states. States routinely contribute to massive health problems in other countries by recognizing the legitimacy of governments that either fail to fulfill their responsibilities regarding the health of their citizens or deprive them of the resources they might otherwise use for securing health care or the better living conditions that are essential for health.

Under the current state system, international recognition of the legitimacy of a government confers two eminently abusable rights: the right to dispose of the country's natural resources and the right to borrow from individual countries or international agencies such as the World Bank.[5] The first right enables corrupt government officials to enrich themselves with wealth that properly belongs to the people and could be used by them to ameliorate their health problems, in part by raising their standard of living. The second right enables state leaders to incur crushing national debts that make it harder for their people to lift themselves from poverty and reap the health benefits of a higher standard of living.

The traditional criterion for legitimacy in the state system is normatively vacuous. The Principle of Effectivity asserts that the basis for conferring the rights of sovereignty, including the right to dispose of resources and the right to borrow, is simply the ability to exercise control over a relatively stable population within a given territory (cited in Buchanan, 2003, chapter 6). On this criterion, human rights-violating, kleptocratic regimes that pillage their peoples' resources and exacerbate their poverty by incurring debts to fund projects that benefit only ruling elite are legitimate, so long as they achieve control. Furthermore, until recently, the recognition of legitimacy has largely been an all or nothing affair because sovereignty has been regarded as indivisible. However, both the normatively vacuous conception of sovereignty and the assumption that sovereignty is unitary are now being challenged (International Commission on Intervention and State Sovereignty, 2001).

States have a moral responsibility not to be accomplices in injustices by conferring predictably abusable rights on bad governments. The question is whether effective international institutions can be devised that reward responsible governments with the full range of sovereign rights and withhold certain rights from those governments that seriously abuse them. If the effective fulfillment of this responsibility requires the creation of new international institutions that "unbundle" the rights of sovereignty and confer rights only when they can be expected to be exercised responsibly, then states have a higher-order responsibility to contribute to their creation.

If more states did a better job of fulfilling their obligations to refrain from committing injustices and from supporting states that commit injustices, the positive impact on health would be enormous. Consider only the obligation not to engage in unjust wars and not to supply weapons and training to states that are likely to engage in unjust wars or use their military forces unjustly against their own people. From 1998–2004, around 3.9 million people have died in the Democratic Republic of Congo (DRC) as a result of the war raging there. It is estimated that for every violent death in DRC's war zone, there are 62 "non-violent" deaths – from starvation, disease and exposure (Lacey, 2005). This is only one instance of the devastating direct and indirect health effects of war.

To summarize: Even if there were no such thing as positive human rights (such as the right to an adequate standard of living, the right to basic health care, the right to basic education), states would still have rather determinate moral obligations to act in ways that would greatly ameliorate the health problems of the world's worst-off people. Simply by refraining from unjust violence and from supporting unjust governments, states could do much to improve global health.

The responsibilities of states: primary guarantors of their own citizens' human rights

So far we have made the case that states have determinate responsibilities whose fulfillment would do much to ameliorate some of the most serious threats to health simply by appealing to relatively uncontroversial standards of justice. Once we expand the moral framework to include states' responsibilities for protecting the human rights of their own citizens, the scope of their responsibilities increases considerably.

The primary "addressees" of human rights claims are states (Nickel, 1987). This is so, not only because historically states have been the major violators of

---

[5] Thomas Pogge has rightly emphasized the role that the recognition of these two rights plays in global poverty (Pogge, 2002, pp. 22–23, 117, 153, 162–66, 238, 258, 264, 266).

human rights, but also because, for better or worse, they are best equipped to specify and apply determinate human rights norms and to achieve the conditions of distributive justice upon which the effectiveness of individuals' rights depends. International and regional human rights institutions have a valuable role to play in specifying the minimal human rights standards that all states should meet; and in providing venues and frameworks of discourse in which domestic and transnational forces can exert pressure on states to live up to them.

Unfortunately, the connection between human rights and health, though important, has not received the attention it deserves from moral theorists. There are at least two ways in which the connection might be made. On the one hand, a right to health could itself be included among the human rights. On the other, one could think of health as a precondition for the enjoyment of various human rights. Let us consider each approach briefly and try to ascertain their implications for the Problem of Concrete Responsibilities.

The idea of a human right to health

Human rights are best understood as high-priority minimal moral entitlements of all persons and as implying both fairly determinate obligations on the parts of states (their primary "addressees") and more indeterminate obligations on individuals to work with others to promote the protection of these rights, if they have the opportunity and resources to do so.[6] In order to integrate global health issues into the human rights framework, the first question to ask is whether the human right in question is a right to health care or to health. The attraction of focusing on a right to health, rather than to health care is obvious: Health depends upon many factors, health care being only one of them – and, in the larger scheme of things – not the most important of them.

However, the idea of a right to health is not without difficulties. First, there is the problem of settling on a defensible definition of what health is. Among the most basic sources of disagreement here is the division between more "objectivist" and more "social constructivist" conceptions of health and disease.

Second, if the notion of health is understood too ambitiously, satisfying the right to health for all will not be possible, simply because there are some people whose health is so poor that they could not be made healthy even if cost were not an issue. The third difficulty is that cost *is* an issue. However, the right to health as a human right is to be understood, it must – as with other human rights – be understood as a moral minimum, not a maximum. Health is not the only good. For one thing, there are other human rights and protecting them requires that not all of our resources be used to satisfy the right to health. In addition, as most moral theories recognize, there are limits on what we owe to others. For these reasons, any approach to global health that relies on the idea of a human right to health must first develop a defensible conception of the limited character of the right. Unless this is done, it will not be possible to make headway on the problem of determining specific responsibilities for seeing that all enjoy the right, if only because the whole idea will be dismissed as unrealistically demanding or as imposing unacceptable restrictions on individuals' freedom and property rights.

Nonetheless, the lack of a fully developed theory of the human right to health is not such a serious problem if our focus is on the most serious health problems of the world's most vulnerable people. Their health problems are undeniable and severe, regardless of which of a broad range of competing conceptions of health and disease one adopts. Furthermore, whatever the full content of the human right to health turns out to be, it is clear that many states are not ensuring that this right is enjoyed by all of their citizens.

At present, the most significant mechanisms for ensuring compliance with human rights standards are domestic. More specifically, individual states that ratify human rights conventions increasingly incorporate them into their domestic legal systems over time, thereby giving individuals and groups standing to appeal to the courts when they believe their rights are being infringed upon.

However, so long as the idea of a human right to health is left vague and therefore subject to the charge that it implies ever-expanding obligations, there is little hope that it will be incorporated in a meaningful way into domestic legal systems. This pitfall can only be avoided by building a broad international consensus on a conception of the human right to health that is sufficiently determinate to allay the worry about an over-expansive entitlement, while avoiding an overly

---

6 For a lucid articulation and defense of this "entitlements plus" conception of human rights, see Nickel, cited in Buchanan (2003), chapters 1 and 2. For the view that there are certain rights that are preconditions for the enjoyment of all other rights, see Shue (1980).

specified right that would not do justice to cultural differences and differences in the resources available to various states.[7]

One way of achieving this goal would be to articulate a minimal conception of the human right to health that consists mainly of two elements. The first is a set of operationalizable standards for what might be called the "negative" right to health, a specification of the responsibilities of states to remove barriers to access to existing health-care resources, to eliminate discrimination in health services, and to ensure that the health needs of all citizens are taken into account both in the development of health services and in the pursuit of policies of economic development that can have serious health effects. The second is a set of operationalizable standards for ensuring that all citizens enjoy a core set of "positive" health entitlements, including, for example, such relatively uncontroversial items as clean drinking water, basic sanitation and shelter, as well as access to basic perinatal care and immunization for the most serious infectious diseases. In both cases, the standards must be operationalizable in the sense that appropriate international and transnational organizations must be able to make publicly defensible judgments as to whether states are complying with them. The chief responsibility for seeing that this two-pronged strategy is successfully executed lies with the leaders of international and transnational human rights organizations and with individuals who are in a position to work with others to influence their own governments to cooperate with these organizations.

Health as a precondition for the enjoyment of human rights

On some accounts, health is not a human right, but rather something that is nonetheless of critical moral importance because it is a necessary condition for the enjoyment of human rights. To advocate human rights without making a commitment to achieving all the conditions for their effective exercise is morally incoherent.

To a large extent, this second approach to global health converges with that according to which health is a human right. Ensuring that the burden of disease does not undercut the effective exercise of human rights does not require equality of health (however that might be defined) nor that all health needs be met. Instead, it requires a collective effort to forge an international consensus on a core set of health entitlements (both "negative" and "positive") that generally protect individuals against the most serious health problems and that are sufficiently concrete to allow states to be held accountable for providing them, either through their own judicial institutions or through formal or informal pressures from international and transnational organizations.

In some cases, states will not be capable of achieving these basic health entitlements for some or even most of their citizens. The most extreme example is that of literally "failed states," in which civil order no longer exists and there is no government capable of providing any services, including those that are important for health. In other cases, there may be a minimally functioning state, but it lacks some capacities that are critical for providing adequate levels of the core public health and health-care services. When this occurs, the people of wealthier states have an obligation to work together to provide aid to help every state discharge its obligations regarding the health of its citizens.

The effective fulfillment of this obligation will generally require the world's wealthier people to act through the institutions of their own states, by pressuring their political leaders to create international institutions that fairly distribute the burden of providing aid, devise benchmarks for progress, and provide incentives for donors to carry through on pledges of support. An example of this type of international institution might be the Global Fund to fight AIDS, tuberculosis and malaria.

The responsibilities of non-state actors

An obligation not to cause harm?

We argued earlier that states have rather direct and relatively uncontroversial obligations that would, if fulfilled, avoid serious harms to health. It might be thought that every organization, whether private or public, has an obligation not to act in ways that are harmful to people's health. However, the notion of acting in ways that are harmful to people's health is so all-encompassing as to be incapable of providing moral guidance. It covers both cases where the causal connection is sufficiently clear and robust to warrant the attribution of responsibility and those in which it is not.

---

[7] For a valuable contribution to the solution of this problem, see Hessler (2001). See also Hessler & Buchanan (2002).

Where the agent in question is itself a significant causal factor in the production of the harm, the attribution of responsibility may be unproblematic. In some cases, there clearly are obligations not to cause harm that non-state actors violate with disastrous consequences for the health of some individuals. For example, a company may dump large quantities of toxic chemicals into a major river, causing death or serious illness not just in one country, but in several.

However, in morality, as in the law, merely making a contribution to the production of a harm is not sufficient for the attribution of responsibility. One difficulty is that some harms result from the cumulative effects of the actions of many individuals, none of which can reasonably be held responsible for the harm. Thus, when global health problems, such as the pollution of the oceans, result from the cumulative effects of the actions of millions of agents, including individuals, corporations, and governments, the attribution of concrete responsibilities on the basis of causality is not possible. Although much more could be done and ought to be done to hold corporations and governments legally liable for harms to health when appropriate standards for liability apply, it is a mistake to rest the case for addressing global health problems on the reduction of moral responsibility to the obligation not to cause harm. To do so not only requires an indefensible understanding of the relationship between causality and responsibility; it also overlooks the responsibility of a wide range of actors to work together to develop institutions that create morally defensible assignments of concrete responsibilities.

Accordingly, in the discussion of the responsibilities of non-state actors that follows, we will focus chiefly on grounds for responsibility other than the more obvious cases in which an agent's actions play an important and direct role in the causation of health-related harms.

"Global governance institutions"

Like the term "global health," the phrase "global governance institutions" is currently in vogue. It is used to refer to a quite heterogeneous collection of different international organizations, from "government networks" comprised of high level bureaucrats from many nations (including judges and regulators networks; Slaughter, 2004) to the World Trade Organization and the United Nations Security Council. Since there are such great differences among these organizations, we should not expect them all to have the same causal role in global health nor the same responsibilities. For this

reason, we do not attempt even to begin the daunting task of providing a theory of responsibility for all "global governance institutions." Instead, we only aim to articulate some of the different grounds for attributing responsibilities regarding global health to them.

Consistency with the public goals of the institution

In some cases, global governance institutions expressly or tacitly assume responsibilities for global health. One example is the World Health Organization (WHO). Less obviously, the WTO recognizes the importance of its activities for global health and welfare in several of its formal statements. A brief tract intended to explain the functions of the organization to the general public states that the WTO's "goal is to improve the welfare of the peoples of its member countries," (World Trade Organization, 2003) and in a joint report with the WHO, the WTO affirms "human health as important in the highest degree" (World Health Organization and World Trade Organization Secretariat, 2002).

Consider the WTO's Agreement on Trade-Related Aspects of Intellectual Property (TRIPS), which was negotiated and agreed upon in the Uruguay Rounds of 1986–1994 (World Trade Organization, 1994). A strong case can be made that this agreement, far from promoting health as being of "the highest-importance," in fact creates a new obstacle to the amelioration of some global health problems, by raising the prices and slowing the introduction of generic drugs in developing countries. When an organization acts in ways that are inconsistent with its own public commitments to global health, the attribution of responsibility is relatively unproblematic.

Of course, it might also be argued that whether or not it explicitly includes health concerns within its public mission statement, the WTO has come to have responsibilities for health in the process of pursuing its primary goal of liberalizing trade. If the predictable consequences of liberalized trade in certain contexts include working conditions that endanger the health of workers, thereby endangering their human rights, then the organization that is the chief instrument for liberalizing trade is obligated to take these consequences into account in its policies and to cooperate with other actors to ameliorate them. Unlike the simple appeal to special responsibilities for health that organizations sometimes assume, this argument requires much more in terms of elaborating responsibility in the complex causal web connecting liberalized trade policies to the endangering of human rights at the individual level. Given that there can be disagreement about the facts that are relevant to the attribution of responsibilities, a credible identification of the special responsibilities of particular organizations may require reliance on the expertise of "epistemic communities," mobilized through the operation of international organizations such as the International Labour Organization (ILO) or various transnational human rights organizations.

Global corporations

The responsibilities of global corporations for global health fall into three main categories: (1) obligations to avoid actions and policies that in themselves are significant causal factors in harms to health; (2) obligations not to support governments engaged in unjust activities that are harmful to the health of their citizens or others; and (3) obligations not to impede the health-promoting efforts of states, labor organizations and legitimate international and transnational organizations that have more direct responsibilities regarding global health.

As we have already noted, the moral basis of the first class of obligations is relatively straightforward. The main problem is not the attribution of responsibility, but rather how to achieve accountability. In developing countries, the state regulatory agencies charged with holding global corporations responsible for the harms are often too inadequately resourced to be effective. In more developed countries, they are often staffed by people who previously worked in, and still have connections with, the very industries they are supposed to regulate. Or the agencies are ordered to go soft on enforcement by higher government officials who seek political support from powerful corporations.

The second class of obligations is extremely important. Like states, global corporations can and often do help corrupt governments stay in power, with disastrous effects on the health and general welfare of individuals. And like states, global corporations can have powerful incentives to provide such support. However, as the case of apartheid South Africa demonstrates, under certain conditions these incentives can be countered by a sustained global campaign to expose the role of corporations in supporting unjust governments and mobilize public pressure and state action against it.

When corporations explicitly embrace a role in helping to ameliorate a global health problem, as some drug companies have done, they assume new responsibilities and ought to be held accountable for fulfilling them. Apart from such self-assigned responsibilities, the extent to which global corporations have obligations to promote health is debatable. However, it is much less difficult to argue that they at least have the obligation not to impede the efforts of others to ameliorate the most serious health problems of the world's worst off. For example, a global corporation violates this obligation when it blocks the formation of labor unions committed to ameliorating hazards in the workplace. Similarly, even though it is problematic to say that drug companies have an obligation to provide essential medicines at prices that even the poorest people can afford, it is clear that they have an obligation not to exert pressure on governments to ratify intellectual property agreements that increase their profits at the expense of preventing poorer countries from having access to less expensive generic drugs.

Conclusion

Global health is increasingly becoming the object of interdisciplinary empirical research, institutional action and moral concern. If this convergence of factors is to result in a significant amelioration of the most serious health problems of the world's most vulnerable people, the abstract commitment to "improving global health" must be translated into concrete responsibilities for action. We have argued that the needed work of specification requires a systematic understanding of the different roles and capacities of a broad range of private and public institutions, with a sensitivity to the different grounds for attributing responsibility. One important result of our inquiry is that the responsibilities of states are much more extensive than is usually assumed. Instead of focusing only on the obligations of wealthier states to transfer resources to poorer ones, we should recognize the full range of state activities – from making war, to according legitimacy to corrupt governments – that are harmful to health and prevent individuals from achieving a standard of living that makes better health possible.

Acknowledgments

The authors are grateful for research support for this paper from Duke University's Center for Genome Ethics, Law and Policy, part of the Duke Institute for Genome Sciences & Policy.

References

Brock, D. W. & Buchanan, A. (1986). Ethical issues in for-profit health care. In B. H. Gray (Ed.), *For-Profit Enterprise in Health Care* (pp. 224–249). Washington, DC: National Academy Press.

Buchanan, A. (1984). The right to a decent minimum of health care. *Philosophy & Public Affairs* **13**, 55–78.

Buchanan, A. (2003). *Justice, Legitimacy, and Self-Determination: Moral Foundations for International Law*. New York, NY: Oxford University Press.

Gray, B. H. (ed). (1986). *For-Profit Enterprise in Health Care*. Washington, DC: National Academy Press.

Hessler, K. (2001). *A Theory of Interpretation for Human Rights*. Ph.D. dissertation, University of Arizona.

Hessler, K. & Buchanan, A. (2002). Specifying the content of the human right to health care. In R. Rhodes, M. Battin & A. Silvers (Eds.), *Medicine and Social Justice: Essays on the Distribution of Health Care*. New York, NY: Oxford University Press.

International Commission on Intervention and State Sovereignty (2001). *The Responsibility to Protect*. Ottawa, ON: International Development Research Centre.

Lacey, M. (2005). Beyond bullets and blades. *The New York Times*. March 20, 2005.

Nickel, J. (1987). *Making Sense of Human Rights*. Berkeley, CA: University of California Press.

O'Neill, O. (2004). Global justice: whose obligations? In D. K. Chatterjee (Ed.), *The Ethics of Assistance: Morality and the Distant Needy* (pp. 242–259). New York, NY: Cambridge University Press.

Pogge, T. (2002). *World Poverty and Human Rights*. Cambridge: Polity Press.

Shue, H. (1980). *Basic Rights: Subsistence, Affluence, and U.S. Foreign Policy*. (2nd edn.) Princeton, NJ: Princeton University Press.

Slaughter, A.-M. (2004). *A New World Order*. Princeton, NJ: Princeton University Press.

Sreenivasan, G. (2002). International justice and health: a proposal. *Ethics and International Affairs* **16**, 81–90.

World Health Organization and World Trade Organization Secretariat (2002). *WTO Agreements and Public Health*. Geneva: World Trade Organization.

World Trade Organization (1994). Agreement on trade-related aspects of intellectual property rights. www.wto.org/english/docs_e/legal_e/27-trips.pdf. (Accessed March 25, 2005).

World Trade Organization (2003). *The WTO in Brief*. Geneva: World Trade Organization.

Chapter

11

Global health ethics: the rationale for mutual caring

Solomon Benatar, Abdallah S. Daar and Peter A. Singer

Introduction

Despite impressive twentieth century scientific and technological progress, massive expansion of the global economy, enhanced methods of communication and transportation, and deepening insights into the forces that shape the lives and health of people, the world is more inequitable than it was 50 years ago both in terms of access to health care for individuals and in relation to the health of whole populations (Benatar, 1998; Marmot, 2006).

While polarizing economic forces operate in a world of gross imbalances of wealth and power between the rich and poor (within and between countries) and are largely driven by the economic interests of wealthy nations, many political realities within developing countries have also contributed to the suffering of whole populations. These include corruption, ruthless military dictatorships, ostentatious expenditure by the ruling elite, under-investment in basic education and health, excessive military expenditures and ethnic strife and civil wars. Appropriate criticism of such deficiencies should be accompanied by acknowledgment that they are promoted by powerful nations pursuing their own economic and geo-political interests, often through collusion with despots who have much to gain in personal wealth and the maintenance of power at the expense of their citizens.

Nevertheless, it is arguable that the primary responsibility for good governance surely must rest largely within individual nations – even the poorest – as good governance, like democracy, cannot be imposed from outside. In an era of growing global awareness and competing economic interests, it would be desirable for poor countries to be able to negotiate for their own interests, either individually or through regional political/economic bodies such as the East African Community, the Economic Community of West African States and the Southern African Development Economic Community. However, this would require that powerful and wealthy nations do not obstruct such endeavors by privileging their own interests (Katz, 2008).

The recent financial crisis also reminds us that the so-called developed world is not immune from corruption, fraud, unbridled profiteering, poor economic regulation and lack of economic common sense (Kakutani 2009; Krugman, 2009), with far-reaching effects on the lives of many globally. Long-standing disparities in wealth and health within and between nations are now being further aggravated by this crisis, which is already affecting developing countries disproportionately (Leahy, 2009; Milner, 2009; WHO, 2009). Although some countries may be on the way towards achieving the Millennium Development Goals, progress in the very poorest countries, especially those dependent on dwindling aid from the West, are undoubtedly being very adversely affected by the crisis (Chan, 2008; Fidler, 2008; Governance and Social Development Resource Centre, 2009).

There have been some promising "green shoots" in global health in recent decades (Fidler, 2008). These include major increases in funding, for example by the Bill and Melinda Gates Foundation for research to address health needs of the poor and the so-called neglected tropical diseases; the Global Fund; greater awareness among European countries and the USA of just how important global health is; more attention to health systems and provision of basic health-care needs; a somewhat late but growing seriousness in addressing global warming that is likely to affect the health of the poor disproportionately; and serious attention to

Two earlier versions of this work have appeared: Benatar, S. R., Daar, A. and Singer, P. A. (2003). Global health ethics: the rationale for mutual caring. *International Affairs* **79**, 107–138 and Benatar, S. R., Daar, A. and Singer, P. A. (2005). Global health ethics: the need for an expanded discourse. *PLoS Medicine* **2** (7), 587–659.

reforming agricultural practices and improving crop yields, particularly in Africa. All these have made the emerging field of global health a priority for major universities around the world. However, this new interest in global health is not without its shortcomings as Laurie Garrett (2007) and David Fidler (2008) have described in their examination and questioning of what lies beyond this so-called revolution in thinking about global health.

Some years ago we proposed that bioethics, an interdisciplinary field, initially focused on the ethics of interpersonal relationships, could act as a bridge and a wedge towards improving health globally through expanded educational and public discourses promoting widely shared foundational values. Today, in the face of an evolving global financial crisis that strikingly reveals the shortcomings of long-standing and blindly accepted economic dogma (Benatar *et al.*, 2009; Krugman, 2009), we believe that there is an even greater need for action on these issues.

Serious reflection on the ethical foundations of global health, and extension of the discourse on ethics towards a more comprehensive approach, could promote the new mindset needed to improve health and well-being globally. Such a mindset requires realization that health, human rights, economic opportunities, good governance, peace and development are all intimately linked within a complex interdependent world. The challenges we face in the twenty-first century are to explore these links, to understand their implications and to develop political processes that could harness economic growth to human development, narrow global disparities in health and promote peaceful co-existence (Benatar *et al.*, 2009).

We begin here by reviewing a set of values that combines meaningful respect for the dignity of all people with a desire to promote the idea of human development beyond that conceived within the narrow, individualistic, "economic" model of human flourishing. Wider expression of these values could hopefully serve to promote peaceful and beneficial use of new knowledge and power. An initial step forward for global health is suggested through five transformational approaches: developing a global state of mind, promoting long-term self-interest, striking a balance between optimism and pessimism about globalization and solidarity, strengthening capacity and enhancing the production of global public goods for health. These approaches, requiring vision and wisdom in the transfer of knowledge, could lead the way towards a fairer global economy characterized by greater cooperation and less exploitation.

Values for global health ethics

While the values we articulate below serve as the basis for global health ethics, none can stand alone, and the most important is solidarity – which can be defined as attitudes and determination to work for the common good across the globe in an era when interdependence is greater than ever and in which progress should be defined as enhancing capabilities and social justice. Without solidarity it is inevitable that we shall ignore distant indignities, violations of human rights, inequities, deprivation of freedom, undemocratic regimes and respect for the environment. If a spirit of mutual caring could be developed between those in wealthy countries and those in developing countries, we see constructive change as being possible.

Respect for all human life

The idea of respect for human life springs partly from the long-standing religious belief common to many cultures that "man is made in the image of God." Given the diversity of religions and the unfortunate tendency to highlight only their differences, imaginative approaches are needed to promote respect for human dignity on common grounds that all religions share (Kung, 1997). These could be used to promote a sense of spiritual kinship while respecting a diversity of customs and rituals. Kung's suggestion of a global ethic for humankind has been a major conceptual advance and it is regrettable that it has not achieved a higher action profile. Indeed it would seem that today we are further away than ever from attaining inter-religious tolerance or cooperation.

In the secular sphere respect for human dignity, expressed through the Universal Declaration of Human Rights (UDHR), has achieved a high profile and many highly significant and valued results. It is difficult to imagine what the world would be like today without the UDHR. Nevertheless we need to regularly examine how it is being applied globally and how it might best be supported to achieve its lofty goals. While its successes are difficult to fully quantify and while some hold these as the highest hope (Farmer, 2008), some others regard them as limited (Falk, 2000) – perhaps because of recent failures and because insufficient attention has been paid to how powerful and deeply entrenched system forces perpetuate human rights abuses on a grand scale (Benatar & Doyal, 2009).

Human rights, responsibilities (duties) and needs

"Human rights," as a secular concept for promoting human dignity, has the potential to transcend religions, national borders and cultures. In the 1990s the human rights movement flourished and more countries seemed to be accepting universal human rights as a "civilizational" standard (Donnelly, 1998) despite the inconsistencies already mentioned.

Although human rights are widely accepted in the rhetorical sense, much argument continues about the nature and extent of rights. Since the early 1990s a complex debate has also emerged regarding the Western bias and origins of human rights, and the extension of human rights from the West to the rest of the world. While superficially successful, this is largely "unfinished business" (Pogge, 2002).

Despite its great achievements in sensitizing humanity and acting as a template for national and international laws that encompass its principles, the UDHR might have achieved even more influence had it not been for some of the insincerity and compromise in its initial formulation (Rieff, 1999). More recent setbacks relate to post 9/11 events in detention prisons (Amnesty International, 2004). Like all great human achievements that require consensus, the UDHR and the movements it engendered are not perfect. There is some disagreement on what qualifies as a right, little actionable awareness that rights must be matched by corresponding duties and differing perspectives of how to reconcile value systems. These challenges have reduced the extent to which the wider benefits of the UDHR might have become part of the "rights revolution" (Donnelly, 1998).

Inadequate attention also has been paid to the fact that rights and responsibilities (duties) are intimately connected – the conceptual logic of rights entails corresponding duties/responsibilities. Thus duty bearers need to be identified to ensure the realization of rights. If we all claim rights but none are willing to bear duties, rights will not be satisfied. Our ability to enjoy rights is thus determined by our willingness to accept and act on our responsibilities.

Audrey Chapman has expressed concern that political debate is impoverished by a human rights discourse in the USA, which "far more than in other liberal democracies, is characterised by hyper-individualism, exaggerated absoluteness, and silence with respect to personal, civic, and collective responsibilities" (Chapman, 1996). She draws attention to three advantages for paying greater attention to the duties related to specific rights: (i) moving the human rights debate in the direction of who has to do what if these rights are to be realized, (ii) more focused and specific discussions of questions of priority among rights and other important social goals, and (iii) discussions of the inadequacies of the contemporary international political and economic order. She also describes the shift required from an excessively liberal human rights paradigm to a social model of human rights that links benefits and entitlements with the acceptance of a series of responsibilities – the starting point for such rights being the principle of respect for all persons in the context of community. The intensity of the recent furor in the USA over the Obama administration's proposals for health-care reform reveals the lack of significant progress towards making such a shift in that society.

Economic policies, whether national or otherwise, that perpetuate and worsen debt, and that frustrate economic growth in many countries, undoubtedly deny billions of people the decent living conditions essential for human flourishing. The imperfect rules underlying many globalizing policies, coupled with the desire by wealthy countries for endless economic growth, and lack of good governance in poor nations, results in sales of valuable national resources in poor countries to global purchasers with little, if any, accountability by political leaders.

Failure to achieve socio-economic rights is thus to a considerable extent the result of powerful systemic upstream forces that control the global economy, support ongoing rule by cruel despots, shape unfair trade rules, facilitate the arms trade and fuel excessive and selfish consumerism – all of which can undermine the achievement of socio-economic rights for billions of people (Benatar 1998, 2005b; Pogge, 2002, 2005; Benatar & Doyal, 2009). It can be argued that because there is, in reality, so little real respect for the lives of the poor, a large proportion of the world's population cannot benefit from the right of access to basic subsistence rights. Vittorio Hosle's description of "the third world as a philosophical problem" (Hosle, 1992) and the implications of the long-lasting impact of colonial and imperial forces on the lives of indigenous people has been supplemented by Thomas Pogge's philosophical argument illustrating how systemic forces operate to sustain human rights abuses (Pogge, 2002, 2005).

> Human rights violations are not accidents; they are not random in distribution or effect. Rights violations are, rather, symptoms of deeper pathologies of power and are linked intimately to the social conditions that so often determine who will suffer abuse and who will be shielded from harm. (Farmer, 2003, p. 7)

The application of human rights must thus extend beyond civil and political rights to include social, cultural and economic rights and their close integration with the reciprocal responsibilities required to ensure that rights are honored and basic needs are met. Just as the concept of "political citizenship" requires non-discriminatory enfranchisement of all, so the concept of "social citizenship" requires access to the basic requirements for survival and potential flourishing – a requirement of modern democracy (vide infra).

Equity

"Equity" is another concept that could transcend national borders and cultures. Equity can be defined as the provision of equal shares for equal needs or the allocation of unequal shares for unequal needs as long as proportionality is maintained. However, proportionality is difficult to assess because of incommensurability. Some inequalities in wealth, health and disease are inevitable aspects of life. Eliminating all inequalities is not possible. In addition not all inequality is inequitable. Inequity refers to those inequalities that are considered to arise from unfairness. Inequitable disparities in health have become a major focus of attention in recent years.

A significant recent contribution to understanding why equity in health is so hard to achieve comes from The People's Health Movement, Medact and the Global Equity Gauge Alliance who have together produced alternative world health reports highlighting the root causes of poor health. These address a wide range of topics on health and development policy from unconventional perspectives that uncover the flaws in the "development paradigm," and suggest new ways of making progress in health care (People's Health Movement, Medact and the Global Equity Gauge Alliance, 2005, 2008).

However, it seems unlikely that disparities or even unfair differences in health will be greatly reduced merely through changes in the health sector alone. As the achievement of good health requires more than the provision of health-care services, attention needs to be directed towards the forces that drive and perpetuate economic inequity and that have also in recent years shifted much of the discourse in international health policy debates away from considerations of equity to an efficiency-driven perspective. While this market influence, which promotes efficiency reflects a narrow, direct approach to health has value, it also has considerable potential to damage the equity valued by more egalitarian approaches (Navarro, 2007). Market-based approaches wrong-headedly applied, as through the "Washington Consensus" of the 1980s and beyond, caused great damage to health by forcing inappropriate "reforms" on countries and health-care systems. If market approaches were to be applied more responsibly (Royal Danish Foreign Ministry for Foreign Affairs, 2000) and tax evasion more effectively prevented (Brock, 2008) potentially great benefits could be achieved. In essence it is unnecessary to think of efficiency and equity as opposites in this debate and if both were valued, efficiencies could make it possible to share scarce resources more equitably.

Instead of taking a direct approach that focuses on equity in health (a difficult concept to define) as an end in itself, Fabiennne Peter has suggested an indirect approach that sees the pursuit of health as embedded in the broader pursuit of social justice (as an important determinant of health) in general (Peter & Evans, 2001). This approach emphasizes the concept of agency and well-being (defined as "having the capabilities that a person can achieve") and the freedom (vide infra) to pursue one's own life goals within a pluralistic world. It also provides space to address the "politics of need (need for food, shelter, education and protection from harm) in the context of the modern welfare state in general and in relation to public health in particular" (Robertson, 1998).

John Rawls' theory of justice (central to which is a "fair system of co-operation" between individuals who all enjoy fundamental equality and freedom within a particular society) offers an appealing vision of a social order that every citizen finds legitimate despite large differences in their personal values. Rawls' Law of Peoples attempts to address issues of global justice by describing how "peoples" (as nations) that hold liberal values, or that are at least decent societies, could agree to structure their international relations. However, criticisms leveled against Rawls' Law of Peoples on several grounds (Buchanan, 2000), seem to make Rawls' set of laws of limited value for a world in which national sovereignty is waning but remains powerful.

Madison Powers and Ruth Faden have provided a rich theory of social justice with guidance on how to think about health inequalities within an approach that places social justice as the foundation of public health and public health policy (Powers & Faden, 2006). Gillian Brock has recently offered a cosmopolitan account of global justice in which she defends the equal moral worth of every person globally without brushing aside all considerations of nationality or other identities (Brock, 2009). Her work takes Rawls' Law of Peoples as its point of departure. After reviewing criticisms and defenses of his position she provides both a nuanced theoretical account of cosmopolitanism and offers practical opportunities to reduce gross global injustices through protection of individual liberties, reduction in poverty and protection of public goods.

Norman Daniels and colleagues have also made significant contributions to bridging philosophical theories and practical realities by proposing benchmarks of fairness for health reform and adapting these for developing countries (Daniels *et al.*, 1996). With James Sabin, Daniels has also made important contributions to setting priorities in health-care institutions by developing a process of decision-making ("accountability for reasonableness") that, in the absence of agreement on substantive issues of justice at least promotes procedural justice (Daniels & Sabin, 2002). These works represent practical attempts to bring theories of justice, with an emphasis on equity, into practice.

Freedom

Freedom, another highly prized value, includes "freedom from ..." as well as "freedom to ..." Good health and satisfying lives are determined both by the freedom from want (of basic subsistence and educational needs) and by the freedom to undertake activities of one's choice to achieve personal goals. In Amartya Sen's view, the opportunities to undertake these activities (defined by him as "capabilities") should be the focus of action, as he believes that equality can be best promoted by enhancing the capabilities of individuals (Sen, 1999).

Freedom from want (dependent at least to some extent on the actions of others) is essential to achieving these goals. Len Doyal and Ian Gough argue on moral grounds that the freedom to develop one's potential must be coupled to "freedom from ..." through security

of person and access to first-order biological needs – food, clean water, shelter, etc. – as the essentials for decent lives. A sense of empowerment and control over ourselves is, in their view, essential for human flourishing (Doyal & Gough, 1991). Respect for the basic needs and dignity of others, respect for the full range of human rights, belief in the rule of just law, the willingness to take responsibility for one's actions and societal well-being, deriving satisfaction from work well done, contributing to new knowledge, and the freedom to develop one's full potential are essential for the achievement of personal fulfillment and human flourishing.

Sen's work draws on both philosophy and economic analysis to provide an eloquent conceptual exposition and ethical defense of modern dominant development thinking. Richard Sandbrook (2000) has labeled this "pragmatic neoliberalism," with a market-orientation but going beyond orthodox neo-classical analysis and macro-economic reforms (although these remain central), to include responsive governance, political freedoms, improved education, health care and safety nets, gender equity and environmental sustainability.

Sen is considered to be among those who have most effectively explicated the value of democratic institutions to obtaining equity in society. For example, his empirical economic work has established the important lesson that democracy and a free press help to prevent famine. Gro Harlem Brundtland, the former Director-General of WHO, proposes that these very same basic institutions are also crucial in improving health and reducing poverty. Sen has further argued strongly for the freedom to achieve one's capabilities. As with most great thinkers, his work has met with some criticism.

For example, Richard Sandbrook has suggested that his work is incomplete or implausible on three grounds (Sandbrook, 2000). First, Sandbrook contests the assumption that market exchange is "a natural and intrinsically valuable pattern." Second, he identifies shortcomings in Sen's conception of democracy, and deficiencies are noted in his analysis of the "challenges facing democracies." Others have also argued that trade liberalism obstructs the achievement of democracy by giving greater weight to freedom of the market than to methods of governance and sustenance of democratic ideas (Girling, 1997; Royal Danish Ministry of Foreign Affairs, 2000; Teeple, 2000). However, it should be noted that it is not implausible to have good governance in association with humane market approaches. Third, Sandbrook suggests that there are major flaws in Sen's conception of "reasoned social progress." These criticisms, if valid, highlight the challenges that need to be faced if human freedom is to be more widely achieved.

Democracy

Democracy, coupled to the "free-market" system, has been an essential and well-recognized feature of "progress" during the twentieth century. Democracy, a concept that has evolved considerably since its inception in Ancient Greece (Dunne, 1992), should be more than either mere procedural democracy ("free and fair elections"), or constitutional democracy (with its focus on legislated civil and political rights). It undoubtedly must include democratic institutions such as a strong, independent judiciary, a free press and many other socially useful institutions such as NGOs. Democracy should also be characterized by greater accountability for decision-making and other mechanisms for dealing with the inequities that are created and exacerbated by social and economic structures and processes.

Although most modern-day democracies have deficiencies, at their best they aim to provide equal rights to a reasonable income, access to education for children and adequate health-care facilities. Few societies can meet these requirements perfectly within the current system of resource distribution. The example in the wealthiest nation (the USA) of exclusion of almost 20% of its population from adequate health coverage reveals the difficulty of achieving the goals of true modern democracy (Wallerstein, 1999). Understanding such failure also requires insight into the fact that democratization at the global level is not always seen as being in the best interests of capitalist countries (Dunne & Wheeler, 1999; Royal Danish Ministry of Foreign Affairs, 2000; Ralph, 2001).

While it has been argued by the Royal Danish Ministry of Foreign Affairs (2000) that the forces of economic globalization are eroding democracy, four reasons are advanced for why the future world community needs to be more equitably and meaningfully democratic: (i) keeping the dangers threatening a globalized world under control requires cooperation and commitment of a maximum number of states and other institutions; (ii) the process of globalization is in need of control and orientation, notably in its financial and economic facets – more freedom does not mean more equity or equality; (iii) peace and cooperation will only prevail over conflict and wars through shared values of greater scope and depth; and (iv) a set of reasons can be advanced justifying the search for a global democratic community as the only morally and politically acceptable form of social organization.

As democratic market regimes have varied enormously geographically and historically, four valid criteria have been offered by the Royal Danish Ministry of Foreign Affairs for assessing the quality of a democracy: (i) economic participation of all in a wide range of productive activities; (ii) economic justice (fair rewards for activities); (iii) economic morality (addressing the behavior of all actors in the market economy – including public authorities); and (iv) economic moderation (regulation) – one of the most difficult virtues to achieve in a market economy. Achieving better quality democracies is a challenge for all countries, including those that already consider themselves to be stable democracies.

It should also be noted that while sustained economic growth has been achieved over many decades in China this has not been associated with increasing freedom, respect for human rights or other features of open societies in the West, but rather with what has been called Leninist corporatism (Hutton, 2008).

Environmental ethics

As realization grows regarding the impact on the planet of the over sixfold increase in world population and the thirtyfold plus increase in annual energy consumption over the past 150 years, we are increasingly coming to accept the vital need to respect and protect our common environment. Globalization of the world economy, coupled with the desire of emerging economies, like China and India, to emulate wastefully consumptive and unsustainable living standards have adversely affected the environment by encouraging the unrestrained use of natural resources and through pollution of rivers, soil and air in countries where legislation is less stringent or is not enforced.

Such environmental abuse has potentially profoundly adverse effects on health and human well-being (Low & Gleason, 1998; Maslin, 2008; McMichael et al., 2008). In this context the perspective of public health ethics must be extended beyond the local to include the global. Environmental and ecological ethics thus have important contributions to make to the study of global bioethics, as originally recognized by Van Renselaar Potter (1998). Indeed bioethics had its origins in these conceptions before it was focused on interpersonal relationships between doctor–patient spheres by dominant American bioethics groups.

Now more than ever before the evolving economic crisis has made it clear that there is a need for cooperation and some economic regulation to supplement the competitive forces that promoted magnificent progress over several centuries but now threaten to annihilate life on our planet. An alteration in the spectrum of concern from one narrowly focused on ourselves (an anthropocentric ethic) towards a broader spectrum that embraces concern for the environment on which all life depends (an ecocentric ethic) has become crucial. The challenge is to prevent an unmitigated, market-driven, global monoculture, that treats life and nature (including animals) as exploitable, from eclipsing a broader moral vision of the good life (Fox & Rolin, 2001).

Solidarity

The emphasis on the US version of strong individualism in association with neo-liberal economic policies in recent decades has deflected attention from the need to belong to, and contribute to communities. However, while there has been considerable erosion of support for the notion of civic society in some quarters, civil society organizations have mushroomed throughout the world and have become very influential in both health and environmental discourses.

A central aspect of the tension between rugged individualism and social democracy relates to the conception of the self – what it means to be a self-determining person. For strong individualists, the conception of the self emphasizes individual rights (especially civil and political rights), unconstrained personal freedom and a society structured on the basis of free association of such individuals. This version of liberty, with responsibility exclusively to the self, contrasts with the view of social democracy that emphasizes individuals as arising from, and being shaped by, their societies with the individual freedom to choose embedded in social attachments; and whose social and economic rights acknowledge solidarity as a balance between rights and responsibilities to themselves and others (Taylor, 1989).

But even solidarity is not a monolithic concept, and does not need to be linked to political philosophies. For example, within the theoretical construct of the African value system, solidarity takes on a perspective that contrasts significantly with the western notion (Louw, 2004). The African conception of democracy embraces a strong desire to deliberate and to reach consensus through dialogue. Canadian First Nations' values resemble African values – and those of other indigenous people – and emphasize holism,

pluralism, autonomy within community, a balance between the mental, physical and spiritual aspects of life, stewardship over nature and respect for the integrity of the human body after death. Healing requires spirituality and relationships between all of the above. The African concept of ubuntu, meaning "I am because we are," epitomizes these values. The real challenge is how to achieve wide adoption of, and adherence, to this concept.

Richard Rorty argues that solidarity is not discovered by reflection and reasoning, but rather by increasing our sensitivity (empathy) to the pain, suffering and humiliation of others. Such sensitivity, he argues, would make it difficult to marginalize "the other" (Rorty, 1989). Progress towards achieving solidarity requires humility. Humility and arrogance involve general attitudes to one's place in the world and to whether or not one considers oneself subject to the same constraints of morality as other rational beings. Superior intelligence, exquisite beauty, great wealth and high social status, as well as fundamentalist religious beliefs, can lead to the arrogant attitudes that allow some to try to impose their will or way of life on others.

In a world characterized more by arrogance than by humility, a world in which the lives of some are considered to be of infinite value while the lives of others are considered irrelevant and dispensable, there is a great need for empathy and humility in order to promote solidarity and mutual caring. More recently solidarity has been advocated as a (new) ethic for global health policy (Harmon, 2006). This realization and the description by Jonathan Glover of how moral imagination is needed to protect our moral identity and to prevent moral, human responses to atrocities from being eclipsed by ideology, tribalism or distance (Glover, 2001) brings us back full circle to the respect for dignity and universal ethical principles with which this section began.

Extending the bioethics discourse in a globalized world

Until the 1960s, discussions about ethics were largely confined to philosophical and theological studies. Advances in technology and medicine, together with increased concern for individual rights and freedoms, led to a new bioethics in which theologians, philosophers, lawyers and other scholars engaged in a public discourse on applied ethics. Initially, this favored

135

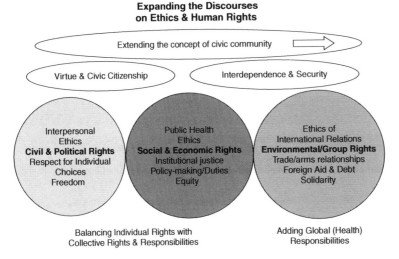

Expanding the Discourses on Ethics & Human Rights

Figure 11.1 Expanding the discourses on ethics and human rights. From Benatar *et al.* (2003).

biomedical issues at the level of individual health – for example death and dying, reproductive medicine and research ethics.

Since the birth of modern bioethics in the 1960s, the world has changed profoundly. Widening economic disparities, rapid population growth, the emergence of new infectious diseases, escalating ecological degradation, numerous local and regional wars, a stockpile of nuclear weapons, massive dislocations of people, advances in science and technology with profound implications for individuals and populations, and, most recently, new terrorist threats to life have demonstrated how interconnected we all are (Singer, 2002). While the bioethics discourse has remained largely focused on interpersonal relationships and is rather parochial, especially in the USA (Fox & Swazey, 2008), new bioethics discourses are emerging in the fields of public health (Nixon *et al.*, 2008) and global health (Green *et al.*, 2008).

Growing global instability and threats from the widening gulf between the world's haves and have-nots call for new ways of thinking and acting. Distinctions between domestic and foreign policy have become blurred, and public health, even in the most privileged nations, is more closely linked than ever to health and disease in impoverished countries. The need for coherence between domestic and foreign policy was acknowledged by President Clinton when he declared HIV/AIDS a global emergency, and also by subsequent endeavors to foster a global response to this pandemic. This has become even more crucial in the face of an impending influenza epidemic and climate change.

Now, more than ever before, local action must be linked to a new global health ethics based on shared values to help make the world a more stable place. Such a new approach could facilitate transformation of current ideas about governance, the global political economy, and relations between countries. A framework that combines an understanding of global interdependence with enlightened, long-term self-interest has the potential to produce a broad spectrum of beneficial outcomes, especially in the area of global health. An extended public debate, promoted by building capacity for this process through a multidisciplinary approach to ethics in education and daily life, could be the driving force for such change. Interest in health and ethics should be extended beyond the micro-level of interpersonal relationships/individual health to include ethical considerations regarding public/population health at the level of institutions, nations and international relations (Figure 11.1)

The way forward for global health ethics – five transformational approaches

A global agenda must thus extend beyond the rhetoric of universal human rights to include greater attention to duties, social justice and interdependence. Health and ethics provide a framework within which such an agenda could be developed and promoted across borders and cultures. The relatively new interdisciplinary field of bioethics, when expanded in scope to embrace widely shared foundational values, could make a valuable contribution to the improvement of global health by providing the space for such a discussion to occur. Our vision, explicated in detail previously and summarized succinctly here, offers a way forward for global health reform through five transformational approaches.

Developing a global state of mind

First, developing a global state of mind about the world and our place in it is perhaps the most crucial element in the development of an ethic for global health. Achieving this will require an understanding of the world as an unstable complex system (Wallerstein, 1999), the balancing of individual goods and social goods, and the avoidance of harm to weak/poor nations through economic and other forms of exploitation that frustrate the achievement of human rights and well-being. Wallerstein predicted that "the first half of the 21st century will … be far more difficult, more unsettling, and yet more open (to change) than anything we have known in the 20th century." He argued that fundamental change towards a substantively rational system would embrace both democratic and egalitarian principles as intimately and inseparably linked to each other.

Michael MccGwire also outlines a rationale for new ways of thinking in a world that has changed so much (McccGwire, 2001a, 2001b). He explicates the context in which the current "Adversarial National Security Program" evolved over the past 60 years and has now "lost its way." He argues convincingly that a paradigm shift is necessary towards what he calls a "Co-operative Global Security Program" – because times and threats have changed – and that progress will only be possible if attitudes about relationships, diplomacy, power and security can be reshaped.

The emergence of a multifaceted social movement, "globalization from below" (in which people at the grassroots around the world link up to impose their own needs and interests on the process of globalization), illustrates additional pathways to constructive change (Brecher et al., 2000).

Promoting long-term self-interest

Second, in arguing that it is both desirable and necessary to develop a global mindset in health ethics, we suggest that this change need not be based merely on altruism, and that promoting long-term self-interest is also essential if we acknowledge that lives across the world are inextricably interlinked by forces that powerfully shape health and well-being. As an example, consider the long-term self-interest and mutual interdependence in the face of emerging new infectious diseases and microbial antibiotic resistance (Garrett, 1994; Benatar, 2001). Acknowledgment that health has important security implications for US Foreign Policy has provided space for an argument that improving the health status of people in developing countries makes both moral and strategic sense (Kassalow, 2001).

Striking a balance between optimism and pessimism

There are both pessimistic and optimistic viewpoints about prospects for achieving widely shared progress through current globalization trends. Both views are valid from different perspectives. As pessimism leads to inaction, and unjustified optimism to ineffectiveness, it is necessary to strike an appropriate balance between these stances. This will require a platform for dialog among stakeholders, and a space where people can share different views about globalization. A broad conception of global bioethics offers a basis for such a space.

The concerns of pessimists are that, in our quest for material possessions and economic "rationality," we have lost the ability to empathize with others and that we no longer value virtue or the spiritual and existential aspects of life. Such skepticism extends to distrust of the free market and to questioning whether democratic values are being appropriately applied. Recent events validate such pessimism.

The optimistic view accepts disparities as the starting point, sees no gap between self-interest and the common good, considers it possible to have empathy without experience, and has faith that minimalist democratic values and free-market forces will inevitably promote public goods. Although optimism is now much reduced some middle path must be identified between polar perspectives.

The problem is not one of pro- and anti-globalization or of individual freedom versus community solidarity within two different languages about politics. As Sandbrook has pointed out globalization cannot be avoided. It is an integral aspect of a world in which the clock cannot be turned back on advances in technology, communication, production and transport. However, a distinction needs to be made between neo-liberal globalization and social-democratic globalization (Sandbrook, 2000).

Developing capacity

Fourth, our vision for promoting an ethic for global health also features the development of capacity and a commitment to a broader discourse on ethics propagated through centers regionally and globally networked in growing and supportive North–South partnerships (Kickbush, 2000; Fidler, 2008). Recognition of responsibility to change our world for the better should also require that multinational corporations and national governments appreciate their new roles in enabling the correct choice of direction (at a time of vital "bifurcation" in world history) to build a better future.

Achieving widespread access to public goods

Fifth, achieving widespread access to education, basic subsistence needs, and work requires collective action, including financing (to make sure they are produced), and good governance (to ensure their optimum distribution and use) (Soros, 2002). Global public goods involve more than one country or region of the world. The current international system is very effective at stimulating the production of private goods (e.g. the role of the World Trade Organization in promoting international trade) but not at the production of public goods – for example education for all children, and the realization of labor rights and human rights.

Conclusions

It would seem that nothing has changed since Lester Pearson noted over 35 years ago that "there can be no peace, no security, nothing but ultimate disaster, when a few rich countries with a small minority of the world's people alone have access to the brave, and frightening, new world of technology, science, and of high material living standards, while the large majority live in deprivation and want, cut off from opportunities of full economic development; but with expectations and aspirations aroused far beyond the hope of realizing them" (Pearson, 1972).

However, it is arguable that there may still be a faint glimmer of hope that such progress is possible. We have argued here that increasing global instability calls for new ways of thinking and acting together with an extended public debate (promoted by building capacity for this process through a multidisciplinary approach to ethics in education and daily life) in the hope that this could be a driving force to make such progress possible.

Developing sustainable well-being for many more people globally requires going beyond economic growth. Constructing new ways of achieving economic redistribution is the key to resolving many global problems. If wealthy people progressively care less for the lives of those whom they relegate to living under inhumane conditions, the lives of the wealthy will become more meaningless and inhuman to the underprivileged masses. This global trap in which neither rich nor poor care if millions of the other group should die is the recipe for ongoing conflict and unnecessary loss of life on a grand scale. While economic equality is an impossible goal, narrowing of the current gap is surely well within our grasp. Fairer trade rules, debt relief, various forms of taxation, such as the Tobin tax on currency trades across borders (that could generate US$100–300 billion per year), prevention of tax evasion and environmental taxes have been suggested as means of facilitating the development of the solidarity required for peaceful co-existence in a complex world.

We propose that global health ethics if combined with political support for cosmopolitan approaches to citizenship and common goods offers the space to pursue imaginative agendas for change towards a fairer, more regulated, economic system that could help catalyze crucial improvements in global health.

Acknowledgments

This chapter is based, with permission, on Benatar, S. R., Daar, A. & Singer, P. A. (2003) Global health ethics: the rationale for mutual caring. *International Affairs* **79**, 107–138 and Benatar, S. R., Daar, A. & Singer, P. A. (2005). Global health ethics: the need for an expanded discourse. *PLoS Medicine* **2** (7), 587–59.

References

Amnesty International. United States of America: Human dignity denied – Torture and accountability in the war on terror. www.amnesty.org/en/library/info/AMR51/146/2004/en (Accessed December 5, 2009).

Benatar, S. R. (1998). Global disparities in health and human rights. *American Journal of Public Health* **98**, 295–300.

Benatar, S. R. (2001). The coming catastrophe in international health: an analogy with lung cancer. *International Journal* LV 1(4), 611–31.

Benatar, S. R. (2005a). The HIV/AIDS pandemic: a sign of instability in a complex global system. In A. Van Niekerk & A. Kopelman (Eds.), *Ethics and AIDS in Africa: the challenge to our thinking* (pp. 71–83). Cape Town: David Philip Press.

Benatar, S. R. (2005b). Moral imagination: the missing component in global health. *Public Library of Science Medicine* **2** (12), e400. www.plosmedicine.org/article/info%3Adoi%2F10.1371%2Fjournal.pmed.0020400 (Accessed December 5, 2009).

Benatar, S. R. & Doyal, L. (2009). Human rights abuses: towards balancing two perspectives. *International Journal of Health Services* **39**, 37–59.

Benatar, S. R., Daar, A. & Singer, P. A. (2003). Global health ethics: the rationale for mutual caring. *International Affairs* **79**, 107–38.

Benatar, S. R., Gill, S. & Bakker, I. (2009). Making progress in global health: the need for new paradigms. *International Affairs* **85**, 347–71.

Brecher, J., Costello, T. & Smith, B. (2000). *Globalisation from Below: The Power of Solidarity*. Cambridge, MA: South End Press.

Brock, G. (2008). Taxation and global justice: closing the gap between theory and practice. *Journal of Social Philosophy* **39**, 161–84.

Brock, G. (2009). *Global Justice: A Cosmopolitan Account*. Oxford: Oxford University Press.

Buchanan, A. (2000). Rawls's Law of Peoples: rules for a vanquished Westphalian world. *Ethics* **110**, 697–721.

Chan, M. (2008) Impact of the global financial and economic crisis on health: Statement by WHO Director-General Dr Margaret Chan. 12 November. www.who.int/mediacentre/news/statements/2008/s12/en/index.html (Accessed December 5, 2009).

Chapman, A. R. (1996). Reintegrating rights and responsibilities. In K. W. Hunter & T. C. Mack (Eds.), *International Rights and Responsibilities for the Future* (pp. 3–28). Westport, CT: Praeger.

Daniels, N. & Sabin, J. (2002) *Setting Limits Fairly: Can We Learn to Share Medical Resources?* Oxford: Oxford University Press.

Daniels, N., Light, D. & Caplan, R. (1996). *Benchmarks of Fairness for Health Care Reform*. Oxford: Oxford University Press.

Donnelly, J. (1998). Human rights: a new standard of civilization? *International Relations* **74**, 1–24.

Doyal, L. & Gough, I. (1991). *A Theory of Human Need*. London: Macmillan.

Dunne, T. & Wheeler, N. J. (Eds.) (1999). *Human Rights in Global Politics*. Cambridge: Cambridge University Press.

Dunne, J. (Ed.) (1992). *Democracy: The Unfinished Journey. 508BC–AD1993*. Oxford: Oxford University Press.

Fact sheet on Tobin taxes. www.ceedweb.org/iirp/factsheet.htm (Accessed December 5, 2009).

Falk, R. A. (2000). *Human Rights Horizons: The Pursuit of Justice in a Globalising World*. New York: Routledge.

Farmer, P. (2003). *Pathologies of Power: Health, Human Rights, and the New War on the Poor*. Berkeley, CA: University of California Press.

Farmer, P. (2008). Challenging opportunities: the road ahead for health and human rights. *Health and Human Rights* **10**, 5–19.

Fidler, D. P. (2008). After the revolution: global health politics in a time of economic crisis and threatening future trends. *Global Health Governance* II (2) http://ghgj.org/fidler2.2afterrevoluton.htm (Accessed November 24, 2009).

Fox, M. W. & Rolin, B. E. (2001). *Bringing Life to Ethics: Global Bioethics for a Human Society*. New York, NY: SUNY Press.

Fox, R. C. & Swazey, J. (2008). *Observing Bioethics*. Oxford: Oxford University Press.

Garrett, L. (1994). *The Coming Plague: Newly Emerging Diseases in a World out of Balance*. New York, NY: Farrar, Strauss and Giroux.

Garrett, L. (2007). The challenge of global health. *Foreign Affairs* **86**, 1–17

Girling, J. (1997). *Corruption, Capitalism and Democracy*. London: Routledge.

Glover, J. (2001). *Humanity: a Moral History of the Twentieth Century*. New Haven, CT: Yale University Press.

Governance and Social Development Resource Centre (2009). *Helpdesk Research Report: The Impact of Financial Crises on Conflict and Social Stability 05.03.09*. www.carleton.ca/cifp/app/serve.php/1231.pdf (Accessed November 24, 2009).

Green, R. M., Donovan, A. & Jauss, S. A. (Eds.) (2008). *Global Bioethics: Issues of Conscience for the 21st Century*. Oxford: Oxford University Press.

Harmon, S. (2006). Solidarity: A (new) ethic for global health policy. *Health Care Analysis* **14**, 215–36.

Hosie, V. (1992). The third world as a philosophical problem. *Social Research* **52**, 227–262.

Hutton, W. (2008). *The Writing on the Wall. China and the West in the 21st Century*. London: Abacus.

Kakutani, M. Inside the meltdown: financial ruin and the race to contain it. *New York Times*, July 21, 2009. www.nytimes.com/2009/07/21/books/21kakutani.html?_r=1 (Accessed December 5, 2009).

Kassalow, J. S. (2001). *Why Health is Important to US Foreign Policy*. New York, NY: Council on Foreign Relations and Milbank Memorial Fund.

Katz, A. (2008). "New global health": A reversal of logic, history and principles. *Social Medicine* **3** (I), 1–3.

Kickbush, I. (2000). The development of international health policies: Accountability intact? *Social Science and Medicine* **51**, 978–89.

Krugman, P. (2009). School for scoundrels. *New York Times*, August 9. www.nytimes.com/2009/08/09/books/review/Krugman-t.html (Accessed November 4, 2009).

Kung, H. (1997). *A Global Ethic for Global Politics and Economics*. Oxford: Oxford University Press.

Leahy, J. (2009). Asia warned of growing poverty. *Financial Times*, June 28. www.ft.com/cms/s/0/3c40ec68-6408-11de-a818-00144feabdc0.html?nclick_check=I (Accessed December 5, 2009).

Louw, D. J. (2004). Ubuntu: An African assessment of the religious other. www.bu.edu/wcp/Papers/Afri/AfriLouw.htm (Accessed November 24, 2009).

Low, N. & Gleeson, B. (1998). *Justice, Society & Nature: an Exploration of Political Ecology*. London: Routledge.

Marmot, M. (2006). Health in an unequal world. *Lancet* **368**, 2081–94.

Maslin, M. (2008). Prognosis for a sick planet. *Clinical Medicine* **8**, 569–72.

MccGwire, M. (2001a). Shifting the paradigm. *International Affairs* 77, 1–28.

MccGwire, M. (2001b). The paradigm that lost its way. *International Affairs* 77, 777–803.

McMichael, A. J., Friel, S., Nyong, A. & Corvalan, C. (2008). Global environmental change and health: impacts, inequalities, and the health sector. *British Medical Journal* 336, 191–4.

Milner, B. (2009). Africa's heavy toll. *Globe and Mail*, Wednesday, June **10**, p. 4.

Navarro, V. (2007). *Neoliberalism, Globalization and Inequalities: Consequences for Health and Quality of Life*. Amityville, NY: Baywood.

Nixon, S. A., Upshur, R., Robertson, A. *et al.* (2008). Public health ethics. In T. M. Bailey, T. Caulfield & N. M. Ries (Eds.), *Public Health Law & Policy in Canada* (2nd edn.) (pp. 39–59). Canada: Lexis Nexis Butterworths.

Pearson, L. B. (1972). Lester B Pearson's public address at St Martin-in-the-Fields, London June 13, 1972 on the occasion of the presentation to him of the Victor Gollancz Humanity Award. www.unac.org/en/link_learn/canada/pearson/speechgollancz.asp (Accessed December 6, 2009).

People's Health Movement, Medact and the Global Equity Gauge Alliance (2005). *Global Health Watch 2005–2006*. London: Zed Books.

People's Health Movement, Medact and the Global Equity Gauge Alliance (2008). *Global Health Watch 2: An Alternative World Health Report*. London: Zed Books.

Peter, F. & Evans, T. (2001). Ethical dimensions of health equity. In T. Evans, M. Whitehead, F. Diderichsen,

A. Bhuyia & M. Wirth (Eds.), *Challenging Inequities in Health: From Ethics to Action* (pp. 24–33). New York: Oxford University Press.

Pogge, T. (2002). *World Poverty and Human Rights*. Cambridge: Polity Press.

Pogge, T. (2005). Recognized and violated by international law: the human rights of the global poor. *Leiden International Law Journal* **18**, 717–745.

Potter, Van R. (1998). *Global Bioethics: Building on the Leopold Legacy*. East Lansing, MI: Michigan State University Press.

Powers, M. & Faden, R. (2006). *Social Justice: The Moral Foundations of Public Health and Public Health Policy*. New York, NY: Oxford University Press.

Ralph, J. (2001). American democracy and democracy promotion. *International Affairs* 77 (I), 129–140.

Rieff, D. (1999). The precarious triumph of human rights. *The New York Times Magazine* August 8, 37–41.

Robertson, A. (1998). Critical reflection on the politics of need: implications for public health. *Social Science and Medicine* 47, 1419–1430.

Rorty, R. (1989). *Contingency, Irony and Solidarity*. Cambridge: Cambridge University Press.

Royal Danish Ministry for Foreign Affairs (2000). *Building a Global Community: Globalisation and the Common Good*. Copenhagen: Royal Danish Ministry for Foreign Affairs.

Sandbrook, R. (2000). Globalisation and the limits of neoliberal development doctrine. *Third World Quarterly* **21**(6), 1071–1080.

Sen, A. (1999). *Development as Freedom*. New York, NY: Anchor Books.

Singer, P. (2002). *One World: The Ethics of Globalisation*. New Haven, CT: Yale University Press.

Soros, G. (2002). *On Globalisation*. New York: Public Affairs.

Taylor, C. (1989). *Sources of the Self: the Making of Modern Identity*. Cambridge, MA: Harvard University Press.

Teeple, G. (2000). *Globalisation and the Decline of Social Reform: Into the 21st Century*. Auroria, ON: Garamond Press.

Wallerstein, I. (1999). *The End of the World as We Know it: Social Science for the 21st Century*. Minneapolis, MN: University of Minnesota Press.

World Health Organization (WHO) (2009). *The Financial Crisis and Global Health: Report of a High-Level Consultation*. Geneva: WHO. January 19 www.who.int/mediacentre/events/meetings/2009_financial_crisis_report_en_.pdf (Accessed December 6, 2009).

Section 3

Analyzing some reasons for poor health

Chapter

12

Trade and health: the ethics of global rights, regulation and redistribution

Meri Koivusalo

Concerns about health are not new aspects of trade policies, but have long been part of trade negotiations. It is also known that failures in public health policies can substantially and adversely affect trade. The economic costs of global epidemics have been rising sharply, but more important is the point that prevention of epidemics requires not only functional public health measures at national borders, but in essence functional health systems.[1] Health policies and trade policies have mutually compatible and strengthening aspects, but there are also crucial and important conflicts of interests. In this chapter I outline ethical issues and questions that relate to these conflicts and the importance of considering trade policies not merely as transnational policies, but also as representing a form of global legal development and governance in relation to rights, redistribution and regulatory measures. These have consequences not only across countries and amongst international organizations and actors, but also for the balance between public policies and interests and those of national and increasingly global corporate actors and interest groups.

In assessing the implications of trade on health policies we can distinguish two different components. The first is the impacts of trade upon determinants of health and health outcomes. The main and core interest here relates to the *magnitude of flows of goods, services, people or capital* with positive and negative implications being assessed in relation to these flows and their influence both on health outcomes and on how national health systems function. The second, and often less clearly articulated aspect of trade, is that of *policy space* and the ways in which decisions and priorities made

in the sphere of trade will affect the regulatory scope and measures applied in health policies and to national health systems. I have earlier addressed this feature of trade policies as "trade creep" (Koivusalo, 1999), and (with Labonté and Schrecker) have defined policy space as the freedom, scope and mechanisms that governments choose, to design and implement public policies to fulfill their aims (Koivusalo *et al.*, 2009). Although policy space is used mostly in relation to national policies it can also be used to address the issue of policy space for health in regional and global level regulatory and policy work.

Two cross-cutting issues

In addition we can identify two important cross-cutting issues concerning the ethics of trade and health policies.

How, by whom and within what kind of framework, are policies and decisions made regarding health and trade?

This issue of governance and politics of health and trade applies not only to where decisions are made, but also raises questions about the legitimacy and accountability of decisions made and those who make them. Health and trade-related concerns have, for example, become heated issues within two recent global negotiation processes under WHO auspices – pandemics (sharing of viruses, and public health), and innovation and intellectual property rights. While health, trade and human rights issues have in particular been considered in the context of access to medicines, crucial and substantially broader governance questions relate to trade and health at both national and global levels in relation to rights, regulation and redistribution as a result of trade policies.

---

[1] The World Health Report 2007 brings up estimates of costs of epidemics as well as further discussing issues that relate to their prevention (WHO, 2007).

An earlier version of this work has appeared: Koivusalo, M. (2006). The impact of economic globalisation on health. *Theoretical Medicine and Bioethics* **27** (1), 13–34.

In terms of redistribution the issue is not merely whether and how trade in health services affects distribution of financing, but also how more systemic implications that result from trade policies and regulatory measures set the conditions of overall availability and use of public resources for health, and how trade relates to social inequalities. Included here are systemic issues in relation to equity aspects of health and health systems, as well as implications of trade policies for social inequalities, social security, social rights and regulation within countries.

Globalization and global trade policies have been promoted under the assumption that "globalization is good for the poor," however the basis of this claim as well as the implications of trade policies on social equity have come under criticism. Birdsall (2006) has emphasized the inherent un-equalizing impact of global markets. The current process of globalization and promotion of trade liberalization and protection of intellectual property rights need to be considered in the context of distribution of resources, impacts on social interventions or poverty reduction measures, and the need for stronger global governance to coordinate social policy measures and interventions.

The World Health Organization (WHO) has legitimacy (in view of successful negotiations on International Health Regulations, the Tobacco Framework Agreement experience and on the basis of its constitutional obligations and scope) to take a more proactive role in global public health law so as to ensure that health considerations remain high on the global agenda (WHO, 2007). Areas of particular concern with respect to governance include pharmaceutical policies, the required relevance of health priorities in research and innovation, control of epidemics, ensuring availability of vaccines, limiting unethical international recruitment practices through binding regulations, and implementing global strategies that would help countries to limit, tax or use public policies to regulate and guide consumption of unhealthy foods and drinks, including alcohol. A crucial governance problem is that while trade policies are implemented on the basis of international legal agreements with the additional power of the World Trade Organization (WTO) dispute settlement process and the potential for trade sanctions, global regulatory measures driven by health considerations have not become strengthened at the same pace, and at worst become further compromised through interest group inclusion and lobbying.

What can be traded and how?

The second cross-cutting aspect deals with more traditional public health issues, such as what should be tradable and how to deal with trade on products hazardous to health. One example of ethically problematic trade is organ trafficking. Anthropological studies have documented the nature and extent of trade and trafficking (Scheper-Hughes, 2000), and a formal United Nations and European Council study has now placed the issue on the United Nations agenda with a call for a new binding international treaty to prevent trafficking in organs, tissues and cells (OTC), protect victims and prosecute offenders. The study draws a distinction between so-called more widespread "transplant tourism" on one hand, and trafficking of humans for this purpose on the other, while calling for the prohibition of financial gain from the human body or its parts as the basis of legislation on organ transplants (Caplan *et al.*, 2009). The line between more acceptable commercialized body enhancement and surgery and that of human cloning, transplants or more ethically problematic areas of trade is likely to be thin. This requires that as part of global trade in services, negotiations regarding the health implications of practices within ethically problematic areas should be considered and taken seriously above mere business considerations within the sector.

A traditional concern with respect to trade in goods is the spread of infectious diseases. Here International Health Regulations set the context of interaction between health and trade (Fidler, 1997). This is also the most traditional and historical context of health and trade relations. However, infectious diseases are not the only concern. Contamination of consumer products or inclusion of substances dangerous to health into products have been of concern in relation to trade in consumer goods, such as toothpaste or toys, where prospects for domestic regulation could become increasingly complex because of international production chains (Ofodile, 2009). In pharmaceuticals and other health-technology products this issue is further complicated by the dangers of not including the correct substances or selling of otherwise substandard products. The large difference between sales price and production cost makes pharmaceuticals an increasingly attractive area for counterfeiters. There is a broader question of how to ensure quality control of global trade in goods, including pharmaceuticals, through regulatory measures both at national and global levels.

However, counterfeiting is also emphasized in the context of patent and trademark infringements and enforcement (Sell, 2008).

Impact of trade flows in goods, services and capital on health outcomes

The general assumption in the sphere of economic and trade policies has been that as long as globalization increases economic growth, it will improve well-being and health. An increase in average income is expected to provide better access to food and care. This assumption remains at the core of claims that economic globalization is beneficial to health. However, the real implications of such expectations are dependent on whether economic growth takes place, how this is distributed within the society, what implications this has for existing public policies and the scope for regulatory measures on health and social determinants of health.

The impact of trade policies on health status of populations differs from the impact of health policies on health systems. In practice a large share of impacts on health takes place outside health systems by influencing the social determinants of health. Food security, access to food and quality of food are all influenced by trade policies, although impacts of trade policies depend on what basis food production is governed and regulated in the first place.

Two main types of ethical concerns can be distinguished: First, those emphasizing insufficient or partial liberalization of trade in agricultural products (including inequities related to unfair trade practices such as unfair use of agricultural subsidies). Second, there are ethical concerns about (a) the impact of the trade liberalization process on agricultural products and food security, (b) the power and roles of commercial interests in the field, and (c) the relative position and roles of consumers, types of farmers, and the food industry in a more liberalized trade regime. While in relation to trade policies it is generally assumed that liberalization brings benefits, in reality the assessment of the consequences of the liberalization of trade range from more positive views (Anderson & Martin, 2005), to critical assessments of winners and losers in more liberalized markets of agricultural products (FAO, 2003). The global food and economic crises have also contributed to the reiteration of rights to food, social security aspects of food security and to efforts to improve global governance on food policy (FAO, 2009).

Food security is an essential concern in the light of an emerging focus on malnutrition and hunger as a result of crises in terms of availability, access to and prices of basic food commodities (FAO, 2009). However, in food policy, changes in agricultural subsidies or policy reforms are not the only areas with trade implications. Powerful transnational actors often benefit more from liberalized trade, as they can reap the benefits of substantial capital investments in technology and other measures that increase output and lower prices. One example is the presence of large agribusiness actors with their bargaining power and influence on lowering producer prices and accumulating profits higher up in the value chain of the final products (Fitter & Kaplinsky, 2001; FAO, 2003). While current global attention has focused more on malnutrition and availability of food, an underlying concern over nutritional quality of products available is also likely to remain an issue. The complex relationship between trade liberalization and dietary transition is not only an issue of market responses to consumer needs, but is also mediated through the impact on supply chain and public policies as well as the role of advertising and promotion of processed and particular types of foods, and changing dietary patterns resulting from the influence and growth of global transnational food processors, fast-food companies and supermarkets (Lang, 2004; Hawkes et al., 2009). Whether and to what extent within a country, or population, transition takes place towards less healthy diets is also dependent on initial quality of diets and on social and public policies that shape access to food and nutritional contents of diets within societies. However, the scope for public policies is in part also dependent on the national and global policy space for health that is possible in a globalizing world.

Increasing mobility of goods tends to include goods of a hazardous nature – in particular alcohol, tobacco and products with high fat and sugar content or low nutritional value. Empirical findings support the expectation of increased domestic consumption of tobacco as a result of increased trade, and suggest that less wealthy countries may be more vulnerable than wealthier countries to the impact of trade liberalization (Bettcher et al., 2000).

The impact of trade policies on health policy

The impact of globalization on health policy is not the same as on health outcomes as the former includes the scope and nature of regulatory measures that governments can impose as well as the implications for costs and availability of health services and treatments. The more individualized and market-led health policies are, the less likely it is that health policies would become restricted by trade policies. Thus, the impact of globalization on national health policies strongly depends on the extent to which such policies regulate or restrict interests and priorities of commercial actors or markets in a more general sense.

Even in a more liberalized and individualized context there remains a role for public regulation in standard setting and labelling of products to promote consumer choice. It is likely that labelling of products will be of greater importance in the context of more consumer-led health policies both in monitoring the accuracy of health claims and adding health-related information or warnings on product packages. Trade concerns over legislation in other countries with respect to health-related issues have also been raised in the Committee on Technical Barriers to Trade, where, for example, the European Commission, USA and Australian delegations raised their industries' concerns over labeling requirements on certain snack foods proposed by the Ministry of Public Health of Thailand to prevent malnutrition among those children with poor eating habits (WTO, 2006, 2008).

The impact of trade policies on health policies further depends on three main channels: first, how health-related standard setting and health-based regulatory measures outside the health sector are affected: second, the regulatory implications for resources and service use within the health sector; and third, access to knowledge and costs of innovation. The realization of these is in part dependent on the ways in which different national interests and trade policy priorities are dealt with in relation to commercial export interests and willingness to utilize provisions of trade agreements or limit the scope of these agreements to allow policy space for health. Examples of this type of effort with respect to TRIPS would include utilizing flexibilities of the agreement to enable access to medicines as well as interpreting the agreement in favor of public health measures. In trade in services this type of measure would include caution with those trade and investment agreements that could exclude health services or limit the extent that health services, health insurance services and respective aspects of state aids or government procurement are included in such agreements.

Health-related regulation and standard-setting

The most traditional context of trade policy implications is within health-related arguments and standard-setting and there are several settlement cases between countries under dispute. The General Agreement on Tariffs and Trade (GATT) covers international trade in goods and includes measures to protect public health. However, the basis for how these policies can be achieved is regulated by the Agreement on Sanitary and Phytosanitary (SPS) Measures (1994). A crucial issue in these disputes is whether measures taken are legitimate and necessary or "protectionism in disguise." It is not surprising that disputes concerning the use of public health provisions have also arisen between Europe and North America – for example in the case of contesting hormone use in cattle raising or the European ban of asbestos. There is also a line of dispute in settlement cases concerning tobacco and alcohol. Although restriction of availability and taxation are known to be effective strategies to reduce consumption of products hazardous to health (Yach & Bettcher, 2000; Babor *et al.*, 2003), these strategies tend to be more vulnerable to trade disputes in comparison to more individualized or less market-restrictive interventions. Another related issue is the role and relevance of the Agreement on Technical Barriers to Trade (TBT), which covers all industrial and agricultural products, and has implications for domestic regulation of quality of products such as toys. There are also broader implications of trade agreements for the implementation of domestic measures; for example, if a country would restrict or ban imports of goods from particular countries or producers on the grounds of health and quality concerns (Ofodile, 2009).

While the sufficient capacity of the SPS Agreement to tackle domestic health protection interests has been emphasized, in the light of the potential hijacking of domestic health-related regulatory measures by national interest groups (Epps, 2008), there still remains a broader concern over problems to regulate some production practices and how to address issues with scientific uncertainty or disagreement. Another analysis emphasizes that, to date, dispute settlement cases have focused on health and environmental considerations without threat to national sovereignty, but that in the settlement process the Appellate Body has been more supportive of these health considerations than the actual Panels (Kelly, 2007). This suggests that in practice the Appellate Body has sought to neutralize the more politically problematic cases. However, the focus on safety of traded products does nothing to help regulatory challenges that relate to inappropriate production practices, which have been part of the hormones-in-cattle dispute settlement case between European Union and USA/Canada (WTO, 1998).

Veggeland & Borgen (2005) have highlighted the problems in the context of the work of the Codex Alimentarius Commission, a joint WHO and Food and Agriculture Organization (FAO) food standard setting organization to which two WTO Agreements refer, as national and commercial trading interests have become reflected more strongly in government stands in Codex since the establishment of the WTO. The question is thus also to what extent strong trading interests have become reflected in the context of national positions and processes with respect to standard-setting. We also need to ask to what extent there might be other conflicts of interests in standard setting and how standards are defined. This perspective is of importance in relation to the role of the International Organization for Standardization (ISO)[2] as a global standard-setting authority, especially if it expands its work further in services, environment and occupational health and safety. In health, attention has already been drawn to the role of the tobacco industry in standard setting for their products within the ISO (Bialious & Yach, 2001).

Health systems and regulation of health services

The General Agreement on Trade in Services (GATS) is of most importance in the field of services negotiations. In terms of health services the impact of GATS has not yet been as visible or as important as movement and migration of health professionals that have taken place as part of a broader globalization process and agenda. In Thailand, for example, external migration of health professionals has occurred without major influence by GATS (Wibulpolprasert, 2004). However, it is clear that this is considered a potential area where services trade could be further liberalized with arguments by proponents of liberalization of services discussing, for example, how in the USA health insurance policies impede trade in health services and the potential savings from sending patients abroad for treatment (Mattoo & Rathindran, 2006).

While the mobility of workforces from poorer countries to rich countries can be seen as a trading opportunity with positive implications for national economies in the form of remittances, the consequences of reduced professional workforces due to external and internal brain drains can be devastating to health systems, in particular in poorer and less resourced areas. A study by the International Labour Organization (ILO) has drawn attention to the role of global recruitment agencies in the process (Kuptsch, 2006). Concerns over the extent and implications of migration for health systems of developing countries has led to the efforts to develop a code within the WHO[3] in addition to the already established several international and national ethical codes with the aim of addressing unethical recruitment practices. An overview on codes of practice and ethical international recruitment has pointed out the limits of ethical codes on their own. Given that despite the introduction of the first ethical guidelines by the Department of Health in the UK in 1999, the outflow increased significantly during the following years, these codes should be viewed more as the initiation of a more ethical process than as a final outcome (Willetts & Martineau, 2004).

Interest in further liberalization of services is now focused in particular on health tourism[4] and mobility of health professionals, in particular provision of services by individuals temporarily in the country.[5] The interest in these areas is currently greater in developing countries, with commercial interests in both health tourism and sending health professionals abroad. Health

---

[2] The ISO is in many ways a hybrid organization that can also be seen as part of global private sector governance with close engagement with business and industries. Its members are national standard-setting agencies, which can be public service agencies or formed by member associations, including companies or representatives of particular industries.

[3] The latest draft code is available as an annex to WHO Executive Board document EB 126/8, available from the WHO website: http://apps.who.int/gb/ebwha/pdf_files/EB126/B126_8-en.pdf.

[4] In GATS Mode 2, consumption of services abroad.

[5] In GATS Mode 4, movement of natural persons from one country to provide a service in another country.

tourism is enabled by the portability of health insurance benefits to other countries, as well as the scope for more commercialized services (such as cosmetic surgery) at the margins, or outside the obligations, of national health systems. Organ trafficking can be seen as the most problematic form of health tourism. Health systems related ethical implications that need to be considered are whether health tourism encourages expansion of the private sector for the use of foreign patients and a decline in services provided for local people or those less able to pay. Unless there is substantial oversupply of health professionals within a country, health tourism tends to draw professionals away from where they are needed and can lead to shortages of those with specific skills because these are in demand in the more commercialized part of the sector.

Another area of interest is cross-border trade[6] in services as new technologies allow images to be transferred through various telemedicine or e-health channels, such as the worldwide web or email. This sector includes selling services in processing and interpretation of scans, X-rays or laboratory samples and specimens. The shifting of clinical trials to developing countries may contribute financial resources and capacities to those countries, but is also likely to draw skilled health personnel to the implementation of clinical trials away from other clinical work. While proponents of the liberalization of trade in health services welcome such developments as a way that developing countries can generate income and the developed world can cut research costs, this process creates both systemic and ethical concerns when health systems become increasingly driven or influenced by the commodification and commercialization of health care.

Trade agreements and in particular GATS also have relevance to domestic policies, including regulation, rights and redistribution within health systems, as a result of what has been agreed on domestic regulation as part of the GATS agreement. However, these implications depend on whether a Member State has included the services sector within its commitments (Fidler *et al.*, 2003; Luff, 2003). The application of requirements for domestic regulation is based on countries choosing to include health services in the context of GATS. Domestic regulation will have implications for licensing of health professionals and regulating health systems more broadly. For example, it is unclear what effect measures for cost-containment would have

in the context of the GATS domestic regulation framework, where these may limit markets or commercial interests. It has been pointed out, for example, that limiting patient choice might be considered as problematic or that cost-containment may not be considered as sufficient grounds for government intervention (Luff, 2003). Concerns over subsidies and in particular equity aspects of health systems have also been raised. While trade in health services is often promoted as a means for more effective health services, a more likely direct consequence is cost escalation as a result of increasing administrative costs, more constrained scope for national regulation and limitations to scope for cost-containment within health systems. The portability of health insurance is one example, where there are pressures to change the basis of reimbursement practices to enable trade (Mattoo & Rathindran, 2006).

Intellectual property rights

Intellectual property rights and their relationship to pharmaceutical policies have been perhaps the most discussed aspect of trade policies globally, and they raise various ethical concerns, including how they relate to human rights. This is reflected in the focus of human rights advocates and special rapporteurs on the terms of particular trade agreements (Hunt, 2006) and in relation to access to medicines in developing countries (United Nations, 2009a). In October 2009 the Human Rights Council unanimously adopted a resolution on access to medicines (United Nations, 2009b). Another issue is how enforcement of intellectual property rights as private rights – as recognized in the preamble of the Trade-Related aspects of Intellectual Property Rights (TRIPS) Agreement – has become an issue within public policies and in the allocation of public resources. In general three main concerns can be raised with respect to health policies and protection of intellectual property rights. The first emphasizes access to knowledge and information; the second focuses on the pricing of new innovations; and the third on incentives that international agreements provide for innovation and, in particular, innovation on the basis of health needs. These are issues that affect health policies in all countries; however, global policies with respect to intellectual property rights are mostly dealt with in relation to the needs of developing countries and increasingly also in relation to bilateral agreements reaching beyond the TRIPS agreement.

While concerns of developing countries have become more legitimate in relation to the TRIPS agreement, bilateral agreements have further changed

---

[6] In GATS Mode 1, cross-border trade in services.

the ground for debates in introducing provisions and measures that were not considered as part of multilateral negotiations (Fink & Reichenmiller, 2005; Roffe & Spennemann, 2006). Ethical issues at the core of both health and trade policies have also been dealt with as part of the WHO Intergovernmental Working Group (IGWG) negotiations on intellectual property rights and innovation as well as on pandemic influenza preparedness: sharing of influenza viruses and access to vaccines and other benefits (WHA, 2008; WHO, 2009a). In the IGWG negotiations a global strategy was finalized, covering a variety of issues, for example, to promote active participation of health representatives in trade negotiations and strengthening mechanisms for ethical review and principles in clinical trials (WHA, 2008). In the area of pandemics, slow progress in negotiations in late 2009 reached the stage where agreement has been gained on sharing viruses, but not yet in terms of access to vaccines and other benefits. A broader ethical concern over access to vaccines and technologies focuses on how burden sharing is implemented. Other considerations include the relevance and scope of intellectual property rights for access, pricing and production of vaccines, and whether burden sharing is based on a voluntary basis or through more obligatory means, which were part of the final negotiations on the matter (WHO, 2009b). In their commentary on sharing of H5N1 viruses to stop a global influenza pandemic, Garret & Fidler (2007) have stated that:

> The deeper problem is, however, that current pharmaceutical strategies for pandemic control basically offer protection to a small number of developed countries. For the rest of the planet, technological solutions are scarce, if not nonexistent.

Another controversial trade and health matter has been counterfeiting. This issue is not new and the WHO has been engaged with it since the 1980s, but has gained more importance due to negotiations affecting enforcement of intellectual property rights. While no one denies the problem of substandard and false medicines, there remains a broad disagreement in terms of appropriate measures and focus of action, particularly because a significant number of health concerns relate to legitimate but substandard products in developing countries (Caudron *et al.*, 2008). The issue of applying measures and procedures for enforcing intellectual property rights in a manner that avoids creating barriers to legitimate trade in medicines was also part of a recent resolution adopted by the Human Rights Council (United Nations, 2009a). The negotiation of the so-called anti-counterfeiting treaty is feared to

further tighten protection of international property rights through enforcement and focus on patent and trade-mark infringements (Sell, 2008), which are not directly health-related, rather than strengthening regulatory oversight and capacities to limit trade in actual hazardous or substandard products.

Governance

Global governance on trade and economic policies has implications for health and social policies as well as for the scope and nature of measures that can be implemented at a national level. Global trade agreements regulate measures that governments can take without impeding trade and those measures they are required to take in order to protect commercial rights. While trade agreements, such as GATS, do recognize governments' right to regulate, this is complemented by the requirement that regulatory measures fit within the scope of given agreements, which, while not limiting regulation as such, implies a modification in *how* governments can regulate.

The shift from trade in goods to trade in services and investment defines different contexts for decision-making and governance, with implications for national policies. In addition to GATS, North American Free Trade Agreement (NAFTA) provisions and bilateral negotiations concerning government procurement and investments also relate to how *risks* are dealt with as part of international agreements and the extent to which the burden of risk is shared between the corporate and the public sectors both within and across countries. This issue is reflected in the Report of the Commission of Experts of the President of the United Nations General Assembly on Reforms of the International Monetary and Financial System (United Nations, 2009b) assessment on capital and financial markets liberalization, GATS and developing countries stating:

> Capital and financial market liberalization, pushed not only by the IMF, but also within certain trade agreements, exposed developing countries to more risk and has contributed to the rapid spread of the crisis around the world. In particular, trade-related financial services liberalization has been advanced under the rubric of the WTO's General Agreement on Trade in Services (GATS) Financial Services Agreement with insufficient regard for its consequences either for growth or stability. Externalities exerted by the volatility in the financial sector have severe negative effects on all areas of the economy and are an impediment to a stable development path. (United Nations, 2009b, p. 103, para 89)

While Member State commitments in GATS can be changed, these changes need to be compensated by extending others. This "locking in" feature has drawn criticism towards GATS in restricting the regulatory scope of governments in sectors that they have included in the agreement and making it more difficult or costly to change this. The potential of WTO provisions in terms of "locking" in and restricting scope for government regulatory intervention were also raised in the context of the financial crisis:

> Agreements that restrict a country's ability to revise its regulatory regime – including not only domestic prudential but, crucially, capital account regulations – obviously have to be altered, in light of what has been learned about deficiencies of this crisis. In particular there is concern that existing agreements under the WTO's Financial Services Agreement might, were they enforced, impede countries from revising their regulatory structures in ways that would promote growth, equity, and stability. (United Nations, 2009b, p. 104, para 94)

The Commission of Experts also draws attention to the fact that the WTO is the only universal body for setting trade rules and resolving trade disputes, but it is also the only universal intergovernmental institution which, at the insistence of major industrial countries, does not have an institutional agreement with the United Nations (United Nations, 2009b, p. 100). While the WTO has separately acceded to coherence commitments with the Bretton Woods institutions, a call has been made that the WTO should be brought into the United Nations system of global economic governance while maintaining its legal and institutional constituency.

The implications of broader global economic governance for global health policies are important as they affect how social determinants of health are shaped and what kind of overall public policies are possible. However, they do not settle issues where major conflicts of interests remain between particular corporate policies and health-policy interests, for example between the interests of commercial health-services providers or the pharmaceutical industry and government health-policy priorities. On the other hand, the relevance and scope for taking into account global health-policy considerations may be much greater within the WTO context than has been assumed. Pauwelyn (2003) has argued that as WTO agreements are framework agreements, their provisions may need to give way to, for example, more specific global agreements in particular areas, such as health or the environment.

In principle a case can be made for exploring the potential to strengthen global regulatory frameworks and rights to regulate a variety of public health

interests and concerns – for example alcohol, pharmaceutical policies, nutritional contents of food, recruitment of a health workforce and ensuring risk and resource sharing in health systems in the context of global health policies. While the Tobacco Framework Convention, alongside the International Health Regulations (IHR), remain the primary examples of implementing a legal public health framework globally (Taylor and Bettcher, 2002), there is substantial scope for strengthening global health governance and legal frameworks in support of health policy aims at national and global levels.

Impact of governance on health

In terms of health more specifically, three aspects of governance and policy-making can be disentangled where more specific arguments and implications can be shown. First, global trade policies and regulation affect the grounds on which, and how, health-related standards are set that affect trade and policies in other sectors both at national and global levels. It is no longer as simple to set health-related standards as part of national (or regional) policy-making without taking into account implications of these for other trading partners. Furthermore, trade interests and increasingly global trade policy interests in standard-setting enhance the tendency to shift decision-making towards more corporate-driven bodies and arrangements that are not appropriate for regulatory decisions for health and consumer concerns.

Second, trade policies and decisions made in the sphere of trade increasingly affect health policies as well as resources and national regulatory policy space within the health sector. This "creeping" impact of economic and trade policy priorities to govern and shape policies in other sectors on the basis of global or regional agreements is of particular importance in areas where national governance is decentralized or regionalized, making it more difficult to observe and recognize "national regulatory interests" in the area. "Trade creep" in health policies has also been cushioned by ignorance, assumed non-relevance and the fact that health-care reforms have changed the more traditional organization of health care within many countries. Governance issues herein relate not only to prospects and potential of Ministries of Health to engage more with trade negotiations, but also affect politics and pressures at the global level and in relation to competence of different international organizations.

The third relates to trade negotiation practices and democratic decision-making. This is of importance regarding lack of clarity both with respect to more specific implications of these agreements as well as with respect to implications from overall negotiation processes. Where agreements are considered as single undertakings, where nothing is agreed until all aspects are agreed, the scope for "horse-trading" across a variety of issues and sectors makes clarity and accountability even more difficult. Yet it is essential to democratic accountability that decisions are made on the basis of understanding the extent and nature of commitments made, in particular if these are enforceable and difficult to renegotiate later.

While GATS provides leeway for governments in terms of deciding the sectors they wish to include and time-bound exceptions, in relation TRIPS policy space needs to be sought for exceptions and provisions made for flexibilities, for example, in the form of compulsory licensing. The Doha Declaration on public health was useful in confirming the scope for compulsory licensing and removing more narrow interpretations, but another concern remains about the relationship between TRIPS provisions on data protection and data exclusivity (Correa, 2002). In GATS the classification of services has been sufficiently unclear to cause unanticipated commitments, as was shown in the dispute settlement case of gambling, where the USA did not interpret gambling and betting services as included with other recreational services in the GATS agreement (WTO, 2005). The so-called "public services exception" in GATS on exclusion of services supplied in the exercise of governmental authority is expressed narrowly and would not, on the basis of current interpretations of the Treaty, include publicly funded but outsourced services (Fidler *et al.*, 2003; Krajewski, 2003).

In addition to interpretational issues and lack of clarity regarding what is implied, trade negotiations also tend to use mechanisms that may deliberately lead to more extensive commitments than would have been sought otherwise. While such practices have also been promoted in the context of multilateral negotiations of GATS, they are more obvious in the field of bilateral negotiations. Bilateral negotiations may utilize different structures and provisions making it harder to understand how commitments have changed in comparison to GATS. This has been the case, for example, with respect to the EU–CARIFORUM partnership agreement (EU-CARIFORUM, 2008). The

EU–Mexico Free Trade Agreement is an example of expansion of commitments as it also covers government procurement and investment and commits the EU and Mexico not to enact legislation that would be more trade restrictive than is presently in force in their service sectors (EU–Mexico FTA, 2001). The legal language and nature of provisions often makes it hard for Ministries of Health to understand particular implications of trade agreements with a higher probability of making more extensive commitments than intended. These inadvertent inclusions in trade agreements "outside own priority setting" can be called "OOPS" commitments as the scope and the extent of commitments are not realized by those to whom they will accrue at the time when they are made (Koivusalo *et al.*, 2009).

Conclusions

In this chapter I have tracked matters concerning trade and health and sought to raise issues that are of importance to the relationship between trade and health, in particular where there are conflicts of interests or priorities. Trade-related requirements may push countries towards compliance and enhance public health aims when regulatory capacity in health is non-existent, inadequate, overwhelmed or captured by strong national industries. However, these situations tend to reflect the failure of health policies to gain sufficient ground in the first place. The real challenge for health and trade policies is the extent to which trade interests and policies sought in the name of these interests may – intentionally or unintentionally – systemically undermine health-related regulatory priorities and practice. Furthermore, the realization of the benefits of economic growth and interconnectedness between countries is not independent of public policies and their capacities to take action.

The required emphasis on the ethics of public policies is too often displaced by more narrow discussion of medical ethics, which is limited to the context of individuals and professional practice. There is therefore failure to address the following ethical dilemmas of public policies:

(1) The ethical consideration of inter-relationships between current global policies concerning commercial rights on the one hand, and realization of human and social rights on the other. This includes (a) cases where trade-related interests of particular interest groups differ or can be in conflict with health policy priorities; (b)

the ethical aspects of the promotion of public or population health and (c) broad notions of health protection and human security.

(2) The ethical basis of current trade policies and expansion of commercial law globally and its relationship to national or regional capacities to address socio-economic inequalities and vulnerability, including measures affecting the social determinants of health; and the ethical basis for the relationship between health and trade policies and governance, legitimacy and accountability.

(3) The ethical dilemmas associated with the implications of trade agreements for cost-containment and equity aspects of health systems and on their organization and financing; the implications of trade policies for private and public sectors and how risks, responsibilities, administrative burdens and burden of proof are shared between public and private sector.

The emphasis on public policies and international aspects of ethical concerns also raises crucial questions about global policy priorities in the context of trade and health and why a better balance between different aims and priorities needs to be sought. Why should intellectual property rights be more important than rights to access to treatment? If health policy concerns would be paramount in pharmaceutical policies, what would this imply for research and development? Are intellectual property rights the appropriate incentives for problem-based research and development? Why should the fair treatment of corporate actors within health services be more important globally than ensuring fair treatment of people within health systems? Why should all products or providers of services be treated similarly if, in practice, this favors global actors over local ones or undermines environmental and labor conditions of production? To what extent are health regulations "hijacked" by important interest groups? What kind of health and public policy assumptions are taken as given in trade policies?

The recognition of conflict of interests between trade and health policies is not a call for unrestricted protectionism, but for better global governance on health and trade, recognition of the systemic implications, conflicting interests, country-specific concerns, and most importantly, a willingness to act upon the challenge at all levels of governance.

References

Anderson K. & Martin, W. (2005). *Agricultural Trade Reform and the Doha Development Agenda*. Washington, DC: World Bank.

Babor, T., Caetano, R., Casswell, S., *et al.* (2003). *Alcohol: No Ordinary Commodity. Research and Public Policy*. Oxford: Oxford University Press.

Bettcher, D. W., Yach, D. & Guindon, G. E. (2000). Global trade and health: key linkages and future challenges. *Bulletin of the World Health Organization* **78**, 521–531.

Bialious, S. A. & Yach, D. (2001). Whose standard is it anyway? How the tobacco industry determines the International Organisation for Standardisation (ISO) standards for tobacco and tobacco products. *Tobacco Control* **10**, 96–104.

Birdsall, N. (2006). *The World is not Flat: Inequality and Injustice in our Global Economy*. Helsinki: World Institute for Development Economics Research.

Caplan, A., Dominiguez-Gil, B., Matesanz, R. & Prior, C. (2009). *Trafficking of Organs, Tissues and Cells and Trafficking in Human Beings for the Purpose of the Removal of Organs*. Joint Council of Europe and United Nations study. Strasbourg: Directorate General of Human Rights and Legal Affairs, Council of Europe.

Caudron, J.-M., Ford, N., Henkens, M. *et al.* (2008). Substandard medicines in resource-poor settings: a problem that can no longer be ignored. *Journal of Tropical and International Health* **13**, 1062–1072.

Correa, C. (2002). *Protection of Data Submitted for the Registration of Pharmaceuticals: Implementing Standards of the TRIPS Agreement*. Geneva: South Centre.

Epps, T. (2008). *International Trade and Health Protection. A Critical Assessment of the WTO's SPS Agreement*. Cheltenham, UK & Northampton, MA: Elgar International Economic Law.

EU-CARIFORUM (2008). Economic partnerships agreement between the CARIFORUM States, of the one part, and the European Union, on the other part. *Official Journal of the European Union* 30.10.2008. L 289/I/3.

EU-Mexico FTA (2001). European Union – Mexico Free Trade Agreement. www.worldtradelaw.net/fta/agreements/eftamexfta.pdf.

Fidler, D. (1997). Trade and health: the global spread of disease and international trade. *German Yearbook of International Law*, 40–200.

Fidler, D., Correa, C. & Oginam, A. (2003). *Legal Review of the General Agreement on Trade in Services (GATS) from a Health Policy Perspective*. Globalisation, Trade and Health Working Paper Series. Geneva: World Health Organization.

Fink, C. & Reichenmiller, P. (2005). *Tightening TRIPS: The Intellectual Property Provisions of Recent US Free Trade*

Agreements (Rep. No. Trade Note 20). Washington, DC: World Bank.

Fitter, R. & Kaplinsky, R. (2001). *Who Gains from Product Rents as Coffee Market becomes more Differentiated.* Brighton: Institute of Development Studies.

Food and Agriculture Organization (FAO) (2003). *Trade Reforms and Food Security: Conceptualising the Linkages.* Rome: Food and Agriculture Organization.

Food and Agriculture Organization (FAO) (2009). *The State of Food Insecurity in the World.* Rome: Food and Agriculture Organization.

Garret, L. & Fidler, D. (2007). Sharing H5N1 viruses to stop a global influenza pandemic. *PLoS Medicine* **4**, 11:e330.

Hawkes, C., Chopra, M. & Friel, S. (2009). Globalization, trade and the nutrition transition. In R. Labonté, T. Schrecker, C. Packer & V. Runnels (Eds). *Globalization and Health. Pathways, Evidence and Policy.* New York, NY: Routledge.

Hunt, P. (2006). The human right to the highest attainable standard of health: new opportunities and challenges. *Transactions of the Royal Society of Tropical Medicine and Hygiene* **100**, 603–607.

Kelly, T. (2007). *The Impact of the WTO. The Environment, Public Health and Sovereignty.* Cheltenham, UK: Edward Elgar.

Koivusalo, M. (1999). *WTO and Trade-creep in Health and Social Policies.* GASPP Occasional Papers 4. Helsinki: STAKES.

Koivusalo, M., Labonté, R. & Schrecker, T. (2009). Globalization and policy space for health and social determinants of health. In R. Labonté, T. Schrecker, C. Packer & V. Runnels (Eds.), *Globalization and Health. Pathways, Evidence and Policy.* New York, NY: Routledge.

Krajewski, M. (2003). Public services and trade liberalisation: mapping the legal framework. *International Journal of Economic Law* **6**, 341–367.

Kuptsch, C. (Ed.) (2006). *Merchants of Labour.* Geneva: ILO.

Lang, T. (2004). *Food Industrialisation and Food Power: Implications for Food Governance.* IIED Gatekeeper Series No 114. London: IIED.

Luff, F. (2003). Regulation of health services and international trade law. In A. Mattoo & P. Sauve (Eds.), *Domestic Regulation and Service Trade Liberalisation.* New York, NY: World Bank and Oxford University Press.

Mattoo, A. & Rathindran, R. (2006). How health insurance inhibits trade in health care. *Health Affairs* **25**, 358–368.

Ofodile, U. (2009). Import (toy) safety, consumer protection and the WTO Agreement on Technical Barriers to Trade: prospects, progress and problems. *International Journal of Private Law* **2**, 163–184.

Pauwelyn, J. (2003). *Conflict of Norms in Public International Law. How WTO Law Relates to other rules of International Law.* Cambridge: Cambridge University Press.

Roffe, P. & Spennemann, C. (2006). The impact of FTAs on public health policies and TRIPS flexibilities. *International Journal of Intellectual Property Management* **1**, 75–93.

Scheper-Hughes, N. (2000). The global traffic in human organs. *Current Anthropology* **41**, 191–208.

Sell, S. (2008). *The global IP upward ratchet, anti-counterfeiting and piracy enforcement efforts: the state of play.* www.twnside.org.sg/title2/intellectual_property/development.research/SusanSellfinalversion.pdf

Taylor, A. L. & Bettcher, D. (2002). International law and public health. *Bulletin of the World Health Organization* **80**, 975–980.

United Nations (2009). *Access to Medicine in the Context of the Right of Everyone to the Enjoyment of the Highest Attainable Standard of Physical and Mental Health.* Resolution adopted by the Human Rights Council. A/HRC/RES/12/24.

United Nations (2009b). *Report of the Commission of Experts of the President of the United Nations General Assembly on Reforms of the International Monetary and Financial System.* September 21, 2009. New York, NY: United Nations.

Veggeland, F. & Borgen, S.O. (2005). Negotiating international food standards: The World Trade Organization's impact on the Codex Alimentarius Commission. *Governance: An International Journal of Policy, Administration and Institutions* **18**, 675–708.

Wibulpolprasert, S., Pachanee, C., Pitayarangsarit, S. & Hempisut, P. (2004). International service trade and its implications for human resources for health: a case study of Thailand. *Human Resources for Health* **2**, 10 doi:10.1186/1478–4491–2–10.

Willetts, A. & Martinea, T. (2004). *Ethical International Recruitment of Health Professionals: Will Codes of Practice Protect Developing Country Health Systems?* January 2004. Version 1.1. www.liv.ac.uk/lstm/research/documents/codesofpracticereport.pdf.

World Health Assembly (WHA) (2008). *Global Strategy and Plan of Action on Public Health, Innovation and Intellectual Property.* World Health Assembly 2008 resolution 61.21. Annex. Geneva: World Health Organization.

World Health Organization (WHO) (2007). *World Health Report.* Geneva: World Health Organization.

World Health Organization (WHO) (2009a). *Pandemic Influenza Preparedness: Sharing of Influenza Viruses and Access to Vaccines and other Benefits.* Report by the Director-General. A/PIP/IGM/13. April 13, 2009. Geneva: World Health Organization.

World Health Organization (WHO) (2009b). *Director-General's Consultation with Member States. Proposals to Finalise Remaining Elements of the "Pandemic Influenza Preparedness Framework for Sharing Influenza Viruses and Access to Vaccines and other Benefits".* Document HSE/GIP/PIP/2009.1. Geneva: World Health Organization.

World Trade Organization (WTO) (1998). *EC Measures Concerning Meat and Meat Products (Hormones). Appellate Body Report.* WT/DS26AB/R. January 16, 1998. Geneva: World Trade Organization.

World Trade Organization (WTO) (2005). *United States – Measures Affecting the Cross-border Supply of Gambling and Betting Services.* WT/DS285/ AB/R. April 7, 2005. Geneva: World Trade Organization.

World Trade Organization (WTO) (2006). *Committee on Technical Barriers to Trade. Notification.* G/TBT/N/THA/215. October 10, 2006. Geneva: World Trade Organization.

World Trade Organization (WTO) (2008). *Committee on Technical Barriers to Trade. Minutes of the meeting of 9 November 2007.* G/TBT/M/43. January 21, 2008. Geneva: World Trade Organization.

Yach, D. & Bettcher, D. (2000). Globalisation of tobacco industry influence and new global responses. *Tobacco Control* 9, 206–216.

13

Debt, structural adjustment and health

Jeff Rudin and David Sanders

Introduction

The debt narrative is encapsulated in the conundrum of why post-apartheid South Africa chose to cripple itself with debts that it could so easily have repudiated. Nelson Mandela described the apartheid debt as "the greatest single obstacle to progress in this country." He explained further

> We are limited in South Africa because our democratic government inherited a debt, which we were servicing at the rate of 30 billion rand a year. That is 30 billion we did not have to build houses, to make sure our children go to schools and to ensure that everybody has the dignity of having a job and a decent income. (ACTSA, 2003; Malala, 2003)

Given that debt accumulated by the apartheid system is an example par excellence of odious debt, the new democratic South Africa had compelling legal and ethical reasons for disowning it (Rudin, 1999, 2000).[1]

Rather than disown the odious debt, the government actively sought to undermine Jubilee South Africa, the campaign founded to repudiate the apartheid debt (*BusinessReport (SA)*, November 8 and 22, 1998).

Moreover, it is arguable that few governments or other creditors would have insisted on Mandela's South Africa repaying odious apartheid debts at the expense of the newly liberated black majority. Additionally, South Africa is far from being a poor country. Being the dominant economic power in Africa also gave the country political influence and both considerations put South Africa in a far stronger position to resist the debt burden than most other peripheral countries.

Before attempting to make sense of this conundrum of South Africa's debt, a few preliminary comments are apposite.

Our own understanding of the world is of a global economic system characterized by interactions between countries of grossly uneven economic development and political power such that the system can be described as having a "core" or center comprising the most developed and powerful countries and a "periphery" made up of all the others.[2] This typology is preferred to geographical terms that are either anachronistic (the "West") or inaccurate (North/South). The idea of a Third World is also anachronistic; while developed/developing suggests that countries that are not "developed" are "developing," even when they are either stagnant or moving backwards mainly as a result of their historical and current position in the global economic architecture. For the purposes of this chapter, the principal core countries are the USA, Canada, the EU countries of Western Europe and Japan – but it should be noted that cores and peripheries also exist within countries.

Numbers that don't add up

To appreciate the magnitude of current debt a comparison should be made with the Marshall Plan, the grants provided by the USA that contributed significantly to the post-Second World War reconstruction of Europe. In today's terms, the Marshall Plan provided aid of some $100 billion. By comparison, in 2007 the total external debt for countries of the periphery was estimated to be $3360 billion. Between 1970 and 2007, this debt increased by 4800% and the amount repaid

---

[1] The Doctrine of Odious Debt reverses normal international law in which in-coming governments unconditionally honor the debts incurred by their predecessors. The Doctrine applies to debts incurred by illegitimate regimes for purposes of defending and/or enhancing their illegitimacy, when, additionally, such illegitimacy is known, or ought to have been known, by the creditors.

[2] The terms center/core/periphery derive from Frank (1967, 1969).

Global Health and Global Health Ethics, ed. Solomon Benatar and Gillian Brock. Published by Cambridge University Press.
© Cambridge University Press 2011.

during this period – $7150 billion – was 102 times greater than what was owed in 1970. In 2007, the latest year for which information is available, the countries of the periphery repaid $520 billion of which $198 billion was public debt.[3] In the same year, the governments of countries in the periphery received $169 billion in new public loans. This translates into a net loss of $29 billion to the countries supposedly benefiting from the very loans that give rise to the debt repayments.

In addition to noting that this difference amounts to a profit of $460 billion to the foreign creditors, this outward flow forces a critical examination of what is universally described as "aid," in its various forms. Official Development Assistance (ODA) from the core and the countries immediately around the center totaled $104 billion in 2007. In the same year, the countries of the periphery spent $800 billion servicing – paying off the amount originally loaned plus interest charges – their external and internal debt (Toussaint & Millet, 2009, pp. 18, 34, 101–109).

Between 1970 and 2007, sub-Saharan Africa, the poorest region in the world, repaid $350 billion in debt. In 2007 it owed $190 billion and repaid $17 billion. The $190 billion owed was more than the total GDP of Africa's 36 poorest countries combined, while the $350 billion that has been repaid is larger than South Africa's 2009 GDP; it is also larger than the combined GDPs of 50 of sub-Saharan Africa's 53 countries. In 2000 Mozambique's per capita external debt was almost seven times the GNP per capita; Angola's was almost four times; and Tanzania's and Zambia's debt were twice their per capita GDP (*BusinessReport* (*SA*), August 8, 2000; Toussaint & Millet, 2009, pp. 102, 107, 108). It is clear that debt of this magnitude can only undermine economic and other developments in these countries.

These sums of money should be contrasted with the almost $13 000 billion the US government alone has made available with its various emergency measures during the current economic crisis (www.Bloomberg.com, March 31, 2009).

The etiology of debt and its morbidity

Too much money

We understand debt to be the result of corporate and geopolitical imperatives, with most individuals

associated with debt probably thinking that what they are doing is beneficial, or perhaps being only dimly aware of what they are implicated in and the harm they were causing. However, there are others who have lost all sense of decency and who are keenly aware of what they do, and who seemingly care little about the consequences for others.

How did we get to the position conveyed by the above data? In recounting the history of poor country debt we will say nothing about the debt crises of the nineteenth and early twentieth centuries, or deal in any depth with what form remedies may take today for the now acknowledged debt crisis. Rather, we shall provide a highly condensed summary of the origins of today's debt debacle with only passing references to how these origins link to the present. Our main focus is on the perversity of debt and the ways in which its effects impact on health (see also George, 1988).

The background causes of the debt crisis of the early 1980s that so adversely affect many countries of the periphery are largely uncontroversial. By the beginning of the early 1970s, Europe was awash with money seeking profitable outlets. The previously mentioned Marshall aid had locked a large amount of dollars into Europe – the Eurodollars. These were followed in 1973 by the "petrodollars" placed in US and European banks by Middle Eastern oil potentates following the super profits from the then huge increase in the price of oil. This "surplus" money was offered at preferential and exceedingly low rates to countries of the periphery, many of which had only recently become independent and were eager to commence with the development denied them during colonialism.

The crisis began in 1979, with a major US policy shift, cemented in 1981 by the election of Ronald Reagan (Margaret Thatcher's election in 1979 marked this shift in Britain), that sharply increased US nominal interest rates to attract foreign investment into the USA. Real interest rates (i.e. minus inflation) jumped from −1% in 1978 to +9% in 1982 (Hanlon, 2000). From a nominal rate (i.e. with inflation) of about 5% in 1973, they shot up to 18.9% in 1981. European banks followed suit to counter what would have otherwise been a US competitive advantage.

Countries of the periphery were adversely affected by two factors. First, interest rates on their foreign debts increased from about 4–5% in the 1970s to 16–18%. Second, because most of their loans were in hard

---

[3] Public debt is defined as is money (or credit) owed by any level of government; either central government, federal government, municipal government or local government.

currencies earned by exports, the collapse of commodity prices, especially oil in 1981, led to a debt crisis in Mexico, a major oil exporter. In August 1982, Mexico was the first country unable to meet its debt obligations. Argentina and Brazil followed in quick succession. All indebted countries in Africa, Latin America and several Asian countries (including Korea) met the same fate. (All interest rates quoted are from Toussaint & Millet, 2009, pp. 53, 55.)

The banks come first

Faced with defaulting debtors, the banks – principally the IMF and World Bank which took over much of the loans made by commercial banks – did what banks always do, regardless of whether their client is a country or a person: they took steps to protect their money. Besides either rolling over the debt or making a further loan to make repayment on the original one possible, these institutions set a number of preconditions before any rescue could happen. To earn the hard currency required for their debt repayment, the banks insisted on priority being given to exports. The banks also insisted on what for them was prudent practice through: (a) reducing government expenditure by minimizing budget deficits and hence the need for government borrowing; and (b) cutting government's social expenditure by removing subsidies on basic foods, introducing user charges for services previously provided free; and freezing civil service pay along with reducing the number of public servants: and all this in order that more could be spent on servicing the debt. The ensuing "fiscal discipline" would additionally address inflation, which had become an additional concern.

The banks, eager to find new investment outlets and accepting the then prevailing Reagan/Thatcher antipathy towards the public sector, with its alleged inefficiencies and predilection to corruption, added privatization to their conditions for helping governments in crisis with their debts. The claimed efficiencies, together with the business practices and ethos of privatization would supposedly create jobs and ease poverty, with the former resulting in greater tax revenue and the latter in reduced government expenditure on the poor, and both would enhance the government's ability to repay its debt. Moreover, privatization would attract foreign investment, which would in turn further stimulate the economy and thereby facilitate debt repayment. However, a precondition for foreign investment was the ending of controls on capital to facilitate its free flow across the globe. Finally, loans to the defaulters or those countries in trouble with their debt repayments would be paid only in installments, after verification that the banks' requirements were being met.

These conditions (and others) are all perfectly explicable in terms of the financial institutions, seeking, not unreasonably, to protect their loans and accordingly placing seemingly reasonable conditions on defaulting governments. The governments, like defaulting individuals, remained at all times free to reject the banks' conditions. All this is standard banking practice. There was no necessary conspiracy involved or ill will intended.

These various banking requirements are the conditionalities, associated with what became known as Structural Adjustment Programs (SAPs), designed to reduce debt to a level repayable by each country. It should be noted that SAPs never addressed questions about development, poverty, health or post-war reconstruction and few were concerned with the ethical implications associated with their implementation. As with any business, the ethics of SAPS was focused on the bottom line.

Structural Adjustment Programs: the wrong medicine

Over time, the conditionalities associated with SAPs were incorporated into a range of other programs: Enhanced Structural Adjustment Programs (ESAPs); Heavily Indebted Poor Countries Initiative (HIPC); Multilateral Debt Relief Initiative (MDRI); Poverty Reduction Strategy Papers (PRSP); and Poverty Reduction and Growth Facilities (PRGF). Indeed, the conditionalities themselves have remained essentially unchanged right up to the present day.

What has been the overall effect of these conditionalities? Structural Adjustment Programs, in whatever form, have failed to reduce the debt burden. All the creditors and their supporting governments recognized this failure; but only implicitly. Explicitly, they have gone no further than acknowledging that the debts could not be paid in full and, therefore, offering to "forgive" part of the debt subject to further formalities. These formalities are SAPs dressed in updated clothing. As Detlef Kotte, of the UN Conference on Trade & Development (UNCTAD) said of HIPC in 2002:

The IMF & World Bank have changed the words, changed the acronyms, changed their methods of consultation, but they have not changed an iota of their creed. (Touissant & Millet 2009, p. 133.)

The failure to ameliorate – let alone cure – the "debt disease" is inherent in the remedy; something that ought to have been apparent at the birth of SAPs in 1982. The main SAPs requirement was then (as now) for each country to prioritize exports. The colonial background of most of the countries of the periphery, however, meant that most of these countries were economically backward, with mining and agriculture being the basis of their economies.

Apart from the enormous subsidies and other protections given by the core governments to their own manufacturing and agriculture, the requirement to concentrate on exports meant the peripheral countries would all be exporting similar products to the core countries which were the main markets. This had three clearly predictable outcomes: (a) the market would be flooded; (b) the countries of the periphery would unavoidably end up competing amongst themselves; and (c) prices would fall – as a result of the first two outcomes. Falling export prices meant economic disaster for poor countries – and a deeper debt trap. In the absence of money to pay off the debt, countries got deeper into debt because they had to borrow new money to pay off old debts.

This obvious prediction is confirmed by the data: between 1977 and 2001 there was a net fall in the price of all raw materials, dropping about 2.8% annually. Minerals and metals were also affected with an annual average fall of 1.9%, while the prices of silver, tin and tungsten dropped by more than 5%. Being so dependent on external markets gravely exposed commodity exporters to the vagaries of what was happening in other countries. Thus, between 1997 (the year when Southeast Asia's financial crisis resulted in large-scale economic collapse) and 2001, commodity prices fell by 53% in real terms. Sub-Saharan Africa's debt crisis of the 1980s was significantly precipitated by a 30% fall in commodity prices between 1980 and 1985 (Hanlon, 2000; Unctad, 2003a, 2003b).

These examples do not, however, convey the depth of human suffering that lies behind the data. Zambia provides egregious examples of the consequences of both enforced privatization and of the more direct human effects of the conditionalities. Copper mining is the Zambian economy. A major test of Zambia's commitment to meet HIPC conditionalities, and thereby have some of its debt "forgiven," required Zambia to privatize its copper mines. In early 2000, it sold ZCCM, the company producing 70% of its copper, to the South African corporate giant, Anglo-American. This privatization was also intended to unlock bilateral loans, principally £20 million from the UK, which had been delayed pending the sale. The privatization resulted in large-scale retrenchment of workers – 30% of the workforce according to the trade union – in a country with already huge unemployment.

Although this forced privatization was to receive debt relief, the World Bank made a further loan available to the Zambian government to finance the layoff of these workers. ZCCM had paid for most social services on the Copperbelt and for Zambia's spending on education and health care. Anglo-American refused to take on any ZCCM-funded local schools and hospitals. For its part, the UK withheld the promised bilateral loan, after the privatization, saying that it then expected Zambia to root out corruption before it would advance the £20 million loan. Shortly after buying ZCCM, Anglo-American changed its mind because the slump in world copper prices made their involvement unprofitable. ZCCM, sold to Anglo at a bargain price, had to be sold again, this time for even less and with other incentives. Besides a low rate of tax, the mines (which use 80% of Zambia's electricity), were guaranteed a fixed price of electricity, at a cost that was 50% below actual cost, and for an extended period. A few years later, the price of copper on the world market went sharply upwards but Zambia was still obliged to provide subsidized electricity to the profitable mines (*BusinessReport* (SA) March 3, 2000, April 6, 2000, April 7, 2000, June 2, 2000; *Mail & Guardian* April 7, 2000; Zulu, 2007).

Noting that Zambia's debt-servicing was exceeding its annual spending on health, welfare, education and sanitation projects combined, South Africa's then Finance Minister, Trevor Manuel stated, in an article titled "G7 has failed in debt relief" in 1999:

> For every dollar that Zambia is able to raise from the Bretton Woods institutions [the IMF & World Bank] they pay out $1.30 in debt settlement. There is something fundamentally wrong with the whole system. (Manuel, *Reuters*, September 20, 1999)

The IMF suspended Zambia from its HIPC relief program in 2003, because the government had overspent on its 2003–04 budget. This forced Zambia to increase income tax to 40% and to impose a pay freeze. The pay freeze was especially difficult for the nearly half a million public service workers because, besides inflation of 17.2%, the government had been unable to honor its 2003 wage agreement, despite having overspent on that year's budget.

As with so many parts of Africa and the world, where poverty and unemployment abound, one worker supports up to ten other people. In 2004, 75% of Zambia's population of 11 million lived below the World Bank's poverty threshold of $1 a day. Before HIPC, the figure was 50% (in 1990) (*BusinessReport (SA)* October 23, 2000).

Education was also affected by the "prudent financial management and fiscal discipline" required by the World Bank, as a condition of Zambia's partial debt "forgiveness." Not only were workers not paid, but the budget ceiling imposed on Zambia meant that some 9000 trained teachers were unemployed while Zambian schools were in desperate need of 9000 extra teachers! Zambia spent $221 million on education in 2004. In the same year it spent $247 million on debt servicing (Reuters, 1999; *BusinessReport (SA)* October 23, 2000; SAPA-AFP February 5, 2004, February 7, 2004, February 14, 2004, February 19, 2004; Oxfam Global Campaign for Education, 2004). Table 13.1 provides some comparative statistics.

In many low-income, highly indebted countries, the low level of spending on social services is explained not only by the high proportion of the budget committed to debt servicing but also by the lack of "fiscal space," constraints on gaining revenue through taxes and managing a government's budget, usually as a conditionality of debt relief, and the low levels of national wealth which reflect inter alia countries' colonial histories and current positions in the global economy. For instance, only a few years ago Ethiopia was spending 22% of its national budget on health and education, but this totaled only

US$1.50 per capita on health. Even if Ethiopia spent its entire budget on health care, it would still not reach the WHO target of US$34 per capita, the amount needed for a basic "package" of health services, as recommended by the WHO's Commission on Macroeconomics and Health (Save the Children UK, 2003). Indeed, per capita health expenditure in most African countries was below $10 per capita in 2006 (WHO 2006, p. 2).

Killing the patient – the health consequences of SAPs

The evolution of debt synoptically described above and the resulting macroeconomic reforms such as SAPs and their later variants undertaken by most peripheral countries have been associated with significant reversals in the welfare and health of large sections of their populations. The mechanisms whereby health has been impacted by such economic changes are through social, environmental and health service determinants of health. These have been recently exhaustively documented in the Report of the Commission on Social Determinants of Health (CSDH) (2008). As the CSDH showed, these factors operate at a local, national and, increasingly, with globalization, at a global level.

Historical and contemporary experiences have shown that there is a definite but complex relationship between economic growth on the one hand and health status on the other. In general, sustained economic growth leads to improved health and nutritional status: in the now-industrialized countries large and sustained decline in mortality, morbidity (disease) and malnutrition paralleled economic growth, and largely preceded any effective medical interventions. However, improved income distribution – even at low income levels – can accelerate improvements in health, well-known examples being China, Sri Lanka, Costa Rica and Cuba (Halstead *et al.*, 1985). In the short term, the inter-relationship is even more complex. There are examples of countries in which high (but unequal) growth has been associated with a decline in health status as reflected by such indicators as infant mortality (Brazil in the 1970s), but there are also cases where economic decline has been associated with significant improvements in health status (Chile, Tanzania). A detailed understanding of these relationships requires study of the particular circumstances in which economic changes take place and the context within which health status is determined. However, issues of provision of services and social equity are of primary importance (Commission on Social Determinants of Health, 2008).

Table 13.1. Percentage of budget allocated to basic social services and debt servicing for the period 1992–1997.

Country	Social services (%)	Debt servicing (%)
Cameroon	4.0	36.0
Côte d'Ivoire	11.4	35.0
Kenya	12.6	40.0
Zambia	6.7	40.0
Niger	20.4	33.0
Tanzania	15.0	46.0
Nicaragua	9.2	14.1

Source: UNDP (2000) *Poverty Report*. Cited by Touissant & Millet, 2009, p. 16.

Although health sector inputs may be the most obvious proximal determinants of health status, the effects of upstream and more distal non-health sector inputs are probably more important. Whilst it is relatively easy to achieve rapid improvements in health as measured by standard quantitative indicators such as infant mortality rates, sustained improvements in the quality of life are more difficult to produce and measure. For instance, certain indicators, such as infant and young child mortality rates, may be rapidly improved by selective primary health-care interventions (e.g. immunization) targeted at these high-risk groups. There is, however, little evidence to suggest that improved nutrition levels, for example, can be maintained by the application of such technical packages in the absence of more general improvements in access to resources.

Further, different time frames apply to the appearance of changes in both sets of indicators. For example, whilst changes in food prices and health service utilization rates may occur quite quickly and be readily assessed and documented, changes in mortality and morbidity rates, and in nutritional status, are both more problematic to monitor, and often become evident only in the medium- to long-term: short-term changes may thus reflect processes operating before the implementation of imposed conditionalities. Another major problem in assessing the impact of SAPs on health is the poor quality and often the unavailability of data on mortality, morbidity and nutritional status, especially in the poorest countries where economic decline has often been most severe and debt most debilitating. Finally, especially in sub-Saharan Africa, it is extremely difficult to disentangle the effects of general economic decline and HIV/AIDS from those of SAPs – although there are analyses that also link the spread of HIV/AIDS in several countries in sub-Saharan Africa to economic crisis and SAPs (De Vogli & Birbeck, 2005).

Given the foregoing, in any assessment of the impact of structural adjustment on health status, it is necessary to analyze the impact of factors operating both within and beyond the health sector, and a range of health indicators must be examined over both the short and long term. The above methodological complexities challenge the attribution of health changes to SAPs themselves, and have been invoked in controversies surrounding the welfare effects of these policies. Several studies conducted in the 1980s that showed an association between reversals in welfare and health were questioned (Cornia et al., 1988) and it was suggested that other contextual factors could explain these phenomena and even that such reversals might have been more dramatic had such economic reforms not been applied (the "counterfactual" argument). A review of the impact of structural adjustment policies on child health therefore suggested that future research on this area should utilize alternative methodologies, including longitudinal study design, to monitor factors likely to impact on health (Costello et al., 1994).

In 1991, Zimbabwe embarked on a structural adjustment program. The reform package contained the typical elements of World Bank/IMF economic strategies: trade liberalization, reduction in social expenditure, devaluation of the currency among others. In the health sector, user fees were introduced. Concerns were expressed early on that this package would have a damaging impact on the health status of the poor, because of reduced access to health care and growing poverty at the household level. The assertion that previous studies had lacked methodological rigor, together with the opportunity offered by Zimbabwe being a "late" adjuster, prompted the initiation of a carefully designed long-term longitudinal study.

A total of about 600 households, equally divided between a rural area and a high-density working-class peri-urban suburb, were enrolled in a longitudinal household study in 1993 and re-interviewed in 1994, 1995, 1996 and 1998. Information was gathered on household economic activity, use of health services and nutritional status of under-5-year-olds. Data based on serial follow-up of rural and urban households suggested that households responded to growing economic hardship by greatly diversifying means of income generation, but these multiple sources of income did not protect households from growing poverty. Rural areas experienced more hardship than urban areas, and there was evidence of significantly increased income inequality even within relatively homogeneous communities. Health service utilization was adversely affected by the introduction of user fees, and a disturbing increase in childhood malnutrition was suggested as well as a deterioration in quality of health care (Bassett et al., 1997, 2000; Bijlmakers et al., 1999).

Notwithstanding the difficulty in separating the effects of structural adjustment from other variables, the weight of research emphasizes that it often preceded increased disparities in health and also exerted both short and long-term effects on health systems (Labonté et al., 2007).

A Canadian study on health systems in Tanzania stated that "The era of structural adjustment may be over, but the effects of earlier damage continue to cast a long shadow" (de Savigny *et al.*, 2004, p. 56).

The most comprehensive review of available studies on structural adjustment and health in Africa, for a WHO commission, stated:

> The majority of studies in Africa, whether theoretical or empirical, are negative towards structural adjustment and its effect on health outcomes. (Breman & Shelton, 2001)

The final word on the health effects of debt is fittingly linked to the most devastating pandemic in human history. The eminent founding executive director of UNAIDS, Peter Piot, noted that Africa spends more on debt servicing each year than on health and education – "the building blocks of the AIDS response" (Piot, 2004).

Making sense of it all

Everyone agrees but …

Structural adjustment programs in all their various forms have remarkably few supporters. The early comments cited below emphasize that the debt of countries of the periphery is a long recognized problem.

In 1969, Nelson Rockefeller alerted the US President of problems accumulating in Latin America:

> Many of the countries are, in effect, having to make new loans to get the foreign exchange to pay interest and amortization on old loans, and at higher interest rates. (Toussaint & Millet, 2009, p. 56)

In the same year, the USA's General Accounting Office (GAO) warned:

> Many poor countries have already incurred debts past the possibility of repayment. (Toussaint & Millet, 2009, p. 56)

Robert McNamara, the then President of the World Bank, noted as early as 1972:

> This situation could not go on indefinitely. (Toussaint & Millet, 2009, p. 56)

In 2000, the Advisory Committee to the US Congress on International Financial Institutions, the Meltzer Commission, informed the President that:

> The IMF [has] a degree of influence over member countries' policymaking that is unprecedented for a multilateral institution. … These programmes have not ensured economic progress. (Toussaint & Millet, 2009, p. 81)

In 2000, the Canadian Prime Minister, Paul Martin, urged the IMF and World Bank to limit the conditionalities. Citing the 160 policy actions required of Sao Tome, the tiny island nation of 140 000 people, to obtain debt relief, he commented:

> This is absurd! (*Cape Times* (*SA*) September 26, 2000)

In 2001, the UN Special Rapporteur was especially forthright:

> Increasing malnutrition, falling school enrolments and rising unemployment have been attributed to the policies of structural adjustment. Yet these same institutions continue to prescribe the same medicine as a condition for debt relief, dismissing the overwhelming evidence that Structural Adjustment Programmes have increased poverty. (Toussaint & Millet, 2009, p. 208)

The UN Conference on Trade and Development (UNCTAD) remarked:

> On any objective assessment of two and half decades of standardised packages of 'stabilization, liberalisation and privatisation', the right kind of growth has simply failed to materialise. (Toussaint & Millet, 2009, p. 208)

The Economist, in its Christmas 1999 edition, asked of the just-announced enhanced version of HIPC:

> Who believes in fairy tales? (Toussaint & Comanne, 2000)

Susan George, author and long-time campaigner against debt, merits the last word. Writing in 2000, she observed

> If I put forward a hypothesis in physics which is proved wrong by an experiment, I must question the theory. … In economics, you can undermine the existence of millions of people, but none of that human evidence will affect the ideology of structural adjustment. (Toussaint & Millet, 2009, p. 82)

Given this unanimity of well-informed opinion, the obvious question to ask in the face of such a wide spectrum of people having long agreed that SAPS are unworkable is: Why is the debt burden still with us? Why has this not been cancelled outright and a long time ago? Or, at least, why has most of the debt of most countries not been recognized as not payable and why has the illegitimacy of the debt mostly not been recognized and debt therefore seen as not payable? Why, in other words, is there still need for a chapter like this one in a book published in 2011? There are three parts to our answer: economic, political and the status of countries of the periphery.

Moral hazard

Before addressing these issues it is necessary to dispose of the argument that debt cannot be cancelled because it would be a "moral hazard" to do so. In this view, letting debtors off is an offence against morality and sets a bad example for future borrowers. The tortuous way morality is invoked is well captured by Horst Kohler, the then managing director of the International Monetary Fund (IMF):

> I doubt that simply writing off debt is the best medicine because it could create a nice and cosy feeling that 'we are now better off' and reduce the awareness of African countries (of the need) to tackle their own problems. (*Cape Times*, July 10, 2000)

So, the debt cannot be written off, according to the head of the IMF, because to do so would mean that African countries wouldn't tackle their own problems. The poor must be tortured for their own good!

However, this issue can easily be disposed of by two considerations. First, core country banks ignored moral hazard when they accepted huge bailouts to prevent their own bankruptcy during the current financial crisis. Second, moral hazard has not prevented debt cancellation when the political will is there. Core countries have cancelled all or large parts of the debt of at least five countries, for example Poland in 1991.

The concept of moral hazard highlights the double standards that plague international debt. Making creditors responsible for their loans is not part of bankers' morality.

Structural adjustment programs as a business opportunity

In 1994, responding to huge pressure from the major transnational corporations (TNCs) of the core countries, the World Trade Organization (WTO) was founded, with most countries as members. The new organization was ostensibly created to provide clear rules in international trade. Additionally, it greatly extended the meaning of trade to include investment and services (the latter through the General Agreement on Trade in Services – GATS). The WTO's real purpose, known to all its members but seldom openly acknowledged, is twofold: to maintain the uneven trade system and to promote a decidedly one-sided understanding of "free trade." More specifically, this means (especially through GATS) liberalization, privatization and the free flow of capital.

The symmetry and synergy between the WTO and SAPs is striking. While it is arguable that SAPs were initially a straightforward banking response to debt-defaulting countries, it would soon have become plain to bankers and others that SAPs had wider "benefits." The enormous growth of finance to its present dominant position within the world economy gives a special importance to SAPs, one that could not have been anticipated in the early 1980s. It would make little sense for the banks to give away with one hand (via debt cancellation) what they are struggling to achieve with the other (via the WTO and more especially GATS). The conclusion is hard to avoid: business has a vested interest in perpetuating the debt trap that fuels SAPs and economic liberalization.

The not so benign bankers

The London Agreement of 1953 between Germany and its creditors provides a striking comparison in the approach to sovereign debt (Rudin, 2003). Germany had been the enemy responsible for the death and destruction resulting from two World Wars. Moreover, Hitler came to power via a democratic election which made the German electorate accountable in a way that does not apply to the people of the countries of the periphery. Yet, the contrast between the London Agreement and HIPC could not be starker.

- Germany was required to pay a maximum of 3.06% of its annual export income on repaying its debt. For the poorest countries on earth, HIPC requires them to use between 20% and 25% of their export income on debt servicing.
- To qualify for consideration for debt-relief opportunities under HIPC, a country's total external debt has to be in the order of 160% of its GDP. The "debt ratio" is usually considered problematic if it is anything between 80–100%, that is, if the debt is equivalent to between 80–100% of what a country generates annually in its own currency from all economic activities. Germany's debt ratio in 1953 was a mere 21.2%.
- To qualify for consideration under HIPC a country's foreign debt has to be at least 280% larger than its national budget. Germany's "fiscal debt ratio" in 1953 was 4.9%.
- A HIPC candidate country has 3 years in which to introduce its particular conditionalities. It then has a further 3 years in which to demonstrate its good behavior before receiving very limited debt relief. The London Agreement placed no similar conditionalities on Germany.
- What the London Agreement did instead was to place significant conditionalities on the creditors. The London Agreement required three major benefits from creditors. First, creditors had to promote

German exports because the debt payments were made entirely from trade surpluses. No trade surplus meant no debt payments; reduced trade surpluses meant reduced debt servicing. Second, Germany had the option of imposing import restrictions if the balance of trade with any of the debtor countries failed to produce a surplus. Finally, creditors were given no sanctions against Germany, in the event of any German infringement of the agreement. The most that the creditors could expect was the convening of direct negotiations with the option of seeking advice from an appropriate international organization. HIPC is entirely free of such demands on the creditors.

The London Agreement shows that SAPs could be very different. HIPC, which in any event applies only to a tiny number of countries and even fewer people when compared with the population of the countries of the periphery, testifies to economic and political interests trumping the needs of the people of the periphery.

The even less benign IMF and World Bank

Politics shape debt as much as finance. The IMF and World Bank make this clear. As the Meltzer Commission, the Advisory Committee to the United States Congress on International Financial Institutions, observed in its 2000 report:

> The G7 governments, particularly the United States, use the IMF as a vehicle to achieve their political ends.

Robert Zoelick, who became President of the World Bank in 2007 but speaking as the then US Trade Representative, was no less forthright:

> Countries seeking free trade agreements with the United States should meet criteria beyond those of an economic and commercial nature. At the very least, those countries should cooperate with the United States in its external policy and its national security objectives.

Debt was a highly advantageous lever that made possible the USA's abuse of the World Bank and IMF; while the undemocratic governance structures of both the IMF and World Bank made these institutions perfect instruments of core country – especially US – control (Toussaint & Millet, 2009, pp. 39–43, 67–73, 99).

Political control

Africa was debt free before the 1960s. This was because sub-Saharan Africa was under colonial rule and, other than Ethiopia, had no independent countries. Core countries learnt that debt was a most useful mechanism of control over countries enjoying nominal independence. This much is alluded to in the previous two quotations.

The threat of the Soviet Union – and now China – added enormously to the political value of creating and maintaining dependency, via debt. Indonesia provides an early example of both how the dependency is created and the connection between that dependency and dictatorships, especially when large loans are involved. In August 1965, Indonesia withdrew from the IMF and World Bank. Shortly afterwards, the army overthrew the president and massacred 750 000 communists. Under the new president, Gen Suharto, Indonesia rejoined both bodies. In December 1966, Suharto was rewarded with a 4-year moratorium on all debt servicing, followed by the renewal of payments limited to less than 6% of export earnings and 0.7% of GDP.

As Joseph Stiglitz, the Chief Economist of the World Bank from 1997 to 1999 noted:

> In many cases, the loans were used to corrupt governments … The issue was not whether the money was improving a country's welfare, but whether it was […] meeting] the geopolitical realities of the world. (Hanlon, 2000, p. 885; Toussaint & Millet, 2009, p. 38)

Governments willing to be corrupted

Why, regardless of country and continent, of race or religion and as a constant since independence, should there be a never-ending supply of political and economic leaders willing to be corrupted, in one form or another? Greed is too simple an answer unless one posits a highly problematic "human nature." A more developed answer is required especially when leaders, like in post-apartheid South Africa, include many who readily risked their lives and made great sacrifices in liberation struggles without any question of material reward.

One explanatory factor is the structural position of countries of the periphery: they are the marginal parts of a world system. This subsidiary structural position profoundly shapes how the bourgeoisie, the elites within the peripheral countries, think, feel and act. This second factor is best captured by Franz Fanon in his classic of 1961, *The Wretched of the Earth*:

> The national middle-class discovers its historic mission: that of intermediary. Seen through its eyes, its mission has nothing to do with transforming the nation; it consists, prosaically, of being the transmission line between the nation and a capitalism, rampant though camouflaged, which today puts on the mask of

neo-colonialism. The national bourgeoisie will be quite content with the role of the Western bourgeoisie's business agent. … But this same lucrative role, this cheap-Jack's function, this meanness of outlook … symbolise the incapability of the middle class to fulfil its historic role … [of national transformation. Instead] the spirit of indulgence is dominant … and this is because the national bourgeoisie indentifies itself with…the decadence of the bourgeoisie of the West. … [The national bourgeoisie] is in fact beginning at the end. It is already senile before it has come to know the petulance, the fearlessness, or the will to succeed of youth. (Fanon, 1961 [1963], pp. 152–153)

How does being a "business agent" become "lucrative;" how does it feed "the spirit of indulgence" other than through the rent-collecting of bribery?

The "historic mission" of the peripheral bourgeoisie that makes them prematurely "senile" explains why governments of the periphery accept SAPs in all their odious forms. Core countries often provide the (legal) pay and perks of peripheral politicians and public officials (Hanlon, 2004). The readiness of the Zambian government to meet the conditionalities of HIPC, regardless of the consequences for the majority of Zambians, is readily explicable when one realizes that almost half of its national budget comes from foreign "aid."

The psychopaths?

As earlier stated, most of the people dispensing aid, including loans, and devising SAPs are probably well-intentioned. There are, however, a smaller number for whom the ethics of decent human relationships seem not to count (Bakan, 2005; Perkins, 2005). Most of them, however, including a core of policy advisers in the World Bank, the IMF, the Pentagon and similar institutions, would claim to be driven by higher – though still moral – considerations involving the national interest or ideologies in which difference (for example communism, socialism, Islam) is seen as dangerous.

There are, however, a few people who make a living buying, at discounted prices, that part of debt that even SAPs recognize as being unpayable, and then squeezing the indebted countries to pay up the full debt. Yet, this unconscionable behavior is perfectly legal. Its name within the financial industry is revealing: "Vulture Funds."[4] This suggests that these human vultures, although reprehensible, hold up a mirror to

the rest of us. What system and what ethical theories or values tolerate such living off the weak and desperate in far-away countries? Being the ultimate form of debt collection, Vulture Funds in their various forms force the rest of us to question our humanity and our society's ethics.

The way forward

Rights-based debt repudiation

Human rights have long been enshrined in both national and international law. More recently social and economic rights complement the more established civil and political ones. Debt clashes most directly with social and economic rights. Health rights clearly compete with debt servicing.

All countries of the periphery can calculate the cost of meeting their still outstanding socio-economic rights. These costs ought to have unquestioned priority over debt servicing. The predictable cry from the creditors that they couldn't afford the cost of putting human rights first rings hollow when set against the almost $13 trillion the USA alone is currently spending saving its selfish and greedy bankers (www.Bloomberg.com, March 31, 2009).

While the moral argument is unassailable, ethics seems to count for little in such matters. The issue is a political one. However, a rights-based approach could provide the ethical, legal and ultimately the political grounds for uniting the peoples of both the core and periphery of our single world. Their united mobilization might enable a challenge to the governments, bankers and peripheral bourgeoisie. The message is a simple one. People come first. Repudiate the debt to make this happen. Ecuador has recently done so.

References

Action for Southern Africa (ACTSA) (2003). *Southern Africa calls for reparations for apartheid.* August.

Bakan, J. (2005). *The Corporation – the Pathological Pursuit of Profit and Power.* London: Constable.

Bassett, M. T., Bijlmakers, L. A. & Sanders, D. M. (1997) Professionalism, patient satisfaction and quality of health care: experience during Zimbabwe's structural adjustment programme. *Social Science and Medicine* 45, 1845–1852.

Bassett, M. T., Bijlmakers, L. A. & Sanders, D. M. (2000). Experiencing structural adjustment in urban and rural households of Zimbabwe. In M. Turshen (Ed.), *African Women's Health* (pp. 167–191). Trenton, NJ: Africa World Press Inc.

---

[4] A vulture fund is a private equity or hedge fund that invests in debt issued by an entity that is considered to be very weak or dying.

Bijlmakers, L. A., Bassett, M. T. & Sanders, D. M. (1999). *Socioeconomic Stress, Health and Child Nutritional Status in Zimbabwe at a Time of Economic Structural Adjustment – A Three year Longitudinal Study.* Research Report No. 105. Uppsala: Nordiska Afrikainstitutet.

Breman, A. & Shelton, C. (2001). *Structural Adjustment and Health: A Literature Review of the Debate, its Role Players and the Presented Empirical Evidence.* WHO Commission on Macroeconomics and Health Working Paper WG 6:6. Geneva: World Health Organization.

Commission on Social Determinants of Health (2008). *Final Report: Closing the Gap in a Generation: Health Equity through Action on the Social Determinants of Health.* Geneva: World Health Organization.

Cornia, G., Jolly, R. & Stewart, F. (Eds.) (1988). *Adjustment with a Human Face: Ten Country Case Studies.* Oxford: Oxford University Press.

Costello, A., Watson, F. & Woodward, D. (1994). *Human Face or Human Facade? Adjustment and the Health of Mothers and Children.* Occasional Paper. London: Institute of Child Health.

De Savigny, D., Kasale, H., Mbuya, C. & Reid, G. (2004). *Fixing Health Systems.* Ottawa: International Development Research Centre. Cited in Labonté, R., Blouin, C., Chopra, M. *et al.* (2007). Towards health-equitable globalisation: Rights, regulation and redistribution. *Final Report of the Globalization Knowledge Network.* Geneva: World Health Organization Commission on Social Determinants of Health.

De Vogli, R. & Birbeck, G. L. (2005). Potential impact of adjustment policies on vulnerability of women and children to HIV/AIDS in Sub-Saharan Africa. *Journal of Health Population and Nutrition* **23**, 105–120.

Fanon, F. (1961) [1963]. *The Wretched of the Earth.* New York, NY: Grove Press.

Frank, A. G. (1967). Capitalism and underdevelopment in Latin America – historical studies of Chile and Brazil. New York, NY: Monthly Review Press.

Frank, A. G. (1969). *Latin America, Underdevelopment or Revolution – Essays on the Development of Underdevelopment and the Immediate Enemy.* New York, NY: Monthly Review Press.

George, S. (1988). *A Fate Worse than Debt: a Radical New Analysis of the Third World Debt Crisis.* London: Pelican Books.

Halstead, S. B., Walsh, J. A. & Warren, K. (Eds.) (1985). *Good Health at Low Cost.* New York, NY: Rockefeller Foundation.

Hanlon, J. (2000). How much debt must be cancelled? *Journal of International Development* **12**, 877–901.

Hanlon, J. (2004). *How Northern Donors Promote Corruption. Tales from the New Mozambique.* The Corner House Briefing No. 33. Sturminster Newton: The Corner House.

Labonté, R., Blouin, C., Chopra, M. *et al.* (2007). Towards health-equitable globalisation: Rights, regulation and redistribution. *Final Report of the Globalization Knowledge Network* (p. 56). Geneva: World Health Organization Commission on Social Determinants of Health. www.globalhealthequity.ca/electronic%20library/GKN%20Final%20Jan%208%202008.pdf

Malala, J. (2003). Mandela: Apartheid debt paralysed ANC. *ThisDay*, October 9.

Oxfam Global Campaign for Education (2004). Undervaluing teachers: IMF policies squeeze Zambian education system. London: Oxfam International.

Perkins, J. (2005). *Confessions of an Economic Hit Man.* London: Ebury Press.

Piot, P. (2004). Plenary Address for Closing Ceremony, XV International AIDS Conference: Getting Ahead of the Epidemic (Bangkok, July 16, 2004). Geneva: UNAIDS. Cited in Schrecker, T., Labonté, R. & Sanders, D. (2007). Breaking Faith with Africa: The G8 and population Health post-Gleneagles. In A. F. Cooper, J. J. Kirton & T. Schrecker (Eds.), *Governing Global Health: Challenge, Response, Innovation* (pp. 181–251). Aldershot: Ashgate.

Reuters (1999). G7 has failed in debt relief – Manuel. September 20. Reuters.

Rudin, J. (1999). *Apartheid Debt: Questions & Answers.* Johannesburg: Jubilee South Africa.

Rudin, J. (2000). *Odious Debt Revisited.* Johannesburg: Jubilee South Africa.

Rudin, J (2003) Forgive us this day our odious debt. *Mail & Guardian*, February 21.

Save the Children, UK (2003). *Submission to the World Development Report 2004: Making Services Work for Poor People.* London: Save the Children.

Toussaint, E. & Comanne, D. (2000). *Debt Relief: Much Ado About Nothing.* Brussels: CADTM Committee for the Abolition of Third World Debt.

Toussaint, E. & Millet, D. (2009) *60 Questions, 60 Answers on Debt, IMF and World Bank.* Brussels: CADTM Committee for the Abolition of Third World Debt.

United Nations Conference on Trade and Development (UNCTAD) (2003a). Economic Development in Africa. Commercial Results and Dependence on Commodities. Geneva: UNCTAD.

United Nations Conference on Trade and Development (UNCTAD) (2003b) Commodity Yearbook. http://ro.unctad.org/infocomm

World Health Organization (WHO) (2006). *Harmonization for Health in Africa: An Action Framework.* Geneva: WHO.

Zulu, M. (2007). Multi-Stakeholder Consultation on Financing Access to Basic Utilities for All. Lusaka, April 23–25. Unpublished.

Chapter

14

The international arms trade and global health

Salahaddin Mahmudi-Azer

Introduction

Despite the superficially friendly and respectable face of the world's current arms business, it remains as murky, secretive and amoral as it has always been. This secretive and destructive network of producers and traders of arms continues to be the driving force, and at times the initiating force, of many modern-day global conflicts in which civilians are the main victims (Burrows, 2002).

Until the Second World War, civilian deaths were a relatively small percentage of total deaths in conflicts (about 14%). But this classical face of conflict was changed by the mass murder of civilians in the Second World War. The genocidal campaigns against Jews, Roma and other distinct groups, together with the bombings of cities such as London, Dresden and Tokyo, and the use of nuclear bombs on Hiroshima and Nagasaki, brought civilians to the forefront of conflicts unlike any other conflicts in previous times. The nuclear bombs alone killed some 200 000 civilians instantly and caused physical and psychological damage to many more which continues even today (Coupland, 1996).

The trend towards mass killing and genocidal campaigns against civilians did not end with the Second World War, and to date civilians continue to be the main victims of conflict around the world.

Since the end of the Second World War, conventional weapons have been responsible for the deaths of more than 30 million people. The ongoing trend in escalating civilian deaths in modern-day conflict is extremely alarming. As a percentage of all deaths in conflict, these have risen dramatically to 67% in the 1970s, 75% in the 1980s, and 90% in the 1990s (Garfield & Neugut, 1991).

Given the destructive power of modern-day weapons and the magnitude of recent conflicts, their indirect impact on civilian lives is also far greater than in the past, with many dying from hunger and disease as an indirect result of crop destruction or being forced to flee their homes to become members of the world's growing refugee population (Judd, 1995).

A grim and sad example of the civilian toll in a modern-day conflict is the war in the Democratic Republic of Congo (DRC). As a result of this war, which started in 1998, 3.3 million people died, of whom only about 200 000 were killed directly through violence. The remaining 3 million deaths were attributed to such war-related causes as rampant infectious disease, hunger, malnutrition and dislocation of the population (Hawkins, 2004).

In 2008, a study carried out by the Iraq Family Health Survey Study Group estimated the number of violent civilian deaths in Iraq from March 2003 through June 2006 to be 151 000. While this survey was able to identify the number of violent deaths of civilians in that period, the number of civilians who lost their lives as an indirect result of the conflict remains unknown (Alkhuzai et al., 2008).

The vast majority of wars since 1945 have taken place in the developing world, many of which were proxy wars between the USA and the former Soviet Union. Furthermore numerous civil wars have arisen from historic, ethnic or religious enmities and resistance to oppressive governments (Sivard, 1993). Sadly, it seems that for the most part, conflicts and poverty go hand in hand. Between 1990 and 2001, there were 57 major armed conflicts in 45 different locations involving 16 of the world's 20 poorest countries (Wiharta & Anthony, 2003). While these conflicts undoubtedly profited the producers and traders of arms, they have also exacerbated and complicated the desperate conditions of the majority of the world.

Increasingly, the arms of choice in civil conflict around the world are anti-personnel weapons.

An earlier version of this work has appeared: Mahmudi-Azer, S. (2006). Arms trade and its impact on global health. *Theoretical Medicine and Bioethics*, 27 (1), 81–93.

Landmines, which are the most notorious and noxious of anti-personnel weapons, have brought about a new dark era in conflicts, resulting in typically severe injuries, often requiring amputation and frequently causing heavy loss of blood. According to the 1980 UN Convention on Conventional Weapons, minefields are to be marked and cleared once fighting has ended and landmines are to be designed so that they self-destruct within a limited period of time. However, in most instances neither obligation is met, and most landmines are accidentally detonated by innocent civilians long after conflicts are officially over. Ironically, it is less expensive to purchase and lay land mines than it is to remove them. In Cambodia, for example, a landmine can be bought on the black market for $10, but once laid, it costs at least $30 to locate and remove (Sidel, 1995).

Over the last few decades a tremendous effort has been made by civil society and non-governmental organizations to ban the use of landmines. In May 2009, the 1997 Mine Ban Treaty (also known as the Ottawa Convention) had been signed by 156 countries. Among the 37 countries who had not signed the treaty were three of the five permanent members of the UN Security Council, namely the USA, Russia and China, which are also known for their disproportionate contributions to the global arms trade. In addition, many countries which are currently at war have refused to sign the ban (Hiffler, 2000). It is estimated that there are currently more than 100 million landmines buried worldwide and another 100–150 million are in stockpiles. More than 60 countries are known to have vast minefields, including Afghanistan, Angola, Cambodia, Iraq, Mozambique and Somalia. Cambodia alone has an estimated 9 million mines (Imperato, 1995).

The global arms traders: who sells, who buys?

Extensive, up-to-date and credible data on who sells and who buys weapons is recorded and summarized in the Annual Yearbook of the Stockholm International Peace Research Institute (SIPRI), an easily accessible source (Anthony et al., 2009).

Between 1997 and 2000, the USA, the UK, Russia, France and China delivered 65–97% of their exported arms to developing countries. In some cases, arms were sold to both sides of a conflict, for example in the Iran–Iraq War and in the ongoing tension between Pakistan and India (Anthony et al., 2009). This disappointing approach by permanent members of UN Security Council is an indication that conflicts are viewed by them as markets for their arms and not as a threat to global security.

Clearly, the more spent on armaments by governments in the developing world, the less will be available to spend on desperately needed health care, education and social services. Pakistan, for example, spends heavily on military equipment, while allocating less than 1% of its gross domestic product to health care (Akram & Khan, 2007). In a June 2005 press release, Amnesty International accused the G8 countries (the USA, the UK, Germany, Canada, Italy, France, Russia and Japan) of undermining their commitments to poverty reduction, stability and human rights with irresponsible arms exports to some of the world's poorest and most conflict-ridden countries (Amnesty International, 2005).

In 2003, the USA transferred weapons worth approximately $1 billion to 18 of the 25 countries involved in active conflicts (Berrigan & Hartung, 2005). In addition, the US government sells arms to countries well known for violating human rights, including Indonesia, Columbia, Uzbekistan and Saudi Arabia. Strikingly, 20 of the top 25 countries to which the USA sells arms are either undemocratic regimes or governments with records of major human rights abuses, or both (Defense Security Cooperation Agency, 2003).

The UK sold $4.7 billion worth of arms in 2003, second only to the $13.7 billion sold by the USA, and since 2003 their arms production and sales have grown to a new record high. The UK Government imposed changes to arms export guidelines and have relaxed controls and oversight requirements, leading to a significant increase in particular areas of the arms trade. Indeed, it seems that since 2003 there has been a several-fold increase in the number of arms components licensed for export by the UK government. According to the latest annual report on weapons-related exports, in 2006 the UK government approved arms exports to 19 of the 20 countries it identified as "countries of concern" for abusing human rights. They included Saudi Arabia, Israel, Colombia, China and Russia. The report also reveals that during 2006 the UK government authorized the export of more than 15 000 sniper rifles to countries including Pakistan, Jordan, Turkey and Saudi Arabia, components for military aircraft and tanks for China, and heavy machine guns for Colombia (Hawley, 2003; Evans & Norton-Taylor, 2008).

In 2004, arms sales to developing countries totaled nearly $21.8 billion (an increase above the $15.1 billion in 2003) and the value of weapons sales worldwide increased to $37 billion – the highest since 2000 (United Nations Development Program, 2004). While countries in the developed world purchase arms from each other, the bulk of the arms trade is destined for the developing world. According to Control Arms, a coalition of NGOs working to stop the arms trade: "an average of $22 billion a year is spent on arms by countries in Africa, Asia, the Middle East and Latin America, a sum that otherwise spent could enable these same countries to be on track in meeting the Millennium Development Goals of achieving universal primary education (estimated at $10 billion a year) and to reducing infant and maternal mortality (estimated at $12 billion a year)" (Grimmett, 2008).

An example of a civil war which clearly showed the role of the arms industry and trade was that of the Democratic Republic of the Congo (DRC), as mentioned earlier. Arms used in the conflict were supplied by multiple sources, including Belgium, China, France, Germany, Israel, Spain, the UK and the USA. Furthermore; arms delivered to the governments of Rwanda, Uganda and Zimbabwe by Albania, China, Egypt, Israel, Romania, Slovakia and South Africa also made their way to the DRC (Hartung & Moix, 2000).

From 1994 to 1997, Saudi Arabia was the largest purchaser of arms among the developing countries, spending $12.4 billion. More recently, its purchases have declined due to the debts and obligations incurred during the first Persian Gulf War. The USA, the UK and Russia supplied Saudi Arabia with arms worth $9.7 billion, $4.0 billion and $3.6 billion respectively (Grimmett, 2002).

Among various major arms suppliers in the world the USA is the only arms supplier with two distinct systems of exporting arms. The first system is similar to that employed by most other countries, that is, government to government exports. This process is closely monitored and statistics are made public. The second is a licensed commercial export system that is neither well monitored nor made public, leaving it open to abuse. In the latter system, an exporting corporation obtains a license from the government stating to whom it plans to export and what it plans to send. However, there is no requirement to disclose what is actually sent (Grimmett, 2002).

Adverse effects of the global arms trade

Fueling conflict and human rights violations

Arms suppliers are regarded as having a direct role in initiating, exacerbating and maintaining conflict (Burrows, 2002). In the majority of conflicts, the most vulnerable victims are children. According to UNICEF, 2 million children were killed in armed conflicts between 1986 and 1996, and 6 million children were seriously injured or permanently disabled (UNICEF, 2002). It is also widely believed that "the trade in arms perpetuates, worsens and legitimizes the systematic abuse of human rights all over the world" (Amnesty International, 2008). In recent conflicts, arms (mostly supplied by industrialized countries) have been widely used to violate the rights of civilians. In a majority of conflict situations, geopolitical and economic interests have trumped the protection of human rights. In its "war on terror" the USA lifted previously existing sanctions from countries it then sought as allies, some of which were well known for their violations of human rights, including Philippines, Turkey, Georgia, Tajikistan, Pakistan and Columbia (Federation of American Scientists, 2005).

Small arms are specifically linked to human rights violations, as they are easier to obtain than larger weapons and can be used by child soldiers, an abuse in and of itself. Small arms are "inexpensive, portable, lethal, long-lasting and easy to operate" (United Nations, 2001). They are more readily accessible on the illicit market than their larger counterparts and are frequently exchanged for cash or such contraband items as diamonds and drugs. It is estimated that some 639 million small arms are currently in circulation and most are in private hands (Bowcott & Norton-Taylor, 2003).

In 2002, the G8 countries allocated $20 billion to programs aimed at preventing nuclear, chemical and biological weapons from falling into the wrong hands. By contrast, considerably less attention and resources have been allocated to address the acquisition of small arms by state actors and armed groups (Berrigan, 2004).

Over the last several years the role of small arms in conflicts has gained the attention of civil society. In 2001, a UN Conference on the Illicit Traffic in Small Arms and Light Weapons developed a plan of action that was followed by a UN Conference on Small Arms in 2006. Despite the tremendous effort from Amnesty International, Oxfam, and the International Network on Small Arms, to convince the participating governments to "outlaw weapons sales involving exportation for use entailing violations of international human rights or humanitarian law," the conference ended without agreeing on an outcome (United Nations, 2006).

Global instability

Stockpiles of armaments are now growing at a rate that would have seemed inconceivable only a decade ago. Instead of limiting the trade in arms, the "war on terror" has likely exacerbated it. Lately, major powers have used arms exports as incentives for allies whose commitment to democracy and human rights is questionable. In 2001, the Philippines received more than $100 million in US military equipment, including helicopters, transport planes and 30 000 M16 rifles (United Nations, 2001). The black market trade in guns is flourishing with stolen, lost or illegally sold arms being acquired by armed insurgent groups. As a result, far from lessening the threat of terrorism, the export of military equipment to such tenuous democracies may only serve to exacerbate human rights abuses, aggravate local tensions and prolong civil conflicts (Amnesty International & Oxfam, 2003).

Environmental degradation

In addition to direct harm to the health and well-being of human societies caused by the arms trade, there are indirect consequences of great concern. One such consequence is the damage to the environment and its ecosystems caused by nuclear weapons, Agent Orange and depleted uranium. While some researchers maintain that the evidence for the harm done by depleted uranium is insufficient, most now concur that it has done serious damage and that its impact will continue for centuries. Environmental pollution associated with nuclear weapons is well documented and the fall-out from nuclear atmospheric testing is projected to cause between 100 000 and 500 000 cancer fatalities by the end of this century (Makhijani, 2008). Nuclear testing fall-out contributes to climate change by creating massive dust clouds that obscure sunlight and lower temperatures. Radiation also contaminates exposed food and water supplies, which can result in debilitating and life-threatening neuromuscular and gastro-intestinal effects (Leaning, 2002).

A study by the US National Cancer Institute examining the effects of the testing of nuclear weapons at the Nevada site during the 1950s found that a significant portion of the milk supply was contaminated with iodine-131, a compound linked to thyroid cancer (Centers for Disease Control and Prevention & the National Cancer Institute, 2001). Chemical weapons such as napalm and herbicide defoliants are linked to environmental degradation and destruction. "Agents Orange, White and Blue" were used by the USA during the Vietnam War to destroy forests, grain crops and rice fields. After many years of debate and denial, it has now been established that the agents cause a wide range of organ and metabolic dysfunctions, such as cancers, birth defects and genetic damage (Environmental Agents Service, 2003).

Efforts to limit the global arms trade

Several campaigns have emerged over the years to expose the negative impact of the arms trade. However, the armaments lobby, led by manufacturing/market interests of the private and public sectors, and other powerful forces have succeeded in limiting their effectiveness (Cornish, 1996).

Several UN Conventions address the arms industry and place limits and controls on certain types of weapons. However, these conventions are not binding on particular countries unless they sign on and ratify each agreement, indeed, each component of each agreement needs to be ratified and signed (Boese, 2004). Perhaps the most comprehensive agreement is the "Convention on Certain Conventional Weapons," also known as the "United Nations Convention on Inhumane Weapons." This Convention, which has been evolving since 1981, applies both to inter-state and intra-state conflicts. Protocol 1 (1983) bans weapons that contain "nondetectable fragments" that evade detection by X-rays and are therefore difficult to remove. Protocol 2 (1983, amended 1996) regulates, but does not ban, the use of landmines and booby traps. This Protocol has been signed by 76 countries, including most of the world's major producers and users of landmines (e.g. China, India, Israel, Pakistan, Russia and the USA). However, these countries have refused to sign the Ottawa convention that bans these weapons completely. Protocol 3 (1983) regulates the use of incendiary weapons, Protocol 4 (1996) prohibits the use of lasers designed to cause blindness and Protocol 5 (2003) deals with unexploded and abandoned ordnance. The signatories are currently debating further items, including adding compliance mechanisms and a provision to ban small caliber bullets, which can cause major injuries by ricocheting or tumbling around inside a body (Boese, 2004).

Numerous other international treaties aim to limit the proliferation of arms. Many of these are UN sponsored, while others are more geographically specific. In 1991, the UN General Assembly adopted a resolution on "transparency in armaments" that set up a voluntary registry of conventional arms transfers. Unfortunately, the majority of manufacturing countries have failed to sign on. The European Union, for its part, has made some limited efforts to control arms trade by introducing a Code of Conduct that monitors major conventional weapons trades and the end use of these weapons. Shortcomings that undermine the effectiveness of this code include weak or non-existent controls on transfers to third parties and increasingly weaker controls on the sale of components (Control Arms, 2004).

In addition to the opposition to conventional arms controls from the manufacturing countries there is opposition from non-manufacturing, non-nuclear countries. As the countries that possess nuclear weapons refuse to abolish them, the non-nuclear countries see no reason to lessen their capacity to defend themselves against stronger opponents (Hawley, 2003).

Despite resistance from arms manufacturers, there have been outstanding efforts by numerous non-governmental organizations in the past 20 years to limit the production and trade of weapons. Organizations such as the International Association of Lawyers Against Nuclear Arms, the World Summit for Social Development, and Control Arms (a campaign jointly run by Amnesty International, Oxfam, and the International Action Network on Small Arms) have made valiant efforts. In October 2003, Control Arms issued a call for effective arms control: Every government in the world has a responsibility to control arms, both their possession within its country's borders and their export across its borders, to protect its own citizens and to ensure respect for international human rights and humanitarian law in the wider world. The world's most powerful governments, who are also the world's biggest arms suppliers, have the greatest responsibility to control the global trade.

The five permanent members of the UN Security Council, France, Russia, China, the UK and the USA,

together account for 88% of the world's conventional arms exports; and these exports contribute regularly to gross abuses of human rights. The challenge to all governments is urgent. They must cooperate to control and limit the flow of arms and the spread of arms production. At the very least, arms-exporting countries must not supply arms where there is a clear danger that they will be used for violations of international human rights and humanitarian law (Amnesty International *et al.*, 2005).

The 1997 Landmines Treaty, made possible by the combination of both active government and civil society support, marks one of the greatest achievements for the global opposition to the arms trade. Although the scourge of landmines has not yet been eradicated, no country has openly traded in these weapons since 1997. Perhaps a similar combination of public pressure and action by sympathetic governments is needed to secure an effective and binding arms trade treaty.

Conclusions

Despite efforts to limit arms production and trade, the arms industry is a formidable economic and geopolitical force that is gaining in strength and impunity. Millions of civilians have paid with their livelihoods and lives for the maintenance of this trade and, given the unprecedented rate of growth for the industry, it is frightening to contemplate future casualties. In order to assure a more stable and peaceful future for our planet and to eradicate the victimization of so many innocent civilians, serious efforts have to be made to limit the manufacture and trade of arms. It must be conceded that "... in the 21st century the applications for newly developed military-related technologies and the difficulty, if not impossibility, of controlling access to such technologies are likely to go far beyond what was experienced, and imagined, in the 1990s" (Cornish, 1996). This is a public health issue that demands serious attention from the bioethicists of developed nations.

References

Akram, M. & Khan, F. J. (2007). *Health Care Services and Government Spending in Pakistan*. Pakistan Institute of Development Economics – Working Papers, 32.

Alkhuzai, A. H., Ahmad, I. J. & Hweel, M. J. (2008). Violence-related mortality in Iraq from 2002 to 2006. *New England Journal of Medicine* **358**(5), 484–493.

Amnesty International (2008). *Blood at the Crossroads: Making the Case for a Global Arms Trade*

Treaty. www.amnesty.org.uk/uploads/documents/doc_18674.pdf (Accessed December 2009).

Amnesty International, Oxfam & International Action Network on Small Arms (2005). *The G8: Global Arms Exporters: Failing to Prevent Irresponsible Arms Transfers.* www.iansa.org/control_arms/documents/g8report/g8-control-arms-paper-en.pdf (Accessed on December 2009).

Amnesty International & Oxfam (2003). *Shattered Lives. The Case for Tough International Arms Control.* www.amnesty.org/en/library/asset/ACT30/003/2003/en/2f38f752-d690-11dd-ab95-a13b602c0642/act300032003en.pdf (Accessed December 2009).

Amnesty International Press Release (2005). AI Index: POL 30/01612005 (Public). News Service No. 159, June 22.

Anthony, I., Bauer, S. & Bodell, N. (2009). *Stockholm International Peace Research Institute (SIPRI) Yearbook. Armaments, Disarmament and International Security.* Stockholm: SIPRI.

Berrigan, F. (2004). *Small Arms? Big Problem.* Common Dreams News Center. www.commondreams.org.

Berrigan, F. & Hartung, W. D. (2005). *U.S. Weapons at War: Promoting Freedom or Fueling Conflict?* Arms Trade Resource Center, World Policy Institute.

Boese, W. (2004). *Convention on Certain Conventional Weapons at a Glance.* Arms Control Association. www.armscontrol.org/factsheets/CCW.asp (Accessed December 2009).

Bowcott, O. & Norton-Taylor, R. (2003). War on terror fuels small arms trade. *Guardian Unlimited.* www.guardian.co.uk/armstrade/story/0,10674,1059843,00.html. (Accessed December 2009).

Burrows, G. (2002). *The No-Nonsense Guide to the Arms Trade.* New York: Verso.

Centers for Disease Control and Prevention & the National Cancer Institute (2001). *Report to Congress: A Feasibility Study of the Health Consequences to the American Population of Nuclear Weapons Test Conducted by the United States and Other Nations.* www.ieer.org/offdocs/falloutprogrpt.pdf (Accessed December 2009).

Control Arms (2004). *Arms Trade: New Report Reveals Major Loophole in British Arms Export Controls.* www.controlarms.org/latest_news/export_loopholes_250204.htm. (Accessed December 2009).

Cornish, P. (1996). *Controlling the Arms Trade: The West versus the Rest.* London: Bowerdean Publishing Co.

Coupland, R. M. (1996). The Effects of Weapons on Health. *Lancet* 347, 450–451.

Deputy for Operations and Administration, Defense Security Cooperation Agency (2003). Foreign Military Sales, Foreign Military Construction Sales and Military Assistance Facts. www.dsca.mil/programs/biz-ops/2003_facts

Environmental Agents Service (2003). Department of Veterans Affairs. Agent Orange Brief. www.publichealth.va.gov/exposures/agentorange/health_effects.asp (Accessed December 2009).

Evans, R. & Norton-Taylor, R. (2008). UK tops world table of weapons sales. *The Guardian,* June 21.

Federation of American Scientists (2005). *United States Arms Sales Policy Related to Counter-Terrorism and Near East/South Asia, Arms Transfers.* www.fas.org/terrorism/at/ (Accessed December 2009).

Garfield, R. M. & Neugut, A. I. (1991). Epidemiological analysis of warfare: a historical analysis. *Journal of the American Medical Association* 226, 688–692.

Grimmett, R. F. (2002). *Conventional Arms Transfers to Developing Nations, 1994–2001.* Report for Congress.

Grimmett, R. F. (2008). *Conventional Arms Transfers to Developing Nations, 2000–2007.* CRS Report for Congress.

Hartung, W. D. & Moix, B. (2000). *Deadly Legacy: U.S. Arms to Africa and the Congo War.* Arms Trade Resource Center, World Policy Institute.

Hawkins, V. (2004). Stealth conflicts: Africa's World War in the DRC and international consciousness. *Journal of Humanitarian Assistance,* 1, 1–16.

Hawley, S. (2003). *Turning a Blind Eye: Corruption and the UK Export Credits Guarantee Department.* Dorset: Corner House. www.thecornerhouse.org.uk/pdf/document/correcgd.pdf (Accessed December 2009).

Hiffler, L. (2000). Banning the antipersonnel landmines: a treaty not too far! *Tropical Doctor* 30, 244–246.

Imperato, P. J. (1995). Clearing the fields: solutions to the global land mines crisis. *New England Journal of Medicine* 332, 1525–1526.

Judd, F. (1995). Conflict, famine and the arms trade. *Medicine and War* 11, 99–104.

Leaning, J. (2002). Environment and health. Impact of war. *Canadian Medical Association Journal* 163(9), 1157–1161.

Makhijani, A. (2008). *A Global Truth Commission on Health and Environmental Damage from Nuclear Weapons Production.* Institute for Energy and Environmental Research. www.reachingcriticalwill.org/legal/nwc/mon2truth.html (Accessed December 2009).

Sidel, V. W. (1995). The international arms trade and its impact on health. *British Medical Journal* 311, 1677–1680.

Sivard, R. L. (1993). *World Military and Social Expenditures.* Washington, DC: World Priorities.

UNICEF (2002). *The State of the World's Children.* Geneva: UNICEF.

United Nations (2001). *Report of the United Nations Conference on the Illicit Trade of Small Arms and Light Weapons in All its Aspects.* http://disarmament2.un.org/cab/smallarms/ (Accessed December 2009).

United Nations (2006). *Report of the Conference to Review Progress Made in the Implementation of the Programme of Action to Prevent, Combat and Eradicate the Illicit Trade in Small Arms and Light Weapons in All Its Aspects.* www.un.org/events/smallarms2006/pdf/rc.9-e.pdf (Accessed December 2009).

United Nations Development Program (2004). *Human Development Report.* New York, NY: UNDP.

Wiharta, S. & Anthony, I. (2003). Major armed conflicts 1991–2000. *SIPRI Yearbook*, 109–125.

Chapter

15

Allocating resources in humanitarian medicine

Samia A. Hurst, Nathalie Mezger and Alex Mauron

Background

Allocating resources in humanitarian medicine is a vitally important and cruelly difficult exercise. In the huge disconnect between severe human needs and limited resources, even asking how allocation can be fair can seem harsh. Do those involved in humanitarian medicine not simply do all they *can*?

Daunting as the questions regarding how to allocate resources fairly and legitimately in humanitarian medicine may be, they are gaining in importance for at least three identifiable and related reasons.

First, one of the primary motivating factors for humanitarian medicine is the rule of rescue, "the imperative people feel to rescue identifiable individuals facing avoidable death," or other plights invoking a shock or horror reaction, "without thinking about the costs too much" (Jonsen, 1986; McKie & Richardson, 2003). As humanitarian medicine successfully raises awareness of urgent health-related needs in poverty-stricken regions of the world, the number of such identifiable victims increases. Indeed, we should expect identified needs to remain greater than the available means as long as there are both pressingly needy sick persons, and advocates raising awareness to their plight. One usual implication of the rule of rescue is that an identifiable, immediate victim should have priority over distant "statistical" lives. From the perspective of a humanitarian organization, persons in need are indeed identifiable, and giving aid to them is saving real, not "statistical" lives. As the number of such identifiable victims, and the diversity of their needs, increase, so does the complexity of allocation decisions. This makes allocation decisions more important, but also harder to think through. Another difficulty is that part of the rule of rescue is that we should not think about the costs involved. This means that even asking how to allocate resources in humanitarian medicine can seem problematic. If humanitarian medicine "must do *something* ..." about each crisis, then allocating resources away from any of them could seem intrinsically wrong. Asking how to allocate resources could seem to reflect a lack of moral concern. Although it could seem obvious that humanitarian medical organizations must, and should, make choices between competing situations of need, this point has indeed needed to be formally defended (Wikler, 2003). This would seem to confirm the difficulty of thinking through allocation when faced with different situations where the rule of rescue could apply.

Second, one of the reasons why many find humanitarian advocacy convincing is an ongoing – though admittedly controversial and incomplete – shift from a charity view to a rights-based view of international health (Hendriks & Toebes, 1998; Katz, 2004). This makes the claim for help more compelling. Humanitarian medical organizations usually originate from the financially richer part of the world, although not all individual humanitarians do. On a rights-based view, it would thus be all the more convincing to assign a share in the duty to fulfill such a right to these organizations. Exactly how much the rich are required to help the poor is controversial. Very generous answers, such that we owe until the need becomes smaller than our own, have been criticized as too altruistic to be required (Scheffler, 1992). But it has also been argued that we do have a collective duty to maximize beneficence to those in need (Murphy, 2000), or that such duties arise in rich countries from shared responsibility in maintaining global rules that harm the global poor (Pogge, 2005), or from a collective duty to rescue which non-governmental organizations enable us to fulfill (Nagel, 2005). Under such views, the basic problem

An earlier version of this work has appeared: Hurst, S. A., Mezger, N. and Mauron, A. (2009). Allocating resources in humanitarian medicine. *Public Health Ethics* 2 (1), 89–99.

becomes practical: most people do not do their share. Even so, we may not be required to do more than our own share (Murphy, 2000). So *how much* humanitarian medicine would be required under this obligation remains unanswered.[1] Any claim to a right to health – for example to assure fair equality of opportunity (Daniels, 1985) on a global scale (Caney, 2001), or to fulfill a human right (United Nations, 1948) – would be likely to lead to an increase in the number of those recognized as requiring assistance, as compared with charity-based views. The importance of fair allocation would consequently be increased as well, as both the need for fairness itself, and the strain on resources, increased. Indeed, this would be the case even if we were to take a more modest view. Minimally, humanitarian medical organizations should offer help when they are the only, or one of the few, who are on the spot and able to offer help or make the emergency known to others, as in the "duty to rescue": if you can save someone at no excessive cost to yourself, then you should (McIntyre, 1994). Nevertheless, this would still mean that as the breadth of their activities increased, so would the number and scope of the situations with which they would be expected to deal, and with it the importance of fair resource allocation.

Third, partly as a consequence of increased recognition of rights-based claims to health care, an increasing number of the situations faced by humanitarian medicine are protracted rather than acute "crises." Such protracted crises simultaneously increase the difficulty and the importance of fair allocation.

In war, or natural disaster, humanitarian medicine intervenes to minimize the effect of the crisis on human health through medical intervention (Birch & Miller, 2005). In acute crises, this is often understood to mean "through any means available at the time." In such situations, the kind of response that can be set up is limited by the severity of the emergency. The crisis is usually limited in time. Finally, although these situations are sadly not rare, they are perceived as exceptional. They are violently different from ordinary life, even when ordinary life is set in precarious circumstances. Even if "the best possible intervention" is far from perfect, humanitarians are indeed doing "the best they possibly can" under very obvious and specific circumstances. They are not allocating resources away from anyone, nor are they setting a precedent or sending a message that the limits used would in any way be appropriate under more normal circumstances.

Increasingly, however, humanitarian medicine's actions extend to more protracted crises (Rougemont, 1995; Michael & Zwi, 2002), such as concerns for primary care in Darfur, and access to antiretrovirals in sub-Saharan Africa. These situations give rise to different technical challenges (Hendrickson, 1998). They also pose different ethical challenges. The kinds of harm they risk inflicting differ. Acute interventions risk diminishing self-sufficiency in specific ways (such as wiping out local food markets, for example) (Redmond, 2005). Interventions of a more chronic kind have raised concerns about "propping up repressive and irresponsible governments" (Michael & Zwi, 2002). The importance of consulting communities, to understand their needs, and show them respect, also becomes more visible in protracted crises (Palmer, 1999; Diallo *et al.*, 2005).

As regards resource allocation decisions, protracted crises differ from acute crises in important ways. The available time-frame no longer quasi-automatically constrains the available resources. Deliberate choices more clearly control the amount of resources that will, in fact, be made available. Defining "the best we can possibly do" becomes fuzzier, and resources will sometimes be allocated away from situations of need. Furthermore, situations of chronic need are not distinct from everyday life. They are part of the daily routine for much of humanity. This is a crucial difference: decisions made in exceptional circumstances do not constitute appropriate precedents for "normal" life. A degree of double standard will set times of acute crisis apart from normal times, and this can be justified by exceptionally strained circumstances. However, the ethical picture changes when that double standard becomes part of everyday life. We may then become used to it. It may even seem to provide an unfortunate justification to an ethically unacceptable situation. Making resource allocation decisions responsibly is both more difficult and more important in protracted crises.

---

[1] An approach based on non-ideal theory does point to one avenue where further enquiry could suggest a threshold, both for the duty of humanitarian medicine, and for the resources that it ought to have. Additionally, since some may do their own share by giving resources to humanitarian medicine, and inasmuch as many people currently do not do their share, this could mean that humanitarians could claim, up to a point, that others could fulfill their share by giving them more resources than they currently do.

This chapter invites further examination of several challenges specific to resource allocation in humanitarian medicine, and proposes one strategy to improve distributive fairness in this context.[2] As experience regarding actual allocation decisions in humanitarian medicine is not widespread, the next section briefly outlines examples. Following that we describe some of the difficulties in allocating resources fairly and legitimately which are either increased in humanitarian medicine or specific to its international context. All of these issues would benefit both from theoretical exploration on specific application to humanitarian medicine, and from empirical research on the impact of different strategies. We then propose that some headway could be made by adapting existing frameworks of procedural fairness for practical use in humanitarian organizations. The penultimate section presents Daniels & Sabin's "Accountability for reasonableness," an influential approach to resource allocation, and the limits to its application to humanitarian medicine. Finally we propose adaptations which could address some of these limits.

A few examples

Allocation decisions in humanitarian medicine can take several forms. Some choices will involve weighing different programs against each other. This was the case in 2005 when the Swiss section of *Médecins Sans Frontières* (MSF) took a very painful decision not to respond to the Pakistani earthquake. At that time, the huge emergency nutritional crisis in Niger was already occupying a large portion of the organization's human resources, as were other difficult crises like Darfur. The annual budget for departures had already been doubled that year. Responding to this new medical crisis would clearly have led to serious neglect of other

missions, and might have pushed the organization over the brink. In this case, priority was given to the more stable missions. Back-up was offered to other MSF sections on site, conditions were defined under which a greater response would have been initiated, and the situation was regularly re-evaluated.

Some choices will address the scope of an organization more generally. An example is the choice of whether to consider HIV a worldwide neglected emergency. *Médecins Sans Frontières* usually provides treatment for acute, medical, often neglected problems, and only deals with chronic diseases such as diabetes or cardiovascular diseases on a case-by-case basis.

Such choices regarding which disease to treat also directly lead to choices between individuals. Strict admission criteria in hospitals can mean that, as a doctor, you may have to send back a young patient complaining of clear inaugural diabetic symptoms. The treatment she needs is obvious (insulin), yet you cannot offer it although you know that she will not find it elsewhere either. Although selection on the basis of the disease a patient suffers from is usually viewed as a public health rather than as an individual criterion in resource allocation, this can be – and in practice often is – understood as choosing one individual over another on the criterion of their diagnosis.

Challenges to fair allocation in humanitarian medicine

In cases like these, and in addition to the difficulties attached to resource allocation in any context (Coulter & Ham, 2000), fair allocation in humanitarian medicine raises specific ethical difficulties regarding non-ideal fairness, the scope of global solidarity, legitimacy in non-governmental institutions and the potential for conflicts of interest.

Fairness in an unfair world

Fair access to medical treatment can be understood in a variety of ways, but sufficientarian, egalitarian and prioritarian views all lead to the same initial conclusion regarding the international context of humanitarian medicine: it is more difficult. If fair access to health care is usually understood to mean that everyone has access to some basic response to their health-related needs (sufficientarian), perhaps even the same access (egalitarian) and that the worse off get at least some priority (prioritarian), how should we face the choice between practicing medicine to a lower standard to share out

---

[2] We recognize that normative controversy could focus on the very existence of humanitarian medicine. For the purposes of this paper, however, we will accept the premise that its existence is justified, to examine the more specific issue of fair resource allocation in its context. This assumption is reasonable. Despite its suggested negative effects, humanitarian medicine saves many lives and improves others, is mostly welcome by its recipients, garners enough support to owe its continued existence to funding by individuals, and more generally exists to help those in the sort of physical need we readily recognize as a valid claim for help. The skeptical reader may perhaps find the empirical premise – that humanitarian medicine actually does exist – sufficient to read on.

resources among more people, or refusing this change and treating fewer people, all of whom are by the way equally needy and certainly among the worse-off globally as regards their health-related needs? Generic antiretroviral therapy, used with simplified follow-up protocols, made treatment available to tens of thousands who would otherwise not have had access to it in poor countries (Calmy *et al.*, 2004). The effectiveness of these drugs is similar to that of others used in industrialized countries (Laurent *et al.*, 2004), however the degree of safety afforded by simplified surveillance may not be the same. This led to heated debate (Dyer, 2004). In addition to the difficulty of either allowing a greater degree of risk or allowing more people to go without treatment, both these solutions still leave many patients without access to life-saving drugs. Thus, it could be said that neither outcome is fair. How to identify a fair decision in such a context? One of the aspects this controversy reveals is that in most circumstances we count on some degree of fairness already existing in the group where issues of resource allocation arise. Humanitarian medicine faces the problem of having to be as fair as possible in an unfair world.

Equity without a community

Health systems usually exist to support a common endeavor to care for everybody's health. We are accustomed to thinking of equity within defined groups, where reciprocity forms the basis for accepting unified standards in access to health care. Humanitarian medicine faces the problem of finding equitable solutions where no community supports reciprocity. Humanity itself could theoretically form such a circle of solidarity, in that there is no presently identified intrinsically insurmountable obstacle to such a situation. However, in practice it is currently clearly not a cohesive group, or even a group united as regards reciprocity in health care. It has been argued that "the extension of economic and cultural relationships beyond national borders" gives us reason for international solidarity, or even social contracts (Beitz, 1975), and that global distributive justice ought to be egalitarian (Hinsch, 2001), at least as regards minimum conditions for a decent human life (Beitz, 2001). Despite our increasingly rights-based view of international health, which grounds itself in the emergence of a human right not only to the conditions of health (United Nations, 1948) but also to health itself (Hendriks & Toebes, 1998; Katz, 2004), such common standards do not extend

to how to allocate health resources fairly. Humanity currently neither supports a system of reciprocity for health care, nor common standards of equity in allocating health-care resources. Thinking about fairness and equity in the context of humanitarian medicine is harder.

This issue has been discussed mostly as regards access to needed drugs in poor countries, especially in the context of antiretroviral therapy in facing the HIV/AIDS pandemic. Macklin, for example, proposed definitions of equity based on priority to those likely to benefit the most, to reducing disparities in health or in access to health care, to the worse off, or to some form of reciprocity (Macklin, 2003). Each of these principles is problematic in some circumstances, and they can conflict with one another. For example, the utilitarian principle can result in our ignoring claims on the part of the most vulnerable, or the worse-off. Giving unlimited priority to the worse-off can result in our pouring resources into situations where we help but little, and ignoring situations where more effective help can be offered. Giving in return to those who have contributed – one form of reciprocity – can sometimes favor the best-off, those capable of contributing in the first place, who are likely to be less needy. A consequence of these problems is that none of these principles seems to be a likely candidate to substitute straightforward application of a theory of justice for the sort of social contract that is lacking.

Legitimacy

Although we may be more likely to accept allocation decisions as legitimate if they are fair, legitimacy in humanitarian medicine poses a distinct problem. First, how is the question of what makes a decision legitimate to be understood in this context? The actions of humanitarian medicine do not represent "coercively imposed collective authority" (Nagel, 2005), so if we are asking about the sort of legitimacy a state requires, any requirement for legitimacy could be questioned upfront. Nevertheless, the extent of humanitarian organizations' actual role in decisions that affect the basic conditions of a decent life, especially "where states are weak" and where "a diversity of agents and agencies … can contribute to justice" is compelling (O'Neill, 2001, p. 194). So questions usually linked to state legitimacy may not be entirely inappropriate here. Minimally, under what conditions can decisions regarding the allocation of international health-care resources be considered legitimate when made by non-governmental organizations? The nature and extent of a duty to provide humanitarian medicine may shape questions regarding legitimacy. If we view humanitarian medicine as charity, and base decisions on which plight we find most poignant, it is not clear that we need give any further reasons. If, however, we have a duty to provide help, including humanitarian medicine, for example because we share responsibility in maintaining international rules that harm the global poor (Pogge, 2005) and their health (Pogge, 2002), this could affect not just what our duty is, but how it should be fulfilled. If "the extension of economic … relationships" gives us reason to share resources internationally (Beitz, 1975), this too will affect what legitimacy in humanitarian medicine might look like. Recognizing a right to health care for any reason has a similar effect. Consequently, the same development from charity-based to rights-based claims to health should be expected to affect the issue of legitimacy as well. A more rights-based approach will require stronger legitimacy in allocation decisions, and would also tend to shift the target of accountability from donors to include beneficiaries.

The second difficulty is that just about any claim for legitimacy in allocating resources in humanitarian medicine seems bound to be incompletely fulfilled. We may for example think that those affected by allocation decisions should have the possibility of understanding and critiquing them (Forst, 2001). This however might include all populations who need the assistance of humanitarian medicine, as well as donors, and those who would implement these decisions: a difficult logistical problem. Fulfilling minimal claims for legitimacy, such as those based on the view that humanitarian medicine is strictly superogatory charity work, does seem more feasible,[3] but does not make such a view any more convincing.

Although procedural fairness could represent some beginning towards greater legitimacy (see following sections), allocation decisions in humanitarian medicine may ultimately never be entirely legitimate under current international circumstances. In any case, philosophical analysis of legitimacy in humanitarian intervention has tended to focus primarily on legitimacy to transgress negative rights in the context of decisions regarding whether or not any intervention was justified.[4] Humanitarian medicine, however, raises issues of legitimacy in resource allocation for positive rights, such as the right to health or health care, and allocation within existing programs, in decidedly non-ideal circumstances. These issues would benefit from further exploration.

Conflicting goals and interests

Justifications used by MSF for allocation decisions are not limited to a single goal, or even to principles of equity (Fuller, 2006). This shows that something richer is going on, but also makes a potential for goal conflicts apparent. One example is the potential for conflict between the goals of *témoignage* – speaking out regarding human tragedies – and care. At first sight, these two goals seem very similar. They arise from the same kinds of motivations and circumstances: being there and able both to help and to speak out, when no – or few – others are. Indeed, *témoignage* may sometimes take up where the possibility of other actions stops. An action remains possible when we are otherwise powerless.

There are, however, two potential tensions there. First, for humanitarians "doing the best they can" in an imperfect world can involve "cutting corners" in individual actions to do the most good overall. For example, using simplified follow-up protocols for antiretroviral treatment has enabled scale-up of programs to reach more patients, but possibly at the cost of a small degree of safety to individuals as some side-effects will be detected later than would have been the case with more intensive laboratory testing. Such expediency, however, should not be perceived as the norm (Harding-Pink, 2004). Second, conducting advocacy and care simultaneously can also lead to conflicts of interest. Speaking out regarding a human tragedy can also be in the interest of the organization itself, at the cost of vulnerable individuals who, for example, might be identified on posters in a victim role that could be detrimental to them individually. In theory, the most important points may be to protect consent and confidentiality in advocacy and to ensure that the goal of benefiting the victims is always present, avoiding situations where a campaign might be purely self-serving. Nonetheless, the implementation of strategies to regulate conflicts of interest could be difficult to verify in self-regulating organizations serving disenfranchised individuals.

---

[3] Legitimacy may then require truthfulness towards donors as to the use of funds, but little else.

[4] For example by intruding on the independence of a state, through force, to protect its citizens from human rights abuses – see for example Buchanan, (1999).

Although this set of issues does not aim to be comprehensive, careful and creative thoughts on any of these points could contribute to better strategies for allocating resources in humanitarian medicine, based on more robust ethical argumentation than could be the case otherwise. The development of more robustly argued ethical conclusions has been called for regarding public health in general (Ashcroft, 2008). At least some specific approaches are likely to be needed in the international non-governmental setting of humanitarian medicine. Although we agree with this call for more substantive solutions, in the following sections we propose that some headway could nevertheless be made by adapting existing frameworks of procedural fairness for practical use in humanitarian organizations. The application and specification of principles of procedural fairness to this context point to a number of areas where governance, but also distributive fairness, could be improved despite the specific difficulties faced there.

Accountability for reasonableness and its limits in humanitarian distribution

As reasonable people will disagree about where the limit ought to be, and about what correct criteria might be, discussion of resource allocation has increasingly shifted from searching for guiding principles to outlining processes for fair decision-making (Coulter & Ham, 2000). One influential process put forward for this purpose, Daniels & Sabin's "Accountability for reasonableness" (Daniels & Sabin, 1997), starts by recognizing that we have no generally accepted principles for setting limits in health care. This poses a problem both for fairness and legitimacy, the latter being especially problematic in instances where democratic control is lacking, such as limitation decisions made by private insurance companies in the USA. It should be noted here that although the context addressed by these authors is very different from humanitarian medicine, the absence of a participative democratic process is a crucial similarity. In their seminal paper, Daniels and Sabin critique three prevalent views regarding fair distribution. First, the market is subject to too many failures to function as a fair limit-setting mechanism (Arrow, 2001), and should not be expected to function to provide us with positive

rights (such as the right to health care; Daniels, 1985) but only with goods which we have a liberty right that no one should prevent us from acquiring them (such as cars). Second, moral philosophy cannot be simply applied to allocation dilemmas, which present us with unresolved issues (Daniels, 1994). Third, democratic decision-making is not the only feasible option. The authors present a process which, so they argue, is able to offer procedural fairness – and with it conditions of legitimacy for these decisions – in resource allocation.

The idea is to make decisions about limits legitimate by accepting that both "winners" and "losers" in allocation decisions will have valid claims, and following a fair process using the following four elements. (1) The publicity condition: decisions regarding both direct and indirect limits to care, and their rationales, must be publicly accessible. (2) The relevance condition: a rationale will be reasonable if it appeals to evidence, reasons and principles that are accepted as relevant by fair-minded people who are disposed to finding mutually justifiable terms of cooperation. (3) The revision and appeals condition: there must be mechanisms for challenge and dispute resolution regarding limit-setting decisions, and, more broadly, opportunities for revision and improvement of policies in the light of new evidence or arguments. (4) The regulative condition: there is either voluntary or public regulation of the process to ensure that conditions 1–3 are met.

In addition to more robust allocation decisions, the authors hope to foster the development of a corpus of argued decisions from which a basis could be drawn for future situations: a sort of case-law, which could help to refine decisions through time. Through the second condition, they aim to recognize that all have an interest in having justifications acceptable to all. The third and fourth conditions aim to connect the process to broader deliberative processes in society.

Using this framework in humanitarian medicine poses specific difficulties. In applying the publicity condition, reaching the beneficiaries of humanitarian medicine with the relevant information is likely to be particularly difficult. The revision and appeals condition will be similarly difficult to apply, as the affected populations are often disenfranchised and less able than most to defend their own interests. Indeed, this is often precisely why they need humanitarian aid. Identifying "evidence, reasons, and principles that are accepted as relevant" could be more difficult across cultural barriers. Lack of public regulation, which sometimes places humanitarian organizations in situations where they assume state duties without state legitimacy, or checks and balances, also limits the ways in which the regulatory condition can be applied. The additional goals pursued by the authors, which form a part of their approach's appeal, also seem more difficult in a humanitarian context. Connection to broader deliberative processes requires a community within which such processes exist. Our common interest in having justifications which are acceptable to all is strongly grounded in reciprocity. Even more pragmatically, where would a corpus of similar decisions be kept? How would it be accessible? Given the tension between distribution in humanitarian medicine and the "rule of rescue," could humanitarian organizations fear that keeping such a corpus would make them seem callous, thus endangering their funding?

Adaptations for use in humanitarian medicine

Some of these obstacles may not be surmountable, at least at present. The first requirement in attempting to adapt accountability for reasonableness to humanitarian medicine is recognizing that doing better is a valid goal, even if problems remain. This should be no surprise. In our unjust world, aiming directly at ideal fairness could be daunting to the point of immobilization. It is already crucial that a lesser goal does not leave us lacking criteria for fair distribution. In other words, immobilization is unnecessary: making a situation fairer is worthwhile even if complete fairness is inaccessible. Neither does fair distribution require that everyone get what they have a valid claim to: it requires that what is available be distributed without discounting anyone's claims. As long as, say, the decision to use generics rather than brand-name drugs to treat HIV avoided such discounting, then, it was a fair decision. Our incapacity to make the world globally fair does not make concerns for fairness moot. We can still judge decisions according to whether they make things *fairer*, even if they cannot make them *fair*. Similarly, increasing fairness in allocation decisions is a valid goal even if a perfect process cannot be implemented. An adapted version of accountability for reasonableness could at least complement other mechanisms in doing so.

Some possible adaptations are outlined in Table 15.1. Despite the difficulty in reaching beneficiaries, the publicity condition would at minimum be a requirement for internal explicitness. As one member of a humanitarian organization put it, there are things that we cannot do if we must write them. Although these examples are purely fictitious, such "things" might include giving priority to a personal friend in a program with limited treatment spots, keeping a program open at the expense of a more urgent one to avoid admitting failure, or siding with individuals belonging to one of several warring factions in allocation decisions. In any case, according to this comment, even strictly internal publicity could sometimes represent an improvement. Attempting to fulfill the publicity condition could also include publicity to donors. Humanitarian organizations depend on their reputation to raise funds from private donors. This could not legitimately replace, but might complement, accountability to beneficiaries themselves. Although such solutions would remain imperfect, decisions could also be made accessible at least sometimes to local staff, community leaders and governments. Reasons for allocation decisions would also have to be accessible to any beneficiaries with whom it happened to be easy to come into contact. For example, individual patients who might ask why a local program was being terminated should receive a frank answer.

The relevance condition poses a particular problem, as different understandings of equity can lead to contradictory conclusions, and different considerations might be deemed more or less relevant across cultural settings. If we admit that there will be no single principle of fairness applicable to all situations, however, we can retain consistency in our decisions by examining all the plausible principles accessible to us, and systematically choosing the "least worse" option *on each principle's own terms*. On this model, decision-makers would examine the conclusions predicted by sufficientarian, prioritarian, egalitarian or utilitarian criteria for reaching the specific allocation decision they faced. They would then estimate how great each available transgression would be. This smallest degree of wrong would not be determined according to yet another principle, but internally, based on the severity of each transgression *on the basis of the principle which it transgressed*. When attempting to make a fair choice based on considerations of equity, we would first evaluate what conclusion each

Table 15.1. Adapting frameworks.

Daniels and Sabin's 'Accountability for reasonableness'	Publicity condition	Relevance condition	Revision and appeals condition	Regulative condition
	Decisions regarding both direct and indirect limits to care, and their rationales, must be publicly accessible	A rationale will be reasonable if it appeals to evidence, reasons, and principles that are accepted as relevant by people who are disposed to finding mutually justifiable terms of cooperation	There must be mechanisms for challenge and dispute resolution regarding limit-setting decisions, and, more broadly, opportunities for revision and improvement of policies in the light of new evidence or arguments	There is either voluntary or public regulation of the process to ensure that conditions 1–3 are met
Obstacles in humanitarian medicine	Reaching beneficiaries is difficult	Different understandings of equity, and no opportunity to discuss them	Disenfranchised populations	No public regulation
Adaptation to practice	Internal explicitness, publicity to donors, local staff, community leaders, and governments, and readiness to explain reason to beneficiaries who are reached	Consistent reasoning strategy to weigh these different views in specific situations	Advocacy within the organization on behalf of those populations	Regulation must be internal, and should itself be publicly accessible

Source: Daniels, N. & Sabin, J. (1997).

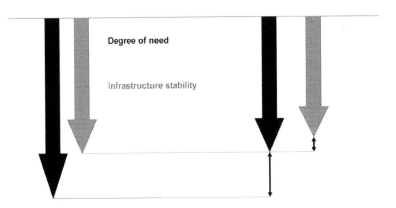

Figure 15.1 Choosing the smallest degree of wrong when evaluating two specific situations (arrows represent two countries, A (darker arrow) and B (lighter arrow)).

definition of equity would point to. Then, we would assess how severe the transgression of the other principles would be with each of these conclusions (Hurst & Danis, 2007). One recurrent dilemma at MSF is when and where to start HIV programs in unstable regions, where the organization may not stay long. Figure 15.1 illustrates how evaluative judgments regarding different parameters of such cases (here, infrastructure stability and the population's

need for the program) could be expressed. In the example presented here, country A is needier than country B, so in a prioritarian framework it is likely to be preferred on grounds of fairness as the target of an intervention. However, its infrastructures are also slightly less stable, making an intervention there less likely to be sustainable and decreasing long-term utility to beneficiaries as compared with an intervention in country B. Such comparisons are rarely straightforward, but they are routinely made. So far, so good. If we apply prioritarian – or egalitarian – principles and start a program in country A, we will thus get a little less benefit as the situation will be less stable in the long term. On utilitarian grounds, and all other things being equal, there will be a degree of wrong involved. If, however, we apply a utilitarian principle and go to country B, we will be disregarding the greater need of the citizens of country A. On prioritarian grounds, there will again be a degree of wrong involved. Inasmuch as each of these principles allows for the existence of greater or lesser wrongs, the respective degree of wrong in each case can be estimated. Comparing them will identify which is the smallest available wrong, as assessed according to the principle being transgressed. In this case, then, the transgression to prioritarianism would be worse if humanitarian medicine used a utilitarian approach and gave priority to the country with the more secure context. Therefore, country A should have priority. This is not the same as choosing the best consequences, which could lead to the opposite conclusion. This approach is limited, as different principles may well be incommensurable. Nevertheless, moral judgment is still necessary in such cases, and reasons must be given where possible. While these evaluations and judgments cannot be spelled out in detail, humanitarian organizations currently do make them: they may often be able to explain why, in a specific case, problems linked to unsustainable infrastructures, say, are minor while the needs at stake are extreme. Although the reasons that can be given on that basis will often under-determine such choices, the exercise in reflective equilibrium which we propose does delimit the sort of choices more likely to be justifiable by setting each principle relevant in a given situation as a partial constraint on the others.

Difficulties linked to the revision and appeals condition would be increased by the very vulnerability of the populations requiring humanitarian assistance. Those affected by allocation in humanitarian medicine are often disenfranchised and less able than most to defend their own interests. Here, however, the increased scope of humanitarian medicine's actions could provide a partial alternative. Given enough competing projects, decisions could be challenged by members of the organization itself. This would require that humanitarians act as advocates for the people they are helping "on the ground": a form of internal *témoignage*.

Given the absence of public regulation of humanitarian allocation decisions, the regulative condition would have to be met voluntarily, or at least through internal regulation. In order to bolster this condition, enforcement mechanisms could themselves be subject to the publicity condition.

The aim to improve fairness in allocating decisions could thus be furthered by using an adapted form of Daniels and Sabin's "Accountability for reasonableness" framework in humanitarian medicine. This application would require internally explicit decisions and rationales, publicity to donors as well as local staff, community leaders and governments, frank answers to any beneficiary – or potential beneficiary – who asked for clarification of decisions and their rationale, a consistent reasoning strategy to weigh conflicting views of equity in specific situations, advocacy within the organization as a mechanism for revision and appeals, and internal regulation according to publicly accessible mechanisms.

The additional goals pursued by the authors, to connect such decisions to broader deliberative processes, fulfill our common interest in having justifications which are acceptable to all, and initiating a corpus of similar decisions, could probably also be reached in an adapted form, at least in part. Given organizations with a strong deliberative tradition, or who are challenged to explain their motives publicly, connection to broader deliberative processes could happen either internally, or externally. It could increasingly take place internationally, as the number of such organizations increases and confront their choices and motivations. Potential disincentives to keeping a corpus of similar decisions could also have a pragmatic solution. As harms to the reputation of humanitarian organizations would mostly accrue in comparisons, a common decision to keep a pooled corpus of allocation decisions could partly address this concern. This would have the added benefit of increasing the size of the corpus available to each organization. Risks to the reputation of humanitarian medicine as a whole could be addressed by visible enhancement of fair allocation decision-making.

Clarity about the needs to make allocation decisions, and to accept imperfect solutions, as well as about the process used to reach such decisions, would be important in forming an evolving base for refining resource allocation decisions in humanitarian medicine. Clarity about these points would also serve an additional purpose. Becoming habituated to making do with very little and coming to perceive this as morally acceptable in general is a very real risk in humanitarian medicine (Harding-Pink, 2004). It should remain clear that such expediency, including the use of imperfect allocation strategies, is only morally acceptable *as long as there is no morally better alternative available*. This kind of clarity must for example be fostered if humanitarians are to speak out against unequal treatment, attempt to make treatment *fairer* by sometimes applying a double standard themselves, and avoid the impression that they are accusing themselves of unfairness in the process.

Conclusion

Allocating resources is difficult in any context, but raises specific ethical difficulties in humanitarian medicine. These difficulties are increasing. Minimally, we believe headway could be made by adapting existing frameworks of procedural fairness for practical use in humanitarian organizations. Despite the difficulties in applying it to humanitarian medicine, Daniels & Sabin's "Accountability for reasonableness" could be adapted to include internally explicit decisions and rationales, publicity to donors as well as local staff, community leaders and governments, frank answers to any beneficiary – or potential beneficiary – who asked for clarification of decisions and their rationale, a consistent reasoning strategy to weigh conflicting views of equity in specific situations, advocacy within the organization as a mechanism for revision and appeals, and internal regulation according to publicly accessible mechanisms. Clarity about the needs to make allocation decisions, and to accept imperfect solutions, as well as about the process used to reach such decisions, would be important both to refine resource allocation decisions, but also to bear in mind the difference between standards to advocate and standards which must currently be accepted. Importantly, the complexity of these challenges should encourage, rather than hinder, broader discussion on ethical aspects of resource allocation in humanitarian medicine.

Acknowledgments

The authors wish to thank Bernard Baertschi, Alexandra Calmy, Maria Merritt, Ulrike von Pilar, Marinette Ummel, Ulrich Vischer, the participants of the ethics and policy workshops of the MSF HIV training programs of Geneva and Berlin, and the editors and anonymous reviewers for useful comments, as well as Christophe Fournier from MSF International, and Isabelle Segui-Bitz, and Christian Captier from MSF Switzerland, for allowing us to use real examples.

This work was funded by the Institute for Biomedical Ethics at the Geneva University Medical School and by the Swiss National Science Foundation (grant 3233B0–107266/1). This paper is based on a background paper written in 2005 by one of the authors (SAH) for *Médecins Sans Frontières* as a contribution to the La Mancha deliberation process. The views expressed here are the authors' own, and not necessarily those of the Geneva University Medical School, of the Swiss National Science Foundation, or of *Médecins Sans Frontières*.

Competing interests: NM is a member of the board of MSF Switzerland. SAH has given workshops for MSF Switzerland, MSF Germany and MSF international.

References

Arrow, K. J. (2001). Uncertainty and the welfare economics of medical care. 1963. *Journal of Health Politics, Policy and Law* **26**(5), 851–883.

Ashcroft, R. (2008). Fair process and the redundancy of bioethics: a polemic. *Public Health Ethics* **1**(1), 3–9.

Beitz, C. R. (1975). Justice and international relations. *Philosophy and Public Affairs* **4**(4), 360–389.

Beitz, C. R. (2001). Does global inequality matter? *Metaphilosophy* **32**(1/2), 97–112.

Birch, M. & Miller, S. (2005). Humanitarian assistance: standards, skills, training, and experience. *British Medical Journal* **330**(7501), 1199–1201.

Buchanan, A. (1999). The internal legitimacy of humanitarian intervention. *Journal of Political Philosophy* **7**(1), 71–87.

Calmy, A., Klement, E., Teck, R. *et al.* (2004). Simplifying and adapting antiretroviral treatment in resource-poor settings: a necessary step to scaling-up. *Aids* **18**, 2353–2360.

Caney, S. (2001). Cosmopolitan justice and equalizing opportunities. *Metaphilosophy* **32**(1/2), 113–134.

Coulter, A. & Ham, C. (2000). *The Global Challenge of Health Care Rationing*. Buckingham: Open University Press.

Daniels, N. (1985). *Just Health Care*. New York: Cambridge University Press.

Daniels, N. (1994). Four unsolved rationing problems. A challenge. *Hastings Center Report* **24**(4), 27–29.

Daniels, N. & Sabin, J. (1997). Limits to health care: fair procedures, democratic deliberation, and the legitimacy problem for insurers. *Philosophy and Public Affairs* **26**(4), 303–350.

Diallo, D. A., Doumbo, O. K., Plowe, C. V. *et al.* (2005). Community permission for medical research in developing countries. *Clinical Infectious Diseases* **41**(2), 255–259.

Dyer, O. (2004). Bush accused of blocking access to cheap AIDS drugs. *British Medical Journal* **328**, 783.

Forst, R. (2001). Towards a Critical Theory of Transnational Justice. *Metaphilosophy* **32**(1/2), 160–179.

Fuller, L. (2006). Justified commitments? Considering resource allocation and fairness in Médecins Sans Frontières-Holland. *Developing World Bioethics* **6**(2), 59–70.

Harding-Pink, D. (2004). Humanitarian medicine: up the garden path and down the slippery slope. *British Medical Journal* **329**(7462), 398–399.

Hendrickson, D. (1998). Humanitarian action in protracted crisis: an overview of the debates and dilemmas. *Disasters* **22**(4), 283–287.

Hendriks, A. & Toebes, B. (1998). Towards a universal definition of the right to health? *Medical Law* **17**(3), 319–332.

Hinsch, W. (2001). Global distributive justice. *Metaphilosophy* **32**(1/2), 58–78.

Hurst, S. A. & Danis, M. (2007). A framework for rationing by clinical judgment. *Kennedy Institute of Ethics Journal* **17**(3), 247–266.

Jonsen, A. R. (1986). Bentham in a box: technology assessment and health care allocation. *Law, Medicine and Health Care* **14**(3–4), 172–174.

Katz, A. (2004). The Sachs report: Investing in health for economic development – or increasing the size of the crumbs from the rich man's table? Part I. *International Journal of Health Services* **34**(4), 751–773.

Laurent, C., Kouanfack, C., Koulla-Shiro, S. *et al.* (2004). Effectiveness and safety of a generic fixed-dose combination of nevirapine, stavudine, and lamivudine in HIV-1-infected adults in Cameroon: open-label multicentre trial. *Lancet* **364**(9428), 29–34.

Macklin, R. (2003). Ethics and equity in access to HIV treatment: "3 by 5" initiative. www.who.int/ethics/en/background-macklin.pdf.

McIntyre, A. (1994). Guilty bystanders? On the legitimacy of duty to rescue statutes. *Philosophy and Public Affairs* **23**, 157–191.

McKie, J. & Richardson, J. (2003). The rule of rescue. *Social Science and Medicine* **56**(12), 2407–2419.

Michael, M. & Zwi, A. B. (2002). Oceans of need in the desert: ethical issues identified while researching humanitarian agency response in Afghanistan. *Developing World Bioethics* **2**(2), 109–130.

Murphy, L. B. (2000). *Moral Demands in Non-ideal Theory.* Oxford: Oxford University Press.

Nagel, T. (2005). The problem of global justice. *Philosophy and Public Affairs* **33**(2), 113–147.

O'Neill, O. (2001). Agents of justice. *Metaphilosophy* **32**(1/2), 181–195.

Palmer, C. A. (1999). Rapid appraisal of needs in reproductive health care in southern Sudan: qualitative study. *British Medical Journal* **319**(7212), 743–748.

Pogge, T. W. (2002). Responsibilities for poverty-related ill health. *Ethics and International Affairs* **16**(2), 71–79.

Pogge, T. W. (2005). Real World Justice. *Journal of Ethics* **9**, 29–53.

Redmond, A. D. (2005). Needs assessment of humanitarian crises. *British Medical Journal* **330**(7503), 1320–1322.

Rougemont, A. (1995). From humanitarian action to international health. *Soz Praventivmed* **40**(1), 3–10.

Scheffler, S. (1992). *Human Morality.* Oxford: Oxford University Press.

United Nations (1948). *Universal Declaration of Human Rights, Article 25.* 2007. www.un.org/Overview/rights.html.

Wikler, D. (2003). Why prioritize when there isn't enough money? *Cost Effective Resource Allocation* **1**(1), 5.

Chapter

16

International aid and global health

Anthony B. Zwi

Introduction

Nancy Birdsall (2008) has described Overseas Development Assistance (ODA) as being guilty of "seven deadly sins." Her critique exposes many weaknesses of the international aid system. How applicable are these "sins" to development assistance for global health? How do we make sense of the contradictions regarding the value and utility of ODA and the critiques of how it operates? And, most importantly, how might "we" do better?

This chapter explores the nature of foreign aid, as it relates to global health, and seeks to assess its value(s) and constraints. The chapter is structured around four key elements: (a) trends in overseas development assistance for health; (b) motivations and influences on aid; (c) an assessment of current aid structures and approaches and (d) emerging issues, considerations and recommendations.

Background

The world's club of wealthy countries, the Organisation for Economic Co-operation and Development (OECD), noted as "outrageous" the ongoing human tragedy of failed development: 9 million avoidable deaths in those under 5 years of age and 536 000 maternal deaths per year (OECD, 2009). Widespread acknowledgment of limited achievements of international aid, a decade earlier, led to agreement at the Millennium Summit to establish global targets for development, the Millennium Development Goals (MDGs). These comprised a set of eight inter-related development goals designed to close the poverty gap between rich and poor countries and to improve the health and well-being of over a billion people living on less than $1 per day (see www.un.org/millenniumgoals/). The MDGs reflect priority development concerns and include

commitments to reduce poverty and gender inequalities, improve access to education, water, sanitation and health care, promote environmental sustainability and enhance partnerships for development. While all are intimately connected to health, three are explicitly focused on health goals and targets: MDG 4 (reducing child mortality), MDG 5 (reducing maternal mortality) and MDG 6 (tackling HIV/AIDS, tuberculosis and malaria).

Scrutiny of the failure to make substantial progress towards achieving the MDGs by 2015 has intensified, along with acknowledgment that many will not be met, in many countries. The African continent has the longest way to go, and in the Asia–Pacific, none of the developing countries are on track to meet the full set of goals, with many struggling to meet these targets. The MDGs are critiqued on many levels, including for establishing a standard, rather than context-specific, set of targets, and for failing to focus attention on inequalities within countries and the right to health. Nevertheless, they remain widely at the core of the current development agenda, despite concerns that they contribute to excessive "Afro-pessimism" and stigmatization of countries that deserve support in achieving more modest context-appropriate targets, rather than opprobrium, for failing to meet those set at the global level (Vandemoortele, 2009).

In recent decades there has been an escalation of interest, commitment and resources for global health, in part reflecting the MDGs being placed center-stage. Many new players have emerged – the Global Fund Against AIDS, Tuberculosis and Malaria, the Global Alliance for Vaccines and Immunizations, and the Bill and Melinda Gates Foundation, amongst them – each mobilizing sizeable funds for interventions across the globe (Figure 16.1). Much of the funding available is channeled to disease-specific interventions, and has

Global Health and Global Health Ethics, ed. Solomon Benatar and Gillian Brock. Published by Cambridge University Press.
© Cambridge University Press 2011.

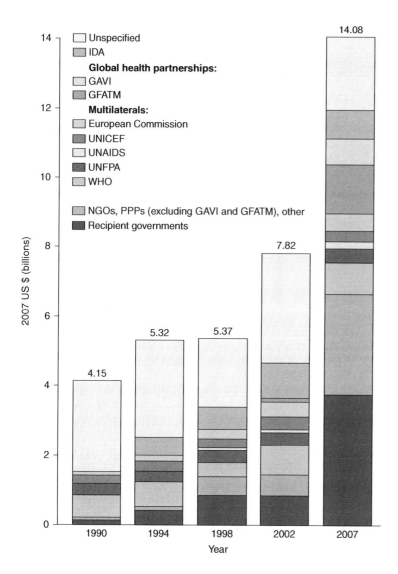

Figure 16.1 Increased funding committed to global health 1990–2007 (Ravishankar, 2009). Note substantial contribution from recipient governments and the emergence of new sources of development assistance for health including GAVI, GFATM, NGOs and public private partnerships.

been critiqued for failing to build the structures and capacity of the institutions of the state to act as guarantor and steward for health advancement. Sustained benefits for general populations have not been achieved (Ravishankar *et al.*, 2009).

While the delivery of health care is primarily the responsibility of national governments, human and financial resources, and systems, are inadequate and have hampered efforts to deliver health care to all. External resources and support have neglected these issues, but are essential to health development in many countries. Overseas development assistance has nearly doubled between 2000 and 2006, while private flows and investments have increased much more rapidly and substantially, starting from a much

higher base (Figure 16.2). While the greatest contribution to health improvement and development will result from the education of girls and the eradication of poverty, ODA can play a valuable complementary role, and indeed may support those two linked objectives. Effective ODA can provide support to the political, economic and social policy improvements which can contribute to improving the lives and livelihoods of the world's population. This is implicit in the interdependent design of the MDGs and specifically MDG 8 which addresses solidarity and partnership between rich and poor countries, through expanded opportunities for trade, cancellation of debt, improved access to technologies, and providing higher levels and more effective ODA.

185

Selected financial flows to developing countries

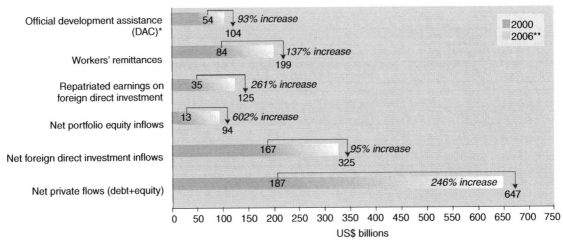

Figure 16.2 Selected financial flows to developing countries highlighting relatively small contribution to developing country economies from overseas development assistance (ODA), 2000–2006. Source: World Bank (2007). Global Development Finance 2007: The Globalization of Corporate Finance in Developing Countries (pp. 37, 55). Washington, DC: World Bank.

The OECD asserts that there is good reason to believe that development assistance for health (DAH) has contributed to improved health outcomes. However, three caveats should be noted: (a) despite improvements many countries are still off-track to achieving the MDGs; (b) the principal determinants of progress on health are domestic – and include public policies and institutions, governance, levels of education and the absence of conflict and (c) enhancing aid effectiveness may improve the quality of DAH, but it remains difficult to measure the specific impact of interventions on health outcomes (OECD, 2009).

In 2002, the World Bank estimated that, if countries improved their policies and institutions, the additional ODA required to achieve the MDGs by 2015 would be US$40–60 billion a year (World Bank, 2002). The UN Millennium Project found that only about 40% of the cost of achieving the Goals could be met by low-income countries themselves, even after taking account of likely increases in domestic incomes and government revenue, and that ODA would be required to fill the gap. More recent estimates have put the figure at a somewhat higher level, with the UN Millennium Project (www.un.org/millenniumgoals) estimating that meeting the MDGs in all countries would cost approximately $121 billion in 2006, rising to $189 billion in 2015, taking into account co-financed increases at country level (Figure 16.3). This assessment assumed also that several countries would "graduate" from the need for ODA to finance investments in achieving

the MDGs before 2015, although this was before the 2008–9 global financial crisis.

The Commission on Social Determinants of Health identifies socio-economic and political context, social position, material circumstances and the health-care system as all influencing the distribution of health and well-being. Development assistance for health can make a valuable contribution, given poor health status, high levels of inequity, poor state capabilities and the need for technical information and support. Many countries are highly dependent on DAH, with more than 30 countries drawing at least 40% of their health funding from ODA (Reinikka, 2008). Particularly for under-resourced and fragile states, a high dependency on ODA is present.

And, while ODA and DAH have the potential to influence every one of the key determinants of health, the value will depend not only on the magnitude of aid, but also on the processes of formulating and implementing it, and on whose interests lie at its core.

What are the trends in ODA for health?

Overseas development assistance is again rising following a trough in the 1980s and 1990s (Figure 16.4). While this rise is welcome, it remains fragile and erratic. In 2008 ODA represented only 0.31% of Gross National Income (GNI) of all Development Assistance Committee (DAC) countries, well below the target of 0.7% of GNI. Only five countries (Denmark, Luxembourg, Netherlands,

Estimated cost
of meeting the
Millennium
Development Goals
in all countries

2003 US$ billions

Note: Numbers in table
may not sum to totals
because of rounding.

Source: 2002 data based
on OECD-DAC 2004.
Projection for 2006-15
are authors' calculations.

Category	Estimated ODA in 2002	Projected for 2006	Projected for 2010	Projected for 2015
MDG support needs in low-income countries				
MDG financing gap	12	73	89	135
Capacity building to achieve the MDGs	5	7	7	7
Grants in support of heavy debt burden	–	7	6	1
Debt relief	4	6	6	6
Repayments of concessional loans	–5	0	0	0
Subtotal	**15**	**94**	**108**	**149**
MDG support needs in middle-income countries				
Direct support to government	4	10	10	10
Capacity building to achieve the MDGs	5	5	5	5
Repayments of concessional loans	–6	–3	–4	–6
Subtotal	**3**	**12**	**11**	**9**
MDG support needs at the international level				
Regional cooperation and infrastructure	2	3	7	11
Funding for global research	1	5	7	7
Implementing the Rio conventions	1	2	3	5
Technical cooperation by international organizations	5	5	7	8
Subtotal	**10**	**15**	**23**	**31**
Estimated cost of meeting the MDGs in all countries	**28**	**121**	**143**	**189**

Figure 16.3 Estimated costs of meeting the Millennium Development Goals in all countries (2003, US$ billions), Source: UN Millennium Project, Final Report, 2006.

Norway and Sweden) contributed above 0.7% of GNI, with some countries such as the USA (0.18%) and Japan (0.18%) way below the proposed target (OECD, 2009). Ireland, France, Spain and the UK have set targets to increase ODA to 0.7% GNI by 2015; others such as Australia and Switzerland have less ambitious targets, around 0.5% GNI by 2015.

Approximately one-third of ODA from OECD countries was destined for the least developed and other low-income countries, one third for lower middle income countries, and one third either unallocated or for upper middle income countries. The largest recipients of ODA were Iraq ($9.46 billion), Afghanistan ($3.48 billion), China ($2.6 billion), Indonesia ($2.54 billion) and India ($2.26 billion), followed by Vietnam, Sudan, Tanzania, Ethiopia and Cameroon. The top five recipients received over 22% of ODA distributed by OECD countries in 2007–2008. The main components

were bilateral development projects, programs and technical cooperation, with lesser contributions to debt relief, humanitarian aid and multilateral agency activities.

The contribution associated with health has risen substantially and comprises a significant proportion of ODA. In 1980–1984, DAH was 5.3% of all ODA; this increased to 7.8% by 2002–2006 (Piva & Dodd, 2009). The precise amounts allocated to global health are not agreed: the World Bank cites a rise from US$2.5 billion in 1990 to almost $14 billion in 2005, but this figure is questioned by *McCoy et al.* (2009a) who suggest that actual disbursements are substantially lower than stated commitments.

The priority given to global health is manifest by United Nations and Security Council debates on health and high-level concerns with the threat of bioterrorism, the risks of emerging and re-emerging

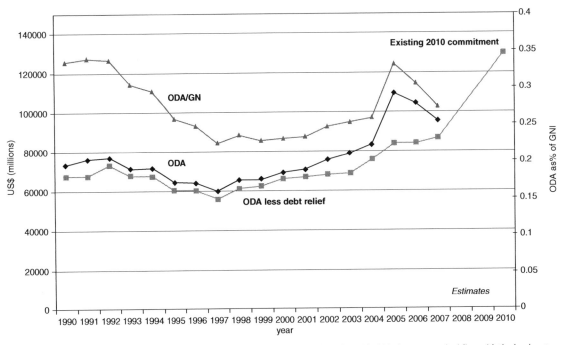

Figure 16.4 Trends in overseas development assistance, highlighting the trough in the mid-1990s, increases coinciding with the lead up to, and after, the Millennium Summit and commitment to the Millennium Development Goals.

infections and other transnational health threats, and recognition of the links between the macro-economy and health. Increased DAH reflects a range of influences: acceptance of the MDGs as an overriding framework for ODA; recognition of health as a core component of governance and nation-building; entry of the range of new actors, notably large-scale private and NGO investment in health development; and the establishment of new modalities for providing aid, such as the Global Fund Against AIDS, TB and Malaria, Global Alliance for Vaccines and Immunization, and the US President's Emergency Plan for AIDS Relief (PEPFAR) amongst others. Such high-profile initiatives seek to attract additional funds and also to channel them in a way which satisfies donors that their investments are being managed more "safely" and with reduced risk. The major increases in DAH are associated, in particular, with massive increases in support to HIV/AIDS, accounting for 32% of DAH from 2002–2006 (Piva & Dodd, 2009).

The availability of additional funds from private sources, notably the Bill and Melinda Gates Foundation, has perhaps stimulated a response by key donors and institutions to exert more agency in shaping the global policy agenda. A recent critique of the Bill and Melinda

Gates Foundation notes, however, that it now funds almost all of the key contributors to global health activity and thinking, including UN agencies, global health partnerships, the World Bank, NGOs and universities (McCoy *et al.*, 2009b). This is of concern, as the substantial funding sums "give the foundation (sic) a great deal of influence over both the architecture and policy agenda of global health" (McCoy *et al.*, 2009b).

McCoy *et al.* (2009a) present a schema which identifies three functions in relation to global health funding: provision, management and expenditure. The providers of global health funding (governments, private foundations, individuals and the corporate sector); those who manage these funds (including bilateral ODA agencies, inter-governmental organizations, global health partnerships, NGOs, private foundations and the corporate sector); and those spending funds (including multilateral agencies, global health partnerships, NGOs, the private sector, and also low and middle income governments and their civil society) differ little in their approaches. The overlapping and messy borders between the many players and their roles, adds complexity and reduces transparency and accountability.

The "fragmented, complicated, messy and inadequately tracked state of global health finance requires immediate attention" (McCoy *et al.*, 2009a). A more detailed analysis of global health funding is required if the efficiency, accountability, performance and equity-impact of these activities is to occur. Development assistance for health is inflated and imprecise (McCoy *et al.*, 2009a) making it difficult to track funding transfers and to facilitate coordination and accountability. Data on private sources of global health funding are especially inaccurate. Furthermore, data from the emerging donors and non-OECD governments such as China and India, as well as a number of wealthy countries from the Middle East, are not as easy to scrutinize as they do not appear in the OECD's Aggregate Aid Statistics and Creditor Reporting System (Piva & Dodd, 2009). New sources of data which extend beyond the OECD are valuable in providing a more complete picture of the patterns of ODA.

Objectives behind ODA – what are the forces (political, economic, ethical) which influence it?

Why does overseas development assistance exist and what purpose does it seek to fulfill? There is widespread recognition of global inequity in health and in all the determinants of health, both within and between countries. This has been well described, including elsewhere in this volume, and needs little reiteration here.

It is clear also that poverty leads to ill-health and ill-health leads to poverty: this is well documented in the peer-reviewed literature. Breaking the vicious cycle between health and poverty and poverty and health, and promoting health gain, both within and between countries, is a broad social policy objective, again, widely agreed.

Addressing these inequities and responding to them can be argued on moral, ethical and practical grounds. Development assistance for health can play some part in reducing these inequalities between and within states. This needs to be addressed at a domestic level as well, where social and health policies, their underpinning values, and their implementation and command of resources, are central. However, for the purposes of this chapter, we focus here on ODA, DAH and their potential role.

Selgelid (2008) sets out the arguments for why wealthy developed nations should be motivated to improve the health situation in developing countries. He identifies 11 potential reasons, which can be

categorized and summarized as egalitarian, utilitarian, libertarian and self-interest. Each has its own rationale and proponents – but together present a compelling case for commitment to addressing health problems in developing countries. Egalitarian arguments are based on the imperatives to ensure that all people should have equal opportunities, that those worst off should have their needs addressed, that the right to health should be fulfilled, and that inequalities in well-being are undeserved and should be rectified. Utilitarian arguments recognize the sacrifices required to address those needs, but argue that overall betterment of the human condition will result. Libertarian arguments stress that historical injustices need redress and that many of the benefits that have accrued to wealthy countries have been at the expense of, and exploitation of, less developed nations and peoples. If these arguments are not sufficiently compelling, others are framed as pure self-interest: addressing developing country health needs reduces threats of emerging infectious diseases, enhances potential for development and new markets, and reduces other costs associated with dealing with health threats. Ultimately such investments are of benefit in promoting security. Selgelid argues that "Those opposed to wealthy government funding of developing world health improvement would most likely appeal, implicitly or explicitly, to the idea that coercive taxation for redistributive purposes would violate the right of an individual to keep his hard-earned income. The idea that this reason not to improve global health should outweigh the combination of rights and values embodied in the eleven reasons enumerated above, however, is implausibly extreme, morally repugnant and perhaps imprudent."

The securitization of ODA and development warrants close observation: countries such as Australia, the USA and the UK have promoted close interaction between their foreign policy, defense and overseas development activities, creating new structures to better coordinate the three "Ds" – development, diplomacy and defense (Howell & Lind, 2009). In so doing, there has been an "almost unnoticed eclipse of the notion 'human security' by more ambivalent notions of 'security'" (p. 1294).

Debate is intensifying. Benatar (2005) highlighted the lack of "moral imagination" in addressing the "deplorable state of global health." He drew attention to how relatively low amounts but high-profile aid eclipses "recognition of the fact that financial, human and other material resources are continuously being extracted from developing countries by wealthy nations striving for their own economic growth," often in collusion with kleptocratic despots who use their power to sell their countries' resources for personal gain. This point is amplified by writers such as Pogge (2008) who critique the notion that global development is about supporting those less fortunate, and should instead be recognized as the result of inequitable global macroeconomic and political structures and policies. He argues forcefully that the constraints to achieving development objectives in many under-resourced countries do not simply reflect poor domestic political choices and policies, but rather global power imbalances. Pogge (2008) argues for a commitment not merely to providing ODA, but much more fundamentally, to reshaping the global political economy.

The emergence of new donors, notably China and India, represents an opportunity to reflect on the development agenda and how it has been framed. Six (2009) argues that the more explicit self-interest driven modes of operation of China, India and other southern donors, enables a more honest debate on the purpose and processes of ODA. More particularly, he argues that western development actors will be forced to drop their "hidden agenda for hegemony" in order to promote an ownership (i.e. country-based) discourse on development and its goals and strategies. Chinese and Indian ODA are framed explicitly in terms of solidarity with other developing countries, pursuing common development, mutual benefits and strategic interests (McCormick, 2008).

A critique of ODA with special emphasis on global health

A critique of ODA needs to take account of the multitude of stakeholders, each playing a part in a global system, each with its own objectives and agendas, each seeking to maximize its own benefit and to minimize risk.

Sumner & Tribe (2008, p. 25) argue that "values are central to disputes about the definition of development – what to improve, how to improve it and, especially, the question of who decides?" They assert that concepts of development are informed by one of three main paradigms – development as a long-term process of structural societal transformation, development as a short- to medium-term outcome of desirable targets and development as a dominant discourse of western modernity. Overseas development assistance reflects

these broader objectives, articulating a given set of values and vision of the future. It is these values, and how they are espoused and promoted by key stakeholders, that influences what role ODA plays and how it is seen by each of the different actors involved.

A political economy perspective is valuable in examining changing trends as it makes more explicit the policy actions of donors, described in terms of their political and economic goals, which in turn are a product of culture, institutions, the distribution of power and the dynamics of competitive interests. Historically, a significant proportion of "aid" (more than 60% between 1980 and 1994) was coercively linked to the purchase of weapons from donor countries; these protected leaders and allowed them unfettered control over the natural resources and people of their countries. Bensimon & Benatar (2006) draw attention to the nearly 15-fold difference in world military expenditure ($839 billion) compared with ODA (around $58 billion) in 2001.

Three political economic approaches can be applied to analyzing ODA: foreign aid as a reflection of the economic interests of powerful groups within donor countries; foreign aid as an effort to maximize benefits to donors working through bilateral or multilateral channels thus enhancing their preferences in the international system; and finally seeing ODA as the result of bargaining among units, notably choice and compromises between donor aid bureaucracies, multilateral aid agencies and recipient government officials, amongst others. The first approach focuses on groups within states, the different political parties, private companies and NGOs, which seek beneficial outcomes as a result of ODA. These groups compete to shape the focus and priorities of ODA. In the second approach the donor state presents a more unified face seeking to promote its international interests, its influence in world affairs, its cultural values, as well as its economic interests. The last approach sees the producers and consumers of ODA as negotiating to maximize their own benefits – for donors this relates to agreement with other nations on broad objectives and values and compliance with any conditions placed on developing country recipients. The recipients also seek to maximize the value of ODA to their own personal or political objectives, while minimizing any conditions or requirements imposed by the donors.

Overseas development assistance has been linked to many other conditionalities and requirements of benefit to the donors. The three biggest donors, USA, Japan and France, have all had noticeable biases in their patterns of aid: the USA targeted one-third of its aid budget to Israel and Egypt; France "gave" overwhelmingly to its former colonies; and Japan favored countries that voted with it in the UN (McCormick, 2008). The emerging donors too, such as China, require endorsement of foreign policy objectives such as the "one China policy," or tie ODA for infrastructure projects to implementation by Chinese companies (McCormick, 2008).

Recognizing the political economy of international aid helps one understand why some of the persistent weaknesses and failures recur and are not effectively addressed. It becomes apparent, also, that maximizing the effectiveness of ODA in development terms may not be the main consideration, nor is addressing poverty or promoting equity on a global level. Influence may also be sought through more subtle means: the World Bank through its role as a "knowledge bank" promotes use of "common language, rhetoric and discourse" which are internalized as ideas, norms and constructs which reinforce the neoliberal paradigm (Das, 2009).

Tandon (2009) argues that there are three things wrong with the present aid and development architecture: the relationship between aid and development is not fully understood or "is deliberately fudged;" as discussed in public discourse there is an assumption that both aid and development are simply "technical" despite the fact that its form and content are clearly based in political considerations; and third that the dominant conceptual framework hides "under the carpet" their "power-political" and historical dimensions.

Seven deadly sins associated with ODA

Birdsall (2008) highlights the "seven deadly sins" associated with the poor quality of much ODA. The seven sins identified were (i) "impatience" – with institution building and having a limited commitment to longer-term support; (ii) "envy" – failure to effectively coordinate and at other times to collude with one another and not necessarily in the interests of the developing countries involved; (iii) "ignorance" and a failure to effectively evaluate development interventions; (iv) "pride" – notably a failure to exit when appropriate; (v) "sloth" – sloppiness with concepts and their application, and in particular pretending that participation is equivalent to developing country ownership; (vi) "greed" – characterized by unreliable and inadequate, or as Birdsall (2008) puts it "stingy" transfers; and (vii) "foolishness" – characterized by inadequate

commitments to funding global and regional public goods. We describe and relate each to global health.

Impatience with institution building

Development can be conceptualized as a process of "creating and sustaining the economic and political institutions that support equitable and sustainable growth." Particular problems arise where states have poor institutions or low capacity, often because they are fragile or conflict-affected, or may not be in a position to promote development.

In the effort to deliver specific services and to promote lines of accountability to donors, the underlying health systems and state institutions have often been neglected, and the intersection of external support and national development activities is poor. Delivering multiple public goods such as disease control, surveillance and information systems, and building local capacity, all depend on a functional health system with adequate infrastructure and human, material and other resources yet investment in these is often missing (see Chapter 5 by McKee).

In conflict-affected and post-conflict countries, initial surges in ODA are channeled through short-term emergency relief funding, with the mobilization of development funding, and the more sustained efforts required to build institutions over the longer term, being more difficult to mobilize and sustain (Health and Fragile States Network, 2009). Furthermore, inflows of aid are often directed to particular programs, typically through NGOs, and donor-funded efforts may suck up the best available human resources thus undermining system building and the strengthening of institutions.

Impatience for "results" may also lead to a focus on highly visible short-run projects where donors can claim successes and avoid the risk of being associated with institutional failures (Birdsall, 2008, p. 518). Impatience for results also leads to longer-term underinvestment in less politically visible (and therefore less attractive) areas such as human resource development. Donors often establish their own project implementation units alongside government bodies, thus further bypassing, and in some cases undermining, government systems.

The historical emphasis on vertical and disease-specific programs (Zwi & Mills, 1995) represents a failure, in health, to commit to addressing long-term institutional constraints. The new donors like the Bill and Melinda Gates Foundation again typically fund alongside, rather than directly to, emerging health systems. The Bill and Melinda Gates Foundation in 2007 spent almost as much on global health as the recurrent budget of the World Health Organization for that year – $1.65 billion dollars (McCoy *et al.*, 2009b).

Envy (collusion and coordination failure)

Recipient countries now deal with dozens of donors and a wide array of agencies – bilateral, multilateral, NGO and private sector. Donors will operate in some sectors and not others, and within those sectors, some areas of activity and not others. Donors typically seek to manage their projects as this increases their visibility and control. For country staff, however, the range of agencies is bewildering with extensive requirements for engagement, hosting missions, visiting the field, procuring materials, monitoring and evaluation and more. Grundy (2010), examining immunization programs in five Asian countries (Bangladesh, India, Indonesia, Sri Lanka, Nepal), found that the Inter-Agency Coordinating Committee structures to manage and coordinate GAVI-related activities were somewhat narrow and should be broadened to include all relevant stakeholders and to facilitate support for the "immunization system," including such matters as coordinating technical support, identifying gaps and evaluating interventions.

Donors compete not only for visibility, but also for local talent and skills – "poaching" staff from each other or from the public sector, at times weakening the institutions they are ostensibly supporting.

Initiatives such as the International Health Partnerships seek to bring donors together to better coordinate and to reduce pressures on recipient governments, often through agreement on broad health strategy, support for a national plan, at times through a Sector Wide Approach (SWAp) for health. The Development Assistance Committee of the OECD is piloting donor harmonization efforts in a number of countries and some benefits are suggested. However, many donors, including the biggest, the USA, often have preferences for bilateral arrangements outside of these "common basket" approaches.

Ignorance (failure to evaluate)

One of the most consistent and damning critiques of ODA is that it is poorly evaluated and that the same mistakes are made time and time again. Policies and reforms are often proposed in the absence of good evidence. Key reforms, such as the introduction of user fees as promoted by the World Bank, were based on theoretical and ideological considerations; when the evidence was collated, benefits were limited and potential harms considerable.

Failure to evaluate may be functional: it reduces the likelihood of exposing development flaws and weaknesses. Careful evaluation is costly and difficult to undertake. Given that there is often more pressure within most donor countries to reduce budgets than to increase them, any negative assessments and damaging information may pose problems to securing longer-term funding. For some of the players – whether or not the ODA is effective is not the main question – rather it is about what resources can be captured and used for the benefit of key stakeholders. Rigorous evaluation of health-system support and its impacts are far less developed. Fiszbein (2006) suggests that development impact evaluation is an international public good, and that more effort should be made to ensure they are undertaken and available.

Pride (failure to exit)

Donors are often reluctant to exit even if there is no evidence of achievement and no clarity that their investments are bringing development gains. At a time when there is some pressure on donors to increase their development aid, as 2015 approaches and the target of 0.7% of GNI for ODA looms, there may be some reluctance to withdraw from programs which absorb large amounts of funding, while closing them down for being ineffective and diverting those funds elsewhere, would require more energy and creativity … and is therefore less attractive.

Sloth (pretending participation is sufficient for ownership)

Engagement is often top-down and hierarchical – reflecting a biomedical and more technocentric approach, with limited local ownership and participation/engagement. Exceptions are present – particularly in relation to HIV/AIDS and participatory approaches to health promotion and prevention – but these are neither dominant nor especially influential. Donors need to much more actively strengthen the critical relationships among policymakers, providers and clients (Reinikka, 2008).

Support to civil society engagement in health deserves more attention. Davis (2009) suggests that donors talk about commitment to consultation, participation and engagement, but their actions are limited. A recent study indicated that DAH, if provided to government, appears to lead to concomitant reductions in government commitment to health expenditure, whereas if directed through civil society structures would leave government expenditure intact (Lu *et al.*, 2010).

Greed (unreliable as well as stingy transfers)

While the total funding for global health has risen substantially, much funding continues in small limited tranches which achieves little alone but requires as much work (negotiation, transaction costs, reporting and monitoring) as for much larger projects.

There are "significant imbalances" in the allocation of aid which run counter to agreed principles of "effective aid" (Piva & Dodd, 2009). Countries with comparable levels of poverty and health receive remarkably different levels of ODA and there are considerable imbalances in relation to which health conditions attract attention. Chad attracts only $1.59 health ODA per capita compared with around $20 per capita in Zambia. Ten countries attract almost 50% of all health ODA globally, and the majority of funding is often allocated to HIV-related activity. The OECD itself has recognized the inefficiencies and inequities that result from unequal commitment of aid to "aid darlings" and those who receive little DAH, the "aid orphans" (OECD, 2009). The vast majority of aid orphans are in Africa, where needs are often greatest. In only seven countries does attention to MDG-5 (improve maternal health) comprise more than 10% of health ODA (Piva & Dodd, 2009).

Piva and Dodd's study of OECD DAH found that there were 13 819 commitments made for activities valued at under $0.5 million each – these small projects represented 67.5% of all DAH but accounted for only 3.6% of total health ODA. A large number of small projects is inefficient, has high transaction costs in negotiating and reporting, requires extensive additional monitoring and implementation capacity, and reflects high degrees of fragmentation of DAH (Piva & Dodd, 2009).

Important areas remain seriously underfunded: health system strengthening, mental health and human resources development. Campaigners argue that health and economic gains for the "bottom billion" of the world's population would result from relatively modest investment in neglected tropical diseases (Hotez *et al.*, 2009). "We live in an almost $100 trillion economy, therefore $2–3 billion … for comprehensive disease control should be considered a modest yet highly effective mechanism for alleviating the poverty of people in the bottom billion," they argue.

Foolishness (underfunding of regional and global public goods)

Around 25% of all DAH is associated with global and regional multi-country initiatives – considerably more than education-related ODA in the same period (2002–2006) (Piva & Dodd, 2009). In part this reflects the high proportion of funds allocated to HIV/AIDS (40% of global and regional multi-country initiatives) and global immunization programs.

In Malawi, in the mid to late 1990s, a "staggering" 10% of DAH was allocated to training (Reinikka, 2008). One of the rationales for this was to provide incentives and additional benefits to health workers with low wages, but at the same time large training commitments meant many health workers were away from their posts. Furthermore, if the same amount of funding was allocated to supporting salaries, health workers on average could have been paid 50% more that year (Reinikka, 2008).

The Bill and Melinda Gates Foundation plays an important role in stimulating new technologies, devoting more than one-third (37%) of its funds to research and development or basic sciences research, but risks under-funding core health system support. McCoy *et al.* (2009b) suggest that the Bill and Melinda Gates Foundation promotes the growth of private provision of health care in low and middle-income countries, further undermining an important role for public and government systems in shaping policies which set the context for health system development. The determinants of health attract relatively little attention or funding, while vertical systems, medical technologies and the private sector are promoted.

General budget support amounts to only 6.4% of health ODA, and Piva & Dodd (2009) draw attention to the lack of support for "systems issues" – management, logistics, procurement, infrastructure and workforce development. They highlight the fact that these "areas may not appeal to donors" but "they will have to be tackled if current progress in disease control is to continue and if the quality and coverage of health services are to improve." Das Gupta & Gostin (2009) note the absolute lack of attention to, and support of, public health systems and capacity in developing countries.

McCoy *et al.* (2009b) critique the global health program of the Bill and Melinda Gates Foundation, drawing attention to the apparent inequities in how such resources are distributed. Significant amounts are allocated to a relatively small number of grantees (e.g. over $1 billion to PATH), large amounts are destined for US-based organizations, and granting decisions seem to be "largely managed through an informal system of personal networks and relationships rather than by a more transparent process based on independent and technical peer review" (McCoy *et al.*, 2009b, p. 1650).

Public–private partnerships have been promoted as a means for mobilizing additional resources and support for health activities, and are widespread. Many focus on combating neglected diseases or on developing new drugs or vaccines. The UN and its agencies have been at the forefront of engaging with the private sector in an attempt to foster collaboration to increase available resources and promote partnerships with civil society organizations, philanthropic foundations, governments and the private sector, to benefit global health. The World Bank suggests that such partnerships could help address specific cost and investment challenges, while the WHO hopes that engaging these wider groups of players will contribute to improving equity in access to essential drugs and to researching neglected diseases.

Concerns about the viability of public–private partnerships to improve global health equity revolve around several issues (Asante & Zwi, 2007). While seeking to be seen as socially responsible and to demonstrate "good corporate citizenship," they may simultaneously take actions that are largely motivated by profit. Several multinational drug companies still engage in policies that restrict universal access to antiretroviral drugs. A number of "unhealthy habits" characterize many global public–private partnerships: they skew national priorities, deprive national stakeholders of a voice in decision-making, are not accountable or transparent in relation to partner selection or grant disbursements, fail to compare the costs and benefits of public versus private systems of delivery, and do not adequately resource the transaction costs (Buse & Harmer, 2007).

The traditional donors from the wealthiest countries, most members of the OECD, have been joined by a number of rapidly growing, and increasingly important, countries such as India, China, Brazil, South Africa and Indonesia. These new donors have their own views of how development should proceed, and of what return they expect from their investment. Their approach to providing ODA without engagement in local politics, but ostensibly in solidarity with other developing countries, is a powerful counter-balance to longstanding offers of assistance from OECD members. China, India and others are actively engaged in a "silent revolution" in development assistance, weakening the bargaining position of western donors, and exposing standards and processes that are out of date or ineffectual, while offering competitive, and in many ways, attractive, alternatives (Woods, 2008).

Efforts, spearheaded by the OECD to enhance the effectiveness of aid include the Paris and Accra Declarations, which aim to address issues of ownership by recipient countries, to ensure greater donor harmonization and alignment with national country priorities. A key issue will be to determine whose agenda(s) lie(s) at the foundation of agreed policies and strategies, and whether "coordination," "harmonization" and "alignment" occur in practice.

Emerging issues, considerations and recommendations

The discussion above highlights numerous problems and weaknesses within the aid environment. Some of these are inherent given the political economy of aid and the desire for each of the stakeholders involved – donors, civil society, multilateral institutions, government and service providers – to secure benefits for themselves and their clients. Given the differing objectives of DAH for different stakeholders, seeking consensus on methods and approach is naïve and likely to be contested.

On the other hand, there is increased, and widespread recognition that ODA should be increased and that a substantial proportion of such funds should be devoted to the social sector – health, education, water and sanitation amongst them. The additional funds mobilized should make possible a far wider engagement and support for longer-term development of the health sector. A key sphere of activity will be facilitating policy analysis, donor coordination, common-basket funding and Sector Wide Approaches, and broad health system strengthening. The OECD (2009) itself highlights the degree of fragmentation present in the global health environment, and suggests that the default position should be to "think twice" before establishing yet another initiative related to DAH, and that a "radical pruning" of the very long tail of small health projects is required. The range of players now operating in the global health arena, and the increased scrutiny, should be followed through by increased accountability, transparency and harmonization.

Ruger (2009), citing as unacceptable that a child born in Afghanistan should be 75 times more likely to die by the age of 5 than a child born in Singapore, proposes a "global health justice" approach. This demands a commitment to promoting universal ethical norms and shared global and domestic responsibilities for health. Tandon (2009) argues that ODA should be based on solidarity, stating that the entire aid industry and its present architecture need to be thoroughly reformed in order to create "a more honest relationship" between donors and recipients. He argues that developing countries are making "heroic efforts to disengage" from the "lock-in situation" through which their development is constrained by the former colonial powers who continue to dominate the processes of globalization and the institutions of global governance. He suggests that not only are the well-documented structural adjustment programs of the IMF and World Bank major "shackles," but so too are the new coordination and harmonization mechanisms which still leave the powerful OECD countries in control.

The big funding schemes such as the Bill and Melinda Gates Foundation and the Global Fund Against HIV/AIDS, TB and Malaria, should also be open to more scrutiny and accountability, developing systems which help support health systems worldwide in an effort to ensure delivery of appropriate, effective and equitable services (Sidibe *et al.*, 2006). While new technologies are desirable, applying what is already known and ensuring that people gain access to effective preventive, promotive and treatment services would make a massive difference to the global health situation.

Institutional development and capacity enhancement generally ought to be prioritized. An independent assessment of ODA activities would be valuable – allowing a range of independent agencies to participate in independent and accountable evaluation and monitoring activities. Greater investment in evaluations is required.

The future should have a much stronger rights-based approach; reasonable health and health services should be seen as the right of all people on the planet,

and both their own governments, and others further afield, are duty-bearers with a responsibility to address these needs and present inequities. "Rights-based development" should bring together the right to development with rights-based approaches, conceptualizing development as, in part, the attainment of economic justice (Davis, 2009).

Cometto *et al.* (2009) identify one of the structural constraints as being the privileging of financial sustainability from domestic revenues as a key consideration – employing Tandon's approach to solidarity and Pogge's identification of developed countries as responsible for much underdevelopment, would turn the tables, substantially. Cometto *et al.* (2009) propose a focus on seeking measurable outcomes in all spheres that affect coverage, quality, equity and access to services that influence health outcomes; that key bottlenecks in health system functioning and delivery should be overcome; disbursements should go beyond the public health sector to other sectors which have an influence on health; more budgetary support through grants not loans; greater engagement of civil society; more transparent governance and accountability for major funding initiatives; and an independent mechanism for assessing proposals, and presumably also, monitoring outcomes.

Conclusion

This chapter has sought to situate DAH within a broader context. It has drawn attention to the opportunities resulting from the increased commitment and resources devoted to global health, and to consider their implications. Trends in ODA were reviewed and the greater attention to global health issues highlighted. Key issues related to the range of players and their interests and how political economy can help us understand performance, effectiveness, and failure within the global health environment. Political economy enhances understanding of the interests at stake and of why and how differences of opinion and approach might arise. We highlighted what Birdsall has termed the "seven deadly sins" and sought to consider their implications for DAH. Other views on the moral and ethical responsibilities to promote global health and of the role of DAH were discussed. Finally, some brief recommendations were made, including more effort to place human rights, social justice and the interests of communities in low-income countries, at center-stage.

In the aftermath of the global financial crisis of 2008–10 and the failed Copenhagen Summit on climate change (2009) a fundamental shift away from blaming governments in low- and middle-income countries to instead acknowledging that wealthy countries should take some responsibility for failed, incomplete and uneven development. Development assistance for health is no panacea, but careful reassessment and critique offers suggestions of how more good than harm can be done – if solidarity with those whose poor health most constrains their lives and livelihoods, is genuine.[1]

References

Asante, A. D. & Zwi, A. B. (2007). Public-private partnerships and global health equity: prospects and challenges. *Indian Journal of Medical Ethics* **IV**(4), 176–180.

Benatar, S. R. (2005). Moral imagination: the missing component in global health. *PLoS Medicine* **2**(12), e400.

Bensimon, C. M. & Benatar, S. R. (2006). Developing sustainability: a new metaphor for progress. *Theoretical Medicine and Bioethics* **27**, 59–79.

Birdsall, N. (2008). Seven deadly sins: Reflections on donor failings. In W. Easterly (Ed.), *Reinventing Foreign Aid* (pp. 515–551). Cambridge, MA: MIT Press.

Buse, K. & Harmer, A. (2007). *Global Health: Making Partnerships Work*. Briefing Paper 15, January 2007. London: Overseas Development Institute.

Cometto, G., Ooms, G., Starrs, A. & Zeitz, P. (2009). A global fund for the health MDGs? *Lancet* **373**, 1500–1502.

Das, T. (2009). The information and financial power of the World Bank: knowledge production through UN collaboration. *Progress in Development Studies*, **9**, 209–224.

Das Gupta, M. & Gostin, L. (2009). *How can donors help build global public goods in health?* Policy Research Working Paper 4907. Washington, DC: World Bank.

Davis, T. W. D. (2009). The politics of human rights and development: the challenge for official donors. *Australian Journal of Political Science*, **44**(1), 173–192.

Fiszbein, A. (2006). Development impact evaluation: new trends and challenges. *Evidence & Policy* **2**(3), 385–393.

Grundy, J. (2010). Country-level governance of global health initiatives: an evaluation of immunization coordination mechanisms in five countries of Asia. *Health Policy and Planning* **25**, 186–196.

Health and Fragile States Network (2009). *Health Systems Strengthening in Fragile Contexts: A Report on Good Practices and New Approaches*. www. healthandfragilestates.org

Hotez, P. J., Fenwick, A., Savioli, L. & Molyneux, D. H. (2009). Rescuing the bottom billion through control of neglected diseases. *Lancet* **373**, 1570–1575.

Howell, J. & Lind, J. (2009). Changing donor policy and practice in civil society in the post-9/11 aid context. *Third World Quarterly* **30**(7), 1279–1296.

Lu, C., Schneider, M. T., Gubbins, P. *et al.* (2010). Public financing of health in developing countries: a cross-national systematic analysis. *Lancet* **375**, 1375–1387.

McCormick, D. (2008). China & India as Africa's new donors: the impact of aid on development. *Review of African Political Economy* **35**(115), 73–92.

McCoy, D., Chand, S. & Sridhar, D. (2009a). Global health funding: how much, where it comes from and where it goes. *Health Policy and Planning* **24**(6), 407–417.

McCoy, D., Kembhavi, G., Patel, J. & Luintel, A. (2009b). The Bill & Melinda Gates Foundation's grant-making programme for global health. *Lancet* **373**, 1645–1653.

Millennium Development Project www.un.org/ millenniumgoals/

OECD (2009). Working Party on Aid Effectiveness. *Aid for Better Health – What are We Learning about What Works and What We Still Have to Do?* An interim report from the Task Team on Health as a Tracer Sector. DCD/DAC/ EFF(2009)14.

Piva, P. & Dodd, R. (2009). Where did all the aid go? An in-depth analysis of increased health aid flows over the past 10 years. *Bulletin of the World Health Organization* **87**, 930–939.

Pogge, T. W. M. (2008). *World Poverty and Human Rights: Cosmopolitan Responsibilities and Reforms*. (2nd edn.) Cambridge: Polity Press.

Ravishankar, N., Gubbins, P., Cooley, R. J. *et al.* (2009). Financing of global health: tracking development assistance for health from 1990 to 2007. *Lancet* **373**, 2113–2124.

Reinikka, R. (2008). Donors and service delivery. In W. Easterly (Ed.), *Reinventing Foreign Aid* (pp. 179–199). Cambridge, MA: MIT Press.

Ruger, J. P. (2009). Global health justice. *Public Health Ethics* **2**, 261–275.

Selgelid, M. J. (2008). Improving global health: counting reasons why. *Developing World Bioethics* **8**(2), 115–125.

Sidibe, M., Ramiah, I. & Buse, K. (2006). The Global Fund at five: what next for universal access for HIV/AIDS, TB and malaria? *Journal of the Royal Society of Medicine* **99**, 497–500.

Six, C. (2009). The rise of postcolonial states as donors: a challenge to the development paradigm. *Third World Quarterly* **30**(6), 1103–1121.

---

[1] The author would like to thank Professor Solomon Benatar for encouragement, support and helpful comments during the writing of this chapter.

Sumner, A. & Tribe, M. (2008). *International Development Studies. Theories and Methods in Research and Practice.* London: Sage.

Tandon, Y. (2009). Aid without dependence: an alternative conceptual model for development cooperation. *Development* **52**(3), 356–362.

Vandemoortele, J. (2009). The MDG conundrum: meeting the targets without missing the point. *Development Policy Review* **27**(4), 355–371.

Woods, N. (2008). Whose aid? Whose influence? China, emerging donors and the silent revolution in development assistance. *International Affairs* **84**(6), 1–18.

World Bank (2002). *The Costs of Attaining the Millennium Development Goals.* www.worldbank.org/html/extdr/mdgassessment.pdf

Zwi, A. B. & Mills, A. (1995). Health policy in less developed countries: past trends, future directions. *Journal of International Development* **7**(3), 299–328.

Chapter

17

Climate change and health: risks and inequities

Sharon Friel, Colin Butler and Anthony McMichael

Introduction

Human-induced climate change will affect everyone, mostly adversely. It will have greatest, and generally earliest, impact on the poorest and most disadvantaged populations on the planet. The emerging disruption to key life-supporting environmental systems, caused by climate change, has been mostly generated by a small fraction of modern society. It is one of the biggest ethical issues and challenges of our time. Climate change – itself a product of great inter-nation disparities in economic status and power and thus associated with profound global social inequities – looks likely to worsen those inequities. More generally it will likely exacerbate existing health inequities within all countries.

This chapter describes the main dimensions of inequity concerning climate change and health, and the implications for policy. Inequities exist on several main axes. There are the underlying inequities in the negotiated international agreements for schedules of greenhouse gas emissions reduction (e.g. the 1997 Kyoto Protocol and its emerging successor). There are inequities in relation to the health impacts of climate change, both because of the accompanying inversely related history of national emissions and because the absolute increments of disease burdens and premature deaths will directly reflect the pre-existing levels of poor health in climate-vulnerable populations – much of which would by now, in a fairer world, have been reduced (including via the Millennium Development Goals program). There is, too, the near certainty of great inequities spanning current and future generations, as we fail currently to respond adequately and equitably to what is increasingly recognized as a pressing, growing and potentially catastrophic process of climate change.

Climate change

There is consensus among international climate scientists that Earth's warming by around 0.6 °C since the mid 1970s is mostly due to the human-induced increase in concentration of greenhouse gases (GHG) in the lower atmosphere (IPCC, 2007b). The resultant additional "greenhouse" absorption of infra-red energy, radiating out from Earth's solar-warmed surface, is the overwhelming cause of current global climate change. As ever, there is a background of natural fluctuation in the planet's temperature – upon which human actions are now imposing an unusually rapid increment. Further, because of the momentum and delay in the climate system, there is already an additional human-induced warming of approximately 0.5 °C to be "realized." Then, given the likely range of future emissions, climate scientists estimate a further total warming within the range of 1.8–4.0 °C by 2100 (IPCC, 2007b).[1]

Carbon dioxide (CO_2), the dominant greenhouse gas, persists in the atmosphere for many decades, some of it for centuries. Its concentration (approaching 390 parts per million by volume, ppmv) is now 38% higher than the preindustrial level (Le Quere *et al.*, 2009). The additional warming effect of the other greenhouse gases, principally nitrous oxide (N_2O) and the far more rapidly removed methane (CH_4) – both of which have much greater warming effects per unit volume– have raised the CO_2-equivalent concentration to around 450 ppmv. This combined impact has already imparted

---

[1] Most of the variation in warming estimates, particularly after mid-century, reflects uncertainty about future patterns of population growth, economic development, social change and technological choices – and hence emissions.

Global Health and Global Health Ethics, ed. Solomon Benatar and Gillian Brock. Published by Cambridge University Press.
© Cambridge University Press 2011.

a high probability that Earth's average surface temperature will rise by more than 2 °C during this century – a rise that is likely to disrupt or destroy many natural environmental assets, species and ecological processes (Rockstrom *et al.*, 2009). Rises will be greater at higher latitudes, with medium-risk scenarios predicting 2–3 °C rises by 2090 and 4–5 °C rises in northern Canada, Greenland and Siberia (Costello *et al.*, 2009).

Further, as Earth's temperature enters this "danger zone" the likelihood of crossing critical thresholds increases. Various critical events and feedback processes will then occur, including the massive release of additional GHGs from tundra and peatlands (Canadell *et al.*, 2006). As the temperature rises there will likely be increased, and more severe, heat waves, droughts, storms and floods. These changes will bring heightened risks to human societies and to human health and survival (McMichael, 2009).

Climate change: an ethical issue

The disruption to the global climate and other life-supporting environmental systems by modern society is perhaps one of the biggest ethical issues of our time and arises from profound global inequities. By the term "inequity" we mean not only an unequal distribution but one that is also unfair and remediable.

We next describe several inequitable aspects concerning climate change and health. We focus on the inequity of GHG emissions contrasted to the social and health risk resulting from GHG concentrations. We show how this inequity is embedded in and consistent with older and more pervasive forms of global inequity.

Imbalance in emissions

Discussion of equity in GHG emissions requires consideration of their source, rate of change, cumulative volume and purpose. Though China has recently overtaken the USA as the largest national emitter of CO_2, its per capita emissions are still only one-fifth of the size. Further, a substantial fraction of China's emissions arise from the manufacture of consumer items destined for consumption in higher-income countries (Guan *et al.*, 2009). Together, the developing and least-developed economies (forming 80% of the world's population) have accounted for less than 25% of global cumulative CO_2 emissions since the mid-eighteenth century (Raupach *et al.*, 2007). Emissions from India are on a rising trend. Even so, its per capita carbon

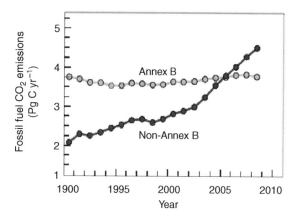

Figure 17.1 Growth rate in carbon emissions of developed and developing countries. Note: Annex B countries are mainly developed countries; Non-Annex B are mainly developing countries. Source (Le Quere *et al.*, 2009). Pg Cyr^{-1} = Billion tonnes Carbon per year.

footprint is less than one-tenth of that in high-income countries. Considering poor populations, rather than poor nations, the carbon footprint of the poorest 1 billion people on the planet is around 3% of the world's total (UNDP, 2007).

Geo-spatial relocation of emissions

From a cursory look at Figure 17.1, we would surmise that developing countries now exceed developed countries in the amount of carbon that they emit annually. While the growth in emissions over the past two decades did indeed occur mainly in developing countries, a quarter of it is attributable to production of goods for consumption in industrialized nations (Le Quere *et al.*, 2009). The modern-day economic system, with globalization of trade and production of goods, thus facilitates more advantaged nations and institutions externalizing their GHG emissions to the producer country.

The Kyoto Protocol's strictly geographical (within-nation) approach to national emissions accounting, and hence mitigation responsibility, introduces a clear dimension of inequity. This results from the incentives, which flow from the Protocol, for developed (Annex B) nations to "outsource" GHG emissions used in the production of GHG-intensive materials which are then consumed in the developed nation – without making any noticeable difference to climate change.

Another example of geo-spatial inequity lies within the food and agriculture sector. The UK livestock sector is responsible for emitting about 36 metric tonne (ton) carbon dioxide equivalents (MtCO$_2$-e) annually. These estimates relate to emissions generated within UK borders only and do not count the embedded emissions in the totality of goods and services consumed nor emissions resulting from global change in land use that is associated with livestock production in the UK (Friel *et al.*, 2009).

Who has the right to emit?

Unless we are blind to the risk of precipitating dangerous climate change, the necessary policy decisions concerning mitigation and the global share of permissible emissions pose a core ethical issue. It could be argued from an ethical perspective that people should have inalienable rights to the minimum emissions necessary to their survival or to some minimal quality of life. Presently, developed countries have largely exhausted the world's capacity to take up, redistribute and sequester carbon in the process of industrializing and so have, in effect, denied other countries the opportunity to use "their shares." Access to a fundamental "global commons" has thus been usurped. Butler argues that there are enough global resources, knowledge and technology to provide an adequate standard of living for most of the world's (current) population (Butler, 2008), but the current imbalance reflects geographic vulnerability and lack of political and economic power on the part of many low- and middle-income countries.

How mitigation of future climate change is addressed raises issues of fair and just economic development among some of the world's poorest countries and communities. Observers in low-income countries point out that the historical activities in rich countries have caused most climate change so far. Since low-income countries have many urgent needs for development, they naturally place mitigation of their own greenhouse-gas emissions at a lower priority. Yet, if the current trajectory of GHG emissions is to be slowed, many low- and middle-income countries indeed will need to take mitigation action, in addition to the urgent and far-reaching emissions reductions needed in high-income countries (Haines *et al.*, 2009).

Delaying action

It is sometimes argued that the uncertainty of the scientist's predictions is a reason for not acting at present, and that we should wait until some further research has been concluded. This argument is poor economics. (Broome, 1992, p. 17, in Gardiner, 2004)

Excessive procrastination on the grounds of alleged scientific uncertainty[2] is another example of injustice. Some nations continue to defer significant reductions in their GHG emissions, partly on the basis of persistent scientific uncertainty about climate change and its impacts. Implicitly, this inaction asks the recipient of climate change impacts to bear the burden of risk until the scientific uncertainties are resolved. Such populations, usually distant in place or time, are forced to accept this risk in exchange for almost no benefit. Citing uncertainty as an excuse for inaction is to either deny the current evidence of the reality and seriousness of climate change or to unfairly offload the risk to other peoples (Gardiner, 2004).

The time frame: intergenerational inequity

Climate change justifies exploration of the moral relevance of decisions taken by previous generations. By analogy, some of the deleterious health effects of past industrialization are being experienced today (e.g. environmental lead and asbestos exposures). Greenhouse gases started to rise at the start of industrialization, but while their theoretical effect on the climate was suggested in the nineteenth century widespread understanding of the scale and risk of GHG-related climate change is far more recent. The impacts of past and continuing climate change will be felt by future people. The effects of climate change on children now and in the future raises another challenging ethical issue. Because of their immature organ systems, neurobiology and dependence on caregivers, children are particularly susceptible to heat stress, gastroenteritis and natural disasters, as well as to family stresses linked to droughts, loss of livelihood and familial dislocation – and this will have long-term health consequences for many children (Strazdins *et al.*, in press).

Climate change: a health issue

Our discussions thus far have been concerned with the science of climate change and inequities and ethical issues raised in the production of greenhouse gas emissions. In terms of consequences, climate change will affect the lives of most populations in the next decade and has been described as one of the greatest threats to human health (Costello *et al.*, 2009). One major, though conservative, estimation, coordinated by

---

[2] The case in November 2009, shortly before the COP 15 conference.

Table 17.1. Major categories of health risks from climate change (McMichael, 2009).

Direct effects

Increased risk of injury or death from extreme weather events such as floods, fires or storms.

Increased morbidity and mortality associated with more frequent and intense heat waves

Increased risk of respiratory illnesses from higher ground-level ozone and other air pollutants.

Exacerbation of asthma and other respiratory allergic conditions from increases in airborne pollens and spores.

Indirect consequences

Increased risk of malnutrition from impaired agriculture (and from associated impoverishment from loss of rural livelihoods).

Increased risk of gastroenteritis (e.g. from salmonella, campylobacter and temperature-sensitive vibrios).

Change in the range and seasonality of outbreaks of mosquito-borne infections such as malaria, dengue fever or chikungunya virus.

Health risks for displaced persons/groups and possible risks for their host populations.

Increased mental health risks such as post-traumatic stress disorder associated with extreme weather events or depression/suicide associated with impoverishment or lost livelihood (e.g. long-term drying in rural regions) or displacement.

WHO, suggested that the extent of climate change that had already occurred by the year 2000 (relative to the 1961–1990 average climate) was directly responsible for the loss of at least 5.5 million disability adjusted life years (DALYs) in that year. However, that assessment of the disease burden attributable to climate change related only to deaths, disease and disabling injuries caused by diarrhea, malaria, accidental injuries in coastal floods and inland floods or landslides, and malnutrition (Campbell-Lendrum *et al.*, 2003).

Changes in climatic conditions and increases in weather variability affect human well-being, safety, health and survival in many ways. Some impacts are direct-acting and immediate. Other effects are less immediate and typically occur via more complex causal pathways (Table 17.1). Although some vector-borne diseases will expand their range and seasonality, and death tolls will increase because of heatwaves, the indirect effects of climate change on basic human needs such as food, water and shelter will be likely to have the biggest effect on global health. Unless there are surprising advances in cultivars and cultivation, a substantially increased fraction of the world's population is likely to face severe food shortages and water insecurity by the end of the century due to climate change. Climate change is likely to impair crops, herds and fish stocks in many ways, especially in low-latitude countries. These mechanisms include through rising temperatures, water stress, extreme weather events, spreading plant and animal diseases, sea level rise and ocean acidification. The health of millions of people will be compromised not only by reduced nutrition, but through an increase in the frequency of intense hurricanes, cyclones and storm surges causing flooding and direct injury, increasing the health risk among those living in urban slums and where shelter and human settlements are poor (Costello *et al.*, 2009). With this will come extensive displacement of people and livelihoods, each with implications for physical and mental health.

All of this climate change-related health risk is on top of pre-existing infectious and non-communicable disease burdens, often in poor countries with already under-resourced health-care systems.

Inequitable health consequences of climate change

In terms of absolute burden, however, it seems clear that it [climate change] most threatens the poorest and most vulnerable populations in all societies, probably in close inverse proportion to income, wealth, and power. The rich will find their world to be more expensive, inconvenient, uncomfortable, disrupted, and colorless – in general, more unpleasant and unpredictable, perhaps greatly so. The poor will die. (Smith, 2008)

Climate change will exacerbate existing social and health inequities. Adverse health outcomes are likely to be greatest in low-income countries and among poor people living in urban areas, elderly people, children, traditional societies, subsistence farmers and coastal populations. In general, the greatest health risks are experienced by those contributing least to the underlying environmental damage i.e. the least economically advanced countries and lower social status groups within rich and poor countries alike (Friel *et al.*, 2008). The conservatively estimated 150 000 additional deaths attributable to climate change in the year 2000 (see the above-mentioned WHO study: Campbell-Lendrum *et al.*, 2003), were almost entirely concentrated in the world's poorer and vulnerable populations (Figure 17.2). In developing countries, diseases transmitted

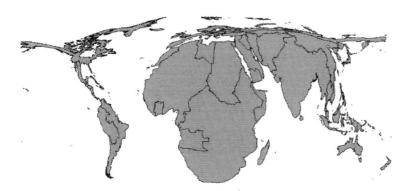

Figure 17.2 Deaths attributable to anthropogenic climate change between 1970 and 2000, displayed as a density-equaling cartogram (Patz *et al.*, 2007).

by water, soil and vectors such as trematode flatworms (schistosomiasis), hookworm and filarial worms (filariasis) are often many times more common among people in the lowest socio-economic category. The phenomenon also occurs in rich countries: in the wake of Hurricane Katrina in the USA, children from lower-income groups were at increased risk of developing severe mental health symptoms (McLaughlin *et al.*, 2009).

Climate change's pathways to health inequities

Much of the currently emerging global variation in health impacts of climate change is due to existing economic, social and health inequities. Some of the variation, of course, is due to geography – for example, as with small island states. This is seen in the regional variation in predicted rates and types of climatic change; differing underlying vulnerabilities (such as existing levels of heat and food stress, and exposure to disease vectors); and differing capacities to adapt to changing conditions. We now describe some of the ways in which climate change will contribute to global health inequities.

Extreme weather events

Climate scientists anticipate that weather patterns will become more variable as global warming proceeds (IPCC, 2007b). A general increase in frequency and intensity of many types of extreme weather events is anticipated.

Weather disasters – such as the cyclones that have struck vulnerable, poor, coastal populations of Bangladesh, Myanmar and Vietnam in recent times – injure and kill. Likewise the hurricanes that frequently impinge on the Caribbean, causing property damage, injury, deaths and distress. Floods in northern Kenya

have had many direct adverse health effects, in addition to causing outbreaks of Rift Valley Fever, affecting both livestock and humans.

Extreme weather events can increase infectious disease spread (e.g. cholera), food shortages, impoverishment and mental health consequences of loss and trauma. In addition to the diverse social, behavioral and mental health impacts of more extreme bushfires, floods and storms, there is a range of risks to social stability and mental health from the longer-term drying trend that is now becoming evident in Australia (Berry *et al.*, 2010).

Sea-level rise

Sea level is rising faster than in the 1980s and 1990s. This is due to two main consequences of global warming: first, thermal expansion of ocean water and second, the melting of land-based glaciers and ice-sheets (particularly the massive Greenland glacier). Some recent estimates indicate that a rise of one meter, or more, could occur by the end of this century (Allison *et al.*, 2009). Even if stabilization of atmospheric concentrations of greenhouse gases were achieved in the next few decades, sea level will continue to rise for many centuries as the slow processes of heat distribution throughout the oceans proceed.

Sea-level rise poses both direct and indirect risks to health and health equity. This manifestation of climate change has profound implications for the one-third of the world's population who live within 60 miles of a shoreline and 13 of the world's 20 largest cities located on a coast (McGranahan *et al.*, 2007). It is a crucial issue for many low-lying small island states in the Pacific and Indian Oceans, the Caribbean, and elsewhere, and also for various low-lying coastal populations (e.g. in Bangladesh) and river delta regions. A rise of one meter would inundate an area of Bangladesh currently inhabited by around 10% of its total population, and would eliminate a significantly greater proportion of the nation's rice production. Much of the Maldives is little more than one meter above sea level.

Coastal inundation, more extensive episodes of flooding, increasingly severe storm surges (especially at times of high tide) and damage to coastal infrastructure (roads, housing and sanitation systems) would all pose direct risks to health. There is, too, a range of indirect risks to health. These include the salination of freshwater supplies – a particular problem for many small islands, as their aquifer "cells" of water are encroached upon – the loss of productive farm land, and changes in breeding habitats for coastal-dwelling mosquitoes. Other indirect health risks include the mental health consequences of property loss, break-up of communities, displacement and emigration, and the possible risks of tension between displaced and receiving groups.

Temperature extremes

Heatwaves kill people, primarily by causing heart attacks, strokes, respiratory failure and heatstroke. The notorious August 2003 heatwave in Western Europe caused an estimated 40 000–50 000 deaths, especially in older persons. Temperature extremes also affect physiological functioning, mood, behavior (accident-proneness) and workplace productivity. The already poorer health outcomes experienced among lower occupational grades will be exacerbated by temperature extremes, especially in outdoor workers and those working in poorly ventilated hot factory conditions (Kjellstrom, 2009).

Drought

Droughts are predicted to become more frequent and severe in many regions of the world under climate change. These cause hunger, starvation, displacement and misery; farming jobs are lost, and suicide rates, especially in farmers, often rise. A similar range of health risks will result from the long-term drying foreseen by climate modelers for the sub-tropical regions. Such drying now appears to be becoming evident in several continents, including southern Australia, parts of southern Africa (e.g. Zimbabwe, South Africa), southern Canada and the Mediterranean region (especially southern Spain). Impoverished rural persons who are displaced by climate-related downturns in farm yields and livelihoods and who move into peri-urban slum-dwelling are at risk of

mental trauma, and are likely to be exposed to infectious disease, including HIV, via transactional (commercial) sex (McMichael *et al.*, 2008).

Food insecurity

The equity implications of climate change appear to be particularly profound for food security. The World Health Organization's above-mentioned estimate of disease burdens already attributable to climate change in the year 2000 identified malnutrition as the pre-eminent component of health loss. Most of that estimated loss (via premature deaths, stunting and disabling infection) was in young children in developing countries.

Food insecurity persists widely; more than 1 billion people worldwide are undernourished (FAO, 2009) – a number that has increased substantially in the last decade. During 2008, as food prices escalated and shortages emerged, concerns were widely expressed about climatic influences on food yields. Modeling studies consistently project that climate change will, overall, have a negative impact on global food yields. However, those impacts will occur very unevenly. In general, countries in the tropics and subtropics, where both warming and reduced rainfall are likely to occur, are at greatest risk. There is a cascade of impacts on food yields, transport and access in southern Africa (including South Africa, Zimbabwe, Botswana, Lesotho and Malawi) (McMichael *et al.*, 2008). Many studies indicate that South Asia is particularly vulnerable, and likely to experience declines in cereal grain yields of the order of 10–20% by later this century (IPCC, 2007a). Meanwhile, temperate zones may benefit – at least before temperature rises exceed threshold levels.

As warming proceeds, various fish populations important to local food security are anticipated to move to higher latitudes. This will affect protein supplies, and livelihoods, in coastal populations in much of Africa, many small island states and large Asian river deltas. The world's fisheries provide over 2.6 billion people with one-fifth of their average annual protein intake. In addition to the widely reported ongoing decline in ocean fisheries, a 2007 report by the World-Fish Center concludes that climate "shocks" such as coral reef damage, warmer waters, acidification (due to increasing uptake of CO_2) and decreased river flows (a crucial source of recycled nutrients for both freshwater and ocean fisheries) will exacerbate the already serious problem of over-fishing. The report names as particularly vulnerable countries Angola, Pakistan, the Democratic Republic of Congo, Russia and – although data were less available – Pacific nations such as Samoa, Vanuatu and the Solomon Islands (World Fish Center, 2007).

In isolated and food-insecure regions, downturns in yields of crops and pastures can quickly turn into hunger, undernutrition, starvation and, on occasion, conflict. A report by the UN Environment Program in 2007 concluded that recent tensions in Sudan between traditional farmers and nomadic herders over declining pasture and evaporating water holes have helped precipitate conflicts (UNEP, 2007).

Water insecurity

Access to water and food is a prerequisite for health and survival. Water scarcity poses multiple risks to health. These include water-borne infectious diseases (cholera, other diarrheal organisms, cryptosporidium, etc.), vector-borne diseases associated with water storage (e.g. malaria and schistosomiasis), exposure to higher concentrations of salt and chemical contaminants in water, impaired food yields (especially irrigation-dependent crops) and conflict situations.

Climate change will exacerbate water insecurity and thereby health inequities. Currently, 450 million people in 29 countries suffer from water shortages and it is estimated that two out of every three people will live in water-stressed areas by the year 2025 (UNEP, 2008). In Africa alone, 300 million people are currently water insecure; climate change will increase this number to an estimated 480 million by 2025.

Concerns are rising in vulnerable regions such as India, Bangladesh, Myanmar and the Mekong River basin and delta, where Himalayan glacier loss is beginning to affect flows, and where there is real prospect of inter-country tensions because of up-stream diversion of flows. China, for example, may well divert much of the headwaters for the great rivers of South Asia and Southeast Asia (Indochina) that come from the northern slopes of the Himalayas.

Infectious diseases

Many infectious diseases are sensitive to climatic conditions. In warmer conditions, bacteria in food and in nutrient-loaded water multiply. Studies in the UK, Australia and Canada have shown a clear relationship between short-term higher temperatures and the rate of occurrence of salmonella food poisoning. Changes in rainfall patterns affect river flows, flooding, sanitary

conditions and the spread of diarrheal diseases, including cholera.

Many vector-borne infections, transmitted by mosquitoes, other insects or rodents, are sensitive to temperature, rainfall, humidity and wind. As temperature rises, infectious agents within mosquitoes (e.g. the protozoan parasite *Plasmodium falciparum* and dengue virus) mature more quickly, while mosquitoes reproduce more efficiently and must feed (blood-meals) more often. Surface water patterns influence mosquito breeding; humidity affects mosquito survival.

Many of the "zoonotic" infectious diseases that spill over into human populations from animal sources are influenced by climate-related changes in density and movement of the "reservoir" animal species. Examples include: West Nile Fever (now in USA and Canada: birds), Rift Valley Fever (Kenya: cattle) and Ross River Virus (Australia: kangaroos).

Some vector-borne infections appear to have increased their geographic range in association with regional warming. This includes the incidence of malaria in some eastern African highlands, tick-borne encephalitis in northern Sweden, Lyme disease in Canada, and schistosomiasis (for which the temperature-sensitive water snail is intermediate host) in eastern China.

Health effects of social and cultural disruption

Some health and health equity effects occur at several removes from the actual change in climate. This is well illustrated by the impacts of the relatively rapid ongoing warming in the Arctic region. The resultant loss of sea-ice and permafrost is disturbing traditional living, hunting and eating patterns in the Inuit communities of northern Canada. This has lessened physical mobility options and has increased reliance on imported energy-dense processed foods, thus amplifying obesity, cardiovascular disease and diabetes.

Climate change is very likely to cause a dramatic increase in human movement, both within states and across international borders (IPCC, 2007a). The predicted increase in frequency and severity of climate events such as storms, cyclones and hurricanes, as well as longer-term sea-level rise and desertification, will lessen people's ability to subsist in some regions. Around one-fifth of the world's population lives in coastal areas affected by rising seas and natural disasters – especially those living in major river deltas (e.g. Bangladesh, Egypt), parts of Central America, eastern China and India, and many small island states. Populations in the Maldives, Tuvalu, Kiribati and parts of the Caribbean face the risk of whole-nation displacement. In his authoritative review, Stern described earlier projections of 200 million displaced persons as "conservative" (Stern, 2007).

The mental health consequences of these social and cultural disruptions, and of associated perceptions of future threats, pose an increasingly important risk to health. This may apply particularly in children. Long-standing expectations, at least in higher-income countries, of continued material gains and ever improving conditions of life should now be superseded by an understanding that environmental and social consequences of climate change associated with endless consumption cannot be ignored.

Common causes of climate change and health inequities

We have described how modern society is fuelling climate change which in turn affects human health and health inequity. Modern society also affects health in other ways. On average, there have been major improvements in health outcomes in most, but not all, countries in the world. However, key elements of our modern global world – asymmetric economic growth between nations and populations, unequal improvements in daily living conditions (access to health care, schools and education, conditions of work and leisure, shelter, communities, towns or cities), unequal distribution of technical developments and suppression of human rights have widened health inequities and, arguably, accelerated dangerous climate change (Friel et al., 2008).

Within this milieu of underlying common causes of climate change and global health inequities lie economic policies, processes of urbanization and global food systems – each overlapping and each identified as playing a major role in population and planetary health. We now describe key elements of each of these large complex drivers and policy areas.

Economic policy

Particularly since the Second World War, the nature of global economic and social policy has changed dramatically. In 1944 the Bretton Woods accords aimed to generate economic growth based on a liberal system of open markets. The General Agreement on Tariffs and Trade (GATT) which arose from these negotiations (and subsequently the World Trade

Organization in 1994) liberalized the market and established general principles of freer trade. During the 1980s and 1990s, the international financial institutions embraced a set of economic policies known as "the Washington consensus." These policies were designed to promote the role of the market (involving deregulation, privatization of public services, measures designed to achieve low inflation rates and stable currencies and mechanisms enhancing the operations of multinational corporations), and propelled the world towards even greater economic integration and deregulation.

This is by way of illustrating how the economic pathway followed since the Second World War has helped create a degree of global interconnectedness and interdependence hitherto unheard of. While beneficial in many respects – facilitating greater transfer of capital, technology, knowledge and people – the gains have been uneven, with asymmetries in power, income, goods, services and health at the global level (Labonté & Schrecker, 2007). Nearly 3 billion people still live on less than $2 per day (ILO, 2008). Around two-thirds of the world's poor are to be found in Asia and every second child on the planet lives in poverty. Some have argued that the structural adjustment policies introduced by the International Monetary Fund to ensure debt repayment and economic restructuring diverted government resources away from public goods like health, education and sustainable development (Messner et al., 2005). Similarly, the prevailing international trade agreements impede government capacity to protect public health, to regulate occupational and environmental health conditions and food products and to ensure affordable access to medications (Shaffer et al., 2005).

The creation of such a global marketplace, demanding ever-increasing volumes of production and, with increasing wealth, encouraging more and more consumption of goods, has helped create a global society that is increasingly dependent on finite natural resources and use of fossil fuels (Hanlon & McCartney, 2008). Compounding the environmental degradation from the activities of mid-nineteenth century industrialization, modern society has destabilized the ecosystem and exacerbated climate change. The global importance of rapidly emerging economies is growing as they become major economic and trade partners, competitors, resource users and polluters on a level that compares to the largest of OECD countries. The primary energy consumption of Brazil, Russia, India and China together is expected to grow by around 70% between 2005 and 2030, compared with about 33% in the 30 OECD countries.

Urbanization

Accompanying globalization, market liberalization and economic integration has been the urbanization of the planet. While urban living has provided many benefits it has also come at some cost, both to population health and to the environment (Knowledge Network on Urban Settings, 2007).

Almost two-thirds of urban dwellers live in developing countries in cities that have grown at breakneck speed with limited investment in infrastructure, housing, human resources and public health. The associated poor urban living conditions, particularly those among the billion people living in low-income urban settlements ("urban slums") are the breeding ground for communicable disease. These high-density settlements with inadequate water and sanitation services increase vulnerability to climate-sensitive infectious diseases such as diarrhea and dengue (Campbell-Lendrum & Corvalan, 2007). And as the degree of urbanization and national income increase so too does the prevalence of new urban health problems including diabetes, heart disease, obesity, mental health problems, alcohol and drug abuse and violence (Ezzati *et al.*, 2005). Road traffic injuries, vehicle-related air pollution and traffic noise cause thousands of cases of poor health and deaths each year, with urban areas by far the most affected. The design of cities – increasingly large sprawling conglomerations – fuels the nutrition transition and associated obesity epidemic, partly through urban planning that ignores the need for walking, cycling and playing in the urban landscape. The unequal nature of urbanization and the resulting built environment impacts more adversely on low-income groups who live in poorer conditions (Knowledge Network on Urban Settings, 2007).

Climate change, amplified by the heat island effect in inner city environments, is causing increased heat stress levels and health risks. Poor neighborhoods with little environmentally friendly infrastructure/buildings/green space are likely to be more exposed to urban heat compared with more affluent neighborhoods, and have less capacity to adapt to the impact. Lower socioeconomic groups are more likely to be those urban workers exposed to working conditions with excess heat and therefore at increased risk compared with higher social status groups (Kjellstrom, 2009).

The current model of urbanization poses significant direct environmental challenges. The same urban landscape promotes use of the car thereby perpetuating air pollution and fossil fuel use (and risk of road traffic accidents). Transport and buildings contribute an estimated 21% of global CO_2 emissions (Confalonieri *et al.*, 2007) – mostly from cities in the developed world. However, the combination of rapid economic development and concurrent urbanization in poorer regions means that developing countries will be both vulnerable to health hazards from climate change and increasing contributors to that problem (Campbell-Lendrum & Corvalan, 2007). Indeed, with improved financial means, particularly among the burgeoning urban middle classes in developing countries, more people – 1.3 billion globally – have moved to the top end of the consumption ladder characterized by more, and more frequent, use of fossil-fuel dependent cars (Myers & Kent, 2003).

Food systems

The food system contributes to health inequities through inequities in global and domestic food availability and nutrient quality, accessibility and affordability (termed here the Triple A_e rating) (Friel *et al.*, 2008; Hawkes *et al.*, 2009). The Triple A_e rating of the food system is partly determined by conditions of trade, agricultural production, food provisioning systems, price and food preparation. Not only does the food system affect health, it is a major contributor to greenhouse gas emissions (~30% globally) and thus to climate change (Garnett, 2008). The food system produces emissions at all stages in its life cycle – from the farming process itself (and associated inputs) to manufacture, distribution and cold storage through to food preparation and consumption and the disposal of waste. IPCC estimates that global agricultural emissions could grow by between 36–63% by 2030 (Smith *et al.*, 2007). And as described previously, food systems are also increasingly affected by climate change causing major disruption to food and nutrition security in the majority of countries worldwide.

Structural adjustment in low- and middle-income countries, coupled with increasing trade liberalization, particularly the agriculture trade agreement in the 1994 Uruguay Round of GATT opened up these countries to the international market. Regional trade agreements soared at a rate of 15 per year in the 1990s and the 1994 Uruguay Round of the GATT pledged countries to reduce tariffs, export subsidies and domestic agricultural support. Although trade can be a mechanism for countries to reduce poverty and improve food security, unilateral trade liberalization and uneven distribution of global food stocks through protectionist trade arrangements have been associated with greater economic insecurity and adverse dietary changes, while the expected benefits to economic growth have not accrued evenly (Elinder, 2005). Many developing countries experienced more than a doubling of food import bills as a share of GDP between 1974 and 2004. Emerging economies, such as Brazil, Russia, India and China, have seen massive increases in their purchasing power, particularly among the urban middle classes, contributing to population shifts from diets based on traditional plant-based staple foods to more expensive and GHG emissions-intensive animal source products.

Blouin and colleagues argue that trade liberalization has distorted the food supply in developing countries in favor of highly processed, calorie-rich, nutrient-poor food, thereby contributing to the double burden of under- and overnutrition in those countries (Blouin et al., 2009). These same foods are water- and fossil fuel-intensive to produce.

The recent global food price rise shows that the global agricultural and food production system is vulnerable to short-term shocks that threaten the sustainability of the food supply chain, especially in low-income countries which rely heavily on food imports. The production of crops for biofuels is impacting on food production, depleting biodiversity and water, worsening climate change (e.g. via deforestation) and contributing to food price increases (Scharlemann & Laurance, 2008). Rising food prices will hit the poorest hardest but it will affect everyone except the super-rich. Some will be able to maintain a healthy diet of fresh produce, fish, lean meat and grains; some will only be able to purchase the cheapest sources of calories – highly processed, long shelf-life products, containing hardened fats and bulk starches, preserved with sugar or salt that increase the risk of obesity and diabetes, and many millions will be unable to afford even that (Lobstein et al., 2008).

Climate stabilization, development and health improvement

Climate change, on top of existing inequities in social conditions, threatens to undermine global action to address long-standing health problems and curtail progress towards the Millennium Development Goals. Addressing the common drivers of climate change and population health will not only improve global health, but advances will also be made in poverty eradication, national economic development and social equity such that people, communities and nations will be better able to resist current climate change and avert further damage to the global environment and climate.

A recent series of studies on climate change mitigation and global health (Haines et al., 2009) illustrate a major health-based incentive to propel the world forward on climate change abatement. The papers highlight how policies to promote mitigation that have strong co-benefits in health and other development needs provide a potential political bridge across the development gap between rich and poor countries. The provision of affordable clean household energy in developing countries can contribute to the attainment of all eight MDGs, both through the co-benefits to health and through contributions to poverty reduction, provision of productive work, reduction of unproductive time and thereby reduction of gender inequities. Climate change mitigation policies may well result in differential rates of health improvement that favor the poorer nations and populations. For example, cleaner-burning cooking stoves in India could bring about 12 500 additional years of healthy life per million population compared with about 850 additional years of healthy life per million population in the UK (Markandya et al., 2009). Similarly, more sustainable transport systems would yield an estimated 7400 additional years of healthy life per million population annually in London, UK, versus approximately 13 000 in New Delhi, India (Woodcock et al., 2009).

The co-benefits arguments show that climate change mitigation can improve health. Beyond this, a global energy transition is clearly required, not only to minimize climate change but also to avert the public health and other costs of oil depletion (Hanlon & McCartney, 2008). Indeed, there is a growing risk that market-based arguments will be used to substitute oil by coal, a policy which would greatly exacerbate GHG accumulation. To prevent these consequences, analysts have for decades been calling for a massive global energy revolution. However, these innovations continue to be impeded by technological obstacles and by the artificially low price of fossil fuels.

Conclusion

Climate change throws into sharp relief many of the issues to do with inequities in living standards, political power, resource use, levels of exposure to environmental stresses and health and life expectancy.

The continuing inability of nations to come to terms with the very unequal history of greenhouse gas emissions between industrialized and non-industrialized countries, and thereby to forge a fair and differentiated schedule of emissions reduction, constitutes a major current political and economic inequity. Climate change itself threatens to increase existing health inequities within and between populations, and to undermine the improved living standards and better health so often assumed to be the destiny of future generations.

In contrast, well-directed emissions reduction (mitigation) policies at national level, and (meanwhile) effective and fairly funded adaptation strategies, each have the potential to safeguard and improve health, and to do so in ways that reduce inequities between populations.

References

Allison, I., Bindoff, N., Bindschadler, R. et al. (2009). The Copenhagen Diagnosis. Updating the World on the Latest Climate Science. Sydney: The University of New South Wales Climate Change Research Centre (CCRC).

Berry, H., Bowen, K. & Kjellstrom, T. (2010). Climate change and mental health: a causal pathways framework. International Journal of Public Health 52(3), 123–132.

Blouin, C., Chopra, M. & van der Hoeven, R. (2009). Trade and social determinants of health. Lancet, 373, 502–507.

Butler, C. (2008). Environmental change, injustice and sustainability. Journal of Bioethical Inquiry 5, 11–19.

Campbell-Lendrum, D. & Corvalan, C. (2007). Climate change and developing-country cities: implications for environmental health and equity. Journal of Urban Health 84, 109–117.

Campbell-Lendrum, D., Corvalán, C. & Ustün, A. P. (2003). How much disease could climate change cause? In A. McMichael, D. Campbell-Lendrum, C. Corvalan et al. (Eds.), Climate Change and Human Health: Risks and Responses (pp. 1543–1649). Geneva: World Health Organization.

Canadell, J., Pataki, D., Gifford, R. et al. (2006). Saturation of the terrestrial carbon sink. In J. Canadell, D. Pataki & L. Pitelka (Eds.), Terrestrial Ecosystems in a Changing World (pp. 59–78). Berlin: Springer-Verlag.

Confalonieri, U., Menne, B., Akhtar, R. et al. (2007). Human health. In M. L. Parry, O. F. Canziani, J. P. Palutikof, P. J. van der Linden & C. E. Hanson (Eds.), Climate Change 2007: Impacts, Adaptation and Vulnerability. Contribution of Working Group II to the Fourth Assessment Report of the Intergovernmental Panel on Climate Change. Cambridge: Cambridge University Press.

Costello, A., Abbas, M., Allen, A. et al. (2009) Managing the health effects of climate change. UCL Institute for Global Health and Lancet Commission. Lancet 373, 1693–1733.

Elinder, L. S. (2005). Obesity, hunger, and agriculture: the damaging role of subsidies. British Medical Journal 331, 1333–1336.

Ezzati, M., Hoorn, S. V., Lawes, C. et al. (2005). Rethinking the "diseases of affluence" paradigm: global patterns of nutritional risks in relation to economic development. PLoS Medicine 2, e148.

Food and Agriculture Organization (FAO) (2009). The State of Food Insecurity in the World. Rome: Food and Agriculture Organization.

Friel, S., Marmot, M., McMichael, A. J., Kjellstrom, T. & Vågerö, D. (2008). Global health equity and climate stabilisation – need for a common agenda. Lancet 372, 1677–1683.

Friel, S., Dangour, A. D., Garnett, T. et al. (2009). Public health benefits of strategies to reduce greenhouse-gas emissions: food and agriculture. Lancet 374, 2016–2025.

Gardiner, S. (2004). Ethics and global climate change. Ethics 114, 555–600.

Garnett, T. (2008). Cooking up a storm: food, greenhouse gas emissions and our changing climate. Guildford: Food Climate Research Network, Centre for Environmental Strategy, University of Surrey.

Guan, D., Peters, G., Weber, C. & Hubacek, K. (2009). Journey to world top emitter: an analysis of the driving forces of China's recent CO2 emissions surge. Geophysical Research Letters 36, L04709.

Haines, A., McMichael, A., Smith, K. et al. (2009). Public health benefits of strategies to reduce greenhouse-gas emissions: overview and implications for policy makers. Lancet 374, 2104–2114.

Hanlon, P. & McCartney, G. (2008). Peak oil: will it be public health's greatest challenge? Public Health, 122, 647–652.

Hawkes, C., Chopra, M. & Friel, S. (2009). Globalization, trade and the nutrition transition. In R. Labonté, T. Schrecker, C. Packer & V. Runnels (Eds.), Globalization and Health: Pathways, Evidence and Policy. New York: Routledge.

International Labour Organization (ILO) (2008). Global Employment Trends. Geneva: International Labour Organization.

IPCC (2007a). *Climate Change 2007: Impacts, Adaptation and Vulnerability*. Contribution of Working Group II to the Fourth Assessment Report of the Intergovernmental Panel on Climate Change. New York: Cambridge University Press.

IPCC (2007b). *Climate Change 2007: The Physical Science Basis*. Contribution of Working Group I to the Fourth Assessment Report of the Intergovernmental Panel on Climate Change. New York: Cambridge University Press.

Kjellstrom, T. (2009). Climate change, direct heat exposure, health and well-being in low and middle income countries. *Global Health Action* 2, 1–3.

Knowledge Network on Urban Settings (2007). *Our Cities, Our Health, Our Future: Acting on Social Determinants for Health Equity in Urban Settings*. Final Report of the Urban Settings Knowledge Network of the Commission on Social Determinants of Health. Geneva: World Health Organization.

Labonté, R. & Schrecker, T. (2007). Foreign policy matters: a normative view of the G8 and population health. *Bulletin of the World Health Organization* 85, 185–191.

Le Quere, C., Raupach, M. R., Canadell, J. G. *et al.* (2009). Trends in the sources and sinks of carbon dioxide. *Nature Geoscience*, advance online publication.

Lobstein, T., Friel, S. & Dowler, E. (2008). Food, fuel and NCDs. *Lancet* 372, 628.

Markandya, A., Armstrong, B., Hales, S. *et al.* (2009). Public health benefits of strategies to reduce greenhouse-gas emissions: low-carbon electricity generation. *Lancet* 374, 2006–2015.

McGranahan, G., Balk, D. & Anderson, B. (2007). The rising tide: assessing the risks of climate change and human settlements in low elevation coastal zones. *Environment and Urbanization* 19, 17–37.

McLaughlin, K., Fairbank, J., Gruber, M. *et al.* (2009). Serious emotional disturbance among youths exposed to Hurricane Katrina 2 years postdisaster. *Journal of the American Academy of Child and Adolescent Psychiatry* 48, 1069–1078.

McMichael, A. (2009). *Climate Change and Human Health. Commonwealth Health Ministers' Update 2009*. Woodbridge, UK: Pro-Brook Publishing.

McMichael, A., Butler, C. & Weaver, H. (2008). *Climate Change and AIDS: a Joint Working Paper*. Nairobi: UNEP & UNAIDS.

Messner, D., Maxwell, S., Nuscheler, F. & Siegle, J. (2005). *Governance Reform of the Bretton Woods Institutions and the UN Development System. Dialogue on Globalization*. Berlin: Friedrich-Ebert-Stiftung.

Myers, N. & Kent, J. (2003). New consumers: the influence of affluence on the environment. *Proceedings of the National Academy of Sciences USA* 100, 4963–4968.

Patz, J. A., Gibbs, H. K., Foley, J. A., Rogers, J. V. & Smith, K. R. (2007). Climate change and global health: quantifying a growing ethical crisis. *EcoHealth* 4, 397–405.

Raupach, M., Marland, G., Ciais, P. *et al.* (2007). Global and regional drivers of accelerating CO_2 emissions. *Proceedings of the National Academy of Sciences USA* 104, 10288–93.

Rockstrom, J., Steffen, W., Noone, K. *et al.* (2009). A safe operating space for humanity. *Nature* 461, 472–475.

Scharlemann, J. & Laurance, W. (2008). How green are biofuels? *Science* 319, 43–44.

Shaffer, E., Waitzkin, H., Brenner, J. & Jasso-Aguilar, R. (2005). Global trade and public health. *American Journal of Public Health* 95, 23–34.

Smith, K. (2008). Mitigating, adapting, and suffering: how much of each? [Commentary]. *Annual Review of Public Health* 29.

Smith, P., Martino, D., Cai, Z. *et al.* (2007). Agriculture. In B. Metz, O. R. Davidson, P. R. Bosch, R. Dave & L. A. Meyer (Eds.), *Climate Change 2007: Mitigation. Contribution of Working Group III to the Fourth Assessment Report of the Intergovernmental Panel on Climate Change (IPCC)*. New York. NY: Cambridge University Press.

Stern, N. (2007). *The Economics of Climate Change: The Stern Review*. Cambridge: Cambridge University Press.

Strazdins, L., Friel, S., McMichael, A. J., Woldenberg-Butler, S. & Hanna, E. (in press) Climate change: an Australian intergenerational health equity analysis. *International Public Health Journal*.

United Nations Development Program (UNDP) (2007). *Human Development Report: Fighting Climate Change: Human Solidarity in a Divided World*. New York, NY: United Nations Development Program.

United Nations Environment Program (UNEP) (2007). *Sudan: Post-Conflict Environmental Assessment*. Nairobi: United Nations Environment Program.

United Nations Environment Program (UNEP) (2008). *Vital Water Graphics: An Overview of the State of the World's Fresh and Marine Waters*. (2nd edn.) Nairobi: United Nations Environment Program.

Woodcock, J., Edwards, P., Tonne, C. *et al.* (2009). Public health benefits of strategies to reduce greenhouse-gas emissions: urban land transport. *Lancet* 374, 1930–1943.

WorldFish Center (2007). *The Threat to Fisheries and Aquaculture from Climate Change*. Penang: WorldFish Center.

Chapter

18

Animals, the environment and global health

David Benatar

Introduction

When people talk about global health, and the ethics thereof, they almost invariably mean global *human* health. This is not because it is impossible to have more expansive notions of global health that include other species. Instead it is because most people who are concerned about global health, like most of those who are concerned about local health, are either not concerned at all, or are much less concerned, with the health of other species. Thus global health ethics, although expanding the reach of health ethics geographically, has not extended moral concern to other species within that global space.

This is unfortunate for at least two reasons. First, there is good reason to think that not only humans but also some other animals, the sentient ones, are worthy of moral consideration. That is to say, they are the sorts of beings to which we have moral duties. I shall not argue for this conclusion here, in part because it has been defended extensively elsewhere,[1] but also because overlooking animal welfare in the way that people generally do, poses a considerable threat to global human health. Thus, even those who fail to recognize the moral standing of non-human animals but do recognize the moral standing of humans should be more attentive to animal well-being on account of its instrumental value for human health.

There are those who think that not only non-human animals but also the natural environment itself – plants, as well as local ecosystems and the global aggregation of these – is worthy of moral consideration.[2] I do not share this view. However, one need not go as far as

attributing moral standing to the environment to think that we have duties to preserve it. Although we may have no (direct) duties *to* the environment, we could still have (indirect) duties *concerning* the environment. The latter duties could be grounded in the interests that sentient beings, either human or non-human or both, have in an environment that is conducive to their own health and general well-being. Global human (and animal) health can be affected by the state of the global environment.

There is now considerable awareness of the impact of the environment on human health and thus of the need to act in environmentally responsible ways. This is so even if most people do not do enough in response to this awareness. Matters are quite different, however, when it comes to the connection between animal and human interests. Indeed, arguably the most common view on this matter is that advancing or protecting human interests regularly requires overriding animal interests. Humans, it is thought, want to eat animals, need to experiment on them to advance medical science, and must cull them when they present a nuisance or a threat. In all these cases, animal and human interests are thought to conflict rather than coincide – a disputable view that I shall not evaluate here.

While people realize that humans pay a price for environmental damage, they often do not realize the human costs of much maltreatment of animals. I propose to rectify this by noting the ways in which human and animal interests coincide. I shall also make reference to the manner in which environmental degradation threatens global human health. Once these facts have been described, albeit briefly, I shall raise and respond to various arguments for the view that we nonetheless have no duty, based on human interests alone, to preserve the environment or to improve our treatment of animals.

---

[1] For example, Singer (1990), Reagan (1983) and DeGrazia (1996).

[2] On this view "global health" takes on an additional meaning. It refers also to the health of the globe, of planet earth.

Global Health and Global Health Ethics, ed. Solomon Benatar and Gillian Brock. Published by Cambridge University Press. © Cambridge University Press 2011.

Animal interests and global human health

Animal interests and human health intersect in a variety of ways, but not all of these are equally relevant for *global* human health. For example, vegetarian diets advance animal interests in not being killed. The humans who benefit most directly from vegetarian diets are the vegetarians themselves. They benefit from not consuming animal flesh. Although these advantages could aggregate to have an impact on global health, the contribution to global health is merely the sum of benefits to individuals.[3] This is unlike other factors impacting on human health, where the harms or benefits to some spill over into affecting others and which are thus more likely to impact on global health.

Consider infectious diseases, for example. They contribute significantly to the global burden of disease. By their nature, they are also the diseases that carry the greatest threat of suddenly spreading and thus, at least for a period, affecting and killing many more people than they usually do. For this reason their capacity to cause fear in addition to illness and death is considerable.

Some have suggested that "[a]ll human viral infections were initially zoonotic in origin" (Weber & Alcorn, 2000) although the precise animal source and route of transmission to humans is often a matter of some dispute.[4] Whether or not it is true that *all* human viral infections have animal origins, it certainly seems that *many* do. Consider some examples. Severe acute respiratory syndrome (SARS) arose in the live-animal (i.e. "wet") markets of China (Guan *et al.*, 2003).[5] Variant Creutzfeldt–Jakob disease probably arose from bovine spongiform encephalopathy (BSE) (Will *et al.*, 1996; Scott *et al.* 1999). And the source of the HIV,

which causes AIDS, is widely thought to be the simian immunodeficiency virus that is found in non-human primates (Gao *et al.*, 1999; Sharp *et al.*, 2001). The animal origins of avian and swine influenzas are reflected in their colloquial names. Although these latter two diseases have not as yet (that is, at the time of writing) killed as many people as was feared, the fears are not without some justification. Influenza epidemics arise periodically. Although not all are equally dangerous the fears of dangerous epidemics and pandemics are grounded both in historical experience of such lethality and in the knowledge that the ongoing process of mutation could yield more deadly strains. The relevant questions therefore, are not whether a new epidemic will arise, but rather *when* it will arise and *how bad* it will be (Osterholm, 2005).

Although some zoonoses are probably unavoidable, much human suffering resulting from zoonotic diseases could probably have been avoided had humans treated animals better. Consider, for example, the wet markets from which an influenza or SARS epidemic could be launched. In these markets live animals of diverse kinds are kept in large numbers and cruelly close quarters ready for sale and fresh slaughter. The concentration of animals, their overlapping sojourns in the markets (allowing disease to spread through vast numbers of animals) and their interactions with humans (facilitating human infection) make these markets ripe for zoonoses (Webster, 2004). Once an epidemic starts among animals, it can also spread to those animals reared in less cruel conditions.[6]

If humans did not eat wet market animals, there would be fewer of them (because fewer would be bred), the animals would not suffer from being housed in close quarters and they would not be slaughtered. Consequently, the risk of zoonoses would be greatly diminished. In the case of variant Creutzfeld–Jakob disease, humans would not have become infected had some humans not killed and eaten cows infected with BSE. Moreover, BSE would not spread among cattle if humans did not process offal, including neural matter from BSE-infected cattle, to produce feed for other cattle, a practice that was prompted by the volume of cattle that humans eat. If the plausible hypothesis that HIV resulted

---

[3] To clarify, vegetarianism does have *indirect* global health benefits, to which I shall turn soon. For now I am only showing that not all human benefits from vegetarianism impact as markedly on *global* health.

[4] This sentence is from David Benatar "The Chickens Come Home to Roost," *American Journal of Public Health*, Vol. 97, No. 9, pp. 1545–6, 2007. Reprinted, with permission of the copyright holder, the American Public Health Association.

[5] This sentence and the next two are from David Benatar "The Chickens Come Home to Roost," *American Journal of Public Health*, Vol. 97, No. 9, pp. 1545–6, 2007. Reprinted, with permission of the copyright holder, the American Public Health Association.

[6] This paragraph and the next are from David Benatar "The Chickens Come Home to Roost," *American Journal of Public Health*, Vol. 97, No. 9, pp. 1545–6, 2007. Reprinted, with permission of the copyright holder, the American Public Health Association.

from simian immunodeficiency virus is indeed true, then the most likely causal route of transmission was through infected simian blood during the butchering of these animals. The butchering itself was most likely for the purposes of providing non-human primate meat ("bushmeat") for human consumption, a practice that continues today.

Now it might be suggested that there is no use closing the barn door once the virus has bolted across the species barrier to humans. That, however, is a myopic view. It sees only the damage that has already been done and ignores the likelihood that unless we close the door on treating animals in the ways they have been treated in the past, new diseases (or new strains of diseases) will still emerge.

Nor are the relevant diseases only viral or prion diseases. Millions of pounds of antibiotics are added to animal feed in so-called "factory farms." The antibiotics have a dual purpose – to prevent the spread of bacterial disease between animals in intensive confinement and also to promote growth (Boyd, 2001, p. 647). This volume of antibiotic use would be unnecessary if animals were not treated as commodities to be fattened as quickly as possible and to be produced in the greatest possible number. The maltreatment necessitates the use of antibiotics, but the widespread use of antibiotics in turn poses a longer-term threat to humans because it can be expected to breed resistant strains of the organisms currently targeted by the antibiotics (Boyd, 2001, p. 650).

The environment and global human health

The impact, both actual and potential, of the environment on global human health is much more widely recognized than is the connection between animal welfare and human health. Nevertheless, the main themes are worthy of mention.

Whereas for most of human history, environmental degradation had only local effects, today things are very different. Many of the effects of environmental damage are now global. There are two broad interrelated reasons for the greater impact humans are having on the environment. First, there are many more humans than there used to be. For most of human history there were no more than a few tens of thousands of humans, and for long periods considerably fewer than this. However, the human population began to increase exponentially just a few hundred

years ago. There were about half a billion humans by the middle of the seventeenth century. This increased to 1 billion by 1804, 2 billion by 1927, 3 billion by 1960, 4 billion by 1974, 5 billion by 1987 and 6 billion by 1999 (McMichael, 2001, p. 188). At the time of writing there are in excess of 6.8 billion (and the number continues to grow).

The second reason why humans are having a much greater impact on the environment now than they did for much of their history is that the per capita consumption of the earth's resources has also burgeoned, attributable in large part to technological developments since the industrial revolution. Non-renewable resources (such as fossil fuels) and slowly renewable resources (such as groundwater, fertile soil and forestation) are being depleted. Current levels of usage are thus not sustainable. Moreover, it is not merely that these resources are being depleted but that their use, particularly at massively increased rates, has effects on the environment. For example, burning fossil fuels increases atmospheric levels of carbon dioxide, one of the major "greenhouse gases" responsible for global warming. The increase in carbon dioxide is exacerbated by the depletion of forests (Houghton et al., 1990, p. xv) because plants remove carbon dioxide from the atmosphere. Concentrations of another greenhouse gas, methane, have also increased significantly. Among the causes of this are biomass burning, coal mining and massive increases in the number of cattle being reared for human use (Houghton et al., 1990, p. xv). Chlorofluorocarbons, which were only invented in the 1930s but which have been widely used since then, are destructive of the ozone layer and thereby another major contributor to global warming (Houghton et al., 1990, p. xv).

Global warming can be expected to have further environmental effects. For example, sea levels would rise as polar ice melts (Houghton et al., 1990, p. 275). This would have devastating effects for low-lying islands and coastal areas (McMichael, 2001, pp. 305–306) and the large proportion of humanity living there. It can also be expected to affect weather patterns and food production, both of which would impact on health. Pathogens that thrive in warmer temperatures could cause outbreaks and the geographical spread of various infectious diseases (McMichael, 2001, pp. 300–303).

Global warming is not the only environmental change likely to impact on global health. Deforestation, in addition to contributing to global warming, also leads to increased flooding. Ozone depletion, while contributing to global warming, also threatens higher levels of skin cancer, adverse effects on vision and possibly also on the immune system (McMichael, 1993, pp. 183–194). Irresponsible use of land can lead to desertification, with a resultant impact on food production and access to potable water.

The dislocation of people caused by rising sea levels, combined with shortages of water and arable land, would likely result in conflicts over scarce resources (McMichael, 2001, p. 300).

Humans tend to think of themselves as a highly successful, adaptable species but they often forget that adaptability is *to an environment* and thus is heavily constrained by the environment. In other words, while humans can adapt to some changes in environment, they cannot adapt to most possible changes. Humans can currently survive in only a very small part of one universe, and it is only relatively recently in the history of our small planet that conditions became conducive to the emergence of humans.[7] Given both how recent the human species is and how many millions of other species have become extinct, any evidence of the resilience of our species is extremely limited.[8]

Responding to arguments that humans have no duty to treat animals and the environment better

So far I have shown that some maltreatment of animals and the environment can impact adversely on global human health. Accordingly, even those who are not concerned about animals or the environment have anthropocentric reasons to avoid the relevant maltreatment. Those who would prefer not to alter their treatment of animals and the environment may nonetheless want to resist the conclusion that we have a duty to make these changes. Sometimes they do this by denying the factual claims I have made. They deny, for example, that humans are contributing to global

warming or otherwise damaging the environment in ways that will cause human suffering. This is not the place and I am not the person to evaluate that challenge. The overwhelming majority of the relevant scientific community accepts the factual claims I have made and thus, while I cannot exclude the possibility that the majority of relevant scientists are mistaken, the dominant scientific view is not an unreasonable starting point. On the assumption that the factual claims are true, I shall, in the following sections, consider and reject three philosophical arguments for the view that humans have no duty to change the way they treat animals and the environment.

The argument from insignificant difference

One commonly advanced argument is that any individual's actions make no noticeable contribution to the unfortunate effects described. For example, even if rearing many animals in cramped conditions makes the emergence of new zoonotic diseases more likely, no individual's purchase of meat makes a discernible difference to the likelihood of the unfortunate outcome.[9] Similarly, even if humans are collectively causing global warming, any individual's actions make no significant contribution to that trend. Thus many are inclined to assume that they are not harming anybody in purchasing their meat or driving their petrol-guzzling cars.

Derek Parfit (1984, p. 75ff) has described this sort of argument as a "mistake of moral mathematics." Others too have noted that there is a difference between making an imperceptible difference to an outcome and making no difference at all.[10] If each person contributing to a harmful outcome is said to inflict *no* harm then the sum of harmless actions should also be zero harm. But it is clearly false that the sum of individual actions is not harmful. Jonathan Glover (1975, p. 174) recommends what he calls the "Principle of Divisibility" – "that the harm done in such cases should be assessed as a fraction of a discriminable unit, rather than as zero." He provides an engaging and helpful example to illustrate the problem that results from rejecting the principle of divisibility:

> Suppose a village contains 100 unarmed tribesmen eating their lunch. 100 hungry armed bandits descend on the village and each bandit at gunpoint takes one tribesman's lunch and eats it. The

---

[7] A. J. McMichael (1993, p. 1) notes that "*Homo sapiens* has existed for less than one ten-thousandth of Earth's lifespan – and, indeed, for less than one-thousandth of the time since animal life ventured from the oceans onto the dry land."

[8] Unlike most, I do not find the prospect of human extinction regrettable in itself (see Benatar, 2006). However, there are better and worse ways for humans to become extinct, and the suffering of masses of people inhabiting an increasingly inhospitable environment is among the worse ways.

[9] This sort of argument, although in a version discussing animal rather than human interests, is advanced by Shafer-Landau (1994).

[10] See, for example, Glover (1975).

bandits then go off, each one having done a discriminable amount of harm to a single tribesman. Next week, the bandits are tempted to do the same thing again, but are troubled by new-found doubts about the morality of such a raid. Their doubts are put to rest by one of their number who does not believe in the principle of divisibility. They then raid the village, tie up the tribesmen, and look at their lunch. As expected, each bowl of food contains 100 baked beans. The pleasure derived from one baked bean is below the discriminable threshold. Instead of each bandit eating a single plateful as last week, each takes one bean from each plate. They leave after eating all the beans, pleased to have done no harm ... (Glover, 1975, pp. 174–175)

Rejecting the principle of divisibility entails that it makes a moral difference whether each bandit takes one plate of food from one tribesman or whether each takes one bean from each tribesman. However, because there is actually no moral difference between these, we should accept rather than reject the principle of divisibility.

The principle of divisibility has clear application to the sorts of harms I have described. The individual consumer's contribution to the harms humans will likely suffer as a result of environmental damage and maltreatment of animals may be indiscernible, but they are not therefore either zero or morally not worth considering.

The argument from insignificant difference, which I have now rejected, should not be confused with an overlapping, but distinct argument: the egoistic argument that I could lack a *self*-interested reason to desist from actions that aggregated with similar actions of others, will cause us all harm. This is the so-called "tragedy of the commons." Every individual has a self-interested reason to consume as much as possible of a common resource, even though everybody's doing likewise will deplete the resource, making everybody worse off in the long run. This is because everybody can reason as follows: "If I desist from consuming, I lose out whether or not others are partaking. If they *are* partaking, I lose the advantage of joining them before the resource is depleted; and if others are *not* partaking, I can benefit without the resource being depleted."

The egoistic argument just sketched can acknowledge that my actions aggregated with similar actions of others will cause us all harm, but it can deny that I have a self-interested reason to desist. By contrast, the argument from insignificant difference can acknowledge that I should consider the interests of others but it denies that the interests of others are negatively affected by the specified actions of an individual.

However, the two arguments do overlap: in both cases the difference the individual makes to bringing about the tragic outcome is too small to be noticeable. This overlap is instructive because we can apply to the argument from insignificant difference a solution that is regularly applied to the tragedy of the commons. This solution, which involves a shift in focus from the individual to the aggregation of individuals, may appeal even to those who were not persuaded by my earlier response to the argument from insignificant difference.

The tragedy of the commons can be avoided by establishing an authority over the commons – an authority that regulates its use and, by penalizing violators, provides a self-interested reason to individuals to comply with the regulations that promote the common good. Similarly, a shift in focus, from individual action to public policy provides a second solution to the argument from insignificant difference. Good public policy will prohibit the *kinds* of actions (as distinct from individual actions) that cause harm. The makers of public policy are not interested in your action independently of the actions of everybody else. They are interested in the aggregated actions of individuals. It is quite clear that the aggregation of certain individual actions causes harm. There is thus good reason to adopt policies that protect global health.

Two kinds of "discounting" argument

I have described a number of ways in which maltreatment of animals and damage to the environment can adversely affect global human health. Some people who think that we have no duty to prevent those adverse affects do so because these effects are not immediate but rather will be felt only in the future. In this section and the next I consider arguments of this kind.

First, in this section, I consider two kinds of "discounting" argument – a radical one and a more moderate one. The radical argument concludes that we need not consider the interests of future people at all. The moderate argument concludes that the interests of future people, although worthy of moral consideration, should not weigh as heavily as the interests of present people. Thus, while the radical version of the discounting argument "discounts" in the sense of "does not count at all," the more moderate argument "discounts" in the sense of "counts less."

Radical discounting

Consider, first, the radical discounting argument. It denies that we have *any* duties to some humans.

According to this view, morality (or justice) should be understood in terms of reciprocity. Morality, on this view, is a contract between parties who undertake to bear the costs of the contract in exchange for the more substantial benefits that the contract yields. On this view, morality is grounded in rational self-interest: You agree not to stab my back and I agree not to stab yours.

One of the implications of such a view is that we have no duties, even no negative duties, to future people.[11] We do nothing wrong if we harm them. This is because there can be no reciprocity with future people. First, we cannot enter into agreements with them. When we exist they do not, and when they exist, we do not. Second, while we can affect their lives, they can do nothing to us.[12] Thus, we would have no self-interested reason to enter into an agreement with them even if we could. This fact is captured in the famous quip "Why should I care about posterity? What has posterity ever done for me?" This view is different from the one embodied in another famous (or, more accurately, infamous) quotation, the imagery of which is particularly apt in our context: "*Après moi, le deluge.*"[13] This latter view expresses an indifference to the interests of future people, whereas the "morality as reciprocity" view goes further and claims that this indifference is morally acceptable.

The reciprocity view of morality is deeply flawed. Not only does it exclude future people from moral consideration, it also excludes some currently existing people. Most obviously it excludes those who, throughout their lives, are sufficiently severely disabled that we either cannot enter into an agreement with them or have no self-interested reason to do so.

This is a difficult conclusion to swallow, and there seems to be good reason not to swallow it. The reciprocity view seems to misunderstand fundamentally what morality is about. Although we have a duty to do what we have agreed to do, it is far from clear that the only duties we have are those we have agreed to.

Moreover, it seems that part of the point of morality is to ensure that we give consideration to people irrespective of their ability to do things for or to us. This is not, as Allen Buchanan (1990, p. 233) says, "mere prejudice or irrational benevolent impulse." Instead it is "a stable, theoretically embedded practical belief" (Buchanan, 1990, p. 233).[14] If we reject this view, we are committed to thinking, among other things, that there is nothing wrong with torturing, for one's own pleasure, a severely disabled person with whom one has no self-interested reason to enter into an agreement.

Moderate discounting

There is a more moderate and arguably more common discounting argument. It does not treat the interests of future people as intrinsically unimportant. Instead it claims that the further in the future costs are expected the less weight they should have in decisions about what we should do. This is the Social Discount view, common in economics. The precise *rate* per annum at which future costs should be discounted is a matter of dispute, but I shall attempt to bypass that specific question and shall instead ask whether future costs should be discounted at all.

Various reasons might be offered for prioritizing current people over future ones.[15] The first and worst reason is that current people exist earlier. There is nothing to recommend this view. The time at which one exists should not, in and of itself, determine how much one's basic[16] interests count. An analogy between geographically and temporally distant people is apt. Although it might be psychologically easier to harm somebody who is far away than somebody who is close by, it is not morally less bad. People's important interests do not count less merely because those people are geographically distant. Nor do they count less merely because they are temporally distant. Consider Joel Feinberg's helpful example of a person who hides a bomb in a kindergarten, setting it to explode six years later, at which time it kills or maims many five-year olds (Feinberg, 1984, p. 97). It is hard to see how this person's act is any less bad than if he[17] had

---

[11] Some people, for reasons that will be implicit in what follows, might wish to restrict this claim to those future people whose lives do not overlap (or do not overlap significantly) with ours.

[12] I leave aside here the things they could do to our remains or the memories or records of us.

[13] "After me, the flood." This is usually attributed to Louis XV, but that attribution may be apocryphal.

[14] These issues are discussed in much more detail in this article.

[15] Simon Caney discusses these issues in more detail than I am able to here. See Caney (2009).

[16] I add this adjective because Simon Caney is correct that one might draw a distinction between more and less important interests with regard to discounting. See Caney (2009, p. 167).

[17] For an argument why using the male pronoun is not sexist, please see Benatar (2005).

set the bomb to explode five minutes after he had left the building.[18]

The problem with the first reason for discounting the interests of future people is that it is arbitrary. The mere fact that people exist later is irrelevant. Other reasons for discounting the interests of future people, therefore, will need to be non-arbitrary. They will need to explain *why* later costs should be counted less. The most common such reason is that a cost should be discounted to the extent that it is less than certain. There can be various reasons to be unsure that a cost will materialize, but one of them is that if it will occur at all, it will only occur later. All things being equal, the later something is projected to occur, the less sure we can be that it will occur. This is because there are so many possible intervening variables that could mitigate or eliminate the outcome. For example, a cost that is projected for the distant future might well never be paid because all life will have become extinct for a reason quite independent of the action that generates the projected cost. Thus, if dangerous increases in global temperature were projected to occur only in a million years time, those concerned about human health should worry less, because the chances of humans having become extinct for other reasons by that time are much higher than the chances of humans becoming extinct by next year. Temporal discounting is thus but one kind of discounting for diminished probability. It is not futurity per se, but the lower probability that explains the discounting.

While this explanation has a certain plausibility to it, it is an unconvincing justification for denying that the current generation has a duty to change the way it treats animals and the environment. This is because at least some of the quite serious consequences of environmental damage for global human health are projected (with degrees of probability ranging from "virtually certain" to "likely") to occur in the very foreseeable future (later in the twenty-first century) (Pachauri & Resinger, 2007, pp. 11–13). As far as I know, similar risk assessments resulting from maltreatment of animals have not been conducted.[19] However, given the historic

frequency of epidemics and pandemics of zoonotic infectious diseases, we have strong inductive reason to think that the next one is not so far off as to be significantly discountable.

Thus, even if social discounting is appropriate, the rate at which we can discount at least some of the serious costs is so minimal as to be practically irrelevant. This is particularly the case because these later costs may be averted without incurring serious costs now. Consuming less need not entail a lower quality of life for current people, or at least for the more affluent among them, who are also the biggest consumers per capita. Shifting to alternative, renewal energy sources, for example, would mean that we could use as much energy without consuming non-renewal resources and polluting the environment. Eating less meat need not lower quality of life. Indeed, it could even raise it by securing the individual health benefits that come from a diet with less meat.

There is a third kind of reason that might be advanced for discounting future costs – one that is compatible with (but which does not require) thinking that later people *will* bear the costs. This kind of reason suggests, following some or other preferred principle of distributive justice, that it would be fairer for future generations to bear the cost.[20] While it is impossible to consider all possible distributive principles that could plausibly justify discounting future costs, any such principles would have to assume that later people were better able to bear the costs, perhaps because they would be wealthier or because they would have the technical capacity to reverse or adapt to the environmental damage.

But even such lines of argument seem doomed. First, this discounting rationale may conflict with the previous one – discounting on the basis of uncertainty. After all, we cannot be sure that future generations will be richer than ours. Indeed, it could be that on account of what we do, they are poorer than we are. (Just think what a deadly pandemic, water scarcity and millions of refugees from rising sea levels and associated conflicts could do to the global economy.) Second,[21] even if future generations are wealthier than ours, it does not follow that all people within those generations will be.

---

18 To be fair, the social discount rate is often set very low – significantly less than 1% per annum – in which case defenders of it would be committed to thinking it is only marginally less bad to set the bomb to explode in 6 years' time. Those who think this is an adequate defense, need only adapt Professor Feinberg's example such that the bomb is set to explode in the significantly further future.

19 This is indicative of the point, made earlier, that there is much greater awareness of the connection between

the environment and global human health, than there is between animal and human well-being.

20 Simon Caney raises this possibility, in order to reject it. See Caney (2009, pp. 170–175).

21 The following responses are either drawn or adapted from Simon Caney (2009).

Because the poorest of future people are most likely to suffer the consequences of our actions, any principle based on ability to pay would assign the costs of our actions to us rather than them. Third, even if all future people were richer or technologically more advanced than we are, they might be insufficiently wealthier or technologically advanced to warrant discounting. The costs may increase at a greater rate than the wealth and technical capacity. It may thus be sufficiently cheaper and easier, all things considered, to prevent the problems than to fix them later.

A policy of prevention has the added advantage of avoiding those harms that will creep up on humans, perhaps springing suddenly, and will thus be felt before they are prevented or mitigated. A zoonotic pandemic is just such a possibility. People keep engaging in the risky behavior. Once the lethal pandemic arrives it will be too late to prevent many deaths. Damage control will be the only option. Similarly, scientists now fear various climate change "tipping points." These are possible major changes that are irreversible (within human rather than cosmic time frames). They could cause quite considerable human suffering that may be immune to financial and even technical solutions. In other words, a policy of prevention could avoid a situation in which a problem arises that cannot be fixed.

The "non-identity" argument

The discounting arguments, I noted earlier, take it to be relevant that the effects on humans of our damage to the environment and of our maltreatment of animals will be felt in the future. The next argument does the same, but in a different way. Instead of arguing that future people should count less or not at all, it allows that future people *could* count equally. However, it questions whether future people really are harmed by our current actions. This might sound to some like an empirical argument, one that denies that our current actions will lead to epidemics or will damage the environment in the way most scientists think. However, the argument at hand is instead a philosophical one, embodying metaphysical, conceptual and ethical features.

The metaphysical component pertains to "personal identity in different possible histories of the world" (Parfit, 1984, p. 351) or, in other words, to the necessary conditions for a particular person's coming into existence. Each one of us emerged from a combination of particular sex cells (a particular ovum and a particular

spermatozoon).[22] Thus, for example, had a different spermatozoon (whether of the same man or a different one) fertilized the ovum from which one developed, one would not have come into existence. Somebody else would have existed instead.

Derek Parfit (1984) has famously argued that when we are choosing between a policy of conservation and a policy of depletion, the identity of which people will exist in the future will likely be affected.[23] This, he thinks, is because following such different policies will affect which people meet and procreate, or at least when they will procreate. Because the identity of future people is contingent upon the conjunction of two specific gametes, choosing between two very different policies could readily affect who comes into existence.

Consider, next, the conceptual component of the argument. Here "harm" is understood as "making somebody worse off than he or she would otherwise have been." For somebody to be "worse off" in some state, it is then suggested, one must be able to compare that state to the alternative state in which he would have been. However, if that person would *not otherwise have been*, one cannot compare the state in which he exists with the alternative.

The problem, then, is that following a policy of depletion instead of a policy of conservation might harm nobody. Nobody who exists at some later time is worse off than they would otherwise have been, because if the alternative policy of conservation had been adopted then different people would have existed. Although the quality of life of those people who exist as a result of a policy of depletion will be worse than the quality of life of those people who would exist as a result of a policy of conservation, it will not be worse than the quality of *their own* lives would have been.

Consider next the ethical component of the argument I am now considering. If the foregoing is correct then we cannot morally require conservation and prohibit depletion on the grounds that the latter *harms* future generations. This poses a problem for those ethical approaches – so-called "person-affecting" approaches – that seek to evaluate actions on the basis of whether they affect people.

Thus, it is said, if we are to claim that conservation is preferable to depletion, we must instead appeal to

---

22 A similar story could be told, *mutatis mutandis*, for clones.
23 In the following paragraphs, I outline the bare bones of his argument.

an alternative moral framework, often known as an "impersonal" approach. Impersonal approaches are not concerned with whether an action makes people worse off. Instead they are concerned with whether one outcome (impersonally considered) is better than the alternative, even if it is not better *for* anybody. Impersonal views can say why we should opt for conservation rather than depletion: the outcome of the former will be better than the outcome of the latter.

Although impersonal views can explain why we should opt for conservation over depletion, such views lead to repugnant and absurd conclusions that call into question whether an impersonal approach is a suitable refuge for those wishing to explain the wrongfulness of depletion policies or practices. In brief, the problems include the following.

Impersonal views that are interested in producing the greatest *total* good must allow, when choosing between two possible outcomes, that an outcome in which the people have a lower quality of life is preferable if there are sufficient additional people that the total happiness is greater than in the alternative outcome. This means that these impersonal total views must prefer a world in which there are billions of people leading lives that are barely worth living to a world in which there are only a hundred thousand people with very good quality of life, as long as there is more happiness in total in the more populous world. Derek Parfit (1984, pp. 381–390) rightly calls this conclusion repugnant.

The more populous world just described might contain more happiness in total than the more sparsely inhabited one, but it nonetheless contains less happiness *on average* – that is the total good divided by the number of people. This might lead some impersonal theorists to seek the outcome with the greatest amount of good on average (rather than in total). But this too is problematic. Consider the following: You are contemplating whether to have a child. On the impersonal average view, you are permitted to have the child if its existence would raise the average quality of life of all people. This means, to use Derek Parfit's memorable example, that the quality of life of the ancient Egyptians can be relevant to whether or not you may have a child. Yet it seems clear that "research in Egyptology cannot be relevant to our decisions whether to have children" (Parfit, 1984, p. 420).

If person-affecting views as well as impersonal ones are problematic, then it is unclear what the grounds are for saying that we should avoid those actions that will lead future people to suffer. This is clearly a problem, even if it is not clear how the problem can be solved.

Various solutions have been proposed, although it is unsurprising that they have proved contentious. If we focus on the person-affecting approach, one could deny that all changes to our behavior would affect the identities of future people. While abstaining from driving might lead to one's meeting and mating with somebody closer to home and thereby affecting the identity of future people, a change from a vehicle that consumes lots of petrol to a more fuel-efficient one or, in time, to a car powered exclusively by renewable energy sources, need not have that effect. Nor is it clear why the choice between rearing animals intensively or not, should affect the identity of (many) future people.

Even if we assume that all such changes would alter the identity of future people, we might take issue with the notion that to harm somebody is to make that person worse off (Benatar, 2006, p. 21). And even if we think that harming somebody is to make him worse off, we might deny that this must involve a comparison between two states of the person (Feinberg, 1992).

However, given how contested these solutions are, I propose to show how we can *bypass* the problem even if we cannot *solve* it. In other words, let us assume, for the sake of argument that we cannot explain why it is wrong to engage in actions that cause later generations to suffer. I contend that we ought still to desist, for purely anthropocentric global health reasons, from damaging the environment and maltreating animals. This is because the evidence suggests that not changing our actions will later harm people who *already* exist. Some of the youngest people on the planet can expect to be around for up to another 80 or 90 years, a time span within which significant effects of our actions are likely to be felt (Pachauri & Reisinger, 2007, pp. 11–13). Our current actions threaten also older people and those disadvantaged young people whose life expectancy is not as long as more advantaged children. The intensive rearing of animals poses an ongoing threat of a deadly zoonotic pathogen emerging and becoming pandemic. The very young and the very old are especially vulnerable, but in the case of very virulent pathogens people in the prime of their lives are also at serious risk. It is thus simply a mistake to think that our actions will have an impact only on the quality of life of future humans – those who have not yet come into existence. Our actions will impact on them and even if these impacts will be more serious than earlier ones, sufficient damage could be done to existing people in order to warrant our desisting from the actions in question.

"The end [of this essay] is nigh"

There have been those, throughout human history, who have predicted "doom soon" – an impending catastrophe and sometimes even the "end of the world".[24] While such doomsayers are *sometimes* (or will someday be) correct, most of them make the mistake of telescoping the future of humanity or some component thereof. Telescopes make things look closer than they really are. A far more common error is either to look through the wrong side of the telescope, making the consequences of our actions look further away, or not looking at the future, but rather focusing myopically on the present. This is one reason why humans act the way they do. Just as smokers pay more attention to their immediate gratification than to the long-term costs to themselves, so do many people maltreat animals and contribute to the destruction of the environment for their immediate gratification without thinking of the longer-term consequences of their actions for themselves and others.

This shortsightedness and attention to more immediate gratification is, of course, but one of many reasons why humans are not doing more to curb their excesses. Another, related, problem is the mistaken perception or assumption of the invulnerability of the human species. This connects with the previous point in that the sense of invulnerability is fed by taking a more immediate view rather than a longer view. But it is also attributable to a widespread faith in the human capacity to adapt. There is a tendency to think that we can find a solution to any problem. Indeed, all too often, the focus is on cures rather than on prevention. This explains, for example, why so little attention has been given to preventing new pandemics by avoiding exploitative treatment of animals, and why so much attention has been given to responding to pandemic threats when they do occur. This attitude increases animal suffering. Having bred them in intensive conditions or otherwise mistreated them, thereby generating the pandemic threat, humans then cull animals in their millions when the threat begins to materialize, or they experiment on them in order to produce vaccines or cures. These reactive instead of proactive inclinations also harm humans. Trying to

nip a pandemic in the bud or, worse still, attempting to curb it once it is in full vigor, is generally less effective than preventing it upstream.

The world is laden with suffering – both human and animal. It will remain that way as long as there is sentient life on the planet. However, there are things we can do to influence just how much suffering there is. I have shown how current human practices damage the environment and bring suffering to animals in ways that can be expected also to cause human suffering. I have rejected various arguments that we need not desist from these practices. In doing so, I have suggested that instead of "killing two birds with one stone" we, in one go, could and should be sparing two kinds of being – human and non-human animals – from suffering.

References

Benatar, D. (2005). Sexist language: alternatives to the alternatives. *Public Affairs Quarterly* **19**, 1–9.

Benatar, D. (2006). *Better Never to Have Been: The Harm of Coming Into Existence*. Oxford: Oxford University Press.

Benatar, D. (2007). The chickens come home to roost. *American Journal of Public Health* **97**, 1545–1546.

Boyd, W. (2001). Making meat: science, technology and American poultry production. *Technology and Culture* **42**, 631–664.

Buchanan, A. (1990). Justice as reciprocity versus subject-centered justice. *Philosophy and Public Affairs* **19**, 227–252.

Caney, S. (2009). Climate change and the future: discounting for time, wealth and risk. *Journal of Social Philosophy* **40**, 163–186.

DeGrazia, D. (1996). *Taking Animals Seriously*. Cambridge: Cambridge University Press.

Feinberg, J. (1984). *Harm to Others*. New York, NY: Oxford University Press.

Feinberg, J. (1992). Wrongful life and the counterfactual element in harming. In *Freedom and Fulfilment* (pp. 3–36). Princeton, NJ: Princeton University Press.

Gao, F., Bailes, E., Robertson, D. L. *et al.* (1999). Origin of HIV-1 in the chimpanzee *Pan troglodytes troglodytes*. *Nature* **397**, 436–441.

Glover, J. (1975). It makes no difference whether or not I do it. *Proceedings of the Aristotelian Society, Supplementary Volume* **XLIX**, 171–190.

Guan, Y., Zheng, B. J., He, Y. Q. *et al.* (2003). Isolation and characterization of viruses related to the SARS coronavirus from animals in Southern China. *Science* **302**, 276–278.

Houghton, J. T., Jenkins, G. J. & Ephraums, J. J. (Eds.) (1990). *Climate Change: The IPCC Scientific Assessment*. Cambridge: Cambridge University Press.

---

[24] That is the *human* world, because the earth itself will survive the fulfillment of many such predictions.

McMichael, A. J. (1993). *Planetary Overload: Global Environmental Change and the Health of the Human Species.* Cambridge: Cambridge University Press.

McMichael, A. (2001). *Human Frontiers, Environments and Disease.* Cambridge: Cambridge University Press.

Osterholm, M. T. (2005). Preparing for the next pandemic. *New England Journal of Medicine* 352, 1839–1852.

Pachauri, R. K. & Reisinger, A. (Eds.) (2007). Summary for policymakers. In *Climate Change 2007: Synthesis Report. A Report of the Intergovernmental Panel on Climate Change* (pp. 1–22). Geneva: IPCC.

Parfit, D. (1984). *Reasons and Persons.* Oxford: Oxford University Press.

Reagan, T. (1983). *The Case for Animal Rights.* Berkeley, CA: University of California Press.

Scott, M. R., Will, R. G., Ironside, J. *et al.* (1999). Compelling transgenetic evidence for transmission of bovine spongiform encephalopathy prions to humans. *Proceedings of the National Academy of Sciences USA* 96, 15137–15142.

Shafer-Landau, R. (1994). Vegetarianism, causation and ethical theory. *Public Affairs Quarterly* 8, 85–100.

Sharp, P., Bailes, E., Chaudhuri, R. R. *et al.* (2001). The origins of acquired immune deficiency syndrome viruses: where and when? *Philosophical Transactions Royal Society London B* 356, 867–876.

Singer, P. (1990). *Animal Liberation.* (2nd edn.) New York, NY: New York Review of Books.

Weber, J. & Alcorn, K. (2000). Origins of HIV and the AIDS epidemic. *Medscape General Medicine* 2, 1–6.

Webster, R. G. (2004). Wet markets – a continuing source of severe acute respiratory syndrome and influenza. *Lancet* 365, 234–236.

Will, R. G., Ironside, J. W., Zeidler, M. *et al.* (1996). A new variant of Creutzfeldt-Jakob disease in the UK. *Lancet* 347, 921–925.

Chapter

19

The global crisis and global health

Stephen Gill and Isabella Bakker

The crisis consists precisely in the fact that the old is dying and the new cannot be born; in this interregnum a great variety of morbid symptoms appear.

(Gramsci, 1971, p. 276)

Introduction

We have previously argued that the present global financial and economic crisis is a clear manifestation of an unstable and contradictory world characterized by a disjunction between: (a) massive economic growth, unprecedented advances in science, technology/medical care; and (b) widening disparities in wealth and health within and between nations. Indeed, modern advances in health are increasingly driven by market forces, and therefore benefit about 20% of the world's population while 44% (about 3 billion people) live under miserable conditions on less than $2 per day, gaining little from conventional science and medicine (Benatar *et al.*, 2009).

To this we would now add:

(1) The present crisis is much more than a crisis of capitalist accumulation or a necessary self-correction aided by macroeconomic intervention and bailouts.

(2) The crisis also reflects contradictions of what we call "market civilization" – an individualistic, consumerist, privatized, energy-intensive and ecologically myopic pattern of lifestyle and culture which is currently dominant in world development (Gill, 1995).

We argue here therefore that to grasp the profound challenges to global health we need to look well beyond the economic and financial crisis to begin to appraise the massive problems the world is facing – an *organic crisis* is the term we use to describe this situation (Gill,

2008). Certainly orthodox economics (or political economy) is limited in making sense of the broader dimensions of such an organic crisis. Indeed, this is a question which is both historical and epistemological. To answer it we need to actually look at the historical evidence and operation of really existing capitalism through intellectual frameworks which are not narrow and abstract but that are broad ranging and realistic enough to be able to grasp the scale and depth of the crisis that we face.

Thus in this chapter we will use the concept of organic crisis to shed light on the links between global health, the financial crisis and what we refer to as new enclosures which undermine public provisioning and access to health care. Here, however, whilst we merely note that there is a complex relationship between the global financial crisis and effects on health, we should underline that there is mounting evidence that as the economic crisis continues to unfold, maintaining funding for global health services in developing countries that rely on foreign aid to provide necessary treatments will be under severe pressure. This compounds the desperate issues of malnutrition discussed at length in this essay.

Indeed, in our *Power, Production and Social Reproduction: Human In/Security in the Global Political Economy*, we hypothesized that we are in a period of global contradiction where on the one hand, we see the intensified power of capital through neo-liberal political and constitutional reforms and on the other hand, a weakening of the conditions for stable and sustainable social reproduction (Bakker & Gill, 2003). This contradiction goes well beyond the global financial and economic crisis of 2007–09.

The deep crisis of global capitalism which the world has experienced in 2007–09 has in fact greatly exacerbated this contradiction, as well as undermined some of the basic conditions of existence of the majority of people, thus endangering their human security and posing intense threats to global health, understood as the health of the global population as a whole.

What many consider to be the deepest crisis of accumulation for global capitalism since the 1930s is apparent through a number of concurrent crises that impact the lives of billions of people on the planet. As world leaders from the G20 countries have focused their activities and huge financial resources in responding to the global banking collapse, simultaneously enormous numbers of people have been pushed towards the brink of starvation, whilst at the same time badly needed resources to bolster public health initiatives and to deal with primary health-care issues were being cut. The public was told that the categorical imperative was restoring the capitalist financial system despite the fact that for several decades political leaders aligned with the Washington Consensus have insisted that public social and health expenditures needed to be curtailed as matters of fiscal prudence. At the same time, the Director-General of the International Labour Organization commented that the huge bail-outs amounted to "billions for the banks and pennies for the people."[1]

This is why we see the wider context for this situation – and the threats to global health that it poses – as part of a *global organic crisis*, one that is simultaneously an economic crisis, a social crisis and a crisis in the relationship between human beings and nature. It is also dramatized by a global food crisis involving over a billion people who are starving, and by threats to the collective future of the planet posed by global warming and ecological degradation. It is a crisis of the dominant development model and thus of what we call *market civilization* on a world scale. In short the global organic crisis is posing fundamental threats to the survival and well-being of billions of people who command very little in the form of economic resources and ownership, in contrast to the very small numbers of super-wealthy billionaire plutocrats who have gained control over the lion's share of global assets (Davies, 2006).[2]

Many of these issues and problems can be connected to the basic logic of the dominant pattern of accumulation in the global political economy – which we call disciplinary neo-liberalism – and in turn to the form of unequal and unjust social development which it fosters. This pattern of social development is also ecologically unsustainable. It is premised upon energy-intensive, consumerist and ecologically myopic patterns of economic activity – a market civilization which by definition is exclusive and can be only available to a minority of the population of the planet, but which is nevertheless serving to consume the vast bulk of global resources.

In this article we outline a number of key concepts and hypotheses to help make sense of some of the characteristics of the global organic crisis, and we link them to a reading of some of the patterns of social development and social distribution associated with what we call a *global enclosure movement*. We then analyze such developments in terms of their implications for global health, both now and in the future. We conclude with some theoretical and practical reflections on public finance, both at local and global levels, and make some proposals for a reorientation of taxation and expenditure policies so that they can better address fundamental human needs, provide for a healthier and more just global society and contribute towards its social and ecological sustainability, and help move us away from the market civilization model.

Key concepts and hypotheses

To advance our analysis, we will introduce here a number of foundational political economy concepts that correspond to some of the dominant historical structures (understood as the patterned or institutionalized forms of human agency) of globalized capitalism. We think these concepts help explain some of the transformations and contradictions to which we have just referred. Three of these key structures can be conceptualized as the *new constitutionalism*, *disciplinary neo-liberalism* and *exploitative social reproduction*. These concepts are intimately connected, on the one hand, to the projects of liberal reform that have increasingly shaped global society and economy over the past 30 years, and, and on the other, to the effects of those reforms on the structures of everyday life associated with communities and caring institutions.

---

[1] "Billions for the banks, pennies for the people" (Juan Somavia, ILO Director in *Financial Times* April 20, 2009).

[2] By the end of 2000, the top 1% of wealth holders owned 40% of total global assets – that is 37 million wealthy people. The bottom 50% of people (approx 3.3 billion) collectively owned less than 1% of total global wealth. Since 2001 the distribution of global wealth has become far more unequal.

Disciplinary neo-liberalism

Disciplinary neo-liberalism is the dominant discourse of political economy which has shaped our times. It is often associated with the so-called "Washington Consensus" of Wall Street, the IMF, World Bank and the US Treasury on economic policy. It refers to the liberal ideas, institutions, political forces and policies that are intended to deepen the power of capital and shape patterns of global economic and social development, partly by extending market values and economic and financial disciplines ever further into politics and society, and into the ways that human beings relate to nature and the basic issues of livelihood. Its wider context is a free enterprise economic system dominated globally by the giant firms that control most large industries (e.g. in food, pharmaceuticals, software). Disciplinary neo-liberalism is politically shaped by (and is intended to be commensurate with) the interests of big corporate capital (especially financial capital) and the state in not only the G8, especially the USA, but also in so-called emerging nations such as China and India. Disciplinary neo-liberalism, whether it is in the form of the Washington Consensus or World Bank structural adjustment and IMF stabilization, or in terms of strictures of the European Union urging the necessity of privatization and liberalization of trade and investment flows, has become central to defining programs of political and economic reform – as well as shaping responses to the economic crises of ever-increasing severity since the late 1970s, originating in the orthodox economic measures that were mandated to deal with the Third World Debt Crises of the 1980s. Indeed, one of the political characteristics of the present deep crisis is the way that most of the debate about the appropriate responses has been dominated by disciplinary neo-liberal forces – by contrast in the 1930s there were a variety of significant political alternatives to capitalism in the form of Soviet Communism and a variety of forms of Nazism and fascism. Opposing forces seem to be relatively weak after three decades of disciplinary neo-liberalism which has reshaped the terrain of political and economic contestability.

New constitutionalism

New constitutionalism is a political–juridical counterpart to disciplinary neo-liberalism, which, in the terminology of the World Bank, is intended to "lock in" liberalization of formerly closed economies and sectors so they are exposed to market disciplines – so that in effect market forces come to govern more and more areas of social, political and economic life, assuming that these are profitable. It does so by means of a variety of legal and constitutional mechanisms – e.g. entirely new liberal constitutions (as in the former communists states as they are transformed into capitalist states) or else by means of treaties which codify new rights and freedoms for investors and firms (such as those that created the World Trade Organization or the North American Free Trade Agreement). Other key new constitutional mechanisms are laws mandating balanced budgets and independent central banks. Such independence means in practice that central banks are independent of democratic pressures, so that they can concentrate on their mandates of fighting inflation. In practice the governance of central banks lies mainly in the hands of private financial interests who have a majority in the governing boards. Such "independence" was crucial in the way that central banks were able to commit gigantic amounts of public funds to bail out the global financial system in 2007–2009.

Thus whilst much of contemporary capitalist development can be very short-term in outlook, and concerned to speed up the turnover time of transactions so as to increase profits (e.g. in the global financial markets), a key characteristic of new constitutionalism is that it is longer-term, and intended to minimize uncertainty in investment calculations, and in the case of independent central banks, serve as a lender of last resort and as an ultimate guarantor of financial capitalism. New constitutionalism is manifested therefore in laws, rules and regulations that are very difficult to change, and that serve to legally reinforce, and to a degree to legitimate the rule of the political economy in ways that tend to favor private power holders such as giant corporations, and wealthy investors. A good example of new constitutionalism is the way that the jurisdiction over intellectual property rights at the global level has shifted to the World Trade Organization, and how such intellectual property rights are now principally considered as commodities that can be privately owned, and therefore bought, sold, licensed and protected over the long term by patents, copyrights and trademarks, etc. In the sphere of health this has very significant implications not only for access to affordable medicines and medical equipment but also for the already highly skewed processes of research and development in the provision of new medicines, a process that tends to focus upon cures and palliatives for the maladies of the richer parts of the world at the expense of those afflicting poorer people, especially those in developing countries.

Social reproduction

Social reproduction can be defined as the social processes, human relations and social institutions associated with the creation and maintenance of communities – and therefore upon which all production and exchange associated with the global political economy must ultimately rest.[3] Social reproduction involves not only state provisions associated with health and welfare and the socialization of risk (e.g. pensions, unemployment insurance, social safety nets, kinship networks), but also structures associated with the long-term reproduction of the socio-economic system such as education. These processes, institutions and ideas shape the way that individuals, families and communities view the social, political and indeed moral order. No economic system can sustain itself without an appropriate set of social, cultural as well as economic values. As we shall argue, these elements change across time and space, and under conditions of disciplinary neo-liberalism and new constitutionalism, they tend to be more privatized and premised upon the ideology of the "self-help society." This is why we refer to the structures of social reproduction associated with this pattern of development as *exploitative* since they involve greater levels of exploitation of both labor and nature.

Such concepts can be used to help generate a number of secondary hypotheses that connect to our central hypothesis of an emerging contradiction between the extended power of capital (and its protection by the state) and the possibility for attaining more progressive forms of social reproduction and increased human security for a majority of the world's population.

Thus one of our secondary hypotheses – which relates directly to health provisioning – is that the trend towards the re-privatization of the governance of social and caring institutions (and thus of more privatized medical and health systems) has gone with a tendency towards deterioration in health and health-care provisioning for a majority of people on the planet. This hypothesis is further connected to an increase in the range, scope and depth of socio-economic exploitation in global capitalism amid wider conditions of *primitive*

accumulation* – as well as increased exploitation of nature or the biosphere in ways that may not be ecologically or physically sustainable.

By primitive accumulation, we refer to a term originally advanced by Marx to explain a process by which large segments of the population are violently divorced from their traditional means of self-sufficiency, e.g. peasants who are forced off their land as it becomes privately owned and fenced in to create larger landholdings. As peasants are forced off the land, they become "free laborers" who have no choice but to sell their labor-power to the private owners of such assets (which are the basic means of production) in order to survive (food, which they may have previously produced for themselves, is now obtained in markets mediated by the ability to pay the "market price").

Moreover as we put it in our earlier work:

> Primitive accumulation is not only reflected in privatization of state assets, a trend that increased massively throughout the 1990s, but also in privatization of parts of the state form itself. There are at least two dimensions to this shift: (a) the privatization of previously socialized institutions associated with provisioning for social reproduction; (b) the alienation or enclosure of common social property which we see as part of a new global enclosure movement. Both of these changes tend to grant more power to capital, while simultaneously undermining socialized forms of collective provisioning and human security. (Bakker & Gill, 2003, p. 19)

Three perspectives on capitalism and the present crisis

Capitalism is, of course prone to crises of a recurring nature, and we can identify at least three perspectives on the nature of capitalism and on capitalist crises. Each has very different implications for the way in which it reads the effects of crises on social reproduction in general, and health in particular.

The first is that of the followers of Ayn Rand, F. A. von Hayek and Milton Friedman, which include Alan Greenspan who was, for many years, the Chairman of the US Federal Reserve System. We can characterize this perspective as that of the "pure" neo-liberals, often associated with the so-called Chicago School of Economics. They see capitalism as the most globally economically efficient system. Indeed they believe that if market forces are allowed full play, with governments simply supporting as opposed to restraining market forces, crises are short term and in effect self-correcting – as such markets should therefore be allowed to self-regulate. In this view market forces and

---

[3] Social reproduction has three components: (1) Biological reproduction of the human species; (2) Reproduction of the labor force; and (3) Reproduction of provisioning and caring needs.

families deliver all that is necessary for social reproduction. We might add that there has never been any system in history that has even vaguely approximated this Hayekian vision, since it would presuppose turning not only human beings and nature but also their cultural and social institutions into saleable commodities to be exchanged on impersonal markets.

A second perspective we might characterize as that of the "compensatory" neo-liberals, a perspective which includes most economists, particularly those of the Keynesian or post-Keynesian persuasions. They believe that, because of uncertainty, capitalist accumulation is unstable and cyclical crises are endemic and as such, they require macroeconomic planning and political intervention to allow for stabilization and the resumption of "balanced growth." It should be added here that over the past three decades a consensus has arisen amongst the most mainstream economists that the problem of crisis management had effectively been solved by modern macroeconomic policy, as well as financial regulation – it was largely assumed that crises could be contained, managed and mastered.

Third is a radical position associated with heterodox economists, particularly those on the left who see capitalism as a system of power riven by the contradiction between capital and labor. This contradiction is associated with crises of overproduction and underconsumption. Individual capitalist firms seek to lower workers' wages in order to maximize profits; however, general downward pressure on the real wages of workers ultimately will mean that they have insufficient income to continue to consume the goods and services capitalist firms produce (i.e. overproduction or underconsumption) so that a crisis ensues. Keynes believed that the shortfall in what he called effective or aggregate demand (i.e. underconsumption) could be dealt with by government macroeconomic policies, with governments expanding the money supply and increasing expenditures, so that in effect consumption is boosted and the oversupply of goods is absorbed. Marx believed by contrast, that ultimately such crises, rooted in the fundamental contradiction between labor and capital, would mark the death knell of capitalism – an eventuality we are yet to witness.

More fundamentally for considerations of health and ecology, the radical view of capitalism is that it does not involve the accumulation of goods for livelihood and social well-being, but accumulation of monetary values which in turn allows for control over society and the labor of others – in short the power of capital pursues profits and seeks to further its power over society, which allows it to extract social surplus, partly by enclosing the social commons. Where the radical perspective has been weak – and where the Keynesian perspective has been stronger – is in acknowledging the instabilities and deeply destructive crises associated with finance, and not simply with struggles between capital and labor reflected in crises of overproduction and underconsumption. The radical perspective has also been weak in making the links between power, production and social reproduction.

This is why in our earlier work we suggested that radical and feminist political economy should pay much greater attention not only to the links between global finance and production, but also to the structures of everyday life, including those of social reproduction. Indeed Gill pointed out in 1998 that the epicenter of a future massive global crisis of accumulation might be not in the indebted developing world but in the hyper-liberalized financial markets of the USA, markets governed by the largely self-regulating system of Wall Street banking with its close connections to Washington, DC. Moreover he argued that any such crisis would reverberate very rapidly throughout the globe since the Wall Street system was interconnected deeply with all other key financial centers throughout the world (Gill, 1997). Wall Street was also interconnected with offshore banking locations which have proliferated over the past several decades, allowing corporations and wealthy individuals to evade taxes and to pick and choose where to locate their profits and losses. Such forgone taxes could be used to fund better public goods and to improve on the institutions' provisions of social reproduction.

More to the point, a careful reading of the history of global finance since the late 1970s indicated its growing vulnerability to collapse due to very risky patterns of increased leverage (borrowing and lending out many multiples of a financial firm's capital base) coupled with an explosive growth in ill-understood financial derivatives and other complex financial products.[4] Both of these trends were the result of so-called "financial

---

[4] Banks had been previously required to maintain leverage levels of approximately 10:1 as a measure of prudence; however new regulations introduced in the Clinton Administration meant that banks were allowed to engage in massive leveraging that was previously prohibited (borrowing against capital base by 30:1 or greater, which of course was subsequently shown to be exceedingly risky).

innovation" and "securitization," or more accurately innovations by banks and other financial institutions involving new ways to make profits by repackaging financial assets and increasing their sales turnover.[5] At the same time there was growing complacency on the part of the relevant public institutions, with key banking figures such as Greenspan and his successor at the Federal Reserve, Ben Bernanke, and with international organizations such as the International Monetary Fund, arguing that the markets knew best, and they concluded that the brave new world of global finance was governed by very prudential policies and that risks has been spread throughout the system in a way that made it more resilient and structurally sound.

The crisis of 2007–2009 proved that this perspective was catastrophically wrong. Indeed, as Gill noted, one possible danger in a systemic sense was that these ill-understood and mathematically complex derivatives *were* ultimately based on the provision of real goods, services, resources and commodities, although often at many times removed from the point of production. This is precisely why the financial crisis interacted with what economists call the "real economy," and in particular the mortgage and housing market in the USA, to produce a real and ultimately global catastrophe (Gill, 1997).

Thus the most severe global economic crisis since the 1930s has produced a combination of gigantic public bailouts for private firms and a rapid decline in the conditions of existence for a majority of the world's population. Originating in 2007 in North America and parts of Europe with the collapse of the so-called sub-prime mortgage market, it has since extended to low- and middle-income countries. It continues to spread and is creating dire pressures on some countries that have already received large-scale emergency funding from the IMF while others continue to be tipped into recession (conventionally defined as successive quarters of negative growth in gross domestic product).

It now appears that the world is in a global economic downturn as large as the 1930s and in some respects is significantly worse in relative terms. From the vantage point of orthodox liberal economic analysis, world industrial production tracks closely the 1930s fall in output. Globally unemployment is rising very rapidly, and world stock markets and world trade have followed paths far below those observed in the Great Depression – despite a stock market rally in 2009 associated with the massive bailouts and stimulus packages (Eichengreen & O'Rourke, 2009).[6] More specifically the financial crisis has involved falling profits for many though not all firms (well-connected Wall Street firms such as Goldman Sachs and JP Morgan have greatly benefited from the crisis). It also meant frozen credit markets – at one point banks refused to lend to each other or to the majority of their borrowers. This meant a string of insolvencies that has threatened the global financial system as presently constituted. Governments responded with worldwide socialization of the losses of capital (e.g. bank losses of $4.1 trillion in total according to an IMF estimate as of April 21, 2009) but of course, not the losses of a majority of citizens – one of the defining traits of neo-liberal capitalism is that the losses of large corporations are socialized, whilst profits are privatized.

By contrast, in the USA since the early 1980s the real incomes of most workers have fallen despite longer hours and more intensive conditions of work (before this the American dream was real in so far as workers' incomes grew consistently after the Second World War). This rising rate of exploitation of labor meant that in order to maintain their standard of living and levels of consumption, American workers went ever deeper into debt. On the other hand, the very low rates of interest fostered by the US Federal Reserve System especially after 2000 under Alan Greenspan meant that borrowing appeared to be cheap, and at the same time it fueled a rapid growth in asset prices, and particularly in real estate including residential properties. American families borrowed equity against the value of their properties as prices rose, although their nominal debts began to rise.

However sooner or later something had to give – average Americans could not simply continue to sustain their consumption and to continue to consistently roll over their debts. Things started to go seriously

---

5 Many of the world's biggest players (and speculators) in the global financial markets are not only large banks but also pension funds and insurers, as well as large hedge funds who compete to increase their post-tax rate of return, to assure fund growth and attract more customers/savers.

6 Barry Eichengreen and Kevin H. O'Rourke, *A Tale of Two Depressions.* Online publication June 4, 2009. http://www.voxeu.org/index.php?q=node/3421. The degree to which this view became the conventional wisdom for orthodox economics is partly reflected in the fact that it shattered all Vox online readership records (30 000 views in two days, over 100 000 in a week, now fast approaching 350 000).

wrong when US house prices began to fall in 2006 which coincided with a collapse in the ability of US workers to continue with their debt-funded overconsumption (US savings ratios turned negative); increasing numbers of borrowers found it difficult or impossible to make their mortgage and credit card payments. This triggered huge losses for the banks who had borrowed at vast multiples of their capital base and this rendered them insolvent. Given the complex interbank lending practices and the centrality of certain key institutions in the financial system, the US financial system as a whole was threatened with collapse. The same is true of other key financial centers, notably London; however the European financial systems were also deeply distressed, as was that of Japan.

As can be seen from Figure 19.1, this elicited a massive response on the part of the governments of the biggest economies of the world, underlining our earlier remark that in the prevailing system of global priorities, rescuing capital comes first as a categorical imperative. Although it is very difficult to specify the aggregate size of the bailouts, according to the International Monetary Fund, these have amounted to at least $11 trillion since 2007, and according to some estimates, the total of EU + US + UK bailout pledges and fiscal stimulus measures amount to about $17 trillion, although of course a proportion of this is likely to be repaid. To put this into perspective, the latter sum is over 22 times larger than the total *planned* funds for the UN's Millennium Development Goals (much smaller sums have actually been delivered by the 176 governments that signed off to these goals); the MDGs seek to provide minimum basic health and education for billions of the world's very poorest people between now and 2020.

Recent evidence seems to be that financial crises produce far more significant declines in overall economic activity than those which are characterized by shortfalls in aggregate demand (crises of overproduction and underconsumption). Partly because of the very rapid growth of the financial sector since the 1970s, particularly in the so-called advanced economies in the capitalist world, recent financial crises seem to radically lower the levels of economic activity by very significant amounts – some estimates suggest as much as 10% of total output or gross domestic product (GDP). For example the *Financial Times* (FT) notes: "There is widespread agreement that the damage done in a recession associated with a financial crisis tends to be twice as severe as one that is not. More important is the finding that much of the loss of output in a severe recession

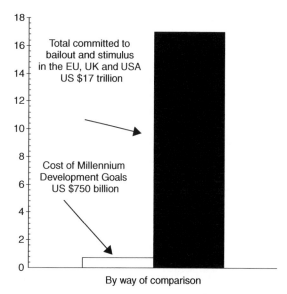

Figure 19.1 Financial bailouts 2008–09 compared with total Millennium Development Goal commitments.

is permanent and that the economy never gets back to its old trend line."[7] Indeed, the FT reports that the IMF now estimates that after a financially induced recession, output is about 10% below its previous trend in the medium term, which it defines as 7 years. There are wide variations to this period. Japan for instance has been stagnating since the Japanese financial and real estate bubble burst in the early 1990s. At one point real estate became so inflated that land values in Tokyo in the late 1980s were estimated to be worth more than those of the whole of the United States (US GDP is currently roughly four times that of Japan).

The FT's leading economist, Samuel Brittan, adds that countries currently experiencing the banking crisis now represent close to one half of real GDP for the advanced economies. He notes that, "This is equivalent to a combined GDP total of about $40 000 bn (€27 050 bn, £24 440 bn) per annum."[8] However, Brittan's estimate understates the scale of the problem – $40 trillion is about two-thirds of *world* total output of $60 trillion ($60 109 bn) at market exchange rates in 2008 according to the IMF. Nevertheless, a financially induced recession in economies totaling $40 trillion would lower global GDP by something in the region of $4 trillion. In 2008, Chinese GDP was $4.327 trillion. So if

---

[7] *Financial Times*, October 29, 2009.
[8] *Financial Times*, October 29, 2009.

one imagines a world without the total economic activity of over 1 billion Chinese, including all the goods produced, sold and exported from China to supply the consumer markets in North America and Western Europe, we can get some idea of the losses of output involved as a result of a massive financially induced global crisis of accumulation.[9]

According to the conventional view – that of the neo-liberal economic orthodoxy of the Washington Consensus, which the *Financial Times* and the International Monetary Fund in their different ways represent – the *opportunity costs* of a financial crisis, understood in terms of output lost or foregone – are much higher for financial crises than with those economic crises caused by overproduction/underconsumption or in Keynesian terminology caused by a lack of aggregate demand due to lack of purchasing power amongst consumers (most of whom are also workers). We might also note that the most vulnerable in this scenario are the unprotected, often non-unionized workers, who lose their jobs first.

However this view of the crisis and the response overlooks several very important things.

First of all, the conventional approach does not really question the qualitative aspects of the situation, and the real nature of the output measured by GDP figures – much of what is produced, including that in China, simply feeds patterns of consumerism and waste, as well as being linked to irrational use of non-renewable resources; indeed much of economic output may not be socially desirable or connected to the health of the population as a whole, or indeed to the sustainability of ecological structures that support life itself.

Second, opportunity costs need not simply be measured in terms of output foregone, but also in terms of the question of the alternative uses of public finance and public expenditure. The massive bailouts and stabilization measures could have involved social, health and educational outlays as well as global redistribution with a qualitative component (e.g. to provide healthier nutrition and basic medical care) which would have led

to a very different path of development to the one that is associated with these trend-lines. The trend-lines associated with the G8 bailouts are connected to restoring, albeit with some effort to use resources more efficiently, much of the very energy-intensive kind of consumerist growth associated with market civilization and the world market in food, which we discuss below.

Morbid Symptoms I: rising hunger and the global food crisis

Sufficient – just enough – nutritious food is a fundamental component of health. Lack of nutritious food has therefore very serious consequences for global health outcomes. Today, partly as a result of the economic and financial crisis, over 1 billion people are eating less, switching to cheaper and lower quality food or forgoing spending on health care and education, simply in order to eat. The longer-term consequences are ominous for human development. Poor nutrition is known to impair mental development, particularly for the young, and it weakens the immune system and the ability to ward off disease. Hunger involves not only class and race but also gender inequalities: 70% of those living in absolute poverty globally are women and more than 60% of those suffering malnutrition are women, and most of them live in the developing world.

Indeed, our world is one where perhaps 50% of the world's population suffers from malnutrition – however 25% of those who are malnourished are in fact overfed, overweight and obese; the other 25% – those just referred to – are underfed or starving. At the epicenter of market civilization, over two-thirds of Americans are overweight, mainly eating unhealthy processed foods that contain many chemicals, hormones and other additives, with their diets based on consumption of too much meat, sugar and salt. This phenomenon is not simply associated with wealthy countries like the USA and the UK; Mexico is second only to the USA in obesity rates and, perhaps not surprisingly, in per capita consumption of soft drinks. This overconsumption of unhealthy foods has been linked to all kinds of diseases and chronic conditions such as diabetes which exact their toll on hard-pressed public health systems (Albritton, 2009, pp. 106–107).

Malnutrition is exacerbated in situations of economic crisis. One reason is that wealthy donor governments tend to cut social expenditures and foreign aid to the poor countries, since these revenue lines do not necessarily have strong domestic political

---

[9] Sources: IMF *World Economic Outlook: Housing and the Business Cycle*. Washington DC: IMF April 2008. Table A1. Summary of World Output p. 241. Global GDP was $60 109 at market exchange rates; Chinese GDP was $4 327 448; http://www.imf.org/external/pubs/ft/weo/2008/01/pdf/tables.pdf. See also International Monetary Fund, *World Economic Outlook Database*, October 2009: Nominal GDP list of countries. Data for the year 2008.

constituencies supporting them. Indeed G8 budget cuts in 2009 included those for emergency food relief, Overseas Development Assistance and the Millennium Development Goals. All of these are intimately connected to questions of human security, global health and of basic humanity.

Thus in the midst of an unprecedented global food crisis which we discuss below, cuts to food aid have put many millions more people at risk of starvation. In 2008 the rich countries gave $5 billion to the UN World Food Program in an effort to avert a worsening of the food crisis; however by 2009 these sums were cut dramatically, so that global food aid reached its lowest level in 20 years, with all the major donors reducing their contributions. This was despite the fact that food prices, already at record levels in 2008, were in many parts of the world, even higher in 2009. As Oxfam's humanitarian policy adviser put it, the shortfall faced by the World Food Program of approximately $2 billion, "will translate into more child deaths, with more than 16 000 children already dying from hunger related causes everyday."[10]

As the *Financial Times* put it in an editorial:

Almost unnoticed behind the economic crisis, a combination of lower growth, rising unemployment and falling remittances together with persistently high food prices has pushed the number of chronically hungry above 1 bn for the first time.[11]

The current food crisis originated with sharp increases in the price of major food grain prices: maize increased in price by more than 50% of its average price in 2003 and 2006; rice prices are 100% higher. Such food price rises have been estimated by the UN as responsible for pushing more than 100 million people back into poverty.

The longer-term trend is even more alarming:

[From 1995] The number of chronically hungry in developing countries started to increase at a rate of almost four million per year. By 2001–2003, the total number of undernourished people worldwide had risen to 854 million and the latest figure is 1.02 billion. Today, *almost one person in six does not get enough food to be healthy and lead an active life, making hunger and malnutrition the number one risk to health worldwide* – greater than AIDS, malaria and tuberculosis combined.[12]

---

[10] John Vidal, "Cuts to food aid millions at risk of hunger and starvation," *Guardian Weekly* October 16, 2009, page 3. See also United Nations World Food Program, "Hungry Get Hungrier As Funding For Food Aid Stutters," www.wfp.org/stories/hungry-hungrier-funding-food-aid-stutters. September 16, 2009.

[11] *Financial Times*, April 6, 2009.

Reflecting the intensification of the global food crisis, world market prices surged further in 2007–08. Overall the UN Food and Agriculture Organization's global food price index rose from 80 in 2000 to 210 in 2008, before it dropped back to 140 in 2009: still almost double the price level of 2000. The disastrous consequences for the 2.8 billion people living on less than $2 a day therefore correlate with these rising world food prices, which have increased in real terms by about 75% since 2005. In other words, the world market has truly become the arbiter of a situation of mass global starvation.

Graphic information on recent price trends is contained in Figures 19.2 and 19.3, mainly from the UN Food and Agriculture Organization.

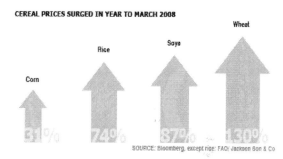

CEREAL PRICES SURGED IN YEAR TO MARCH 2008

SOURCE: Bloomberg, except rice: FAO/ Jackson Son & Co

Figure 19.2 World cereal prices 2007–08. The figure can be accessed at: http://news.bbc.co.uk/2/hi/7284196.stm

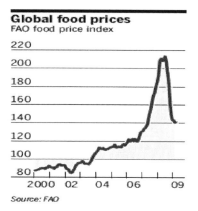

Figure 19.3 Global food prices 2000–09.

---

[12] United Nations World Food Program, "What is hunger?" www.wfp.org/hunger/what-is (Accessed November 14, 2009). Our emphasis added.

ENERGY AND FOOD PRICES, 1992-2008

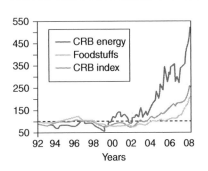

Years

US ETHANOL PRODUCTION 1995-2006
Liters (billions)

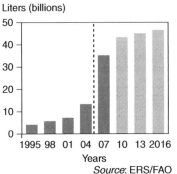

Years

Source: ERS/FAO

Figure 19.4 Energy, food and ethanol. Note: CRB energy is the index of energy prices compiled by the Commodity Research Bureau. The CRB index combines all commodities including energy and food. The figures show how the take off in energy prices at the turn of the twenty-first century preceded that in foodstuffs. The figure can be accessed at: http://news.bbc.co.uk/2/hi/7284196.stm

So what explains this "spike" in global food prices? The conventional explanation is that it has been caused by a "perfect storm" of long-term factors including the declining productivity of land and climate change, resulting in bad harvests in the USA and the EU as well as those caused by the long-term drought in Australia, a shift from grains for food to grains for biofuel production (see Figure 19.4 regarding US ethanol production), plus short-term factors such as hoarding of grains by consumers as well as big grain producers such as Argentina and the Ukraine; producer governments are concerned that riots would be provoked if they had insufficient supply to feed their own populations.

A deeper explanation is complex and it is beyond the scope of this essay to discuss it in any detail. However, in our view, the explanation would involve recent trends towards greater centralization of ownership and control, and greater enclosure of global food supplies by large corporations, and the influence on global food prices as a result of government and corporate strategies. Of particular importance in this latter regard are the global effects of the shift to biofuels production, which correlates with rises in energy prices over the past 7 years (see Figure 19.4). US ethanol production rose rapidly after 2001 and is projected to increase massively; by 2008 approximately 33% of all US corn production went to ethanol production.

In effect the structure of the current world market in food dates back to changes in US policies some 40 years ago and it relates to the changing ways in which developing countries have become integrated into the capitalist world market for food. Of course this was done forcibly into an imperial world market during the colonial era; after the Second World War however, linked to the ideology and practice of self-determination there was a trend in the developing world towards relative self-sufficiency in agriculture and food sovereignty. A

very important change took place in US strategy however in the 1970s – previously US policy mainly concerned the regulation (restriction) of supply. The new policy was its opposite – it gave subsidies to farmers for increasing yields to improve the US balance of trade. This had powerful consequences including rapid concentration of control, the undermining of agricultural systems in developing countries, and it was part of a general shift towards an oil- and pesticide-dependent food production system.[13] Food also became a geopolitical as well as an economic issue at that time, particularly since food prices rose rapidly as a result of massive Soviet grain purchases from the US – a process overseen by the US Department of Agriculture and huge agribusinesses such as Cargill. Since then the market has been dominated by a small number of corporations (oligopolies) – such as the large agricultural conglomerates, Cargill and Archer Daniels Midland. Nevertheless, until the turn of the twenty-first century this has largely meant an era of stable food prices.[14]

One reason for this was the growth in global production. Partly as a result of bad harvests and rising prices in the 1970s, agricultural producers in the developing world were encouraged to use new seed hybrids and other new technologies associated with

---

[13] The release of greenhouses gases from nitrogen-based fertilizer use is, according to Albritton (2009, p. 151), roughly 296 times more potent than carbon dioxide.

[14] The concentration of power in this market rests on a close and strategic relationship between the big agribusinesses and the US and EU governments. In most of the rest of the world, particularly in poor developing world nations, however, firms are much smaller and tend to be less subsidized – emerging large food exporters such as Brazil are partial exceptions to this rule. Thus there is oligopolistic domination of global food production.

the so-called "green revolution," and to gradually move towards a more export-oriented agriculture. These developments were further encouraged by capitalist global organizations such as the World Bank. The result was a shift towards cash crops and a general reorientation of agriculture towards the world market. This shift also included, as noted, more pesticide-intensive and other industrial methods to increase the turnover time of crop and livestock yields linked to sales for the world market.

Thus an era of cheaper food emerged with the result that at some point during the early 1990s the prevailing discourse concerning "food security" came to be redefined as access to food by relying on an "efficient" global market. This seemed to make sense with respect to grains, since abundant American production of heavily subsidized products flooded the world market, and thus prices were kept low. However since the global market was now dominated by American production, itself controlled by a small number of giant corporations, this had the side-effect of wiping out many small producers in not only the USA but also in the developing world, concentrating capital in agriculture, further undermining local self-sufficiency as well as promoting a general shift towards crop monocultures and larger farms. Production by independent and small farmers in both the USA and throughout the world became more integrated into the global corporate system, with crops often based on the use of so-called "terminator" seeds which are disease resistant and produce higher yields. However they need to be obtained on an annual basis from the seed companies (the corporations) since they cannot be used in future crops. The seeds therefore need to be repurchased annually; the seeds are the intellectual property of the corporations that own them, rather than the farmers who may actually grow the crops.

An example shows how this process of centralization, control and enclosure is also intimately connected to new constitutionalism. Mexico entered into the new constitutional North American Free Trade Agreement (NAFTA) in 1994 which guaranteed the right of American producers to sell their grain in Mexico, and vice versa. However since market prices in the USA were much lower than the cost of production not only in the USA but also in Mexico due to large US production subsidies, this had obvious consequences in terms of the competitiveness of Mexican production on the local market, production which, by contrast, was not subsidized. Indeed, once Mexico had signed NAFTA

it was legally obliged to continue with this arrangement, despite the fact that, since the Revolutionary Constitution of 1917, it had maintained its own constitutional protections for small farmers (*eijidos*) and their right to livelihood on the land. Mexico made at least 30 constitutional amendments in order to legally comply with the strictures of NAFTA. Some of these amendments abolished these rights to livelihood with the result that over 1 million Mexican farmers were displaced from agriculture following trade liberalization: they simply could not compete with cheap grains from the USA. Now Mexico, like all other countries, is not only faced with very high real food prices, but also prevailing diets have shifted towards the relatively unhealthy US model.

The structural background still leaves us with the question of how specifically did prices spike, particularly in the period 2004–08? The answer to this is almost certainly the way that the increased cost of basic foods that is triggering global famine is caused by the ongoing switch of grain production, particularly away from wheat towards corn for ethanol production and biofuels. Indeed this may be an ongoing shift, since the development of biofuels has been connected to issues of energy security and the finite supply of fossil fuels. Much of the cause is due to large government subsidies, for example Robert Albritton notes that biofuel production in USA receives "an incredible $7.14 in subsidies for the energy equivalent of 1 gallon of gas" (Albritton, 2009, p. 152). It is well-known that the USA has some of the lowest gasoline prices in the world. The most expensive gas in the USA is in California, where the automobile and suburbanization are a part of the way of life. California's average retail gas prices were $2.981 a gallon in early November 2009, up 40 cents from the previous year.[15]

Jean Ziegler, the UN Special Rapporteur on the Right to Food, has called the diversion of food crops into agrofuel production a "crime against humanity;" indeed the US government tried to pressure the World Bank to suppress a 2008 report that was leaked to the press which showed that biofuels accounted for as much as 75% of the global rise in food prices (Albritton, 2009, p. 152).

---

[15] US Department of Energy, *US Retail Gasoline Prices* (Accessed November 15, 2009). www.eia.doe.gov/oil_gas/petroleum/data_publications/wrgp/mogas_home_page.html

Albritton adds that corn, the main crop used for ethanol, consumes more chemical fertilizers and pesticides than any other crop in the USA; most ethanol refineries are powered by coal producing toxic emissions and greenhouse gases; and biofuel production elsewhere has been linked to deforestation and expanded crop monocultures that have driven the poor from the land as new enclosures are formed, for example in Brazil.[16] Finally, speculation has played a large and highly controversial role: food has become "the new gold" for ethanol producers as well as for investors seeking greater profits as they fled Wall Street for the Chicago Board of Trade and other commodity futures markets during the stock market collapse of 2007–08 to speculate on food and the new forms of energy supply.[17]

Thus one of the many consequences of the intersection between higher food prices and global poverty is the destruction of livelihoods and the creation of new enclosures – the *ejidos* of Mexico have lost their means of livelihood – this is precisely why the Zapatista rebellion was announced on January 1, 1994, to coincide with the official starting date of NAFTA. In much of Africa, even in locations where harvests have been good, because prices of food are so high many very poor people have been selling off their livestock, such as goats which are used for milk, to livestock dealers, in order to pay for food or seeds, to the point where they have nothing left to sell. Another example is in West Africa, where the governments of poorer countries have sold off their industrial fishing licenses to European industrial fishing fleets in order to be able to provide funds to the public revenues – for example in Mauritania 30% of its budget comes from such licenses. However the result is not only long-term depletion in regional fishing stocks, but also the exclusion of local fishermen from what were previously common fishing grounds – a classic example

of primitive accumulation, or accumulation by dispossession. The best fish is exported to the markets of North America, western Europe and Japan; local people who used to eat very good fish, are now simply excluded or priced out of the market.[18]

Not surprisingly, in a world where one in seven people is severely malnourished or starving, in 2007 and 2008 food riots broke out throughout the world – at least 37 nations were experiencing intense food crises. And understandably, people throughout the world questioned the wisdom of defining food security in terms of access to the world market. Indeed throughout the world grassroots movements associated with different conceptions of production, consumption and distribution have been strengthening over the past decade. Important examples include the international organization of farmers, Via Campesina, as well as the Landless Workers' Movement in Brazil (MST) which has taken advantage of clauses that remain in the Brazilian constitution which allow the landless access to the use of land which is not being productively deployed by its owners (large landowners control the vast majority of the land in Brazil, and much of it is not used for farming or for pasture).

These and other grassroots peoples' organizations continue to press for *food sovereignty*, which is a concept of self-sufficiency in food based upon more organic production, on more diverse crop varieties, and involves production relations that are based upon new forms of more egalitarian social organization and distribution – as well as hybrids of both traditional and modern concepts of environmental stewardship and sustainability. Some of the pressure from the grassroots movements has been significant in the developing world. For example in April 2009, 58 developing world governments agreed to engage in programs that would seek to redirect agriculture to support small-scale farmers, especially poor women, to support local knowledge and to do so in ways that would counter global warming. So it would appear that the trend towards relatively autonomous and self-sufficient agricultural production may be gaining momentum, and this, one would hope, will not only alleviate hunger but produce more environmentally and socially sustainable

---

[16] Samantha Pearson, "A perfect storm of troubles: sugar and ethanol," *Financial Times Special Report: Investing in Brazil*, November 5, 2009; Albritton, 2009, p. 151 ff.

[17] As farmers switch their production to grains for ethanol plants, global food and fuel prices are increasingly linked. Lester Brown, President of the Earth Policy Institute in Washington, DC has observed "the price of grain is now directly tied to the price of oil. We used to have a grain economy and a fuel economy. But now they are beginning to fuse." Quoted in Steven Mufson, "Siphoning off Corn to Fuel our Cars," *Washington Post* April 30, 2008.

[18] Anthony Faiola, " Where Every Meal Is a Sacrifice." *Washington Post* April 28, 2008.

patterns of agriculture, creating a nutritional base for the populations.

Indeed the leaders of the G8 countries have become aware of the fact that the ethical and political debate is slipping away from them and that the food crisis has posed enormous issues of legitimacy for global capitalism. The political leaders in the G20 are concerned at being accused of being responsible for (or doing nothing to alleviate) a global humanitarian disaster. In 2009 the G20 therefore offered to invest $20 billion in the developing world to increase agricultural productivity; it remains to be seen whether it will deliver on its promises despite the fact that $20 billion is a drop in the ocean compared with the amounts of money already spent on the bailouts of the big banks. Moreover wealthy private interests such as reflected in the Bill and Melinda Gates Foundation and the Clinton Global Initiative are equally concerned and they also have decided to prioritize the world food crisis in their agendas for action. Nevertheless it needs to be pointed out that the mechanisms they support for doing so still seek to preserve the world market as the principal means of "food security;" they assume that the market and business innovation can find ways to deliver food more efficiently and in so doing alleviate hunger.

A good example of the thinking of giant agri-business interests was reflected in comments made by Paul Conway, senior vice-president at Cargill and responsible for the firm's food security initiatives, ahead of the 2009 UN World Summit on Food Security in Rome, the first to be held since 2002. Conway said the drive towards self-sufficiency in food will fail, adding that the idea that nations "can be self-sufficient in every single food is a nonsense." Conway also warned that "rising populations and wealth in developing countries and governments' targets for biofuel production were likely to continue to put upward pressure on food prices for years to come."[19]

---

[19] Javier Blas, "Food self-sufficiency 'is a nonsense.'" *Financial Times* November 9, 2009. Blas adds: "In the US, the food security agenda, usually left to the Department of Agriculture, has become one of secretary of state Hillary Clinton's strategic projects. Archer Daniel Midland, Bunge, Cargill and Louis Dreyfus – the world's top food trading houses – are at the centre of agricultural trade and their wide business and government relationships allow them to see changes in food policy."

New enclosures of the social commons

Here we outline in more detail the concept of new enclosures that was discussed in the previous section in relation to land and food. The concept of the social commons also enables us to show that access to health systems is coming to be defined by the ability to pay, in a much more commodified system in the era of disciplinary neo-liberalism.

As Marx and more recent critical thinkers have noted, capitalist disciplinary processes are not something that emerge spontaneously but are rather made possible through active strategies of enclosure of commons that in turn increase people's dependence on capitalist markets for their social reproduction including their livelihoods (DeAngelis, 2007, p. 133). Marx's concept of "so-called primitive accumulation" has been subject to debate within the critical literature. For some, the concept signals the historical process that gave rise to the development of capitalism as a mode of production, following feudalism. The focus on "primitive" designates this temporal dimension. For others, the process of primitive accumulation is a precondition for a fundamental aspect of capitalism: the separation of workers from the ownership of the conditions of the realization of their labor (Marx, 1976, p. 874; DeAngelis, 2007, p. 136). In this sense, primitive accumulation is a historical and ongoing process of divorcing producers from the means of production and livelihood.

Enclosure of the commons is a concept that originates from medieval England where the commons describes parcels of land that were used "in common" by peasant farmers whose lives depended on access to and use of shared land to pasture livestock, obtain water from streams, ponds and wells and wood and fuel from forests. Landowners had ownership of these lands but the importance of the commons to the survival of populations was recognized through the courts via strict rules that required landowners to ensure access to the commons by peasants. However, landowners began to bar the use of these lands with the idea of removing commoners and using the land themselves. These "enclosures" were eventually sanctioned by British Parliament who passed the Enclosure Acts stripping commoners of their property rights so that by 1795, about 0.5% of the population of England and Wales owned almost 99% of the land (Bocking 2003, p. 26). Deprived of their access to livelihoods, peasants were forced to move to the cities where some became laborers in the factories of the Industrial Revolution, others were forced into vagrancy, prostitution and destitution.

Rather than this being a moment in the development of capitalism, we argue that enclosures are a continuous characteristic of capital logic that makes the world through commodification and enclosure thereby fragmenting and destroying "commons" that represent social spheres of life which provide various protections from the market. The term social commons relates to capitalist enclosures of social spending, taxation and entitlements (Bakker & Gill, 2003; DeAngelis, 2007, pp. 135, 148).

In addition, as DeAngelis notes, all strategies and types of enclosure share the common character of forcibly separating people from whatever access to social wealth they have, thus leaving them only with access to livelihoods mediated by capitalist markets and money as capital (2007, p. 144). We would agree with DeAngelis then that the enclosing force we have described is not simply an outcome of neo-liberalism but represents an immanent drive of capital that is common to different historical periods. This drive may be part of a conscious strategy such as the English enclosures or more recently, privatization and liberalization of trade and investment regimes (Gill & Bakker, 2006).

In the sub-section below we illustrate how modes of enclosure relate to key aspects of global health financing that typify the move away from a social commons which allowed access to public wealth without a necessary corresponding access to paid work nor the mediation of provisioning through private markets.

Morbid Symptoms II: global health financing

The realignment of social institutions, including those of the care sector (e.g. health and education), involves a shift in the regulative principles that marked much of the post-Second World War period, including the development "project." What has been taking place involves a shift away from public and authoritative regulation that was coupled with socialized provisioning for the broader population. There is thus a retreat from the idea of extended health provisioning as a public good in both rich and poor countries. As with the financial, food and energy markets, there is a parallel shift towards a more market-oriented system where health becomes a commodity. In health care, often on the advice of the World Bank, the IMF and wealthy donor countries, there has been a shift

towards a pay-as-you-go system involving user fees and other forms of self-provisioning. These changes have been complex, but have narrowed the framework of access and entitlements according to level of income and ability to pay.

Continuing pressures to download the costs (and risks) of health financing to individuals has particularly negative consequences for the 84% of the world's population that carries 90% of the global disease burden. These same countries only account for 20% of the global GDP and 12% of global spending on health. The result is that more than half of the health spending in poor countries is paid out-of-pocket. This burden is further illustrated by the gap in spending on health globally: after adjusting for the cost of living differentials, persons in rich countries spend 30 times more on health than those in poor countries (Sen, 2009).

These developments reinforce our argument set out in the previous section that the new enclosures of the social commons represents a shift to private provisioning (privatization), the imposition of commercial norms on the state and removal of more and more of the population from access to social wealth, in this case health services including vital medicines.

For example, a recent study in the *Lancet* on mass privatization in the post-communist countries in the early 1990s point to a significant increase in adult male mortality. The authors of the study conclude that increased unemployment rates during this time "were strongly associated with mortality in countries of the former Soviet Union" (Stuckler *et al.*, 2009, p. 321). They note that four of the five worst countries in terms of life expectancy had implemented programs of mass privatization leading to substantial lay-offs. Yet unemployment, the authors argue, was not the singular mediating relationship between mass privatization and rising mortality. They note that the wider institutions and relations of social reproduction from the former Soviet Union such as provisioning of housing, education, childcare and preventative health care should be considered as important mechanisms that helped people live longer and healthier lives (Stuckler *et al.*, 2009, p. 322).

There is warranted concern that pressures on global health and social financing will now increase due to the financial crisis. For example, the Global Fund to Fight AIDS, Tuberculosis and Malaria announced in 2009 that it is facing a $5 billion dollar funding gap in 2010. Foreign aid appears to be an early and vulnerable target as it only makes up a small percentage of most high-income countries' spending. Yet for many developing nations, especially the most aid-dependent countries in sub-Saharan Africa, more than half of the total public health spending comes from aid commitments. Many other developing countries also do not have any social safety nets in place. As Dr. Margaret Chan, the Director-General of the World Health Organization (WHO) has pointed out there are substantial increased risks for families in many low-income countries where the majority of health services are paid out of pocket. This squeezes public services or leads to a neglect of preventative care entirely (WHO, 2009).

Echoing these concerns, the Director of UNFPA, the United Nation's Population Program, points out that maternal mortality represents the largest health inequality in the world. Yet of all the Millennium Development Goals, progress on MDG 5 which seeks to improve maternal health, is lagging the farthest behind. She notes that with the financial crisis and the reduction in budgets for health, this goal will be even more difficult to realize.[20]

Summarizing some of the global trends, Gita Sen identifies three potential pathways that link health financing to the impacts of the financial crisis (Sen, 2009). The first is related to lower economic growth; the second to growing dependence on IMF borrowing for countries with balance of payments problems; and the third relates to increased dependence on external sources for health financing.

Lower economic growth

We have already noted the deep and long-term effects of a financial recession on economic growth, which may mean as much as a 10% reduction from the previous trend-line of output. In the context of the developing countries where the global health crisis is most profound and immediate, there are therefore additional difficulties for developing world governments because of a loss of tax and other revenues due to the decline in demand and the collapse of trade finance. A loss of export revenues is likely due to both trade protectionism related to agricultural subsidies in the rich countries and their fiscal stimulus packages that reinforce buying domestically (Sen, 2009). In addition, low levels

of economic activity means falling remittances back to developing world countries from their nationals who work abroad. Remittances (estimated at $240 billion in 2007) represent more than twice the total of Official Development Assistance. Whilst the precise amount from remittances spent on health is uncertain, the WHO notes that one survey from Mexico reported that 56% of remittances covered health expenses, so as remittances fall in systems that have shifted to pay-as-you-go, real overall health expenditures will plunge (WHO, 2009, pp. 26–27).

Fiscal restraint and IMF conditionality

A recent WHO high-level consultation on the financial crisis and global health notes that the economic crisis will more generally exert a downward pressure on total health spending. There are countries that are able to maintain spending levels but a good deal of the response depends on government policy and the fiscal space that government has to maintain spending levels, which will of course be constrained as remittances fall in developing countries. At the same time, IMF loan packages for countries in financial distress come with conditions that may actually limit governments' ability to spend on health – particularly if loan repayment is prioritized so that spending restrictions are put into place to limit fiscal deficits to 1%. The WHO also suggests that delaying capital spending on, for instance, infrastructure and equipment is a common short-term response by governments to a crunch in health budgets, despite increasing pressure on service provisioning by the public sector as individual abilities to pay disappear. This can lead to longer-term problems as reductions in maintenance, medicines or other operating costs will have an immediate and negative effect on service delivery (WHO, 2009, pp. 26–27).

External dependence on financing for health

Many developing countries greatly rely on external sources for their health financing. For example in 2006, 23 lower-income countries had more than 30% of total health expenditures funded by external sources. In Ethiopia and Rwanda, more than 50% of government expenditure is financed by donors (WHO, 2009, p. 17). This can take the form of official development assistance (ODA), bilateral financing or increasingly, through Global Funds and private foundations

---

[20] Thoraya Ahmed Obaid, Executive Director, UN Population Fund (UNFPA) "Statement at the World Bank, Washington DC: The Global Economic Crisis in Health: Why Investing in Women Is a Smart Choice." June 29, 2009.

such as the Bill and Melinda Gates Foundation. The WHO notes that ODA tends to fall during periods of recession but this may not always be the case. Yet there is agreement that rhetorical commitments made to ODA of 0.7% of gross national income are rarely achieved, and even if they were they would fall far short of targets set to meet the MDGs; and that much of the ODA is in the form of tied aid, which mandates that technical assistance is supplied from the donor country which receives the benefits so that the bulk of the funds never reach the poorest people (WHO, 2009, p. 28). Also, much of the increase in ODA in recent years has been due to debt relief (for example in strategically significant locations such as Iraq) and for humanitarian assistance related to natural disasters, rather than for additional program spending in areas such as health in national budgets. There are also signs that bilateral donors and private foundations are reducing their financial assistance due to the effects of the financial crisis.

All of these trends come at a time when, according to Dr. Margaret Chan, The Director-General of the World Health Organization, the most ambitious global effort is underway to tackle the root causes of poverty and reduce gaps in health outcomes. The knock-on effects of crisis are known to have particularly harsh effects on women and young children who are the first to be affected by a deteriorating financial situation and food availability.

Public finance and support for the social commons

We have argued that enclosures of common social property are an ongoing process. However, enclosures are also continuously being contested. Many of the public institutions related to social provisioning such as health and education for example, are a response to such resistances. These institutions, structures and social relations represent an ongoing struggle over the limits and uses of democratic control over economic life especially in its distribution of social wealth. In the context of the pressures to liberalize cross-border transactions in money, goods, services, people and information, a "fiscal squeeze" (Grunberg, 1998) in terms of state finances has arisen that has created increasing pressure for further enclosures of the social commons through, for instance, the selling of state assets to achieve fiscal balance (*fiscal squeeze of the social commons*).

A recent example of this, related to health, is connected to the fiscal pressures on the Swedish government occasioned by the financial crisis, which created conditions for the sell-off of parts of the Swedish national health system. For example there was a recent buy-out by private equity groups of the large Apoteket pharmacy chain, a Swedish public health, government-owned entity, which since 1970 has held a monopoly on pharmaceutical sales in that country. At the time of its establishment, the socialist government argued that the supply of medicine was a public good; similarly, state monopolies over the betting and alcohol markets were established to reduce gambling addiction and alcoholism. The current center-right administration has moved to dismantle state-run corporations based on its 2006 electoral platform of cutting state influence in the economy.[21]

These and other developments highlight the importance of focusing on ways of reversing these privatizing trends so that we can consider how to strengthen progressive state financing of the social commons, so as to counter new enclosures of entitlements and social spending. However, it is also important to identify some of the obstacles to realizing change. These obstacles, we argue, are more long term and diverse than the financial crisis and represent the ongoing legacy of the strategies of disciplinary neo-liberalism and new constitutionalism we have outlined in our earlier discussion of global organic crisis.

Factors contributing to the fiscal squeeze of the social commons

The most fundamental forces which have constituted the fiscal squeeze relate to how disciplinary neo-liberalism has become entrenched within the governing structures of the capitalist world, and locked in legally by new constitutionalist measures. Thus intellectual property rights have come to be redefined as a commodity, covered in the World Trade Organization, rather than technical and scientific knowledge being treated as part of the global commons, derived as it necessarily is from the broad intellectual heritage of humankind. Increasingly various forms of social and scientific knowledge are becoming privately owned,

---

[21] Andrew Ward, "Buy-out groups see off Apoteket's peers." *Financial Times*, November 10, 2009.

and protected by patents and other mechanisms, in short as commodities that can be bought and sold on the market place – a form of enclosure of the "knowledge commons."

This process therefore affects knowledge systems more generally, as the thrust of privatization increasingly enters into the world's education systems, and as more and more universities and schools turn to private sources for funding. Of course private funding for research often comes with a price.[22] In this way the conception of education as a public good to be made universally accessible to all, comes under pressure, and inequalities develop between institutions on the basis of their ability to raise private funds, and not simply their capacity to attract the best brains in the world. Harvard University has an endowment which is bigger than the gross domestic product of many countries.

There are a number of more specific mechanisms that are connected to the problem of protecting and financing the global commons, not least of which is the prevailing trend towards increasing liberalization of trade and finance which allows for many corporations and wealthy investors to avoid taxes, and thus their contribution to financing the commons, undermining the tax base of governments. This is why the French call tax havens *les paradis fiscaux* since they allow for tax evasion on a truly monumental scale. Transnational corporations also have a long history of evading taxes through complex accounting measures such as transfer pricing which locate the losses and profits of their activities in the most favorable jurisdictions where taxes are lowest. At the same time there has been intense tax competition between different jurisdictions as capital has become more mobile. To attract such capital companies must provide a favorable investment climate, which inevitably means lower corporate tax rates as well as enormous subsidies and tax holidays for new investments. As a means of broadening the tax base under these circumstances, many governments throughout the world have shifted to indirect taxes, such as value added taxes which are

"regressive" insofar as they exact the same amount of tax per transaction on each consumer irrespective of that person's income level, whether that person is a low-income worker or a billionaire. These taxes are also regressive since poorer people spend a greater proportion of their income on everyday necessities such as food, fuel and housing.

Grunberg links these more global trends and developments in the USA. She notes that the 1986 US Tax Reform influenced all OECD countries in a number of significant ways: (1) The US tax base was broadened in ways that simultaneously removed many tax privileges and exemptions but also included low-income families in the tax base; (2) The very top direct tax rates were reduced dramatically; (3) Fewer tax brackets were created, with the result that the income tax structure overall became much less progressive (Grunberg, 1998, pp. 595–596).

Despite desperately needed public finance requirements to pay for restructuring, retraining workers, the social safety nets and for health care, the fiscal situation of many developing world countries is desperate. As we noted long ago, in addition to tax losses due to falling remittances, transfer pricing, capital flight to tax havens and declining tax revenues due to trade liberalization, many developing world countries (as well as many wealthy ones) lose billions of dollars of potential income each year due to: (1) ineffective domestic tax systems that do not reach landowners, foreign corporations and wealthy individuals; and (2) regressive tax cuts and tax exemptions for foreign investors (for example, there are currently more than 3000 export processing zones, which have similar effects to offshore financial centers insofar as they allow for lower taxes or indeed tax evasion) (Gill & Law, 1988, pp. 191–223). Also, one of the characteristics of the last three decades has been the further growth of the so-called covert or informal economy, which is a nationally and globally widespread means of evading taxes. Estimates of tax evasion vary but are on the rise. According to the *OECD Observer*: "No-one knows exactly how much public money is lost illicitly to tax havens – after all, if it could be measured, it would already be taxed."[23] We discuss taxes and related issues in Chapter 29, on the need for new paradigms – or a new "common sense" – to address the challenges for global health.

---

[22] The medical profession is well known for the way in which pharmaceutical and other medical corporations routinely engage medical scientists in their accumulation strategies, and there have been many controversies concerning the degree to which impartial research and testing on the quality and safety of new drug technologies has been adequately carried out as new drugs are introduced.

---

[23] *OECD Observer*, May–June 2008.

References

Albritton, R. (2009). *Let Them Eat Junk: How Capitalism Creates Hunger and Obesity*. London: Pluto Press.

Bakker, I. & Gill, S. (2003). *Power, Production, and Social Reproduction: Human In/Security in the Global Political Economy*. Basingstoke: Palgrave Macmillan.

Benatar, S. R., Gill, S., Bakker, I. *et al.* (2009). Making progress in global health: the need for new paradigms. *International Affairs* **85**(2), 347–372.

Bocking, R. (2003). Corporatism, privatization drive enclosure of the commons. *The Canadian Centre for Policy Alternatives Monitor* **October**, 26–28.

Davies, J. B. (2006). *The World Distribution of Household Wealth*. Helsinki: United Nations University – WIDER.

De Angelis, M. (2007). *The Beginning of History: Value Struggles and Global Capital*. London: Pluto Press.

Gill, S. (1995). Globalisation, market civilisation, and disciplinary neoliberalism. *Millennium* **23**(3), 399–423.

Gill, S. (1997). Finance, production and panopticism: inequality, risk and resistance in an era of disciplinary neo-liberalism. In *Globalization, Democratization and Multilateralism* (pp. 51–76). New York: Macmillan.

Gill, S. (2008). *Power and Resistance in the New World Order*. Basingstoke: Palgrave Macmillan.

Gill, S. & Bakker, I. (2006). New constitutionalism and the social reproduction of caring institutions. *Journal of Theoretical Medicine* **6**(4), 1–23.

Gill, S. & Law, D. (1988). *The Global Political Economy: Perspectives, Problems and Policies*. Baltimore, MD: Johns Hopkins University Press.

Gramsci, A. (1971). *Selections from the Prison Notebooks of Antonio Gramsci*. New York: International Publishers.

Grunberg, I. (1998). Double Jeopardy: Globalization, Liberalization and the Fiscal Squeeze. *World Development* **26**(4), 591–605.

Marx, K. (1976). *Capital: A Critique of Political Economy*. Volume 1. New York: Penguin.

Sen, G. (2009). SRHR and Global Finance – Crisis or Opportunity? *DAWN Informs* October: 5–6.

Stuckler, D., King, L. & McKee, M. (2009). Mass privatisation and the post-communist mortality crisis: a cross-national analysis. *Lancet* **374**(9686), 315–323.

World Health Organization (WHO) (2009). *The Financial Crisis and Global Health: Report of a High-level Consultation* (pp. 1–34). Geneva: World Health Organization.

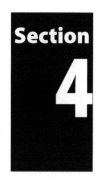

Section 4

Shaping the future

The Health Impact Fund: how to make new medicines accessible to all

Thomas Pogge

Introduction: severe poverty persists on a massive scale and could be greatly reduced at low cost

Many more people – some 360 million – have died from hunger and remediable diseases in peacetime in the 20 years since the end of the cold war than have perished from wars, civil wars, and government repression over the entire twentieth century. And poverty continues unabated, as the official statistics amply confirm: 1020 million human beings are chronically undernourished (FAO, 2009), 884 million lack access to safe water (WHO & UNICEF, 2008, p. 30), and 2500 million lack access to improved sanitation (WHO & UNICEF, 2008, p. 7), while 2000 million lack access to essential medicines (Fogarty Center for Advanced Study in the Health Sciences, n.d.), 924 million lack adequate shelter (UN-Habitat, 2003, p. vi) and 1600 million lack electricity (UN-Habitat, n.d.). About 774 million adults are illiterate (UNESCO, 2008) and 218 million children are child laborers (ILO, 2006, p. 6).

Roughly one-third of all human deaths, 18 million annually, are due to poverty-related causes, straightforwardly preventable through better nutrition, safe drinking water, cheap rehydration packs, vaccines, antibiotics and other medicines. People of color, females and the very young are heavily over-represented among the global poor, and hence also among those suffering the staggering effects of severe poverty. Children under 5 account for half, or 8.8 million, of the annual death toll from poverty-related causes (UNICEF, 2009). The over-representation of females is clearly documented (UNDP, 2003, pp. 310–330).

With the poorest half of humanity now reduced to under 3% of global household income[1] and needing only another 1% to make ends meet, it is clear that we could eradicate most severe poverty worldwide if we chose to try – in fact, we could have done so decades ago. Citizens of the rich countries are, however, conditioned to downplay the severity and persistence of world poverty and to think of it as an occasion for minor charitable assistance.

This widespread lack of attention to the world poverty problem becomes morally indefensible once we understand that its human cost is enormous, that its economic magnitude is pathetically small by comparison, and that it has barely diminished during recent periods of healthy global economic growth. This clearly is a problem that any moral person must pay serious attention to.

Those who begin to pay attention often easily content themselves with the thought that we simply cannot avoid world poverty, at least not at reasonable cost. In this vein, many think of the millions of poverty deaths each year as necessary to avoid an overpopulated, impoverished and ecologically unsustainable future for humanity. While this view once had prominent academic defenders (Hardin, 1974), it is now discredited by abundant empirical evidence across regions and cultures, showing that, when poverty declines, fertility rates also decline sharply (Sen, 1994). Wherever people have gained access to contraceptives and associated knowledge and have gained some assurance that their children will survive into adulthood and that their own livelihood in old age will

---

[1] Data from Branko Milanovic, World Bank, spreadsheet on file with author.

An earlier version of this work has appeared: Pogge, T. (2008). Healthcare reform that works for the U.S. and the world's poor. *Global Health Governance* **2** (2).

be secure, they have substantially reduced their rate of reproduction. We can see this in the dramatic declines in total fertility rates (children per woman) in areas where poverty has declined. In the last 60 years, this rate has dropped from 5.42 to 1.72 in Eastern Asia, for instance, and from 3.04 to 1.38 in Portugal and from 3.18 to 1.83 in Australia. In economically stagnant poor countries, by contrast, there has been little change over the same period: total fertility rates went from 5.50 to 5.36 in Equatorial Guinea, from 6.23 to 5.49 in Mali, from 6.86 to 7.15 in Niger and from 5.52 to 5.22 in Sierra Leone.[2] The correlation is further confirmed by synchronic comparisons. Currently, the total fertility rate is 4.39 for the 50 least developed countries versus 1.64 for the more developed regions, and 2.46 for the remaining countries.[3] The complete list of national total fertility rates also confirms a strong correlation with poverty and shows that already some 95 of the more affluent countries have reached total fertility rates below 2,[4] foreshadowing future declines in population. Taken together, these data provide overwhelming evidence that poverty reduction is associated with large fertility declines.

These data also discredit the claim that we should accept world poverty for the sake of the environment which would be gravely damaged if billions of presently poor people began consuming at the rate we do. The short-term ecological impact of eradicating world poverty would be dwarfed by its long-term ecological impact through a lower human population. Eradicating poverty with all deliberate speed would make a huge contribution to an early peaking of the human population which would bring enormous ecological benefits for the rest of the third millennium and beyond. At current projections, massive eradication of severe poverty can achieve, by 2100, a declining population of 7 billion human beings as compared to a still rising population of 10–14 billion otherwise. It should also be noted that the short-term harm from poverty eradication is often overstated. It is true that, if the poorest half of humankind had an additional 1% of global household income (i.e. 4% instead of 3%) at market exchange rates, then their ecological footprint would expand. But it is also

true that the richer half would then have 1% less (i.e. 96% instead of 97%) of global household income with a consequent contraction of their much larger ecological footprint. There is still a net harm to the environment as ecological footprint per unit of income tends to decline with rising income. But this effect is very small compared with the long-term ecological benefit of poverty eradication. And it can be avoided by small incremental reductions in the ecological burdens the more affluent impose.

What do we owe the world's poor, and what are the grounds of these obligations?

Having disposed of the claim that world poverty is a necessary evil, we more affluent confront the question of what, and how much, we are duty-bound to "sacrifice" towards reducing severe poverty worldwide. Most of the more affluent believe that these duties are feeble, that it is not very wrong to give no help at all. Against this view, some philosophers have argued that the affluent have positive duties that are quite stringent and quite demanding: if people can prevent much hunger, disease and premature death at little cost to themselves, then they ought to do so even if those in need are distant strangers. Peter Singer (1972) famously argued for this conclusion by likening the global poor to a drowning child: affluent people who give no aid to the hungry behave no better than a passer-by who fails to save a drowning child from a shallow pond in order not to muddy his pants.

One problem with Singer's view is to work out how much an affluent person is required to give when there are always yet further urgent needs she might help meet. On reflection, the assumption of such a cut-off point seems odd. It seems more plausible to assume that, as an affluent person expands her assistance, the moral reason to give even more becomes less stringent. We tend to talk in binary terms, to be sure, about whether some effort is morally required or else beyond the call of duty. But there is no plausible formula that would allow us to compute, from data about a person's financial situation, exactly how much she is required to give toward helping those to whom an extra dollar would bring much greater benefit.

Still, as she keeps giving, the moral reasons to give yet more do become weaker, less duty-like and more discretionary. The strength of these moral reasons may fade in this way on account of three factors. First, the

---

[2] esa.un.org/unpp/index.asp?panel=2 (Accessed December 21, 2009).

[3] *Ibid.*

[4] https://www.cia.gov/library/publications/the-world-factbook/fields/2127.html?countryName=&countryCode=&regionCode=%C2%BA (Accessed December 21, 2009).

needs of the poor may become less urgent. Second, giving an extra dollar becomes more of a burden as the donor's income declines. Third, what she has given continuously builds a case that she has already done a lot. These three factors are not in precise harmony. The relevance of the third factor is sensitive to whether her current financial situation reflects the fact that she has already given a lot. Singer and his followers have no algorithm for assessing the relevance of these factors or for determining with any precision whether someone has done her duty or not. Nonetheless, they have a plausible case for concluding that we ought to relieve life-threatening poverty so long as we can do so without giving up anything really significant.

Other philosophers have challenged the terms of this debate and, in particular, the shared suggestion that people in affluent countries are as innocent in regard to world poverty as Singer's passer-by is in regard to the child in the pond. This challenge can be formulated in different ways (Pogge, 2008, pp. 205–210). One can question the legitimacy of the existing highly uneven global distribution of income and wealth, which has emerged from a historical process that was pervaded by grievous wrongs (genocide, colonialism, slavery) and has left many of our contemporaries without a fair share of the world's natural resources or an adequate equivalent. One can criticize the negative externalities affluent populations are imposing upon the world's poor: greenhouse gas emissions that are spreading desertification and tropical diseases, for example, or highly efficient European fishing fleets that are decimating fish stocks in African waters.[5]

One can also critique the increasingly dense and influential web of global institutional arrangements which foreseeably and avoidably perpetuates massive poverty. It does so, for example, by permitting affluent states to protect their markets through tariffs and anti-dumping duties and through export credits and huge subsidies to domestic producers that amount to some $300 billion annually in agriculture alone. It does so by requiring all World Trade Organization (WTO) members to grant 20-year product patents, thereby causing important and cheaply mass-producible new medicines to be priced out of reach of a majority of the world's

population. The existing international institutional order also fosters corrupt and oppressive government in the poorer countries by recognizing any person or group holding effective power – regardless of how they acquired or exercise it – as entitled to sell the country's resources and to dispose of the proceeds of such sales, to borrow in the country's name and thereby to impose debt service obligations upon it, to sign treaties on the country's behalf and thus to bind its present and future population, and to use state revenues to buy the means of internal repression. This practice of recognition is beneficial to many a putschist and oppressive ruler, who can gain and keep political power even against a large majority of his compatriots and thereby greatly enrich himself at their expense. This practice is also beneficial to affluent countries which can, for instance, buy natural resources from a strongman regardless of how he came to power and regardless of how badly he rules. But this practice is devastating for the populations of such countries by strengthening their oppressors and also the incentives toward coup attempts and dictatorial rule. Bad governance in so many poor countries (especially those rich in natural resources) is a foreseeable effect of the privileges our international order bestows upon any person or group that manages to bring a country under its control.

The common conclusion suggested by these various considerations is that the moral challenge world poverty poses to the affluent is not merely to help more, but also to harm less. They are not merely failing to fulfill their positive duties to assist and protect, but also violating negative duties: the duty not to defend or take advantage of an unjust distribution of holdings, or the duty not to contribute to or take advantage of unjust international practices and institutional arrangements that foreseeably and avoidably keep billions trapped in life-threatening poverty.

A violation of the latter duty presupposes that it is reasonably possible for the affluent collectively to shape the international practices and institutional arrangements they design and uphold to be more poverty-avoiding. This presupposition is hard to deny in regard to the examples just provided: it is reasonably possible for us *not* to deplete African fish stocks, *not* to distort world markets through massive subsidies and other protectionist measures that hamper exports from poor countries, *not* to insist on pharmaceutical monopolies that deprive the poor of access to cheap generic versions of advanced medicines, *not* to recognize and arm rulers who oppress their poor

---

[5] The predatory fishing practices of heavily subsidized European fleets in West African waters are described, for instance, in Sharon Lafraniere, "Europe Takes Africa's Fish, and Boatloads of Migrants Follow," *New York Times*, January 14, 2008.

compatriots and steal their resources. Insofar as alternative, more poverty-avoiding practices and rules are reasonably available, the existing international practices and global institutional order must count as unjust and their continued imposition as a harm done to the world's poor.

There is no agreement on how much inequality and poverty just international practices and institutional arrangements may maximally engender. But no precise answer to this question is required for concluding that existing levels of poverty and inequality are excessive. When the basic human rights of a large proportion of humanity are avoidably unfulfilled, then international practices and institutional arrangements must count as unjust insofar as they contribute to this human rights deficit. Especially the more powerful countries then have a responsibility to reform these practices and institutional arrangements so as to make them more human-rights compliant – a responsibility that falls, in the last analysis, upon these countries' citizens. None of us can reform international practices and institutions single-handedly, to be sure, but we can work politically toward such reform and we can also make individual efforts to protect poor people from the effects of the unjust arrangements imposed upon them. Such efforts, though active, are required by our negative duty not to harm: insofar as one contributes to and benefits from the imposition of unjust arrangements, one is responsible for a share of the harm these arrangements cause unless one takes compensating action that prevents this share of the harm from materializing (Pogge, 2005, pp. 60–62, 68–75).

Focusing directly on global health

How, then, might affluent countries go about reforming the global institutional architecture? I noted at the outset the 18 million deaths each year from poverty-related causes. Using the World Health Organization's Global Burden of Disease (GBD) studies, we can break down this figure into some of the more prominent categories of mortality. In 2004, there were about 57 million human deaths. The main causes highly correlated with poverty (WHO, 2008, p. 54, with death tolls in thousands) were: diarrhea (2163) and malnutrition (487), perinatal (3180) and maternal conditions (524), childhood diseases (847 – measles is about half), tuberculosis (1464), malaria (889), meningitis (340), hepatitis (159), tropical diseases (152), respiratory infections (4259 – mainly pneumonia), HIV/AIDS (2040) and sexually transmitted diseases (128).

This huge death toll would come down if global poverty were reduced, but it is also possible to make substantial progress against the GBD directly: existing huge mortality and morbidity rates can be dramatically lowered by reforming our system of funding for the research and development of new medical treatments. I will sketch a concrete, feasible and politically realistic reform plan that would give medical innovators stable and reliable financial incentives to address the diseases of the poor. If adopted, this plan would not add much to the overall cost of global health care spending. In fact, on any plausible accounting, which would take note of the huge economic losses caused by the present GBD, the reform I propose would actually save money. Moreover, it would distribute the cost of global health-care spending more fairly across countries, across generations, and between those lucky enough to enjoy good health and the unlucky ones suffering from serious medical conditions.

Medical progress has traditionally been fueled from two main sources: government funding and sales revenues. The former – given to universities, corporations, other research centers and governmental research facilities such as the US National Institutes of Health – has typically been *push* funding focused on basic research. Sales revenues, usually earned by corporations, have mostly funded more applied research resulting in the development of specific medicines. Sales revenues, by their nature, constitute *pull* funding: an innovation has to be developed to the point of marketability before any sales revenues can be realized from it.

With medicines, the fixed cost of developing a new product is extremely high for two reasons: it is very expensive to research and fine-tune a new medicine and then to take it through elaborate clinical trials and national approval processes. Moreover, most promising research ideas fail somewhere along the way and thus never lead to a marketable product. Both reasons combine to raise the research and development cost per new marketable medicine to somewhere around half a billion dollars or more. Commencing manufacture of a new medicine once it has been invented and approved is cheap by comparison. Because of this fixed-cost imbalance, pharmaceutical innovation is not sustainable in a free market system: competition among manufacturers would quickly drive down the price of a new medicine to near its long-term marginal cost of production, and the innovator would get nowhere near recovering its investment.

The conventional way of correcting this market failure of undersupply is to enable innovators to apply for patents that entitle them to forbid others to produce or distribute the innovative product and to waive this entitlement in exchange for a licensing fee. The result of such market exclusivity is an artificially elevated sales price that, on average, enables innovators to recoup their initial investment through selling products that, even at prices far above marginal cost, are in high demand.

Monopolies are widely denounced by economists as inefficient and by ethicists as an immoral interference in people's freedom to produce and exchange. In regard to patents, however, many believe that the curtailment of individual freedom can be justified by the benefit, provided patents are carefully designed. One important design feature is that patents confer only temporary market exclusivity. Once the patent expires, competitors can freely enter the market with copies of the original innovation and consumers need thus no longer pay a large mark-up over the competitive market price. Temporal limits make sense, because additional years of patent life barely strengthen innovation incentives: at a typical industry discount rate of 11% per annum, a 10-year effective patent life generates 68%, and a 15-year effective patent life 82%, of the profit (discounted to present value) that a permanent patent would generate.[6] It makes no sense to impose monopoly prices on all future generations for the sake of so slight a gain in innovation incentives.

During the life of the patent, everyone is legally deprived of the freedom to produce, sell and buy a patented medicine without permission from the patent holder. This restraint hurts generic producers and it also hurts consumers by depriving them of the chance to buy such medicines at competitive market prices. But consumers also benefit from the impressive arsenal of useful medicines whose development is motivated by the prospect of patent-protected mark-ups.

When everyone has access to vital new medicines as needed, the loss may seem to be dwarfed by the benefit. But billions of human beings are too poor to afford medicines at monopoly prices and thus cannot share the benefit of a patent regime. This benefit of pharmaceutical innovation thus cannot be used to justify *to them* that they should be cut off from medicines at competitive market prices.

This moral point was largely respected so long as expansive patent protections were mostly confined to the affluent states while the less developed countries were allowed to have weaker ones or none at all. The situation changed in 1994, when a powerful alliance of industries (software, entertainment, pharmaceuticals and agribusinesses) pressured the governments of the richest states to impose globally uniform intellectual property rules as enshrined in the TRIPS Agreement.[7] The poorer states agreed to institute TRIPS-compliant intellectual property regimes in order to qualify for membership in the World Trade Organization which (they were then promised) would allow them to reap large benefits from free trade.[8]

The global poor have a powerful objection to the pharmaceutical patent regime imposed on them by the world's governments: "If the freedom to produce, sell and buy advanced medicines were not curtailed in our countries, then the affluent would need to find other (for them perhaps less convenient) ways of funding pharmaceutical research. Advanced medicines would then be available at competitive market prices, and we would have a much better chance of getting access to them through our own funds or with the help of national or international government agencies or non-governmental organizations (NGOs). The loss of freedom imposed through product patents thus inflicts on us a huge loss in terms of disease and premature death. This loss cannot possibly be justified by any gain such patents may bring to the affluent." However morally compelling, this objection is ignored by the more affluent states which have relentlessly pursued the globalization of uniform intellectual property rights – with devastating effects, for instance, on access

---

[6] Patent life is counted from the time the patent application is filed. Effective patent life is the time from receiving market clearance to the time the patent expires. My calculation in the text assumes constant nominal profit each year. In reality, annual profit may rise (due to increasing market penetration, rising disease incidence or population growth) or fall (through reduced incidence of the disease or through competition from "me-too drugs" developed by competing firms). For most drugs, sales decline after they have been on the market for six years or so, and this strengthens the reasons for limiting patent life.

[7] Trade-Related Aspects of Intellectual Property Rights.

[8] The promise was not kept as the high-income countries continue to sabotage the export opportunities of poor countries through protectionist tariffs and anti-dumping duties as well as through huge subsidies and export credits to their domestic producers.

to second-line AIDS therapies and hence on the course of the AIDS epidemic.

The world responds to the catastrophic health crisis among the global poor in a variety of ways: with the usual declarations, working papers, conferences, summits and working groups, of course; but also with efforts to fund delivery of medicines to the poor through intergovernmental initiatives such as 3 by 5,[9] through governmental programs such as the US President's Emergency Plan for AIDS Relief (PEPFAR), through public–private partnerships like the Global Alliance for Vaccines and Immunization and the Global Fund to Fight AIDS, Tuberculosis and Malaria, and through medicine donations from pharmaceutical companies; and with various efforts to foster the development of new medicines for the diseases of the poor, such as the Drugs for Neglected Diseases Initiative, the Institute for One World Health, the Novartis Institute for Tropical Diseases, and various prizes.[10]

Such a busy diversity of initiatives looks good and creates the impression that a lot is being done to solve the problem. And most of these efforts are really doing good by improving the situation relative to what it would be under TRIPS unmitigated. Still, these efforts are not nearly sufficient to protect the poor. It is unrealistic to hope that enough billions of dollars will be collected year after year to neutralize the cost imposed on the world's poor by the globalization of pharmaceutical product patents. It makes sense then to look for a more systemic solution that addresses the global health crisis at its root. Involving institutional reform, such a systemic solution is politically more difficult to achieve. But, once achieved, it is also politically much easier to maintain. And it pre-empts most of the huge and collectively inefficient mobilizations currently required to produce the many stop-gap measures, which can

at best only mitigate the effects of structural problems they leave untouched.

Seven failings of the present pharmaceutical innovation regime

The quest for such a systemic solution can start from an analysis of the main drawbacks of the newly globalized monopoly patent regime.

High prices. While a medicine is under patent, it will be sold near the profit-maximizing monopoly price which is largely determined by the demand curve of the affluent. When there are plenty of affluent or well-insured people who really want a drug, then its price can be raised very high above the cost of production before increased gains from enlarging the mark-up are outweighed by losses from reduced sales volume. With patented medicines, mark-ups in excess of 1000% are not exceptional.[11] When such exorbitant mark-ups are charged, only a few of the poor can have access through the charity of others.

Neglect of diseases concentrated among the poor. When innovators are rewarded with patent-protected mark-ups, diseases concentrated among the poor – no matter how widespread and severe – are not attractive targets for pharmaceutical research. This is so because the demand for such a medicine drops off very steeply as the patent holder enlarges the mark-up. There is no prospect, then, of achieving high sales volume and a large mark-up. Moreover, there is the further risk that a successful research effort will be greeted with loud demands to make the medicine available at marginal cost or even for free, which would force the innovator to write off its initial investment as a loss. In view of such prospects, biotechnology and pharmaceutical companies predictably prefer even the trivial ailments of the affluent, such as hair loss and acne, over tuberculosis and sleeping sickness. This problem of neglected diseases is also known as the 10/90 gap, alluding to only 10% of all pharmaceutical research being focused on diseases that account for 90% of the GBD (Global Forum for Health Research, 2004).

Bias toward maintenance drugs. Medicines can be sorted into three categories. Curative medicines remove the disease from the patient's body; maintenance drugs

---

9 Announced in 2003, this joint WHO/UNAIDS program was meant to provide, by 2005, antiretroviral treatment to 3 million (out of what were then estimated to be 40.3 million) AIDS patients in the less developed countries. In fact, it extended such treatment to about 900 000.

10 A prize is a specific reward offered for the development of a new medicine that meets certain specifications. It need not take the form of a cash payment. The successful innovator may also be rewarded by subsidizing the sale of (advance market commitment), or by buying at a preset high price (advance purchase commitment), a certain large number of doses of a new medicine that meets certain specifications. Or the successful innovator may be granted an extension on any of its other patents.

---

11 In Thailand, Sanofi-Aventis sold its cardiovascular disease medicine Plavix (clopidogrel) for 70 baht ($2.20) per pill, some 6000% above the price at which the Indian generic firm Emcure agreed to deliver the same medicine. See Oxfam (2007, p. 20).

improve well-being and functioning without removing the disease; and preventative medicines reduce the likelihood of contracting the disease in the first place. Under the existing patent regime, maintenance drugs are by far the most profitable, with the most desirable patients being ones who are not cured and do not die (until after patent expiration). Such patients keep buying the medicine, thereby delivering vastly more profit than if they derived the same health benefit from a cure or vaccine. Vaccines are least lucrative because they are typically bought by governments, which can command large volume discounts. This is highly regrettable because the health benefits of vaccines tend to be exceptionally great as vaccines protect from infection or contagion not merely each vaccinated person but also their contacts. Once more, then, the present regime guides pharmaceutical research in the wrong direction – and here to the detriment of poor and affluent alike.

Wastefulness. Under the present regime, innovators must bear the cost of filing for patents in dozens of national jurisdictions and then also the cost of monitoring these jurisdictions for possible infringements of their patents. Huge amounts are spent in many jurisdictions on costly litigation that pits generic companies, with strong incentives to challenge any patent on a profitable medicine, against patent holders, whose earnings depend on their ability to defend, extend and prolong their patent-protected mark-ups. Even greater costs are due to the deadweight loss "on the order of $200 billion" that arises from blocked sales to buyers who are willing and able to pay some price between the marginal cost and the much higher monopoly price.[12]

Counterfeiting. Large mark-ups also encourage the illegal manufacture of fake products that are diluted, adulterated, inert or even toxic. Such counterfeits often endanger patient health. They also contribute to the emergence of drug-specific resistance, when patients ingest too little of the active ingredient of a diluted drug to kill off the more resilient pathogenic agents. The emergence of highly drug-resistant disease strains – of tuberculosis, for instance – poses dangers to us all.

Excessive marketing. When pharmaceutical companies maintain a very large mark-up, they find it rational to make massive efforts to increase sales volume, often by scaring patients or by rewarding doctors. This produces pointless battles over market share among similar ("me-too") drugs as well as perks that induce doctors to prescribe medicines even when these are not indicated or when competing medicines are likely to do better. With a large mark-up it also pays to fund massive direct-to-consumer advertising that persuades people to take medicines they don't really need for diseases they don't really have (and sometimes for invented pseudo diseases).[13]

The last-mile problem. While the present regime provides strong incentives to sell even unneeded patented medicines to those who can pay or have insurance, it provides no incentives to ensure that poor people benefit from medicines they urgently need. Even in affluent countries, pharmaceutical companies have incentives only to sell products, not to ensure that these are actually used, optimally, by patients whom they can benefit. This problem is compounded in poor countries, which often lack the infrastructure to distribute medicines as well as the medical personnel to prescribe them and to ensure their proper use. In fact, the present regime even gives pharmaceutical companies incentives to disregard the medical needs of the poor. To profit under this regime, a company needs not merely a patent on a medicine that is effective in protecting paying patients from a disease or its detrimental symptoms. It also needs this target disease to thrive and spread because, as a disease waxes or wanes, so does market demand for the remedy. A pharmaceutical company helping poor patients to benefit from its patented medicine would be undermining its own profitability in three ways: by paying for the effort to make its drug competently available to them, by curtailing a disease on which its profits depend, and by losing affluent customers who find ways of buying, on the cheap, medicines meant for the poor.

A structural reform: The Health Impact Fund

All seven drawbacks can be greatly mitigated by supplementing the patent regime with a complementary source of incentives and rewards for developing new medicines. With an international interdisciplinary team, I have been detailing such a pay-for-performance

---

[12] Personal communication (November 14, 2007) from Aidan Hollis, based on his rough calculation. He had earlier quantified the deadweight loss in the region "of $5 bn–20 bn annually for the US. Globally the deadweight loss is certain to be many times this figure, because in many markets drug insurance is unavailable and so consumers are more price-sensitive" (Hollis, 2005, p. 8).

[13] See the special issue on disease mongering, edited by Roy Moynihan and David Henry: *PLoS Medicine* 3(4), (2006), 425–465.

mechanism in the form of the *Health Impact Fund*.[14] The HIF is a proposed global agency – financed mainly by governments – that would give pharmaceutical innovators the option to register any new product. They would guarantee to make it available, wherever it is needed, at the lowest feasible cost of production and distribution. In exchange, each registered product would, during its first 10 years on the market, participate in the HIF's annual reward pools, receiving a share equal to its share of the assessed health impact of all HIF-registered products.[15]

The requisite health impact assessment could be conducted in terms of some version of quality-adjusted life years (QALYs), a metric that has been deployed for about two decades by academic researchers, insurers, NGOs and government agencies. The assessment would rely on clinical and pragmatic trials of the product, on tracing (facilitated by serial numbers) of random samples of the product to end-users, and on statistical analysis of correlations between sales data (including time and place of sale) and variations in the incidence of the target disease.

In view of the great cost (in the hundreds of millions of dollars) of bringing a new medicine to market, and to take advantage of economies of scale in health impact assessment, the annual reward pools should be at least $6 billion (which is less than 1% of current global pharmaceutical spending and about 5% of current global investment in pharmaceutical research). If all countries were to join up, each would need to contribute about 0.01% of its gross national income (GNI). If countries representing only a third of the global product participated, each would need to contribute a still-modest 0.03% of its GNI – mitigated by the massive cost savings their governments, firms and citizens would enjoy from low-cost HIF-registered medicines. If the HIF were found to work well, it could be scaled up to attract an increasing share of new medicines.

To provide stable incentives, the HIF would need guaranteed financing some 15 years into the future to assure pharmaceutical innovators that, if they fund expensive clinical trials now, they can claim a full decade of health impact rewards upon market approval. Such a solid guarantee is also in the interest of the funders who would not want the incentive power of their contributions to be diluted through skeptical discounting by potential innovators. The guarantee might take the form of a treaty under which each participating country commits to the HIF a fixed fraction of its future gross national income (GNI). Backed by such a treaty, the HIF would automatically adjust the contributions of the various partner countries to their variable economic fortunes, would avoid protracted struggles over contribution proportions, and would assure each country that any extra cost it agreed to bear through an increase in the contribution schedule would be matched by a corresponding increase in the contributions of all other partner countries.

The HIF has five main advantages over conventional innovation prizes, including advance market commitments and advance purchase commitments. First, it is a structural reform, establishing an enduring source of high-impact pharmaceutical innovations. Second, it is not disease-specific and thus much less vulnerable to lobbying by firms and patient groups. Third, conventional prizes must define a precise finish line, specifying at least which disease the new medicine must attack, how effective and convenient it must minimally be, and how bad its side effects may be. Such specificity is problematic because it presupposes the very knowledge whose acquisition is yet to be encouraged. Since sponsors lack this knowledge ahead of time, their specifications are likely to be seriously suboptimal: they may be too demanding, so that firms give up the effort even though something close to the sought medicine is within their reach, or they may be insufficiently demanding, so that firms, to save time and expense, deliver a medicine that is just barely good enough to win even when they could have done much better at little extra cost (Hollis, 2007, pp. 15–16). The HIF avoids this problem of the finish line by flexibly rewarding any new registered medicine in

---

[14] See www.healthimpactfund.org for details about the team and its work, which have been generously funded by the Australian Research Council, the BUPA Foundation, the European Commission, and the Canadian Social Science and Humanities Research Council. Much critical discussion of the proposal by Gorik Ooms and Rachel Hammonds, Thomas Faunce and Hitoshi Nasu, Devi Sridhar, Michael Selgelid, Aidan Hollis, and Michael Ravvin can be found in a special issue of *Public Health Ethics* **1**(2), (2008), 1–192.

[15] Ten years corresponds roughly to the profitable period of a patent. Under TRIPS, WTO members must offer patents lasting at least 20 years from the patent filing date which is typically many years before the medicine receives market clearance after clinical trials. Because some patents may outlast the reward period, HIF registration requires the registrant to offer a royalty-free open license for generic versions of the product following the end of the reward period.

proportion to its global health impact. Fourth, formulated to avoid failure and in ignorance of the true cost of innovation, specific prizes are often much too large and thus overpay for innovation. The HIF solves this problem by letting its health impact reward rate adjust itself through competition: a high reward rate would correct by attracting additional registrations (producing an increase in the number of registered medicines) and an unattractively low reward rate would correct by deterring new registrations (producing a decrease in the number of registered medicines). Fifth, the HIF gives each registrant powerful incentives to promote the optimal end-use of its product: to seek its wide and effective use by any patients who can benefit from it.

Because HIF-registered medicines would be cheaply available everywhere, there would be no cheating problems as commonly attend any differential pricing schemes aimed to make a medicine more affordable to poor patients or in poor countries. The HIF's global scope also brings huge efficiency gains by diluting the cost of innovation without diluting its benefits.

There is no space here to discuss the design of the HIF in full detail (see Hollis & Pogge, 2008). Let me conclude then by sketching how it would, without revision of the TRIPS Agreement, provide systemic relief for its seven failings outlined above.

High prices would not exist for HIF-registered medicines. Innovators would typically not even want a higher price as this would reduce their health impact rewards by impeding access to their product by most of the world's population. The HIF counts health benefits to the poorest of patients equally with health benefits to the richest.

Diseases concentrated among the poor, insofar as they contribute substantially to the GBD, would no longer be neglected. In fact, the more destructive among them would come to afford some of the most lucrative research opportunities for biotechnology and pharmaceutical companies.

Bias toward maintenance drugs would be absent from HIF-encouraged research. The HIF assesses each registered medicine's health impact in terms of how its use reduces mortality and morbidity – without regard to whether it achieves this reduction through cure, symptom relief or prevention. This would guide firms to deliberate about potential research projects in a way that is also optimal for global public health, namely in terms of the expected health impact of the new medicine relative to the cost of developing it. The profitability

of research projects would be aligned with their cost effectiveness in terms of global public health.

Wastefulness would be dramatically lower for HIF-registered products. There would be no deadweight losses from large mark-ups. There would be little costly litigation as generic competitors would lack incentives to compete and innovators would have no incentive to suppress generic products (because they enhance the innovator's health impact reward). Innovators might therefore often not even bother to obtain, police and defend patents in many national jurisdictions. To register a medicine with the HIF, innovators need show only once that they have an effective and innovative product.

Counterfeiting of HIF-registered products would be unattractive. With the genuine item widely available near or even below the marginal cost of production, there is little to be gained from producing and selling fakes.

Excessive marketing would also be much reduced for HIF-registered medicines. Because each innovator is rewarded for the health impact of its addition to the medical arsenal, incentives to develop me-too drugs to compete with an existing HIF-registered medicine would be weak. And innovators would have incentives to urge a HIF-registered drug upon doctors and patients only insofar as such marketing results in measurable therapeutic benefits for which the innovator would then be rewarded.

The last-mile problem would be mitigated because each HIF-registered innovator would have strong incentives to ensure that patients are fully instructed and properly provisioned so that they make optimal use (dosage, compliance, etc.) of its medicines, which will then, through wide and effective deployment, have their optimal public health impact. Rather than ignore poor countries as unprofitable markets, pharmaceutical companies would, moreover, have incentives to work with one another and with national health ministries, international agencies and NGOs toward improving the health systems of these countries in order to enhance the impact of their HIF-registered medicines there.

Conclusion

This chapter has shown that, thinking morally about global health in a constructive way, we must bear in mind three important points. First, in parallel to the institutional order of a country, global institutional arrangements have a profound effect on the welfare of people everywhere. Second, the present rules governing the world economy, designed and imposed to serve powerful corporate and political interests, could be adjusted in minor but highly effective ways to better serve the interests of all. Third, small changes to the rules that incentivize pharmaceutical research and development would produce large health gains in poor and affluent countries – gains that, over time, would easily cover the economic cost of the scheme. Creating the Health Impact Fund would be a large step toward fulfilling Obama's pledge to "wield technology's wonders to raise healthcare's quality and lower its cost."[16]

Acknowledgment

The author would like to thank Matt Peterson for substantial research and editorial assistance.

References

Fogarty Center for Advanced Study in the Health Sciences (n.d.). *Strategic Plan: Fiscal Years 2000–2003*. Bethesda, MD: National Institutes of Health. www.fic.nih.gov/about/plan/exec_summary.htm (Accessed December 21, 2009).

Food and Agriculture Organization (FAO) (2009). 1.02 billion people hungry: One sixth of humanity undernourished – more than ever before. Press Release, Rome, June 19. www.fao.org/news/story/en/item/20568/icode/ (Accessed December 21, 2009).

Global Forum for Health Research (2004). *The 10/90 Report on Health Research 2003–2004*. Geneva: GFHR. Also available at www.globalforumhealth.org.

Hardin, G. (1974). Lifeboat ethics: the case against helping the poor. *Psychology Today* **8**, 38–43, 123–26.

Hollis, A. (2005). *An Efficient Reward System for Pharmaceutical Innovation*. Working paper, Department of Economics, University of Calgary, econ.ucalgary.ca/fac-files/ah/drugprizes.pdf (Accessed December 21, 2009).

Hollis, A. (2007). *Incentive Mechanisms for Innovation*. IAPR Technical Paper. www.iapr.ca/iapr/files/iapr/iapr-tp-07005_0.pdf (Accessed December 21, 2009).

Hollis, A. & Pogge, T. (2008). *The Health Impact Fund: Making New Medicines Accessible for All*. New Haven, CT: Incentives for Global Health. Also available at www.healthimpactfund.org.

International Labour Office (ILO) (2006). *The End of Child Labour: Within Reach*. Geneva: International Labour Office.

Oxfam (2007). *Investing for Life*. Oxfam Briefing Paper. www.oxfam.org/en/policy/bp109_investing_for_life_0711 (Accessed December 21, 2009).

Pogge, T. (2005). Severe poverty as a violation of negative duties. *Ethics and International Affairs* **19**, 55–84.

Pogge, T. (2008). *World Poverty and Human Rights*. (2nd edn.) Cambridge: Polity Press.

Sen, A. (1994). Population: delusion and reality. *New York Review of Books* **41**, 62–71.

Singer, P. (1972). Famine, affluence, and morality. *Philosophy & Public Affairs* **1**, 229–243.

United Nations Development Program (UNDP) (2003). *Human Development Report 2003*. New York: Oxford University Press.

UNESCO Institute for Statistics (2008). *Literacy Topic*. December 1. www.uis.unesco.org/ev.php?URL_ID=6401&URL_DO=DO_TOPIC&URL_SECTION=201 (Accessed December 21, 2009).

UN-Habitat (2003). *The Challenge of Slums: Global Report on Human Settlements 2003*. London: Earthscan.

UN-Habitat (n.d.). *Urban Energy*. www.unhabitat.org/content.asp?cid=2884&catid=356&typeid=24&subMenuId=0 (Accessed December 21, 2009).

United Nations Children's Fund (UNICEF) (2009). Global child mortality continues to drop. Press Release, New York, September 10. www.unicef.org/media/media_51087.html (Accessed December 21, 2009).

World Health Organization (WHO) (2008). *The Global Burden of Disease: 2004 Update*. Geneva: WHO Publications.

World Health Organization (WHO) and UNICEF (2008). *Progress on Drinking Water and Sanitation: Special Focus on Sanitation*. New York and Geneva: UNICEF and WHO. Available at www.who.int/water_sanitation_health/monitoring/jmp2008/en/index.html (Accessed September 30, 2010).

---

[16] Barack Obama, Inaugural Address, January 20, 2009, www.whitehouse.gov/blog/inaugural-address.

Chapter 21

Biotechnology and global health

Hassan Masum, Justin Chakma and Abdallah S. Daar

Introduction

As the branch of science concerned with the application of biological processes for industrial, health and agricultural purposes, biotechnology joins nutritional science and biomedical engineering as a major application of science and technology for improving human health. But every new technology poses ethical issues. What are the current and potential benefits of the technology, and what are the risks? How can the profit motive be harnessed for technology development, while keeping humanitarian technologies affordable? How much should be invested in developing the technology, and how much in scaling up existing techniques?

This chapter shines a light on these ethical issues by describing how biotechnology might be employed to improve global health, and discussing factors to consider when thinking about risks and implementation. We begin with the example of smallpox and vaccines, and continue on to biotechnologies for applications such as diagnostics, micronutrients, clean water, bioremediation, drug delivery systems and therapies. (It is important to note that the potential longer-term health applications of biotechnology extend far beyond the current and near-term applications which are the focus of this chapter.)

The eradication of smallpox through the advent of vaccination is one of the great success stories of modern medicine and public health (Barquet & Domingo, 1997; Andre, 2002). Although the process of exposing a healthy person to infected materials, known as variolation, was commonly practiced in China, India and Turkey before the mid-fifteenth century, a significant proportion of those treated died from serious infection. It was not until 1789 that an English physician, Edward Jenner, observed that milkmaids who developed cowpox, a less serious disease, did not develop the deadly

smallpox. He extracted pus from blisters of milkmaids infected with cowpox, and inoculated first an 8 year old boy and subsequently a series of 23 subjects. Lack of modern microbiological methods, and caution on the part of the medical establishment, led to tolerance of variolation until free vaccinations could be provided by the British government in 1840.

In the following decades, governments around the world adopted and coordinated vaccination efforts. By 1979, the World Health Organization declared smallpox an eradicated disease. Since then, an estimated two million lives have been saved each year. Though no other major diseases have yet been eradicated, the global spread of vaccination for other diseases has saved millions more.

The story of smallpox illustrates the potential for a simple scientific observation to result in a novel technology that can save millions of lives. That it took over 500 years to scientifically ground and adapt the traditional medicinal approach of variolation, 50 years for the medical establishment to accept the findings, and almost another 150 years to finally coordinate eradication efforts, illustrates the magnitude of the challenges that face good health technologies during their translation and implementation. During that lag time, tens of millions died unnecessarily.

Today, we face the same challenges in many areas of global health. Roughly two million people died in 2008 from HIV/AIDS, many for lack of access to antiretroviral therapies (UNAIDS, 2009). While there has been significant progress in global vaccination prevalence, more millions still die from lack of access to basic childhood vaccinations (Lawn *et al.*, 2005).

The policy options and considerations required to overcome the challenges of developing, validating and delivering good health technologies are complex

Global Health and Global Health Ethics, ed. Solomon Benatar and Gillian Brock. Published by Cambridge University Press. © Cambridge University Press 2011.

(Singer *et al.*, 2007). To fund the discovery and development phases, drug and vaccine developers must be able to recoup their development costs. To enable delivery, health systems must be strengthened in the developing world, and logistics established in order for new health technologies to reach rural and high-risk communities. Across the discovery, development and delivery phases, successful translation of new technologies from "lab to village" requires coordination among multiple and diverse stakeholders.

Biotechnologies, which we define broadly as the use of biological processes for health, industrial and other purposes, clearly have the potential to make a positive impact on health. Yet the historical record shows that achieving a positive health outcome is more difficult than it appears. Evaluating risks for participants in scientific studies that validate health impact, achieving a consensus in the medical community to compel government action, creating the right funding incentives for affordable and low-cost biotechnology innovation and ensuring that delivery channels are effective are among many challenges. In the next section, we further explore these challenges, along with the potential of biotechnology for global health.

The potential of biotechnology for global health

Challenges and opportunities

A seminal year in the development of biotechnology as a scientific discipline was 1973, when two Californian scientists, Herbert Boyer and Stanley Cohen, building on the work of Paul Berg and others, discovered a method to create the first recombinant DNA organism – thus introducing "genetic engineering" to the modern lexicon (Russo, 2003). The biotechnology industry was born three years later in 1976 when Genentech, the first biotech company, was founded after Boyer's chance encounter with venture capitalist Robert Swanson. Since then the biotechnology industry has produced therapies for cancer, diabetes and many lesser-known ailments.

In agriculture, identification of mutant genes for staple crops such as rice has led to increasing yields and disease resistance, even when fertilizer, pesticides and irrigation are limited. The global biotech industry's revenue grew to almost $200 billion for health and agriculture combined by 2008, and the health of millions has benefited from its advances

(Ernst & Young, 2009). Indeed, the hyperbolic mantra adopted by the Biotechnology Industry Organization in recent years has been 'Heal, fuel, feed the world" (Marshall, 2008).

However, these benefits have not been equally enjoyed by those in the South. Most research in biotechnology focuses on the needs of industrialized nations, which is a manifestation of the "10/90 gap" whereby 90% of health research dollars are spent on the health problems of 10% of the world's population. In the first decade of the twenty-first century, traditional players in global health began to recognize this inequity of benefit. In 2002, the World Health Organization released a report titled "Genomics and World Health" that recommended that the WHO should develop capacity "to evaluate advances in genomics, to anticipate their potential for research and clinical application … and to assess their effectiveness and cost in comparison to current practice" (WHO, 2002).

In a separate project, scientific experts from the developing world were surveyed to identify the biotechnology applications potentially most suited to improving health in developing countries (Daar *et al.*, 2002). Biotechnologies were evaluated on the basis of impact, appropriateness, meeting the health burden, feasibility, knowledge gap and indirect benefits such as environmental improvement or economic development.

The most highly rated category was for "Modified molecular technologies for affordable simple diagnosis of infectious disease." The choice is illustrative. First, early, accurate diagnosis of disease can result in prompt treatment, limitation of spread of disease and customization of treatment regimes. Second, these molecular diagnostic technologies already exist in the industrialized world, incorporating sophisticated techniques such as polymerase chain reaction or monoclonal antibodies at centralized laboratories – but the technologies are inappropriate for low-resource settings. The technologies can be made more relevant to the developing world and global health indications by designing the system to employ simpler processes, less expensive materials, and platforms more easily adaptable to settings without running water, refrigeration or electricity (Yager *et al.*, 2008).

The second most highly rated category was for "Recombinant technologies to develop vaccines against infectious diseases." Recombinant vaccine technologies have been critical for disease management in developing countries. Prevention of disease through vaccination can save many times the health-care costs that would be required for treatment. Vaccines do not require sophisticated staff to administer, and are portable. The principal barrier to the adoption of recombinant vaccines has been pricing.

These vaccines can be made more relevant to the developing world by manufacturing the vaccines at lower cost in the developing world itself, thus providing a cheaper alternative to the standard imported vaccines. In the 1970s and 1980s, the price of imported recombinant hepatitis B vaccine was as high as $23 per dose, in countries like India where the majority of the population earned under $1 a day (Frost & Reich, 2009). Few had considered sourcing vaccines from the "global South." Shantha Biotechnics, an Indian biotech firm founded in 1993, saw a market opportunity and developed its own hepatitis B vaccine – one of the first home-grown recombinant products in India. Shantha's vaccine was pre-qualified by the World Health Organization, and triggered a price drop in the Indian market to $0.25 (Chakma et al., 2010).

These two examples of molecular diagnostics and recombinant vaccines show that biotechnology can be highly relevant to the needs of the world's poor. The control of infectious disease can be considerably facilitated by molecular diagnostics and recombinant vaccines. Other biotechnologies such as immunotherapies can aid the treatment of chronic non-communicable diseases – a class of illness which accounts for roughly 60% of all deaths worldwide (Daar et al., 2007).

The main challenge for the top two biotechnologies discussed above was not in basic science, but in adapting existing technology to a low-resource setting, or sourcing the technology more cost-effectively. Given these challenges, it may be that developing countries are advantageous locations for biotechnology innovation because of their geographic proximity to the problem at hand, and lower development and labor costs. By adapting biotechnology solutions locally, developing countries can not only increase the chances of successful adaptation to their own needs, thereby reducing health costs – they can also build a talented base of human capital, attract increased investment capital, and promote economic development (Frew et al., 2007, 2008; Al-Bader et al., 2009; Rezaie et al., 2008).

A recent precedent is Shantha Biotechnics, which was acquired by Sanofi-Aventis in 2009 at a valuation of ~US$784 million. Since its successful introduction of low-cost hepatitis B vaccine in the late 1990s, the firm has brought 11 products successfully to market, and now maintains a product pipeline that includes

pentavalent vaccines for which UNICEF has given a 350 million dose order in 2009. Shantha achieved this international valuation and market success by first focusing on the local health needs of India, and then on health needs elsewhere in developing countries.

Potential for curing disease

Beyond vaccine development, biotechnology has produced new therapies in infectious disease, cancer and autoimmune disorders, and developed recombinant versions of biologics for diabetes and growth disorders. However, it has yet to deliver on the promised cures of genetic therapies, or even the wide adoption of molecularly targeted medicine, with a few exceptions such as Novartis' Gleevec for chronic myeloid leukemia. Its record in the developing world is also mixed, with successes in the Green Revolution leading to increased food production juxtaposed with failures thus far to deliver cures for neglected tropical diseases.

A background question that looms is how much emphasis should be placed on improving access to high-quality and low-cost health care using existing technologies, and how much on investing in new technological advances that may improve health capabilities in the long term. Aravind Eye Hospital, for example, performs low-cost or free cataract surgeries for poor Indians (Miller, 2006). Through the construction of a lens factory and innovative management and business models, Aravind Eye Hospital is able to profitably serve thousands of very poor Indians. Aravind performs 300 000 eye surgeries per year, including cataract surgeries that cost as much as $3000 per procedure in the USA. By simply adapting and streamlining existing surgical strategies, and coupling them to smart, low-cost business practices and enabling technologies such as telehealth to reach rural communities, Aravind achieves a significant health impact.

That said, the question of investing in scaling up proven solutions versus investing in innovation is not an either–or one – both can be done. Although there have been no blockbuster successes for global health to date aside from vaccines, there is a promising pipeline of biotechnology-based platforms. We describe three with broad applicability below.

Molecular diagnostics

Diagnosis is the first step to treatment. The developing world does not have access to many of the best medical diagnostic technologies (Yager et al., 2006). Such technologies were designed assuming air-conditioned laboratories, refrigerated storage of chemicals, a constant supply of calibrators and reagents, stable electrical power, highly trained personnel and rapid transportation of samples. Microfluidic systems coupled with biotechnology have allowed for point-of-care diagnostics that can evaluate patients without the need for an expert operator. Moreover, they are being developed to return same-day test results so that patients can receive appropriate therapy while they are still at the clinic. Immunochromatographic strips (ICS) have been one of the very few diagnostic technologies to be successfully used in the developing world. They are stable at ambient temperatures for more than a year, and can be shipped without refrigeration. The ICS tests developed by PATH with support from the United States Agency for International Development (USAID) can diagnose diphtheria toxin, and a number of sexually transmitted infections (STIs), including gonorrhea, syphilis, chancroid, and chlamydia, and *Plasmodium falciparum* malaria (Yager *et al.*, 2006).

Efficient drug and vaccine delivery systems

More efficient drug and vaccine delivery systems could help to reduce costs and improve health outcomes (Vogelson, 2001; Salamanca-Buentello *et al.*, 2005). From both financial and global health care perspectives, finding ways to administer currently injectable-only medications in oral form is needed, as is finding ways of delivering costly, multiple-dose, long-term therapies in inexpensive, potent, and time-releasing or self-triggering formulations. The promise of administration methods that allow patients to safely treat themselves is significant, particularly in developing countries where doctors, clean syringes, sterile needles and sophisticated treatments can be in short supply.

Recombinant process innovations

A key barrier to the adoption of new therapeutics is the high cost associated with the intellectual property of not only the active compound itself, but also of manufacturing processes for actually producing the compound. By employing novel methods of manufacturing that may be more efficient and cost-effective, firms are able to reduce the cost of the drug. For example, Shantha implemented a process innovation to produce interferon alpha 2-b in *Pichia pastoris*, enabling inexpensive commercial production of this molecule in yeast rather than the traditional bacterial system (Shekar, 2008). Shantha was one of the first biotechnology companies

to produce erythropoietin in serum-free media, which quelled safety concerns regarding serum use in manufacturing. This opened the door for more affordable and higher quality therapeutics accessible to the poor.

Potential for preventing disease

A less expensive way of improving health outcomes compared with curing disease is to take preventive measures through biotechnologies that facilitate vaccination, clean water supplies and nutrition. Improvements in these areas have the potential to ameliorate living conditions in low-income regions worldwide, and their importance is recognized in the Millennium Development Goals.

Vaccines

Vaccines have been one of the main success stories for biotechnology. Many millions of doses of vaccines are dispensed every year for polio, rotavirus, Hepatitis B and others in developing countries. Many of these doses are dispensed as a result of efforts of Southern manufacturers to reduce costs. Millions of lives have been saved as a result (Levine & Kinder, 2004), and vaccines have been valuable to individuals and societies in a variety of ways (Andre *et al.*, 2008). More recent advances have allowed multivalent vaccines that increase efficiency by inoculation for multiple diseases in a single dose. Efforts are underway to develop vaccines for malaria, tuberculosis and HIV/AIDS. The most promising advance to date occurred in 2009 with Phase 3 human clinical trials commencing for RTS,S/AS02, or Mosquirix, which was originally developed by GlaxoSmithKline in the mid 1980s (Malaria Vaccine Initiative, 2009). The vaccine seemed to significantly reduce severe malaria (49%) and clinical disease (35%) in African children. These trials will involve seven African countries, including 11 medical research institutes and 16 000 infants younger than 17 months. Results will be available in 2012, and if positive the vaccine may be available for widescale use by 2015.

Clean water

Bioremediation has become one of the most rapidly developing fields of environmental restoration, utilizing microorganisms to reduce the concentration and toxicity of various chemical pollutants (Dua *et al.*, 2002). Many pesticides once used in massive amounts have long half-lives. For example, DDT has a half-life of 3–10 years. In developing countries with poor systems or unenforced regulations for controlling chemical pollutants, microorganisms can remove the large quantities of waste that are continually introduced into soil and water systems. Microorganisms have the potential to be genetically engineered to improve their efficiency and effectiveness in degrading or absorbing this waste to reduce water pollution. Biotechnology techniques such as biosurfactants, which are surface-active microbial products, have also been incorporated into production processes to lower energy and water consumption, improve productivity and reduce the number of processing steps. Many diseases of the South such as cholera spread through water systems, and low-cost technologies for providing clean water will thus have an immediate positive health impact.

Micronutrients

Deficiencies of micronutrients such as iron, zinc and vitamin A afflict over 2 billion people – most of them women and children in resource-poor families in the developing world. Over 1 million children die each year as a result of vitamin A and zinc deficiencies alone (Micronutrient Initiative, 2009). This global crisis is the result of dysfunctional food systems that do not consistently supply enough of these essential nutrients to meet the nutritional requirements of high-risk groups. Deficiencies of micronutrients result in increased morbidity and mortality rates, lost worker productivity, stagnated national development, permanent impairment of cognitive development in infants and children, and large economic costs and suffering to those societies affected (Welch & Graham, 1999). Breeding strategies coupled to genetic modification can be used either separately or in combination to improve the utilizable micronutrient content in staple food crops, by increasing the total content in the plant portion eaten, decreasing the amounts of antinutrients present in the plant food, and increasing the amounts of promoter substances in the plant food to counteract the negative effects of antinutrients such as phytic acid.

Golden Rice provides a cautionary tale in using biotechnology to address micronutrient deficiencies. It is a variety of rice engineered to produce beta-carotene (pro-vitamin A) to help combat vitamin A deficiency, and it has been predicted that its contribution to alleviating vitamin A deficiency would be substantially improved through even higher beta-carotene content (Paine et al., 2005). Vitamin A deficiency is a major problem in the developing world that can result in permanent blindness, and increased incidence and severity of other diseases. In Asia, vitamin A deficiency is associated with the poverty-related predominant consumption of rice, which lacks pro-vitamin A in the edible part of the grain (endosperm). Providing pro-vitamin A could complement supplementation programs focused on micronutrients. However, Golden Rice experienced a backlash when introduced due to cultural factors and public concerns (Enserink, 2008).

This section explored the potential of biotechnology for global health. The next section discusses factors to consider when thinking about biotechnology's risks and implementation.

Considerations in thinking about biotechnology

Cautions

The promise of biotechnology comes with many caveats. Bioremediation technologies are still in early stages of development, and there are concerns regarding the safety of introducing new microorganisms into the environment with their potential to disrupt ecosystems. Although there are hundreds of thousands of hectares of genetically modified (GM) crops being grown around the world, they are not yet fully addressing key agricultural problems for poor farmers, such as salinity, desertification and drought. Nor have they yet achieved their potential in addressing problems such as malnutrition. For the moment, there are only a handful of GM strains available for staple foods widely cultivated in developing countries, other than corn. Many nations in Africa have a ban on GM seeds.

For health care, health education is integral to the control of the AIDS pandemic, as is the provision and use of male condoms. Improvements in sanitation can markedly reduce the incidence of water-borne diseases, and basic nutritional education can help prevent nutrient deficiencies. These tools are available now, whereas new biotechnologies are in varying stages of development.

Still, there is increasing evidence of the potential of these biotechnologies for improving the health of people in developing countries, accompanied by significant calls for policy support. The report "Freedom to Innovate: Biotechnology in Africa's Development" brought together an eminent panel at the request of heads of state to explore how "to harness and apply biotechnologies to improve agricultural productivity, public health, industrial development, economic competitiveness, and environmental sustainability" (Juma & Serageldin, 2007). It suggested the important role that biotechnological innovation can play in both health impacts and economic transformation.

We ought, therefore, to strive to achieve an appropriate balance between developing such technologies and utilizing conventional strategies. This is not an easy task, but to ignore the potential of biotechnology is not the answer, when there is strong evidence of its usefulness. Part of this balance will involve the appreciation that these technologies can be used to improve conventional public health strategies such as vaccines and sanitation. We cannot conceive health as a product of technical interventions divorced from economic, social and political contexts.

Below we discuss three tensions to keep in mind when thinking about biotechnology.

Safe versus risky

"Safe biotechnologies" such as the vaccines for childhood diseases discussed earlier are accepted by a large majority of populations. (However, this acceptance is far from universal, as recent experiences in polio eradication campaigns show (Jegede, 2007).) In contrast, "risky biotechnologies" are perceived by broad segments of the public to include agricultural biotechnology (Grace, 2006) and germline therapy (Stock, 2003).

The essential distinction is that safe technologies have benefits much greater than their costs, and risks which are low relative to benefits. Risk levels can also reasonably be bounded based on past experience. For example, the experience of vaccination over the past several decades, along with an understanding of the basic science relevant to vaccines, shows that vaccinating a population does not lead to unexpected side effects like mysterious illnesses and plagues – at least, not in significant amounts. In contrast, for some agricultural biotechnologies, it is not clear what risks are posed for ecosystems. A similar tradeoff between cost, benefit and risk is playing out with other technologies like robotics and nanotechnology.

The precautionary principle has been one approach to dealing with technologies perceived as risky. It has been formulated in a variety of ways. One states that uncertainty in the consequences of a technology should not automatically preclude regulatory action; another that, when threats of serious or irreversible consequences exist, scientific uncertainty should not postpone cost-effective mitigation or risk-assessment measures. Many historical examples have been documented where acting on the precautionary principle would have mitigated technological harms (Harremoës et al., 2002).

One helpful tool to make rational judgments would be the availability of honest, comprehensible and accurate risk analysis for new biotechnologies. This might be accompanied by the development of "dashboards" which visually summarize the forces shaping the development and adoption of health technologies, and the collective use of such dashboards by interested parties and the public at large (Masum & Singer, 2007).

Affordable versus profitable

The affordability of drugs to combat common diseases of the poor has become a major international policy issue over the last decade, with aspects including funding options (Hecht et al., 2009) and intellectual property policies (Netanel, 2009). Both humanitarian impulses and governmental responsibilities demand that health care be made available to all.

At the same time, the development of new drugs and therapies is a long and complex process, and thus often expensive. Absent donor or government funding, which has not alone been successful in taking many new therapies from concept all the way to market, private investment is required – and investors naturally consider the risk and profitability of potential investments.

The affordability versus profitability debate plays out in many ways in the development of new biotechnology. In the development of new biotechnology, the question of how to incentivize private investors has had a profound impact on intellectual property regimes, with biotechnology companies and industry associations advocating the necessity of strong legal protection for the products of the investments they make. Others have argued that overly stringent intellectual property protection can hinder short-term affordability and the long-term "intellectual commons" on which new product development rests (Heller, 2008). In the delivery of existing biotechnologies to those who need them, companies which have invested large amounts of capital naturally wish to recoup their investments through what they consider fair pricing – but NGOs, Southern governments, and commentators have advocated for reduced pricing and compulsory licensing for therapies needed to combat "humanitarian emergencies."

There is no simple answer to this debate. However, options exist to advance the debate itself to focus on shedding more light than heat. In the short term, advocates of each point of view might do well to understand the point of view of the other. In the longer term, there might be value in common and transparent cost–benefit tools which clarify the costs various parties would pay under differing regimes, and the corresponding short- and long-term benefits to all parties. More could be learnt from experiments with novel intellectual property and licensing arrangements (Brewster et al., 2005). A better understanding of the effects and processes of the intellectual property regime itself could also help all parties to benefit from it (Krattiger et al., 2007).

In considering costs and affordability of biotechnology, one must consider who benefits: individually, between organizations and between regions. This leads to the concept of the "social value" of a technology, i.e. the aggregate value a population gains from a technology as measured not financially, but with reference to some commonly accepted set of human well-being measures. Social value is difficult to measure, but very real – for example, society is better off with Wikipedia and other quasi public good technologies, even if no one is making large profits out of them (Benkler, 2006).

Social value is distinct from the monetary value typically counted in income and GDP statements. Monetary value (as measured, for example, by the profits of a biotechnology company) measures only the transactional value of a technology, and does not directly consider its other impacts on human well-being. An ethical approach to investing in biotechnology that starts with equity as a core principle might aim to maximize social value, while recognizing that monetary value and profits are not negative in and of themselves. Indeed, technology investments motivated by monetary profits can lead to social value both through the new technologies they generate, and though macroeconomic benefits from the employment and investments they create.

This line of thinking suggests that the motivations of those who partake in biotechnology innovation are relevant to the kinds of biotechnology that are encouraged and developed. Salk's retort when asked who owned the patent for his polio vaccine was, "There is no patent. Could you patent the sun?" (Mahoney et al.,

2004). While such pure altruism may be difficult in an era when biotechnology advances require large infusions of private funds, many for-profit institutions have seen the value and motivational potential of devoting part of their efforts toward global health issues on a cost-recovery basis (BVGH, 2009). The increasing availability of R&D funds targeted toward research in diseases of the poor also helps researchers to "do well by doing good."

Present versus future

At any given point in time, human society possesses a stock of technological know-how – a toolkit which can be drawn from to solve problems and improve the human condition. Knowing how to make effective vaccines makes the average human life today markedly longer and more healthy than in past generations.

Yet the stock of technological know-how is not implemented or distributed evenly. Many technologies that are known today have not been developed into practical health solutions, and many such solutions are unavailable to the bulk of the global population. How much of society's focus should be on making known health solutions more available, and how much on researching new health solutions that might improve the toolkit of future generations? (This same question is present in many areas outside of health, and perhaps most starkly in sustainability dilemmas: how much should be invested in climate change reduction today, and how much in potential new low-carbon technologies for the future?)

The development of Southern health innovation capacity illustrates one way in which the question of relative focus is being answered. While one might think that developing countries should focus most of their energies on scaling up the delivery of existing treatments to meet immediate needs, increasing resources are being invested into the development of indigenous innovation capacity. This is being done for a variety of reasons, including the availability of partnerships and research funds from wealthy countries, a desire to create local research capacity and skilled jobs, concerns about dependence on foreign suppliers for critical health supplies and a recognition that local investments today can lead to less expensive treatments in the near future. Local investments into "affordable innovation" are increasingly taking place in China, India, Brazil, South Africa, Kenya and elsewhere (Frew et al., 2009).

The eradication of smallpox is paying back "innovation dividends" forever on our past investments into health research and delivery – investments which seemed large at the time, but which in hindsight no one would claim were wasted. Polio is experiencing a similar debate today with respect to paying for complete elimination as compared with effective control. Looking back at our past may be a guide to how to think about investments into our future well-being.

Conclusion

Biotechnology has already shown its value for global health, and has considerable potential for developing better therapies in the future. At the same time, the pursuit of biotechnology does not automatically lead to health benefits, and may indeed risk harms. Three aspects of this tension have been discussed, to suggest principles for how to think about the potential health benefits of new biotechnology.

Biotechnology is far from being a panacea. It should be considered as one tool in a larger public health toolkit, which runs the gamut from simple methods like popularizing handwashing to high-tech solutions at the frontier of science. Social determinants of health, economic and political equity, and a variety of other factors considered in this book all play a role.

At the same time, biotechnology has a special status as the branch of applied science which deals most directly with manipulating the constituent elements of life itself for human benefit. The development of vaccines has dramatically improved and will continue to improve the health status of entire societies – initially in the developed world, but now worldwide through global initiatives like GAVI (the Global Alliance for Vaccines and Immunization).

The broader potential of biotechnology can be tapped for further advances in human well-being, if ethical principles guide the development, implementation and distribution of new solutions. Along with the considerations discussed above, there may be principles to be learned from other new technologies. Nanotechnology, water filtration, robotics, LED lights, solar stoves ... the list of new technologies relevant to health is long, and ranges from simple to disruptive advances. By understanding the ethical debates and tensions of each, transferable lessons may be learned for biotechnology (and indeed for dealing with new technologies in general). An example of this cross-technology learning is the consideration of a spectrum of technology-driven "catastrophic risks," along with mitigating policies (Bostrom & Cirkovic, 2008).

The achievements of biotechnology in global health to date, while significant, are only a foreshadowing of its future potential. Genomics may lead to both personalized treatment and a much-improved understanding of disease mechanisms. Developments in stem cell biology and regenerative medicine could introduce a wide range of new therapies and cures. Energy-efficient bio-manufacturing and production of biofuels can mitigate both climate change and pollution. Given the relentless march forward of science, developing answers that guide the development of biotechnology in humane directions is both a practical necessity and a moral imperative.

References

Al-Bader, S., Frew, S. E., Essajee, I. *et al.* (2009). Small but tenacious: South Africa's health biotech sector. *Nature Biotechnology* **27**, 427–445.

Andre, F. E. (2002). Vaccinology: past achievements, present roadblocks and future promise. *Vaccine* **21**, 593–595.

Andre, F. E., Booy, R., Bock, H. L. *et al.* (2008). Vaccination greatly reduces disease, disability, death and inequity worldwide. *WHO Bulletin* **86**(2), 81–160.

Barquet, N. & Domingo, P. (1997). Smallpox: the triumph over the most terrible of the ministers of death. *Annals of Internal Medicine* **127**(8), 635–642.

Benkler, Y. (2006). *The Wealth of Networks: How Social Production Transforms Markets and Freedom*. New Haven, CT: Yale University Press.

Bostrom, N. & Cirkovic, M. M. (Eds.) (2008). *Global Catastrophic Risks*. Oxford: Oxford University Press.

Brewster, A. L., Chapman, A. R. & Hansen, S. A. (2005). Facilitating humanitarian access to pharmaceutical and agricultural innovation. *Innovation Strategy Today* **1**(3), 203–216.

BVGH (2009). *Global Health Innovators: A Collection of Case Studies*. Washington, DC: BIO Ventures for Global Health Report.

Chakma, J., Masum, H., Perampaladas, K., Heys, J. & Singer, P. A. (2010). India's billion dollar biotech in the developing world. *Nature Biotechnology* **28**, 783.

Daar, A. S., Thorsteinsdottir, H., Martin, D. K. *et al.* (2002). Top ten biotechnologies for improving health in developing countries. *Nature Genetics* **32**, 229–232.

Daar, A. S., Singer, P. A., Persad, D. L. *et al.* (2007). Grand challenges in chronic non-communicable diseases. *Nature* **450**, 494–496.

Dua, M., Singh, A., Sethunathan, N. *et al.* (2002). Biotechnology and bioremediation: successes and limitations. *Applied Microbiology and Biotechnology* **59**, 143–152.

Enserink, M. (2008). Tough lessons from golden rice. *Science* **320**(5875), 468–471.

Ernst & Young (2009). *Beyond Borders: Global Biotechnology Report*. London: Ernst & Young.

Frew, S. E., Rezaie, R., Sammut, S. M. *et al.* (2007). India's health biotech sector at a crossroads. *Nature Biotechnology* **25**(4), 403–417.

Frew, S. E., Sammut, S. M., Shore, A. F. *et al.* (2008). Chinese health biotech and the billion-patient market. *Nature Biotechnology* **26**, 37–53.

Frew, S. E., Liu, V. Y. & Singer, P. A. (2009). A business plan to help the "global south" in its fight against neglected diseases. *Health Affairs* **28**(6), 1760–1773.

Frost, L. J. & Reich, M. R. (2009). *Access: How do Good Health Technologies get to Poor People in Poor Countries?* Cambridge, MA: Harvard University Press.

Grace, E. S. (2006). *Biotechnology Unzipped: Promises and Realities*. (2nd edn.) Washington, DC: Joseph Henry Press.

Harremoës, P., Gee, D., Macgarvin, M. *et al.* (Eds.) (2002). *The Precautionary Principle in the 20th Century: Late Lessons from Early Warnings*. London: Earthscan Publications.

Hecht, R., Wilson, P. & Palriwala, A. (2009). Improving health R&D financing for developing countries: a menu of innovative policy options. *Health Affairs* **28**(4), 974–985.

Heller, M. (2008). *The Gridlock Economy: How Too Much Ownership Wrecks Markets, Stops Innovation, and Costs Lives*. New York: Basic Books.

Jegede, A. S. (2007). What led to the Nigerian boycott of the polio vaccination campaign? *PLoS Medicine* **4**(3), e73.

Juma, C. & Serageldin, I. (2007). *Freedom to Innovate: Biotechnology in Africa's Development*. Report of the High-Level African Panel on Modern Biotechnology, African Union and NEPAD (New Partnership for Africa's Development).

Krattiger, A., Mahoney, R. T., Nelsen, L. *et al.* (Eds.) (2007). *Intellectual Property Management in Health and Agricultural Innovation: A Handbook of Best Practices*. MIHR (Oxford), PIPRA (Davis, CA), Oswaldo Cruz Foundation (Fiocruz, Rio de Janeiro) and bioDevelopments-International Institute (Ithaca, NY).

Lawn, J. E., Cousens, S. & Zupan, J. (2005). 4 million neonatal deaths: When? Where? Why? *Lancet* **365**(9462), 891–900.

Levine, R. & Kinder, M. (2004). *Millions Saved: Proven Successes in Global Health*. Washington, DC: Center for Global Development.

Mahoney, R. T., Pablos-Mendez, A. & Ramachandran, S. (2004). The introduction of new vaccines into developing countries, III: The role of intellectual property. *Vaccine* **22**(5–6), 786–792.

Malaria Vaccine Initiative (2009). World's largest malaria vaccine trial now underway in seven African countries. www.malariavaccine.org/files/1122009_RTSSP3PressRelease_FINAL.pdf. (Accessed on January 15, 2010, archived at www.webcitation.org/5mnFJzDkk on December 15, 2010).

Marshall, A. (2008). Join the dots. *Nature Biotechnology* **26**, 837.

Masum, H. & Singer, P. A. (2007). A visual dashboard for moving health technologies from "lab to village". *Journal of Medical Internet Research* **9**(4), e32.

Micronutrient Initiative (2009). *Investing in the Future: A United Call to Action on Vitamin and Mineral Deficiencies*. Micronutrient Initiative. www.unitedcalltoaction.org/documents/Investing_in_the_future.pdf (Accessed January 15, 2010, archived at www.webcitation.org/5n1h45iUy on January 15, 2010).

Miller, S. (2006). McSurgery: a man who saved 2.4 million eyes. *Wall Street Journal* (August 5, 2006). www.aravind.org/tribute/A%20Man%20Who%20Saved%202.4%20Million%20Eyes.pdf (Accessed December 8, 2009, archived at www.webcitation.org/5lrXwNm8B on December 8, 2009).

Netanel, N. W. (Ed.). (2009). *The Development Agenda: Global Intellectual Property and Developing Countries*. Oxford: Oxford University Press.

Paine, J. A., Shipton, C. A., Chaggar, S. *et al.* (2005). Improving the nutritional value of Golden Rice through increased pro-vitamin A content. *Nature Biotechnology* **23**, 482–487.

Rezaie, R., Frew, S. E., Sammut, S. M. *et al.* (2008). Brazilian health biotech – fostering crosstalk between public and private sectors. *Nature Biotechnology* **26**, 627–644.

Russo, E. (2003). The birth of biotechnology. *Nature* **421**, 456–457.

Salamanca-Buentello, F., Persad, D. L., Court, E. B. *et al.* (2005). Nanotechnology and the developing world. *PLoS Medicine* **2**(5), e97.

Shekhar, C. (2008). Pichia power: India's biotech industry puts unconventional yeast to work. *Chemistry and Biology* **15**(3), 201–202.

Singer, P. A., Berndtson, K., Tracy, C. S. *et al.* (2007). A tough transition. *Nature* **449**, 160–163.

Stock, G. (2003). *Redesigning Humans: Choosing our Genes, Changing our Future*. Boston, MA: Houghton Mifflin.

UNAIDS (2009). *AIDS Epidemic Update: November 2009*. Joint United Nations Programme on HIV/AIDS (UNAIDS) and World Health Organization (WHO). Geneva: UNAIDS.

Vogelson, C. T. (2001). Advances in drug delivery systems. *Modern Drug Discovery* 4(4), 49–50.

Welch, R. M. & Graham, R. D. (1999). A new paradigm for world agriculture: meeting human needs – productive, sustainable, nutritious. *Field Crop Research* **60**, 1–10.

World Health Organization (WHO) (2002). *Genomics and World Health: Report of the Advisory Committee on Health Research*. Geneva: World Health Organization.

Yager, P., Edwards, T., Fu, E. *et al.* (2006). Microfluidic diagnostic technologies for global public health. *Nature* **442**, 412–418.

Yager, P., Domingo, G. J. & Gerdes, J. (2008). Point-of-care diagnostics for global health. *Annual Review of Biomedical Engineering* **10**, 107–144.

Chapter 22

Food security and global health

Lynn McIntyre and Krista Rondeau

Introduction

Food is a basic human right.[1] It is also a lens through which we can observe and measure progress in health as well as the protection of human dignity. In 2000, the United Nations (UN) agreed to eight Millennium Development Goals (MDGs). The first goal (MDG 1) was the eradication of extreme poverty and hunger by 2015. To achieve the food security dividend, as we have called it, we need to think about the world as it is in terms of hungry people and about what is most needed if global food security is to be achieved. This chapter examines the issue of food security and global health. The link between the two is obvious – if we achieved food security for all, we would advance the prospects of global health for all, arguably beyond any other single intervention.

What is food security?

It is helpful to begin with clarification of terms. The 1996 Rome Declaration on Food Security states, "food security exists when all people, at all times, have physical and economic access to sufficient safe and nutritious food to meet their dietary needs and food preferences for a healthy and active life." Food insecurity is a lack of food security. The Food and Agriculture Organization (FAO) uses the words "hunger," "undernourishment," and "food insecurity" interchangeably (FAO, 2009a).

Food insecurity is a term that is applied at a range of levels from the individual through to global. At least for the individual, household, and community levels, food insecurity is intimately tied to inadequate income for acquiring food – those who are hungry are so because they cannot afford to buy the food they need. National food insecurity is often discussed in association with food sovereignty – the ability of a nation state to feed its citizens. Although food insecurity exists in all countries, rich and poor, global food security is primarily concerned with its disproportionate existence in lower-income countries, where poverty is deep and hunger and malnutrition are pervasive and often lethal.[2]

This chapter begins with a brief historical context for the goal of global food security and highlights the situation of hunger today. We then present five "Grand Challenges" to food security, followed by an analysis of the ethical dilemmas that accompany the most promising interventions to combat these challenges, and recommendations to achieve global food security. In so doing, we try to provide a balanced view, rather than persuade the reader on the merits of one set of perspectives over another.

A modern historical account of global food insecurity

In October 1945, the Food and Agriculture Organization of the United Nations was formed with its key objective being the elimination of hunger and

---

[1] The right to food is found in article 25 of the United Nations' (UN) Universal Declaration of Human Rights: "Everyone has the right to a standard of living adequate for the health and well-being of himself and of his family, including food, clothing, housing and medical care and necessary social services, and the right to security in the event of unemployment, sickness, disability, widowhood, old age or other lack of livelihood in circumstances beyond his control."

[2] We prefer the terms higher-income countries (rather than "developed" countries) and lower- and middle-income countries (rather than "developing" countries).

Global Health and Global Health Ethics, ed. Solomon Benatar and Gillian Brock. Published by Cambridge University Press.
© Cambridge University Press 2011.

starvation throughout the world. At the end of the Second World War, it was reported that approximately two-thirds of the world's population was undernourished (Waggoner, 1945), and this was perceived as a serious impediment to the maintenance of lasting world peace. A historical account of the occurrence of global food insecurity reveals that during the first half of the twentieth century, the world's most industrialized and wealthy countries experienced food shortages as a result of "crop failures linked to droughts, rising demand for food as a result of income growth, commodity and currency speculation, inflation, trade constraints (in the form of steep tariffs imposed by governments to deal with the crisis), and low productivity due to widespread lack of access to credit, limited use of fertilizer (due to supply constraints), and scarce investments in the seeds, extension, or technology used by [lower-income] country smallholders" (Webb, 2010, p. S1).

From the 1950s onward, imminent food crises spurred significant innovation and investment in research, policies, and practices (notably improved seeds, fertilizers, pesticides and heavy agricultural equipment) that favored intensification over expansion as the primary production growth strategy (Hazell & Wood, 2008).[3] Increased food production through scientific innovation, efficient distribution, and the elimination of global trade barriers were perceived to be important ways to move forward on the FAO's objective. By the end of the twentieth century, a first for the history of humankind, famines – widespread food shortages linked to insufficient production (as opposed to income inequalities) – were largely eliminated due to improvements in agriculture, infrastructure, technology and globalized markets (Hazell & Wood, 2008).

Movement towards the achievement of the FAO's objective greatly accelerated during the first half of the 1970s during what was called the Green Revolution. Large and significant public investments in the agricultural sector for scientific research, rural roads and irrigation translated into increased yields, decreased food prices, and a subsequent decrease in number and proportion of people who were chronically undernourished and food insecure (McMichael et al., 2007; FAO, 2009a; Webb, 2010). Improvements in maternal and child nutrition and health status, as well as increases in life expectancy followed in many regions as a result of the food security dividend of this time period (McMichael et al., 2007). What is noteworthy is that these gains were achieved even as the world's population was growing.

Because of decades of significant public investments in scientific research for agriculture (McMichael et al., 2007; Hazell & Wood, 2008) and attention to global food security, those living in higher-income countries generally enjoy a safe, stable and affordable food supply complemented with comprehensive social welfare policies designed to ensure that those who cannot afford to buy food are provided with some protection.[4] However, since the mid/late 1990s, the number of people who are chronically hungry has been slowly rising, attributed in large part to worldwide reductions in official development assistance devoted to agriculture – from approximately 19% in 1980 to 3.8% in 2006 (FAO, 2009a, 2009b; United Nations, 2009; Webb, 2010). Accordingly, there has been a reversal of global food security gains and an increase in the prevalence of hunger (FAO, 2009a).

Overview of the state of global food security

At the end of 2009, the FAO (2009a) released its tenth report on the state of food insecurity in the world since the adoption of the MDGs. Projections for 2009 estimate that 1.02 billion people, or nearly one-sixth of the world's population, are hungry and undernourished.[5] Figure 22.1 presents the distribution of global food insecurity today, and Figure 22.2 presents the trend in hunger since the nadir of the 1970s.

---

[3] Historically, countries addressed increased food demands through expansion (Hazell & Wood, 2008). The most proximal and fertile lands were cultivated first, and as these became scarce, cultivation expanded to less productive lands and fallow-based cultivation techniques were used (Hazell & Wood, 2008). Eventually, more area was required to acquire food for growing populations, and colonization became a way for many European nations to expand their supply of food (Hazell & Wood, 2008).

[4] Despite social welfare policies and programming, food insecurity does exist in higher-income countries. For example, 9.2% of Canadian households were food insecure in 2004 (Health Canada, 2007) and 14.6% of American households were food insecure in 2008 (Nord et al., 2009).

[5] The FAO uses the terms hunger and undernourished to refer to the condition when an individual's caloric intake is below their minimum dietary energy requirement (FAO, 2009a).

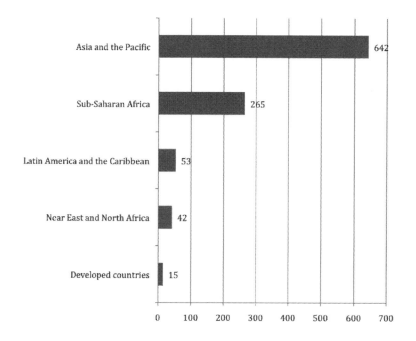

Figure 22.1 Undernourishment in 2009, by region (millions). *Source*: FAO (2009a, p. 11).

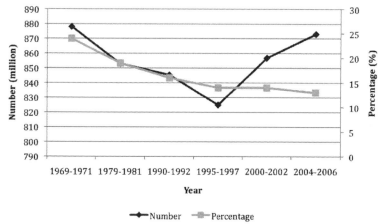

Figure 22.2 Number and percentage of undernourished persons in the world, 1969–71 to 2004–06. *Source*: FAO (2009c).

At the present time, global food insecurity is largely a result of the lack of affordability of food for the poor. The Economic Research Service (ERS) of the United States Department of Agriculture (USDA) compiled household consumption expenditures spent on food consumed at home (ERS/USDA, 2008). Consumers in lower- and middle-income countries devote a considerably greater proportion of their household income to food than consumers in higher-income countries. Residents of the USA, Canada, and the UK, for example, devote less than 10% of their household income to food. Conversely, in Nigeria, Indonesia and Pakistan, more than 40% of household income is dedicated to food. Consequently, these households have less income for essential expenditures such as health care, housing, education and fuel and are, in the end, much more vulnerable to income shocks.

Indeed, the recent world food crisis (2006–08) and the subsequent global economic recession (2008) pushed many people into deep poverty and, inevitably, hunger because they were unable to buy even the most basic food staples. Although the world as a whole currently produces enough food to feed its entire population, more than 1 billion people are hungry because they cannot afford to purchase available food. The UN has estimated that between 55 and 90 million additional people will be living in extreme poverty in 2009 (less than $1.25/day [2005 purchasing power parity]) because of these crises. Furthermore, provisional estimates indicate an increase in the prevalence of food insecurity in lower-income countries in 2008 (17%) compared to 2004–06 (16%) (United Nations, 2009).

In the face of the 2006–08 world food crisis and global recession, impoverished households were indeed obliged to decrease the amount of money spent on health care, education and other non-food items (FAO, 2008). They have also coped by compromising the quality and quantity of food they can buy, increasing their consumption of nutrient-poor grains and starchy staples and decreasing their intake of more expensive, nutrient-rich foods such as milk, meat, fruits and vegetables. As shown in Figure 22.2, the result is the largest number of hungry and undernourished people in the world since 1970 (FAO, 2009a), with concurrent implications for poor health.

Global food insecurity and health

The World Food Program (WFP) asserts that "hunger and malnutrition are … the number one risks to health worldwide – greater than AIDS, malaria and tuberculosis combined" (WFP, 2009a). Because diverse and nutritionally balanced diets are largely unaffordable for the world's poor, malnutrition stemming from chronic undernourishment is the main contributor to disease in lower-income countries (Müller & Krawinkel, 2005). Malnutrition due to excessive reliance on limited, nutrient-poor food staples (e.g. grains, rice and other starchy foods) and failure to achieve minimum daily energy and nutrient requirements leads to increased susceptibility to and severity of infectious diseases, protein-energy malnutrition and micronutrient deficiencies (especially iron, iodine, vitamin A and zinc) (Müller & Krawinkel, 2005; FAO, 2008). Underweight, wasting and stunting are obvious and serious manifestations of severe and chronic malnutrition.

In children, malnutrition results in compromised growth, impaired motor and cognitive development, and poor immune system development and function. Further to this, children's vulnerability to malnutrition is evidenced in its long-term implications. Health and cognitive development deficits that occur in childhood due to malnutrition tend to persist into adulthood and consequently affect long-term health status, educational attainment, and, in the end, diminish opportunities and earning potential throughout the lifetime (FAO, 2009a). Pregnant women have also

been identified as particularly vulnerable to malnutrition as poor nutritional status in pregnancy results in increased risk of intrauterine growth retardation and giving birth to a low birthweight baby, who is then prone to increased risk of growth failure, morbidity and mortality (Blössner & de Onis, 2005). Moreover, all women and men who suffer chronic undernourishment are susceptible to "hidden hunger," i.e. subclinical nutrient deficiencies and malnutrition. Women's vulnerability to malnutrition is increased as well because they tend to sacrifice their own intake for that of their children. Moreover, given recent decreases in real household income due to the rising cost of food staples, men and women have likely increased their time spent working on income-generating activities. These activities are typically labor-intensive (e.g. road work, agricultural field work, etc.) and consequently place increased energy demands and dietary needs on men and women at a time when food and income are scarce.

The achievement of MDG 1, i.e. halving the number of people in the world who are hungry, requires in the first instance halving the number of people living on less than one (1990) dollar per day (World Trade Organization [WTO]/World Health Organization [WHO], 2002). However, economic measures alone will only undo the harm of the global food crisis, not sustain hunger alleviation in the long term. In order to eradicate poverty and hunger, short- and long-term solutions that address immediate hunger relief (e.g. emergency food aid) as well as sustainable long-term strategies that support national and household food security for all are needed (FAO, 2009d). We turn next to the Grand Challenges for global food security.

Grand Challenges for global food security [6]

We suggest that the five Grand Challenges that need to be addressed for global food security are: climate change and environmental concerns; pockets of famine; population growth; agricultural production and sustainability; and dietary transition. We provide

---

[6] This is modeled after the Grand Challenges in Global Health, "fourteen major global health challenges with the aim of engaging creative minds across scientific disciplines – including those who have not traditionally taken part in health research – to work on solutions that could lead to breakthrough advances for those in the developing world" (www.grandchallenges.org/about/Pages/Overview.aspx, 2).

an overview and consideration of concepts that are important for reflection on the ethical implications of addressing global food security; a detailed and comprehensive discussion of each challenge is beyond the scope of this chapter.

Climate change and environmental concerns

Over the next century, climate change is expected to result in higher average temperatures, changing rainfall patterns and rising sea levels. In terms of impacts on agriculture, drought and flooding will be more frequent and severe, growing seasons will be diminished, and yields for both rain-fed and irrigated crops in the poorest regions are expected to decline (McMichael et al., 2007; Consultative Group on International Agricultural Research [CGIAR], 2009). The agricultural sector accounts for approximately one-fifth of total global greenhouse gas emissions, a key contributor to climate change (McMichael et al., 2007). Climate change and its impact on agriculture is expected to be felt most acutely by smallholder farmers in lower- and middle-income countries and will be especially pronounced in the lowest-income countries and those that are already vulnerable due to the centrality of agriculture to their economy and the livelihood of many of their citizens (CGIAR, 2009; FAO, 2009b). Furthermore, future environmental shocks (among other factors) are expected to result in higher food prices, further reducing food security for the world's poor (CGIAR, 2009; Webb, 2010).

Agriculture and agricultural practices are intimately tied to the health of the environment, with subsequent implications for public health and future agricultural productivity (Tilman et al., 2002; McMichael et al., 2007). Concerns associated with agriculture include the conversion of natural ecosystems to agriculture, biodiversity losses, deforestation and forest degradation, the pollution of aquatic and terrestrial habitats and groundwater by agricultural nutrients (e.g. phosphorus, nitrogen), degradation of irrigation lands, the accumulation of pesticides (especially persistent organic agricultural pollutants), and regional and global climate change (Tilman et al., 2002; McMichael et al., 2007; Hazell & Wood, 2008).

Pockets of famine

As previously mentioned, the twentieth century largely saw the elimination of worldwide famine. However, in sub-Saharan Africa (the world's most food-insecure region; FAO, 2009a), parts of South Asia, and throughout North Africa and West Africa, per capita production of cereal has either stalled or reversed (Dyson, 1999, cited in Webb, 2010, p. 2S). Indeed, per capita food production in Africa is reportedly 10% lower today than it was in 1960 (Pretty, 2008) and Africa is the only continent that has not achieved food surpluses to meet the needs of a growing population (Hazell & Wood, 2008). As a result, many countries and regions in Africa still rely on emergency external food aid to feed their people (Hazell & Wood, 2008). In 2008, more than 3.1 million tonnes of emergency food aid were delivered to sub-Saharan Africa (WFP, 2009b).

The HIV/AIDS epidemic in Africa has also heightened the risk and impact of famine in Africa. Those infected with HIV/AIDS are often left weakened and consequently unable to work and maintain agricultural productivity. Many households revert to subsistence farming, which reduces household income and heightens the risk of food insecurity. Furthermore, many are left without the skills, knowledge or labor required to farm when the key person who farmed succumbs to HIV/AIDS.

Population growth

By 2050, the world's population is expected to exceed 9 billion (FAO, 2009b). In order to ensure food security for all, it is estimated that world food production will have to increase by 70% (FAO, 2009b). World population increases result from increased life expectancy and therefore signify increased per capita income. Economic development in recent times has increased demand for, and heightened consumption of, processed foods, sweetened beverages and meat and dairy products (Tilman et al., 2002; Webb, 2010). As a result, global grain requirements, the major agricultural input for the production of these commodities as well as the main food staple in the poorest regions of the world, are expected to double in order to meet heightened demand (Tilman et al., 2002).

Traditional Malthusian principles regarding population growth and food production state that population growth eventually becomes unsustainable when per capita food production is unable to keep pace with population growth due to inherent limits of arable and productive land (Malthus, 1993, cited in Hazell & Wood, 2008). However, this assumes limited innovation in agricultural production (Hazell & Wood, 2008). The Green Revolution rescued the world previously, but world food production has faltered or reversed, leaving a new set of agricultural production challenges for food security locally, nationally and globally (Hazell & Wood, 2008; Webb, 2010).[7]

Agricultural production and sustainability

Global investment in agriculture for lower- and middle-income countries has decreased dramatically since the 1990s with concomitant "shrinking and, in some cases, disappearing [of] national agricultural research systems, public extension, seed multiplication, and rural credit" (Webb, 2010, p. 2S), as well as decreases in yield growth in lower- and middle-income countries (Hazell & Wood, 2008). Increased agricultural production is an important strategy for overall economic growth, alleviating poverty and enabling lower-income countries to become more self-sufficient (FAO, 2009a; Pretty *et al.*, 2003). Furthermore, increased agricultural productivity typically leads to a corresponding decrease in the price of food (FAO, 2009a) and a subsequent increase in domestic food consumption (Pretty *et al.*, 2003).

The world has reason for cautious optimism: in November 2009, the international community met in Rome at the World Summit on Food Security, and declared its intention to "reverse the decline in domestic and international funding for agriculture, food security and rural development in lower- and middle-income countries, and promote new investment to increase *sustainable* [emphasis added] agricultural production and productivity, reduce poverty and work towards achieving food security and access to food for all" (FAO, 2009b, section 7.3). Indeed, the need for sustainable agricultural growth that considers environmental impacts and public health risks is of critical importance (Tilman *et al.*, 2002; Hazell & Wood, 2008; Pretty, 2008).

Past growth in agricultural production due to increased application of fertilizers, the use of some agricultural machinery and irrigation, and expansion of agricultural land area played a direct role in increased per capita world food production (Pretty, 2008). However, it has also resulted in considerable environmental harm (Pretty, 2008). In the future, similar world food production gains, both in magnitude and rate of increase, are unlikely (Tilman, 1999). Even

today, environmental harm to key ecosystems and natural resources has meant that agricultural systems themselves have suffered (Pretty, 2008). Consequently, future agricultural practices and production gains must be sustainable, i.e. "meet current and future societal needs for food and fibre, for ecosystem services, and for healthy lives, and [do] so by maximizing the net benefit to society when all costs and benefits of the practices are considered" (Tilman *et al.*, 2002, p. 671).

Dietary transition

Dietary transition refers to nutritional and food consumption shifts that occur as income increases and populations become more urbanized (Drewnowski, 2000). It is characterized by shifts away from whole grains, vegetables and legumes towards diets that are increasingly comprised of processed and animal source foods that are high in added sugar and fats (Drewnowski, 2000; Popkin, 2006). Typically, dietary transition occurs first in the most affluent groups, but eventually, low-income groups will experience transition as sugar and fat become plentiful and affordable and are subsequently incorporated into the local diet (Drewnowski, 2000). In addition to dietary changes, physical activity patterns typically decrease during leisure, transportation and work (Popkin, 2006). Dietary transition is associated with increased life expectancy, decreased fertility rates, and fewer infectious and nutrient-deficiency diseases, but higher rates of childhood obesity, coronary heart disease, type 2 diabetes mellitus and some types of cancer, which are collectively referred to as nutrition-related non-communicable diseases (NR-NCD) (Drewnowski, 2000; Popkin, 2006).

Lower- and middle-income countries are experiencing increases in NR-NCD associated with dietary transition at a much faster rate than that experienced in the higher-income countries (Popkin, 2006). Industrialization of much of Asia, North Africa, the Middle East, Latin America and some areas of sub-Saharan Africa has occurred in as little as 10–20 years, versus decades or centuries for the higher-income nations (Popkin, 2006). These increases have been linked to globalization and the rapid proliferation of modern food processing, marketing and distribution techniques, widespread trade of technology innovations that impact energy expenditure and vast expansion of the global mass media, resulting in a convergence in global food consumption patterns (Popkin, 2006).

---

[7] For an extensive discussion of the future of global agriculture, including future challenges and drivers of change at a global, country, and local level, see Hazell & Wood (2008).

Controversies in addressing global food security

Several ethical considerations intersect with the Grand Challenges: the use of technology in sustainable agricultural production; food sovereignty versus the globalized market; and micronutrient supplementation versus access to food.

Technology and sustainable agricultural production

There is no disagreement that in order for the world to achieve global food security, agricultural production needs to be increased, and such increases should be sustainable, but there is polarization around the role that biotechnology should play in achieving this goal. Technology in agricultural production refers to innovations and practices that enhance the productivity of agriculture without the need to rely on expansion of cultivated area (Tilman *et al.*, 2002). In the past, agricultural technology encompassed practices such as plant breeding, soil management, the application of fertilizers and pesticides, irrigation and the use of agricultural machinery. The result has been sustained food surpluses for most regions of the world, with the exception of Africa (Hazell & Wood, 2008). It is noteworthy that Africa's inability to produce enough food to feed its population has occurred in tandem with the lowest uptake of modern technological inputs (e.g. use of inorganic fertilizer, share of irrigated cropland, use of tractors) of any region (Wood *et al.*, 2000). Furthermore, technological advances in production are being adopted much faster in higher-income countries that are able to spend money on research and development (Hazell & Wood, 2008).

Despite these overall important gains in food production, the agricultural sector has been criticized for the broader environmental damage that has occurred as a result of the use of agricultural technology. There are some who view past transgressions of the agricultural sector as impetus for the rejection of the role of technology for meeting future increases to agricultural productivity, for fear of increased damage to the environment and diminishment of the productivity of natural agro-ecosystems. However, technology is an invaluable tool for allowing agriculture to adapt to ongoing and future production challenges by making the best use of natural, social, human, physical, and financial capital without damaging them (Hazell & Wood, 2008; Pretty, 2008).[8] As such, technology and agricultural sustainability are not mutually exclusive. As suggested by Pretty (2008), "Agricultural sustainability does not … mean ruling out any technologies or practices on ideological grounds (e.g. genetically modified or organic crops) – provided they improve biological and/or economic productivity for farmers and do not harm the environment" (p. 453).

One of the greatest polarizations confronting the aim of increased agricultural production comes from biotechnology, particularly genetically modified foods. Genetically modified crops are feared because of potential risks and unknown impact to the environment and human health.[9] Genetic modification aside, sustainable agriculture is comprised of many important innovations and techniques that enable it to be both resilient and persistent. These include integrated pest management, integrated nutrient management, conservation tillage, crop rotations and mixed farming (including integration of trees and livestock into the farming system), nutrient- and water-use efficiency, landscape management, aquaculture and water harvesting (Tilman *et al.*, 2002; Hazell & Wood, 2008; Pretty, 2008). A review of the effects of sustainable agriculture on yield (Pretty *et al.*, 2006) revealed significant and promising increases to food production in the poorest regions. This is important given evidence that the increased adoption of subsistence farming in Africa and parts of Asia due to declining yields contributes to more than 60% of deforestation worldwide (Hazell & Wood, 2008).

There is some consensus among proponents of sustainable agriculture for the role of agro-ecology, biochemistry and biotechnology in sustainable agriculture (e.g. Tilman *et al.*, 2002; Pretty, 2008), especially for lower- and middle-income countries (Nuffield Council on Bioethics, 2004). There is also evidence to show that farmers and farming communities are driven to respond to environmental degradation with innovative agricultural techniques and regulations (Wood *et al.*, 2000). Adjustments to agricultural technologies and practices to ensure enhanced sustainability will not be uniform; for most lower- and middle-income countries, the focus will remain on food production,

---

[8] For a full discussion on the principles of agricultural sustainability, see Pretty (2008).

[9] For further discussion on the ethical considerations of genetically modified crops, see Nuffield Council on Bioethics (2004).

while other regions may require additional adjustments to compensate for environmental degradation (Pretty, 2008).

Food sovereignty versus the globalized market

Since the inaugural meeting of the FAO in 1945, the role of international trade in the attainment of global food security has been debated. Agriculture has traditionally, and continues to be, a highly distorted sector of the global economy due to export subsidies and domestic support for the producers in the Organisation for Economic Co-operation and Development (OECD) countries, concurrent with high export tariffs imposed on food items produced in lower- and middle-income countries (Clapp, 2006). Trade liberalization and the elimination of agricultural protectionism is consequently a crucial and important step in enhancing the economic well-being of lower-income countries, which are often heavily dependent on agriculture (Clapp, 2006; Hazell & Wood, 2008).

The 1994 Uruguay Round Agreement on Agriculture of the World Trade Organization was meant to enhance market access through cuts to domestic support subsidies and export tariffs. Instead, subsidies in the OECD countries increased; as a result, world commodity prices for food staples decreased and the domestic markets of lower- and middle-income countries were flooded with subsidized imported products from industrialized countries (Clapp, 2006). Although low food prices are good for (urban) consumers, small-scale farmers are often adversely affected because they are unable to compete in domestic and regional markets (e.g. staples, livestock) or international markets (Hazell & Wood, 2008). The Doha Round of agricultural trade talks is currently underway to address the inequities created by the Agreement on Agriculture and further minimize trade barriers.[10]

Hazell & Wood (2008) have written a balanced critique of the role of trade in agriculture. They argue that in some respects, lower- and middle-income countries have benefited from the internationalization of agricultural trade, particularly in the trade of flowers, fruits, wine and fish. Trade between lower-income countries has also increased. However, many regions have lost market share (both export and domestic) for traditional crops, including staples, following increased competition from both higher-income and lower- and middle-income countries. In addition, regions that are unable to keep pace with yield levels as well as those faced with extraordinary transport costs are at a particular disadvantage in world trading. The rapid pace of globalization has also meant that farmers in lower- and middle-income countries are required to adapt to the new globalized agricultural system very quickly, a task that originally led to current "expensive and market-distorting agricultural support programmes" in most OECD countries (Hazell & Wood, 2008, p. 503).

In addition, adjustments to public sector policies in the 1980s and early 1990s to allow the private sector to play an enhanced role as the "more efficient supplier" led to a decline in public investment in agriculture in lower-income countries, and have generally been unfavorable for poor, small-scale farmers (especially those in Africa and South Asia), while benefiting large agribusiness (Anderson, 2008; Hazell & Wood, 2008, p. 504). In particular, profits paid to large agribusiness corporations have increased, while prices paid to farmers for commodity crops decreased.

While trade liberalization has resulted in some important economic outcomes, it has not led to widespread elimination of poverty and alleviation of food insecurity. In response to these failures, alternative agricultural systems based on *food sovereignty* have gained traction among segments of consumers in lower- and middle-income and higher-income countries alike. Via Campesina, a global network of peasants, small- and medium-sized producers, landless rural women, indigenous people, rural youth and agricultural workers, first introduced the concept in 1996 as a precondition to genuine food security. Since 1996, the definition of food sovereignty has evolved, but at its core are "direct democratic participation, an end to the dumping of food and the wider use of food as a weapon of policy, comprehensive agrarian reform, and a respect for life, seed, and land" (Patel, 2009, p. 665). Food sovereignty aims to shift control of food access and production from large agribusiness and financial institutions, which are typically focused on shareholders and profit, back to local people. Admittedly, food sovereignty and other alternative food systems have drawn attention to the challenges associated with achieving global food security when the products of modern agriculture are viewed primarily as a traded commodity on world markets,

---

[10] As of publication of this chapter, Doha trade talks are ongoing/stalled.

with the market's proclivity for unequal distribution of benefit.

Multinational agribusiness has been greatly criticized for its apparent disregard of people's right-to-food in their unfettered pursuit of profits. Moreover, agricultural protectionism in OECD countries has enabled agribusiness to operate in this manner through tax-breaks, failure to apply anti-trust regulations to agricultural companies, and the elimination of supply controls that drive down the cost of raw inputs and significantly decrease farmers' income (Anderson, 2008). Consequently, ongoing efforts of the Doha Round of agricultural trade talks to eliminate sector-distorting practices are vital to ensure that lower- and middle-income countries have fair access to international markets.

In order to address current shortcomings and inequities, proponents of food sovereignty have proposed many solutions that have already been discussed in this chapter (e.g. support for the poorest consumer, enhanced domestic food production, sustainable use of natural, human, and social capital, mixed farming, etc.). However, it is worth noting that they also consistently reject the use of biotechnology, particularly genetically modified crops.

Without using the term "food sovereignty," Hazell & Wood (2008) have argued that, "left to market forces alone, many small farmers and poorer regions are likely to be left further behind … Public interventions are needed to help distribute the benefits of the new agricultural growth more widely. These should include policies and investments to help integrate small farmers into modern market chains and to promote the long-term development of more remote and less-favored regions" (p. 510). Similarly, Pretty (2008) proposes that agricultural policies encompassing both sustainability and poverty reduction should emphasize the small farmer and local markets, small business and export-led business development, agro-processing, urban agriculture and local livestock markets. Small-scale farmers in lower- and middle-income countries need access to more than fair prices to increase productivity and income; they also need access to affordable inputs, credit and transport and market infrastructure. These are vitally important in enabling poor farmers to generate an adequate income (FAO, 2009d). Therefore, sustainable agriculture, with its focus on increased agricultural production through the judicious use of human, social and natural capital, together with the establishment of a fair international market for agricultural commodities and the integration of small-scale farmers, is likely the more balanced approach to achieving food security.

Micronutrient supplementation versus access to food

Interestingly, one technological "fix" that seems to be unlinked with discussion of agricultural yield is the correction of malnutrition, particularly, the micronutrient-related nutritional deficiencies, in order to mitigate the health harms of insufficient food. Largely the purview of the health domain, the administration of such remedies as vitamin A capsules, and packets of multi-vitamin and mineral supplements is an attractive policy alternative to enhancing the access to food.

The consumption of a varied and balanced diet is the best and most sustainable way to prevent and eliminate malnutrition but as we have emphasized, those who are food insecure are largely unable to afford sufficient or adequate food, relying instead on a limited diet that is based primarily on starchy staples and limited in nutrient-rich foods. Diets that are deficient in one micronutrient are almost certainly deficient in others (Müller & Krawinkel, 2005).

Micronutrient supplementation is clearly one way to *manage* major micronutrient deficiencies, just as emergency food outlets in wealthy countries (e.g. food banks, soup kitchens) have become a primary way of managing domestic food insecurity. Undoubtedly, supplementation has had an important role in the immediate alleviation of clinical and subclinical malnutrition, especially in communities where food supplies are limited (Müller & Krawinkel, 2005). However, because supplementation programs are typically distributed through existing health services, they face issues relating to cost and prioritization, as well as access, as many vulnerable populations are often unable to access health services, even those that are delivered at no cost (Müller & Krawinkel, 2005). Other considerations include synergistic and antagonistic interactions between micronutrients in the formulation of supplementation therapy (Müller & Krawinkel, 2005).

A second approach to addressing micronutrient deficiencies is through the production and subsequent consumption of nutrient-rich staple crops. Indeed, "diet-based strategies are probably the most promising approach for a sustainable control of micronutrient deficiencies" (Müller & Krawinkel, 2005, p. 283). For those who are highly dependent on the consumption of staple crops, enhancing their nutritional profile through biotechnology (e.g. Golden Rice) may alleviate considerable subclinical and clinical conditions resulting from malnutrition, inasmuch as these crops are affordable and accessible to low-income populations. Unlike pharmaceutical interventions (in this context), diet-based strategies raise the ugly specter of genetically modified foods.

In the end, however, access to food through affordable food and poverty alleviation (i.e. political, social and economic reform) remains the most important and durable therapy for addressing the health implications of food insecurity. How then shall Global Food Security be achieved? We conclude with final thoughts and recommendations to move towards the achievement of food security for all.

Moving forward towards global food security

The provision of food and the alleviation of hunger will always improve health and lessen human suffering. Although the state has a moral and legal responsibility to ensure human rights, including the right to food, "people hold their governments accountable and are participants in the process of human development, rather than passive recipients" (FAO, 2004, p. 3). Global solidarity and support for the elimination of poverty and hunger is therefore of critical importance. Inadequate income and its unequal distribution remain the primary drivers of hunger today (Hazell & Wood, 2008); the disparity that exists between lower- and middle-income and higher-income countries is unacceptable when ideas, technology and resources can be exchanged rapidly and relatively unfettered. Furthermore, higher-income countries have a role to play in conditions that have affected the food security status of lower- and middle-income countries (e.g. climate change, agricultural protectionism); they therefore also have a responsibility to act on behalf of the more than 1 billion people who are hungry.

At a minimum, those who are malnourished need access to affordable food, with an explicit aim to balance nutrient density, nutrient cost and social norms (Drewnowski & Eichelsdoerfer, 2009). The FAO (2009a) has recommended a number of strategies to help those who are hungry now, including the creation of sustainable and resilient safety nets and social protection programs that not only reach those in need, but stimulate the local economy through job creation

and increasing agriculture. Local, small-scale farmers must also be provided with access to affordable modern inputs, technologies, resources and infrastructure (e.g. high-quality seeds, fertilizers, feed and farming tools and equipment, electricity, roads and ports) to boost productivity and production (FAO, 2009a). Furthermore, training in the proper use of modern and sustainable agricultural techniques is important, especially in lower-income countries where agricultural extension programs have been underfunded (Hazell & Wood, 2008; Pretty, 2008). Together, these will help to generate wealth for farmers, while decreasing the price of food to consumers (FAO, 2009a). Indeed, per capita income and agricultural productivity are most strongly correlated to food security (Hazell & Wood, 2008).

Reinvestment in agriculture

Reinvestment in agriculture to at least the level of support seen in the 1970s is essential to combat food insecurity, especially in countries where per capita food production has stalled and decreased. Moving forward, agricultural policies, research and technology must address productivity and poverty alleviation in a sustainable manner so that long-term capacity for food production is improved, rather than damaged, and achievements in food security are sustained and resilient, despite future shocks (Tilman et al., 2002; Hazell & Wood, 2008).

How a country directs its investments in agriculture will differ based on the current state of agricultural development and local priorities. For example, middle-income countries will typically require assistance to ensure small-scale farmers are integrated into modern market chains, especially in remote regions (Hazell & Wood, 2008). Furthermore, with increasing economic development and population growth, meeting demand for high-value crops and livestock represents a significant opportunity for agricultural producers (Hazell & Wood, 2008). To meet these demands, producers will require access to technology to cope with the associated production and environmental challenges, e.g. water management, waste disposal, pesticide use and monitoring of health risks (Hazell & Wood, 2008). Conversely, agricultural output in lower-income countries is still focused primarily on staple food crops; therefore, growth in these markets remains the most viable economic prospect for rural populations (Hazell & Wood, 2008). Consequently, public investment should be focused on enabling market access, affordable transport costs, increased access to affordable inputs (e.g. seeds, fertilizer, credit), and increased access to technology to enhance the sector's competitiveness (Hazell & Wood, 2008).

Unreflexive localism

DuPuis & Goodman (2005) coined the term "unreflexive localism," which we use to refer to the preoccupation of some citizens of higher-income countries to further complicate our already inequitable food system by striving to consume from alternative food systems that reject both global-scale food systems and agricultural technology (in particular, biotechnology). Despite good intentions, there is a real risk that a preoccupation with ideologically based alternative food systems will detract from meaningful and timely improvements to global food security. Ironically, the most vocal opponents to the global food system live in countries whose wealth and prosperity are directly linked to the agricultural development that occurred in the twentieth century. And, to be fair, those who reject the global food system are likely responding to real concerns regarding environmental damage and the proliferation of income disparities between small-scale farmers and large agribusiness.

As argued above, sustainable food systems do not preclude technology (Nuffield Council on Bioethics, 2004; Hazell & Wood, 2008; Pretty, 2008). Scientific research and innovation have a crucial role to play in alleviating hunger today and achieving the productivity increases needed in the future to meet demands imposed by population growth, environmental concerns, climate change and energy prices. Rejection of food systems that are global in scale has recently gained significant traction. The dichotomy is such that local systems have come to be seen as "good" or benevolent, whereas global systems are "destructive" (Hinrichs, 2000). Increasingly, local food systems are conflated with sustainability, justice and democracy (Born & Purcell, 2006).

It is a fallacy that local-scale food systems are inherently desirable; instead, the outcomes of any food system – local or global – are embedded within the context and agenda of its key players (Hinrichs, 2003; Allen, 1999; Born & Purcell, 2006). Indeed, a food system approach that is predicated on the local scale on the basis of ideology provides limited opportunity for creating a food system that is sensitive and responsive to environmental concerns, fair and just practices, as well as the need to feed a global community (Allen, 1999). The valuing of local

foods, produced by relatively wealthy local farmers in Europe and North America, discourages the purchase of foods produced from distant, lower-income countries, subsequently limiting economic gains to particular groups (Hinrichs & Allen, 2008). Others have gone as far as to claim that valuing local foods "may be less about the radical affirmation of an ethic of community or care, and more to do with the production of less positive parochialism and nationalism, a conservative celebration of the local as the supposed repository of specific meanings and values" (Holloway & Kneafsey, 2000, p. 294 cited in Anderson, 2008).

Concluding thoughts

In the end, the failures and shortcoming of the global food system create multiple opportunities to achieve a food system that is just and sustainable. Achieving MDG 1 will require a concerted effort on behalf of the entire global community to ensure that the most vulnerable are protected from hunger and malnutrition. The previous century saw numerous advancements and positive improvements towards food security (e.g. the Green Revolution, elimination of famines). The future's challenges should therefore not be seen as insurmountable: "If [the world] is prepared to make the necessary investments, it can reap a food security dividend that enriches all of society with payoffs in health, social capital, sustainability of our physical and social environments, justice, and both cost savings and wealth creation" (McIntyre & Rondeau, 2008, p. 202). We hope that there is time and the will to do so.

References

Anderson, M. D. (2008). Rights-based food systems and the goals of food system reform. *Agriculture and Human Values* 25, 593–608.

Allen, P. (1999). Reweaving the food security safety net: mediating entitlement and entrepreneurship. *Agriculture and Human Values* 16, 117–129.

Blössner, M. & de Onis, M. (2005). *Malnutrition: Quantifying the Health Impact at National and Local Levels.* WHO Environmental Burden of Disease Series, No. 12. Geneva: World Health Organization.

Born, B. & Purcell, M. (2006). Avoiding the local trap: scale and food systems in planning research. *Journal of Planning and Education Research* 26, 195–207.

Clapp, J. (2006). *Developing Countries and the WTO Agriculture Negotiations.* Working Paper No. 6. The

Centre for International Governance Innovation. www.cigionline.org (Accessed November 27, 2009).

Consultative Group on International Agricultural Research (CGIAR) (2009). *Climate, Agriculture and Food Security: A Strategy for Change.* Alliance of the CGIAR Centers. www.cgiar.org/publications/index.html (Accessed December 15, 2009).

Drewnowski, A. (2000). Nutrition transition and global dietary trends. *Nutrition* **16**, 486–487.

Drewnowski, A. & Eichelsdoerfer, P. (2009). Can low-income Americans afford a health diet? *CPHN Public Health Research Brief,* March 2009. Center for Public Health Nutrition, University of Washington. http://depts.washington.edu/uwcphn/ (Accessed December 30, 2009).

DuPuis, E. M. & Goodman, D. (2005). Should we go "home" to eat?: Toward a reflexive politics of localism. *Journal of Rural Studies* **21**, 359–371.

Economic Research Service/United States Department of Agriculture (2008). *Food CPI and Expenditures: 2007 Table 97.* www.ers.usda.gov/briefing/cpifoodandexpenditures/data/Table_97/2007table97.htm (Accessed December 11, 2009).

Food and Agriculture Organization (FAO) (2004). *Implementing the Right to Adequate Food: The Outcome of Six Case Studies.* www.fao.org/DOCREP/MEETING/008/J2475E.HTM (Accessed December 20, 2009).

Food and Agriculture Organization (FAO) (2008). *The State of Food Insecurity in the World 2008. High Food Prices and Food Security – Threats and Opportunities.* www.fao.org/docrep/011/i0291e/i0291e00.htm (Accessed December 30, 2009).

Food and Agriculture Organization (FAO) (2009a). The state of food insecurity in the world 2009. Economic crises–impacts and lessons learned. www.fao.org/publications/sofi/en/ (Accessed November 16, 2009).

Food and Agriculture Organization (FAO) (2009b). *Declaration of the World Summit on Food Security.* World Summit on Food Security. Rome: FAO.

Food and Agriculture Organization (FAO) (2009c). *FAO: Hunger.* www.fao.org/hunger/en (Accessed 30 December 30, 2009).

Food and Agriculture Organization (FAO) (2009d). *The State of the Agricultural Commodity Markets 2009.* www.fao.org/docrep/012/i0854e/i0854e00.htm (Accessed December 20, 2009).

Hazell, P. & Wood, S. (2008). Drivers of change in global agriculture. *Philosophical Transactions of the Royal Society B* **363**, 495–515.

Health Canada (2007). *Canadian Community Health Survey, Cycle 2.2, Nutrition (2004) – Income-Related Household Food Security in Canada.* Ottawa, ON: Office of Nutrition Policy and Promotion, Health Products and Food Branch.

Hinrichs, C. C. (2000). Embeddedness and local food systems: notes on two types of direct agricultural market. *Journal of Rural Studies* **16**, 295–303.

Hinrichs, C. C. (2003). The practice and politics of food system localization. *Journal of Rural Studies* **19**, 33–45.

Hinrichs C. C. & Allen, P. (2008). Selective patronage and social justice: Local food consumer campaigns in historical context. *Journal of Agricultural and Environmental Ethics* **21**, 329–352.

McIntyre, L. & Rondeau, K. (2008). Food insecurity. In D. Raphael (Ed.) *Social Determinants of Health: Canadian Perspectives.* (2nd edn.) (pp. 188–204). Toronto, ON: Canadian Scholars' Press.

McMichael, A. J., Powles, J. W., Butler, C. D. & Uauy, R. (2007). Food, livestock production, energy, climate change, and health. *Lancet* **370**, 1253–1263.

Müller, O. & Krawinkel, M. (2005). Malnutrition and health in developing countries. *Canadian Medical Association Journal* **173**, 279–286.

Nord, M., Andrews, M. & Carlson, S. (2009). *Household Food Security in the United States, 2008.* ERR-83. United States Department of Agriculture, Economic Research Service. www.ers.usda.gov/Publications/Err83/ (Accessed November 30, 2009).

Nuffield Council on Bioethics (2004). *The Use of Genetically Modified Crops in Developing Countries.* London: Nuffield Council on Bioethics.

Patel, R. (2009). What does food sovereignty look like? *Journal of Peasant Studies* **36**, 663–703.

Popkin, B. M. (2006). Technology, transport, globalization and the nutrition transition food policy. *Food Policy* **31**, 554–569.

Pretty, J. (2008). Agricultural sustainability: Concepts, principles and evidence. *Philosophical Transaction of the Royal Society B* **363**, 447–465.

Pretty, J. N., Morison, J. I. L. & Hine, R. E. (2003). Reducing food poverty by increasing agricultural sustainability in developing countries. *Agriculture, Ecosystems and Environment* **95**, 217–234.

Pretty, J., Noble, A., Bossio, D. *et al.* (2006). Resource conserving agriculture increases yields in developing countries. *Environmental Science & Technology* **40**, 1114–1119.

Tilman, D. (1999). Global environmental impacts of agricultural expansion: The need for sustainable and efficient practices. *Proceedings of the National Academy of Sciences USA* **96**, 5995–6000.

Tilman, D., Cassman, K. G., Matson, P. A., Naylor, R. & Polasky, S. (2002). Agricultural sustainability and intensive production practices. *Nature* **418**, 671–677.

United Nations (2009). *The Millenium Development Goals Report 2009*. www.un.org/millenniumgoals/ (Accessed November 10, 2009).

Waggoner, W. H. (1945). Sir John Orr suggests a world wheat pool with stabilized price. *The Globe and Mail*, **30** October, 1.

Webb, P. (2010). Medium- to long-run implications of high food prices for global nutrition. *The Journal of Nutrition* **140**(1), 143S–147S. First published November 18, 2009; doi:10.3945/jn.109.110536.

Wood, S., Sebastian, K. & Scherr, S. J. (2000). *Pilot Analysis of Global Ecosystems: Agroecosystems*. International Food Policy Research Institute and the World Resources Institute. Washington, DC. www.wri.org/publication/ pilot-analysis-global-ecosystems-agroecosystems (Accessed December 30, 2009).

World Food Program (WFP) (2009a). *Hunger*. http://wfp. org/hunger (Accessed December 20, 2009).

World Food Program (WFP) (2009b). *Quantity Reporting*. www.wfp.org/fais/reports/quantities-delivered-two-dimensional-report/run/cat/All/recipient/SUB-SAHARAN+AFRICA+%28aggregate%29/year/2008/ donor/All/code/All/mode/All/basis/0/order/0/ (Accessed December 30, 2009).

World Trade Organization/World Health Organization (2002). *WTO Agreements and Public Health*. www.wto. org/english/res_e/booksp_e/who_wto_e.pdf (Accessed December 9, 2009).

International taxation

Gillian Brock

In previous work I have argued that reasonable indicators of our progress towards global justice include the extent to which: (1) all are enabled to meet their basic needs; (2) people's basic liberties are protected; and (3) social and political arrangements are in place to support these two goals, that is, that enable us to meet our basic needs and protect our basic liberties (Brock, 2005, 2009). How do we get from where we are now to where we should be? The issue of transitioning to any of our ideals of global justice has not received as much attention as it should. In this chapter I examine some measures that would close the gap between our current state of affairs and better enabling people to meet their basic needs. Current global poverty must be one of the most pressing obstacles to realizing global justice. The way in which we are depleting and destroying the global commons is another pressing and related issue. Failing to protect the global commons has a bearing not only on current and future global poverty, but indeed, on the capacity of the planet to provide a life-sustaining environment, and thus on everyone's ability to meet their basic needs. In the second part of the chapter I discuss how concern in this area can also ground a case for global taxation reforms.

Introduction to some key issues

Global poverty remains at high levels. At least 1.4 billion people live below the international poverty line (Chen & Ravallion, 2008). How can we help those in poverty and, especially, how can we help those in poverty to help themselves? There is enormous evidence to suggest that institutions (or practices) matter greatly, whatever other factors are also significant (Rodrik, 2003; Brock, 2009). A number of these have been highlighted as crucially needing reform; in particular,

international institutions can dramatically influence the quality of domestic ones. Thomas Pogge argues for changes to be made to the International Resource Privilege and the International Borrowing Privilege (which I say more about shortly). Others focus on inadequacies with the World Trade Organization, the International Monetary Fund, and so on (Stiglitz, 2002). Clearly there is much work to be done here and the necessary work cannot all be done by one person, let alone in the scope of one chapter. I concentrate here on the practices that currently regulate taxation in our world today and the reforms that are necessary in that area if we are to create a world order that supports the goals of global justice.

Reform to our international taxation and accounting regime must be part of any genuine solution to help those who we want to position to help themselves. I focus here on modifications to the tax and accounting regime for two reasons. First, I think it has thus far been somewhat neglected by political theorists. Our current arrangements contribute greatly to the global poverty problem and allow vast amounts of taxable income to escape taxation. Even modest changes in global tax policy will mobilize revenue that is badly needed in developing countries. Second, notable among the positive policy proposals that are offered, is Thomas Pogge's Global Resources Dividend, a tax on the extraction of natural resources to be set at 1% of world product. The reforms I propose could potentially have a more dramatic effect on global poverty than Pogge's (as I explain). Furthermore, I believe Pogge's Global Resources Dividend proposal can probably only be effective if the more fundamental reforms I suggest are implemented. In order to see why this is the case, I now discuss key aspects of Pogge's view.

An earlier version of this work appeared: Brock, G. (2008). Taxation and global justice: closing the gap between theory and practice. *Journal of Social Philosophy* **39** (2), 161–184.

Pogge on global injustice and some solutions

Pogge argues that there are a number of relevant connections between people in affluent, developed countries ("us") and those in absolute poverty in developing nations ("them").[1] For instance, our positions and theirs "have emerged from a single historical process that was pervaded by massive grievous wrongs" (Pogge, 2001b, pp. 14–15). Historical injustices have a role to play in explaining both our affluence and their poverty. Furthermore, we all rely on a single natural resource base. We have fostered international arrangements concerning the distribution of these resources which benefit us and disadvantage them enormously. More generally, we all "coexist within a single global economic order that has a strong tendency to perpetuate and even to aggravate global economic inequality" (Pogge, 2001b, p. 15). By failing to take steps to reform the international order, we may certainly be failing in some of our positive duties to help those in acute distress. However and more significantly, we may be "failing to fulfill our more stringent negative duty not to uphold injustice, not to contribute to or profit from the unjust impoverishment of others" (Pogge, 2001a, p. 60).

According to Pogge, two international institutions are particularly worrisome: the international borrowing privilege and the international resource privilege. Any group that exercises effective power in a state is recognized internationally as the legitimate government of that territory, and the international community is not much concerned with how the group came to power or what it does with that power. Oppressive governments may borrow freely on behalf of the country (the international borrowing privilege) or dispose of its natural resources (the international resource privilege) and these actions are legally recognized internationally. These two privileges have enormous implications for prosperity in poor countries, as (for instance) these privileges provide incentives for coups, they often influence what sorts of people are motivated to seek power, they facilitate the stability of oppressive governments, and, should more democratic governments gain power, they are saddled with the debts

incurred by their oppressive predecessors, thus significantly draining the country of resources needed to firm up its fledgling democracy. All of this is disastrous for many poor countries.

Because foreigners benefit so greatly from the international resource privilege, they have an incentive to refrain from challenging the situation (or worse, to support oppressive governments). For these sorts of reasons, the current world order largely reflects the interests of wealthy and powerful states. Local governments have little incentive to attend to the needs of the poor as their continuing in power depends more on the local elite, foreign governments, and corporations. Pogge maintains that we (in affluent, developed countries) have a responsibility to stop imposing this unjust global order and to mitigate the harms we have already inflicted on the world's most vulnerable people. If we make no reasonable efforts at institutional reform, benefiting from unjust institutional schemes implicates us in them. Pogge offers suggestions concerning reforming the two international privileges, the thrust of which is that we should only bestow these privileges on democratically elected governments (Pogge, 2002).

However, the main positive proposal that he focuses on in his work is the introduction of a global tax – which he introduces as "a moderate proposal" – that aims to make a start on better discharging this negative duty that we have, the duty not to uphold injustice. The proposal is to implement what he calls "The Global Resources Dividend" (GRD) (Pogge, 2001a). For any resources states or governments decide to use or sell, they must share a very small part of the value of those resources, and as an initial suggestion he proposes the GRD be set at about 1% of the global product. These costs can be passed on to the consumers of these resources, they need not be borne by governments or citizens. The 1% tax would, he estimates, raise about $300 billion annually and this could make an enormous difference to helping the poor if it is well spent. The projects that should be given high priority in funding are those that try to ensure "all human beings will be able to meet their own basic needs with dignity" (Pogge, 2001a, pp. 67–68).

Why more fundamental reforms are also needed

The reforms I discuss are more fundamental and could potentially have a greater effect on global poverty than Pogge's GRD, for several reasons. First, they

---

[1] I continue to use Pogge's terminology here as a shorthand, since it is widely used in the literature and does generally pick out the relevant groups, even though there are clear exceptions.

target some of the central and underlying issues more effectively, blocking several paths now open to corrupt leaders to siphon money away from developing countries. Second, the amounts of money that would become available are far more significant, though the proposals discussed here are also clearly moderate ones. (While simply making more money available is not necessarily going to translate automatically into poverty alleviation, it improves these prospects enormously and at least removes one obstacle currently facing our efforts to alleviate poverty.) Third, the reforms suggested also have the advantage of being more easily implemented, as some of these proposals converge with proposals and plans already gathering momentum and, in some cases, actually being implemented in various ways (as I discuss later). Fourth, arguably, if Pogge's proposals are to be successful, it is necessary in any case to implement some of the reforms I suggest. In the next section I argue for reforms governing transparency, accountability, more openness in financial transactions, less opportunity to evade tax, and importantly, less opportunity to invent prices for goods. Why are these required for Pogge's proposals to be successful?

Consider, for instance, the reforms Pogge recommends to the International Resource Privilege. Even if we succeed in transforming the International Resource Privilege along the lines Pogge would like, so that only democratic governments may sell the country's resources, if there are no disclosure requirements concerning the sale prices of resources, as I go on to discuss, there will not necessarily be any progress, where non-disclosure simply allows corruption to flourish. Citizens will need to know more about the price at which assets are sold and the revenue thereby generated, if they are to hold governments accountable.

Also, if Pogge's major policy proposal, the GRD is to succeed, we will need an international framework against the background of which we could fairly impose the GRD. However, that background framework does not yet exist. Note that Pogge's proposals assume there is open disclosure about how much of the natural resource base is actually being used, and the price at which resources are sold. So, for instance, Pogge's proposal presupposes that we can keep close tabs on how much oil is being extracted and the amounts of money paid for those resources. If there are no requirements to report how much of various resources are being used or extracted, we can enforce a GRD based

only on estimates of how much of a resource is being extracted and also, if we do not know the prices at which resources are traded, again we will need to estimate value. However, both these estimates may be quite unreliable, given our lack of public knowledge in these areas. More importantly, *if there is wide scope to artificially construct or manipulate prices for goods* (as is the case with transfer pricing schemes I discuss), *many can effectively escape the GRD tax*. Indeed, if there are ample opportunities to shift products through various arrangements, so that they are (technically rather than actually) *sold at a loss*, those operating such schemes might argue *there is nothing to tax*.

In the next section, I explore our current situation to show why we need reforms to our tax regime in the areas of more transparency, openness, accountability, less opportunity to invent prices for goods and less opportunity to evade tax.

Global poverty and some taxation issues

It seems to be easy to avoid paying taxes in the world we live in today. It is estimated, for instance, that one-third of total Gross Domestic Product (GDP) is held offshore in tax havens, or effectively beyond the reach of taxation (Boston Consulting Group, 2003; Baker, 2005). It is further estimated that *about half of all world trade* passes through tax haven jurisdictions, as profits are shifted to places where tax can be avoided (Christensen & Hampton, 1999). The policy of "transfer pricing" and other complex financial structures (that I discuss shortly) reduce transparency, thus facilitating tax evasion. It is estimated that through such schemes developing countries lose revenue greater than the annual flow of aid (Oxfam, 2000; Baker, 2005). According to Ray Baker's analysis of the figures (2005), for every dollar of aid that goes into a country, $6–7 of corporate tax evasion flows out of it.

Tax avoidance threatens both development and democracy, especially in developing countries (Christian Aid, 2005; Tax Justice Network, 2005). Because large corporations and wealthy individuals are effectively avoiding taxation, the tax burden is frequently shifted onto ordinary citizens and smaller businesses. Governments often thereby collect much-reduced sums insufficient to achieve minimal goals of social justice, such as providing decent public goods and services. Cuts in social spending are inevitable, and these cuts can have a dramatic effect on other goals such as developing or maintaining robust democracies (Vigueras, 2005; Cobham, 2007).

Furthermore, because most developing countries are in competition in trying to attract foreign capital, offering tax-breaks or tax havens may seem to provide an attractive course. However, as states compete to offer tax exemptions to capital, the number of tax havens increases, thereby making all developing countries worse off. Corporations pay much reduced, if any, taxes, and ordinary citizens have to bear more of the cost of financing the social and public goods necessary for sustaining well-functioning communities (Mitchell & Sikka, 2005).

Some problems with tax havens, transfer pricing schemes and tax evasion

Microsoft reported a $12.3 billion profit in 1999, but paid no tax at all for that year (Citizens for Tax Justice, 2002). How do companies such as Microsoft get to do this?

The use of tax havens is an important channel for tax evasion and constitutes a significant reason why many corporations pay very little or even no income tax. Economic activity is often declared as occurring in places where taxes are low, rather than accurately recorded where it actually took place. "Transfer pricing" is a recognized accounting term for sales and purchases that occur within the same company or group of companies. Because these transactions occur within the company, there is wide scope to trade at arbitrary prices instead of market-attuned ones. Here is a simplified example. A multinational company has a factory in one country, F. The factory produces products, say, microwave ovens for $50, and sells these to a subsidiary in the same group that is based in another country, T, which is a tax-haven. The price of the transfer might be defined by the accountants as the cost of production, so in this case $50. Then the subsidiary in T sells the product to a foreign subsidiary in a further country, S, for (say) $200. If the price of the good to consumers in that third country, S, is $150, the good has then been sold at a loss of $50, technically. Because the cost of the good from the tax-haven country, S, is $200 and the sale price is $150, a net loss of $50 may be recorded in country S, a loss that can be offset against other taxes to be paid (in country S). Despite a real profit of $100 ($150–$50, the actual sales price less the actual cost of production), the company may declare a net tax loss. These kinds of accounting schemes and variations on these

general themes are extremely widespread and many of them are currently perfectly legal.

> You only have to look at the miraculously low global tax payments by many multinationals through the 1990s, or at the vast amounts of crude oil which are traded in a mountain village in landlocked Switzerland, to suspect that this is both well organised and widespread. The aggregate figures for world trade confirm it: around 60% of all trade takes place within multinational corporations, and around 50% appears to pass through tax havens, even though there is scant productive activity occurring there. Evidence from the USA suggests that accounting practices masquerading as transfer pricing "policies" are having a bigger impact on wealth transfers from ordinary people to corporations than any of the headline financial scandals (e.g., Enron, WorldCom). (Tax Justice Network, 2003b)

Quite simply, less revenue taken in, means less is available to spend on public services, which could affect the funding of social programs. Significant cuts to social programs – such as cutting back on police officers and health services – may well have to be made, and some argue that this has resulted in worse crime and poorer health in those areas (Furman, 2006).

International double standards: why we should aim for consistency

Foreign aid, though desirable, is by no means always necessary to finance improvements for the worst off. In many cases, the revenue from resource sales, if actually received and properly spent, would be more than enough to finance the necessary provisions for helping people to meet their needs. This is especially clear if we look at the case of oil and the crippling corruption that sometimes surrounds its sale.

Consider how, for instance, more than $4 billion in oil revenue disappeared in Angola between 1997 and 2002, which equals the entire amount the state spent on social programs during the same period (Human Rights Watch, 2004). As the international oil companies refuse to disclose how much money they paid for oil in Angola, it is impossible for Angolans to monitor where money paid for oil actually went. Natural resources should be held in trust by the state for the benefit of (at least) all citizens of a country. Citizens thus should be entitled to information concerning the sale of their resources. Moreover, recognition of ownership of these resources is acknowledged in the law of developing countries. If they do so belong, those people are entitled to information about how their resources are being managed. Such information helps citizens keep governments accountable for the sale of their resources and the management of revenues that are thereby generated. This information is standardly disclosed in the developed world and the extension to the developing world is long overdue.

The lessons we learn about the case of oil are quite generalizable (Brock, 2009, chapter 5). More transparency in payments and in the flow of money to less-developed countries more generally would eliminate the ease with which corruption can flourish, and would ensure that payments intended to benefit the citizens of a country actually do so. Regulation is clearly needed. Relying on voluntary disclosure tends to punish the more scrupulous and risk their business being transferred to less scrupulous operators. Required payment disclosure is the only fair option, since it levels the playing field for all and eliminates the current international double standard between required levels of transparency in the developed and developing world. Companies can be made to publish what they pay by various mechanisms; for instance, it could easily be made a condition for the listing of oil companies on major stock exchanges (such as London or New York) that they adopt the transparency practice.

Some solutions to the problems of double standards and tax evasion

As I have argued, global standards for taxation and "best accounting practices" need reworking. Lack of transparency, financial secrecy and general lack of information, create serious obstacles to doing the research necessary for suggesting reforms. However, with the information currently available, a number of suggestions can be made. It is instructive to look at what actual proposals are being floated by various non-governmental organizations (NGOs) and other agencies mobilizing for change in this area.

The Tax Justice Network calls for the initiation of a democratic global forum, comprised of representatives from citizen groups and governments across the world, that should engage in widespread debate on these issues and the possibility of implementing policies such as the following:

(1) We should develop systems of unitary taxation for multinationals to put a stop to the entirely false shifting of profits to countries with low or no taxes.

(2) It would be helpful to harmonize tax rates and policy for capital (that is currently highly mobile).

(3) States should cooperate with each other to reduce the destructive effects of tax competition between themselves.

(4) They should consider the possibility of "establishing regional and global tax authorities that can represent the interests of citizens" (Tax Justice Network, 2003a).

Because some economies, especially those in certain less developed countries and some small island economies, depend heavily on their tax-relief practices, reforms aimed at better accounting practices might be harmful to them in the short-term. Multilateral support will be needed to assist with re-structuring.

Whereas such reforms might have seemed quite out of the question pre-September 2001, since 9/11 there is considerable interest in phasing out tax havens. Loopholes in international taxation greatly assisted in financing terrorist organizations. In light of this (and other recent events), there is substantial support for setting international standards for transparency in accounting and for better monitoring of all flows of money (Kochan, 2005). I return to further discussion of arrangements to address tax avoidance and related issues below, after considering other reforms in more detail.

Global taxes, fees or dues to protect global public goods and tackle global poverty

Some justification

Not only should we prevent businesses from avoiding tax but, moreover, additional taxes on businesses should be implemented for the benefits they receive from a number of public goods on which they rely, but for the use of which they do not adequately contribute. There are a number of global public goods that enable and facilitate trade and without which it could not flourish. Examples include: peace, social and political stability, stability of the international and financial monetary system, protection from organized crime, effective law enforcement, populations that enjoy adequate health, an environment that continues to be reasonably life-sustaining, (sustainable) development and the absence of poverty. Businesses profit from the enjoyment of such global public goods. And yet they are not currently required to contribute adequately to the costs of sustaining these goods. Requiring businesses to pay their dues in the form of global taxes of (say) 1% (though I shortly discuss a range of options), would ask no more of them than is required for minimal reciprocity and fairness.[2]

In fact, a number of proposals have been made for various global taxes. In the next section I discuss some of these proposals and some potential implementation issues. Two taxes, in particular, have gained attention: a tax on the carbon content of commercial fuels, commonly referred to as a carbon tax, and a currency transaction tax, often referred to as a Tobin tax, after James Tobin who first floated the idea in the 1970s.

Global taxes: some possibilities

In fact, we do have some global taxes, for instance, on deep seabed mining, which were incorporated in the UN Law of the Sea Convention in the 1980s. Furthermore, recommendations for global taxes have a fairly long history (Paul & Wahlberg, 2002). Research on various taxes has been done, including on how they could be fairly implemented and their predicted effects. Not inconsiderable support for various taxes has been expressed. However, powerful interest groups in many rich countries have reacted negatively towards some of these ideas. At the request of Senator Jesse Helms, the US Congress considered and passed a bill making payment of UN dues conditional on it refraining from promoting any global tax proposals, and this effectively stifled all discussion of the issue (US Senate Bill 1519, 1996). Because of the dire financial position of the UN at that time, all discussion of global taxation then stopped. However, interest in the topic remains, even in the USA, as citizens become increasingly aware of various global problems and their effects on people's lives (Kay, 1995). Support for such taxes is strong in the European Union, and taxes on air travel and energy use have been implemented (to be covered below). I begin by discussing the two proposals that have enjoyed the most serious consideration so far and have enjoyed a small measure of implementation success: the carbon tax and the currency transaction tax (Wahlberg, 2005).

The carbon tax

A carbon tax would tax energy sources that emit carbon dioxide. Current fossil fuel use patterns and the release of greenhouse gases (such as carbon dioxide from fossil fuels) exacerbates global warming and climate change, thereby undermining the environment's ability to continue to be life-sustaining. Climate change can greatly affect agriculture and thereby the world's ability to produce adequate food. Other irreversible damage is predicted, such as dramatic rises in sea levels, which would increase demand for habitable land.

Depending on how high the tax rate is set, a carbon tax could provide incentives to move to more sustainable energy forms. With a $200 tax on every ton of carbon, it is projected there would be a 50% decrease in carbon emissions from current levels and this could generate $630 billion per year (or about 1% of gross world product for the year) (Paul & Wahlberg, 2002). Such a tax might raise the costs of cooking food or transportation quite significantly for poor people. In order to ensure they were not disproportionately burdened by this tax, we need to consider what complementary policies are also needed, perhaps through differential tax rates for different countries, or rebates that are made to low-income households (or others who would have severe difficulties transitioning to the new arrangements) (Carbon Tax Center, 2009).

We could levy carbon taxes directly at the point of sale of carbon fuels, just as value-added taxes (VAT) or sales taxes currently are levied. Since VAT and sales taxes are already widely in use and most fuel sales are computerized, adding an additional 1% carbon tax would not impose much extra cost or difficulty in implementation (Baumert, 1998). Several countries have enacted a carbon tax including: Sweden, Finland, Germany, the Netherlands and Norway. There is some notable support for this in other countries.

Currency transaction tax or Tobin tax

It is estimated that well over half (on some estimates 95%) of the $1.8 trillion in currency transactions that occur every day are speculative and as such are potentially destabilizing to local economies (Wahl & Waldow, 2001). Local currencies can devalue rapidly, causing major financial crises such as occurred in East Asia in 1997/1998, Brazil in 1999 and Argentina in 2001. When the local economy is in the grip of such crises, millions of people can be significantly harmed. In the 1970s, James Tobin suggested a small tax on currency trades to ward off such eventualities, to "throw sand in the wheels" of the markets, slowing down speculation and promoting more long-term investing (Tobin, 1974). The purpose of such a tax

---

[2] For a more extended treatment of these issues including consideration of, and responses to, objections, see Brock (2009, chapter 5).

would be to reduce destabilizing trades, and the order of magnitude proposed is considerably less than 1% on each trade. The tax would promote more stability and better conditions for development.

The USA, Japan, the European Union, Switzerland, Hong Kong and Singapore account for 90% of currency exchange transactions. It is hard to believe we could not collect the tax effectively from such countries if the will was mobilized to do so, as the tax could easily be imposed at the point of settlement and could be levied through computer programs installed in banks and financial institutions (Ul Haq *et al.*, 1996; Wahl & Waldow, 2001; Spahn, 2002). Currency deals already carry an administrative charge in most countries, certainly in the main currency exchange countries, so the administrative feasibility of such a tax is already plain. A tax of just 0.2% is predicted to raise about $300 billion annually.

The tax has had considerable support not just from NGOs but also gained mass backing from politicians and others, including George Soros who himself made billions through speculative trades, and more than 800 members of parliament from five continents who signed an international declaration in support of the tax. Several countries (such as Canada, Belgium and France) have committed to enacting the tax if there is additional support from the international community.

Despite the long history of discussion over the carbon and Tobin taxes, one tax that was only proposed more recently has, arguably, been more successful in terms of widespread implementation than these other two, namely the air-ticket tax, which I discuss next.

Air-ticket tax

President Jacques Chirac first officially proposed this tax. The idea with this tax is that it is a "solidarity contribution" levied on airplane tickets to finance global health programs. An international conference took place in Paris to mobilize support and 13 governments agreed to introduce the tax, namely: Brazil, Chile, Congo, Ivory Coast, France, Jordan, Luxembourg, Madagascar, Mauritius, Nicaragua, Norway and Cyprus, though others have subsequently agreed as well. In addition, 38 countries have established a group to investigate "solidarity contributions" to promote development.

On the current arrangements, in France, the tax amounts to 1 euro per domestic ticket and 4 euros for an international, economy class flight, with slightly more charged for business and first-class flights (Schroeder, 2006). Other ticket taxes involve similar or smaller amounts. The proceeds are being spent on assisting poor countries struggling with malaria, AIDS and tuberculosis. The WHO operates the fund and (among other things) uses bulk ordering to purchase necessary drugs at low cost.

The breakthrough of an air-ticket tax has given the discussion about finding sources of finance that can fund development some momentum. There are many other proposals that pre-date this victory that deserve some discussion as well (Baumert, 1998; Paul & Wahlberg, 2002; Walker, 2005). I discuss some of these next.

E-mail taxes

The idea with this tax would be to raise revenue that could be used to bridge the "digital divide" between rich and poor by improving computer, e-mail, and web-access to those in low-income communities and countries. According to one common suggestion, sending 100 e-mails per day each with a kilobyte document attached would incur a tax of 1 cent. Telecommunication carriers and internet service providers could be charged with the responsibility of collecting the taxes. Consumers in the developed world only would be charged. In 1996, such a tax would have raised $70 billion and the figure would be much bigger today (United Nations Development Program, 1999). It is also possible in this age of out-of-control spam, that a 1% tax on e-mail would gain more support as a way to discourage high traffic in unwanted emails. A problem with this tax is that the global communication possibilities opened up by e-mail are one of the most positive aspects of the current period of globalization, so this tax is unlikely to garner widespread approval.

Tax on world trade

This tax does not explicitly seek to discourage the activity on which it is imposed. The idea, instead, is that the tax would be a fee or contribution for protecting the underlying conditions necessary to sustain international trade, such as peace and well-being (Evans, 1997). In 1998, the volume of world trade was $7.3 trillion and a tax of 0.5% on the trade of goods and services would have raised $37 billion (Paul & Wahlberg, 2002).

Tax on the international arms trade

Arms imports can constitute a significant obstacle to development (Independent Commission on International Development, 1980). Proposals to implement a tax on the international arms trade have been circulated from several sources over a number of years (Independent Commission on International Development, 1980; Mendez, 1992; Paul & Wahlberg, 2002). The idea is to reduce the level of arms trading, but also to raise money for development, to compensate victims of wars, and to promote disarmament. In January 2004, Brazil and France re-launched the idea of an international tax on arms sales and financial transactions, the so-called "Lula Fund" (after Brazil's President Luiz Inacio Lula da Silva), to give it some much-needed momentum. About 70% of world arms exports come from the USA, France and the UK (data from 1993–2000) (European Commission, 2002). Because of this concentration in the weapons production industry, and the fact that all these countries are in favor of controlling arms exports, some initiatives are already underway which could facilitate collection of this tax, such as the UN register for conventional arms and the European Code of Conduct on Arms Exports (European Commission, 2002).

Aviation fuel taxes

Unlike the air-ticket tax which aims at fostering development, the target of this tax is to off-set harmful carbon emissions. Airplane travel is one of the fastest growing sources of carbon emissions and by 2050 it is predicted to cause about 15% of all such emissions (ENDS, 1999). Increased fuel costs would create good incentives for airlines to use more fuel-efficient aircraft and more efficient air-traffic control systems, but would have little effect on passenger demand (Intergovernmental Panel on Climate Change, 2001).

Some other ideas and proposals

Other proposals for global taxes have been suggested including fees for satellites that orbit the earth, fees on the use of the electronic spectrum for radio, mobile phones and television and taxes on international advertising (Walker, 2005). Perhaps a tax on consumption, such as a global sales tax or VAT is also worth considering, especially on luxury goods. A 1% tax on income from businesses in developed countries that engage in international activities is also worth consideration.

While the cases for the carbon, tobin, air-ticket, arms trade and aviation fuel taxes seem quite compelling, further research may be needed to determine whether such taxes might be (unavoidably) regressive or harmful in other ways. (Elsewhere I argue that the case for the Tobin tax is especially strong; Brock, 2010.)

Some issues concerning global taxes for here and now

At the moment, the way global taxes could gain legal standing is through agreements between nation states in an "internationally-harmonized tax regime" (Paul & Wahlberg, 2002). The idea would be for each nation to raise the particular global taxes through its regular tax authority. Each nation would pass on an agreed amount or percentage to an international organization for spending in line with the specified global objectives. More developed countries may be allowed to retain (say) 75% of what they raise, while developing countries may be permitted to keep a much higher percentage, to be spent on public goods or tackling poverty in line with the taxes' objectives. No dramatic changes to international law would be required on this model. The international body that coordinates, collects and disburses revenue must conform to high standards, and people would want such an organization to be representative and accountable. Clearly specifying the goals of revenue collection and how proceeds will be spent (such as is the case with the air-ticket tax) could considerably allay fears about wastage or abuse.

Would we need global taxes to be universal? Not necessarily. Of course, it is desirable if global taxes are levied universally. In the absence of universal support, however, some considerable success is still possible. As we have already seen with the air-ticket tax, substantial progress is possible with even just a few countries' cooperation. We need to get away from the idea that without universal agreement no progress is possible. After all, we do not have universal support and agreement for the International Criminal Court, but that has not stopped enough of us (around 110 countries at the time of writing) from establishing the court and proceeding with its core activities. Progress with respect to the goals of global justice is still quite possible even when powerful players refuse to assist or comply with well-supported agreements. We do not need universal agreement to take significant steps in the right direction. Furthermore, in due course, non-participating states may eventually join a tax regime for several reasons.

Citizens of non-participating states may pressure their governments to join. Non-participating states might lose influence in policies related to spending revenue raised. Plus, once a successful scheme is in place, there might be pressure from the international community to join as well. Most states have now come to appreciate that it is in their interests to agree on common standards in financial and taxation arrangements. For one thing, opaque tax and financial systems, and lack of cooperation, make it difficult to stop money laundering, financing of terrorist organizations and tax evasion (Kochan, 2005). Many fora that aim to eliminate harmful tax practices have been put in place, including the Financial Stability Forum of the G7, the Forum on harmful tax practices of the OECD and the Financial Action Task Force. Since September 11, 2001, action to target terrorist financing has given these initiatives further support.

Financing global public goods properly will be best promoted by establishing an International Tax Organization. Other reasons support such an organization, for instance, the taxes that countries can impose (especially on transportable goods and mobile factors) are significantly constrained by the tax rates others impose, so tax avoidance, tax evasion and other harmful policies can best be addressed if tackled collectively. Furthermore, the reforms suggested in Section II concerned with eliminating tax evasion (or practices resembling this) would boost poor countries' abilities to collect domestic taxes. States are not usually able to collect all the taxes they are owed, especially from powerful multinational corporations, which results in substantial losses in revenues. Receiving more of the taxes poor developing countries are owed will allow these countries enormous sources of funds with which they could do much to address some of the structural causes of local poverty, which might include having more resources for education, job training, health care, infrastructural development, capital investment and so on. In this way, we would be enabling those in poor countries to help their own citizens better. The good news is that, as part of the "War on Terrorism," we in affluent nations seem to have acquired a new "Can Do!" attitude. We apparently now have ways to track money linked to terrorism and money laundering. These same measures will allow us to track the very revenue streams that it was previously thought we could not keep track of for taxation purposes. Indeed, better international financial cooperation is not only feasible; it's happening.

One major worry that may concern readers is that there is a risk that any international tax regime will possess too much power, which it might abuse. What measures could ensure that an international tax regime is democratically run? What measures would limit its power?

These are big issues that deserve extended treatment (but for a start, see Brock, 2009, chapter 5). I have space for only a couple of remarks here. It is worth noting that we already have recently formed some international bodies that do the sort of work recommended in this chapter, notably the Organisation for Economic Co-operation and Development (OECD) Global Forum on Taxation. This OECD body generally provides a good forum for the exchange of ideas about policy with some tangible results, such as the development of proposals for unitary taxation formulae, which could be used in devising better arrangements to replace current transfer pricing practices (OECD, 2001). The OECD body does not, however, have the power to levy taxes directly, nor does any currently existing international tax organization have such power. However, were an international organization to be empowered to collect revenue, it is not clear why such an organization could not be as accountable as other international organizations that we believe do an adequate job of being held accountable, or be modeled along similar lines (such as the World Health Organization or International Labour Organization). It is also worth noting that we have smaller versions of some of these problems at the domestic level as well and have several measures in place to deal with worrisome aspects, which could be applied internationally.

Summary of main conclusions

In this chapter I examined how reform of our international tax regime could be especially important in realizing global justice. Ensuring all, including and especially multinationals, pay their fair share of taxes is crucial to ensuring that all countries, especially developing countries, are able to fund education, health care, job training, infrastructural development and so forth, thereby enabling poor countries to help themselves better. Eliminating tax havens, tax evasion and transfer pricing schemes that do not reflect fair market pricing, are all important to ensure accountability and to support democracies, as is requiring disclosure of revenues paid for resources.

While the taxation ideas discussed in this chapter can certainly happily co-exist with Pogge's (they are not meant to be construed as competitors, as such), I suggested that the collection of proposals concerning taxation reform considered here are likely to be more beneficial, not just because the amounts of money they would release are more significant, but also because they target some of the central issues more effectively, for instance, ensuring more transparency and blocking important avenues currently open to corrupt leaders which facilitate the siphoning of money away from developing countries. The reforms suggested also might have more chance of being implemented, as some of these converge with plans already underway and, in some cases, actually being implemented.

As I also discussed, many particular proposals for global taxes have already been floated and, there is relevant and not inconsiderable support for implementing such proposals. A small number of countries have also introduced some of these taxes. It would not take much to start closing the gap between theory and practice in the area of global taxation, and in that way to make progress toward tackling global poverty and the conditions that sustain it. What is needed is just a bit more of the kind of leadership France has already shown in mobilizing support for, and implementing, the air-ticket tax.[3]

References

Baker, R. (2005). *Capitalism's Achilles Heel: Dirty Money and How to Renew the Free-Market System*. Hoboken, NJ: John Wiley and Sons.

Baumert, K. (1998). *Global Taxes and Fees: Recent Developments and Overcoming Obstacles*. www.globalpolicy.org/component/content/article/216/45849.html (Accessed November 16, 2009).

Boston Consulting Group (2003). *Winning in a Challenging Market: Global Wealth 2003*.

Brock, G. (2005). Egalitarianism, ideals, and cosmopolitan justice. *Philosophical Forum* **36**, 1–30.

Brock, G. (2009). *Global Justice: A Cosmopolitan Account*. Oxford: Oxford University Press.

Brock, G. (2010). Reforming our taxation arrangements to promote global gender justice. *Philosophical Topics* **37**, 141–160.

Carbon-Tax Center (2009). *Managing Impacts*. www.carbontax.org/issues/softening-the-impact-of-carbon-taxes/ (Accessed November 16, 2009).

Chen, S. & Ravallion, M. (2008). *The Developing World is Poorer than We Thought, But No Less Successful in the Fight Against Poverty*. World Bank Policy Research Working Paper No. 4703. Washington, DC: World Bank.

Christensen, J. & Hampton, M.P. (1999). All Good Things Come to an End. *The World Today, Royal Institute of International Affairs* **55**, no.8/9, 14–17.

Christian Aid (2005). The Shirts off their Backs. www.christianaid.org.uk (Accessed November 15, 2009).

Citizens for Tax Justice (2002). *Surge in Tax Welfare Drives Corporate Tax Payments Down to Near Record Low*. Washington, DC: Citizens for Tax Justice.

Cobham, A. (2007). The Tax Consensus Has Failed! *Oxford Council on Good Governance Economy Recommendation, no. 8*. www.oxfordgovernance.org.

ENDS Environmental Daily (1999). Aviation climate effect could grow four fold. June 3. www.globalpolicy.org/component/content/article/216/45842.html (Accessed November 22, 2009).

European Commission (2002). *Responses to the Challenges of Globalization: A Study on the International Monetary and Financial System and on Financing Development*. www.globalpolicy.org/component/content/article/213/45756.html (Accessed November 15, 2009).

Evans, W. (1997). To help the UN, a tax on trade. *New York Times*, July 6.

Furman, J. (2006). Closing the tax gap. www.cbpp.org/4–10–06tax3.pdf (Accessed November 16, 2009).

Human Rights Watch (2004). Angola: account for missing oil revenues. www.hrw.org/en/news/2004/01/11/angola-account-missing-oil-revenues (Accessed November 16, 2009).

Independent Commission on International Development (1980). *North-South. A Programme for Survival. Report of the Independent Commission*. London: Pan Books.

Intergovernmental Panel on Climate Change (2001). *Aviation and the Global Atmosphere*. www.grida.no/publications/other/ipcc_sr/?src=/climate/ipcc/aviation/index.htm (Accessed November 16, 2009).

Kay, A. (1995). Reforming the UN: the view of the American people. In H. Cleveland, H. Henderson & I. Kaul (Eds.), *The United Nations: Policy and Financing Alternatives*. Washington, DC: The Global Commission to Fund the United Nations.

---

[3] This chapter is a significantly shortened version of "Taxation and Global Justice: Closing the Gap between Theory and Practice." *Journal of Social Philosophy* (2008), 161–184, published by Wiley-Blackwell. I am grateful for permission to reprint it here. I am also very grateful for comments and assistance received from Christian Barry, Alex Cobham, James Coe, John Christensen, Stephen Davies, Carol Gould, Nicole Hassoun, Rachel McMaster, Darrel Moellendorf, Richard Murphy, Thomas Pogge, Don Ross and Clark Wolf.

Kochan, N. (2005). *The Washing Machine: How Money Laundering and Terrorist Financing Soil us.* Texere, Thomson.

Mendez, R. (1992). *International Public Finance.* New York: Oxford University Press.

Mitchell, E. & Sikka, P. (2005). *Taming the Corporations.* Basildon, UK: Association for Accountancy and Business Affairs.

Organisation for Economic Co-operation and Development (OECD) (2001). *Transfer Pricing Guidelines for Multinational Enterprises and Tax Administrations.* Paris: OECD.

Oxfam (2000). *Tax Havens: Releasing the Hidden Billions for Poverty Eradication.* http://publications.oxfam.org.uk/ oxfam/display.asp?K=002P0036&aub=Oxfam&sort= sort_date/d&m=99&dc=113 (Accessed November 15, 2009).

Paul, J. & Wahlberg, K. (2002). *Global Taxes for Global Priorities.* www.globalpolicy.org/socecon/glotax/general/ glotaxpaper.htm (Accessed November 16, 2009).

Pogge, T. (2001a). Eradicating systematic poverty: brief for a global resources dividend. *Journal of Human Development* **2**, 59–77.

Pogge, T. (2001b). Priorities of global justice. *Metaphilosophy* **32**, 6–24.

Pogge, T. (2002). *World Poverty and Human Rights.* Cambridge: Polity.

Rodrik, D. (2003). *In Search of Prosperity: Analytic Narratives on Economic Growth.* Princeton, NJ: Princeton University Press.

Schroeder, F. (2006). *Innovative Sources of Finance after the Paris Conference.* Briefing Paper. Friedrich Ebert Foundation/Stiftung (FES).

Spahn, P. (2002). *On the Feasibility of a Tax on Foreign Exchange Transactions.* Report to the German Federal Ministry for Economic Cooperation and Development, Bonn.

Stiglitz, J. (2002). *Globalization and its Discontents.* London: Penguin.

Tax Justice Network (2003a). *Declaration of the Tax Justice Network.* www.taxjustice.net/cms/front_content. php?idcat=3 (Accessed November 16, 2009).

Tax Justice Network (2003b). Transfer Pricing. *Tax Justice Focus (Quarter 4).* www.taxjustice.net/cms/front_ content.php?idcat=75 (Accessed November 16, 2009).

Tax Justice Network (2005). *Tax us if you Can.* www. taxjustice.net/cms/front_content.php?idcat=30 (Accessed November 15, 2009).

Accessed Tobin, J. (1974). *The New Economics, One Decade Older. The Eliot Janeway Lectures on Historical Economics in Honor of Joseph Schumpeter, 1972.* Princeton, NJ: Princeton University Press.

Ul Haq, M., Kaul, I. & Grunberg I. (1996). *The Tobin Tax – Coping with Financial Volatility* (pp. 109–158). New York: Oxford University Press.

United Nations Development Program (1999). *Human Development Report* (p. 66). New York: Oxford University Press.

US Senate (1996). US Senate Bill 1519, 104th Congress, 2nd Session.

Vigueras, J. H. (2005). *Tax Havens: How Offshore Centres Undermine Democracy.* Spain: Akal.

Wahl, P. & Waldow, P. (2001). *Currency Transaction Tax – a Concept with a future – Chances and Limits of Stabilising Financial Markets through the Tobin Tax.* Bonn: WEED.

Wahlberg, K. (2005). *Progress on Global Taxes?* www. globalpolicy.org/component/content/article/216/46020. html (Accessed November 16, 2009).

Walker, J. (2005). *Alternative Financing for the United Nations.* www.globalpolicy.org/un-finance/alternative- financing-for-the-un-5-14.html (Accessed November 16, 2009).

Chapter

24

Global health research: changing the agenda

Tikki Pang

Background

In the face of multiple, diverse and emerging global health threats, global health research has a central role to play in developing effective interventions and sustainable policies to deal with these challenges, especially in the context of reaching the targets set by the health-related Millennium Development Goals (MDGs). As recently stated, "research is a major driver of social and technological innovation that can lead to health and equity improvements through a knowledge-to-action process" (Coloma & Harris, 2009) and, through global health science, "we will never have a better opportunity to improve public health globally" (Farrar, 2007).

The world today faces not only threats from pandemics of infectious disease, e.g. pandemic influenza H1N1, but has to contend with the emergence of resistance to antimicrobial agents, chronic diseases, an aging population, fragile health systems and the health impacts of globalization, e.g. those related to climate change, travel and migration, food insecurity, lack of clean water and the global spread of harmful lifestyles and substances. It is also a reality that it is the developing world that is bearing the brunt of the global disease burden.

Despite increasing amounts of resources spent on global health R&D, an estimated $160 billion in 2005 (Global Forum for Health Research, 2008), there are concerns with the impact of the current financial crisis on the funding of health research, continued weaknesses and constraints in research capacity in developing countries, the inadequacies of the current modes of global health research governance, and the way resources are currently distributed to various areas and types of health research. In addition, global health problems are becoming increasingly inter-sectoral in nature and appropriate strategies are needed to meet

such challenges in order to help redress the gross inequities in health which exist between rich and poor countries. In times of competing priorities and limited resources, good governance, institutional capacity building and devising methods to evaluate the returns on investments in research, and its impact on health outcomes, are some of the important priorities for the future.

In this broad context, is the current global health research agenda adequate and sufficient to meet these daunting challenges? Can the barriers be overcome and is a new research agenda needed? How will a new agenda be developed and implemented? This chapter will explore these important questions.

Current status of global health research – why is a new research agenda needed?

The present section will analyze and describe five current challenges and barriers in global health research and provide a justification for the need of a new research agenda.

Imbalances

First, we are witnessing continued imbalances and gaps in health research which are resulting in market failures for needed interventions and limited access to the benefits of research, especially for populations living in the developing world.

It has been reported, for example, that of 1556 new drugs developed between 1975 and 2004, only 21 (1.3%) were for tropical diseases of the developing world (Chirac & Toureele, 2006). More recently, in an analysis of funding patterns and allocations of major health research agencies, Moran *et al.* (2009) found that

76% of research funding was allocated to only three diseases, HIV/AIDS, TB and malaria. In a recent analysis of the grant-making program of the Bill and Melinda Gates Foundation, concerns were expressed that 40% of all funding was given to supranational organizations and that over a third of funding was allocated to R&D (mainly for vaccines and microbicides), or to basic science research (McCoy *et al.*, 2009). In what he describes as a "three bucket" analogy to represent the tasks of medicine, where the first bucket is understanding the biology of disease, the second about finding effective treatments and the third to ensure effective delivery of the treatments, Pronovost highlighted the existence of the imbalance by suggesting that "we spend a cent on the third bucket for every $1 we spend on the first two" (Laurance, 2009).

These unbalanced patterns of distribution of research grants, of course, ignore the fact that more than 70% of the current global disease burden is linked to chronic diseases with most of the burden being borne, once again, by the developing world. It also neglects other important areas of concern to many developing countries, e.g. the neglected tropical diseases (Hotez *et al.*, 2009) and the burden associated with violence and road traffic injuries.

With regards to the type of research being supported, a study linking current priorities in health research funding to impact on the number of child deaths, found that 97% of grants were designed for developing new technologies which can reduce child mortality by 22%. If, instead, research was done on how to fully utilize existing technologies, this could reduce child mortality by up to 66% (Leroy *et al.*, 2007). It has also been highlighted that the research funding approach of the Bill and Melinda Gates Foundation is heavily weighted towards the development of new vaccines and drugs (Black *et al.*, 2009), and that only 23% of its funding and 3% of NIH funding were for research on delivery and use of existing, proven interventions (Leroy *et al.*, 2007). In a similar vein, an analysis of the research supported by the major UK funding agencies indicated that, on average, only 1% of funding was allocated to health services research (Rothwell, 2006). A view has been expressed that these trends reflect a more general problem with "donor culture" where, since the 1990s, there has been a shift away from funding public health research and research to strengthen health systems to more disease-targeted approaches.

Importantly, there is also a general perception that research agendas are largely dictated by the donor agencies, often with little regard for what may be national health research priorities. Recipient countries are largely without a voice in major funding decisions made by the major donors in the developed world, and, for example, are poorly represented on the boards of major health-related public–private partnership (PPP) organizations which are attempting to develop key interventions for developing world health problems (Tucker & Makgoba, 2008). This has resulted in a concern for the existence of "scientific imperialism" and a question as to whether the current model of PPP's has "… in fact, perpetuated research disparities and power inequities and possibly accentuated the dependency relationship of developing country researchers rather than contributing to correcting the disparity" (Tucker & Makgoba, 2008).

Tensions also continue to exist between the need to promote and protect innovation through intellectual property laws and a more open, equitable sharing of research results. Indonesia's recent refusal to share influenza virus strains with the World Health Organization is a case in point where developing countries fear the possibility that vaccines derived from such strains may be developed by pharmaceutical companies in the developed world – and then sold back to them at prices they cannot afford. In this context, calls have been made at the World Health Assembly that a possible mechanism or instrument for essential health and biomedical R&D would be a health and biomedical R&D "treaty." This proposes an international system which: "(1) ensures sustainable investments in medical innovation, (2) provides a fair allocation of the cost burdens of such innovation, (3) creates mechanisms to drive R&D investment into the areas of the greatest need, and (4) provides the flexibility to utilize diverse and innovative methods of financing innovation while protecting consumers and ensuring access" (CPTech, 2008). This trend towards more formal regulatory approaches also reflects a similar trend in global health governance more generally in relation to the increasing use of "harder" instruments (Gostin, 2008).

Capacity for research

Second, there are continued problems and concerns with research capacity in developing countries (Coloma & Harris, 2009). Low- and low- to middle-income countries contributed only 7% of the global output of scientific literature between 1992–2001 (Paraje *et al.*, 2005) although recent findings are suggesting improvements in the situation. A study by Hofman *et al.* showed that between 1995–2004, the annual number of articles from sub-Saharan Africa indexed in MEDLINE grew 41% from 2073 to 2929 and the number of MEDLINE-indexed journals nearly doubled from 10 in 1995 to 19 in 2004 (Hofman *et al.*, 2009). The indicator used, however, which is the number of scientific publications, does not reflect other important factors such as the appropriate balance between different types of research skills (e.g. between biomedical and health services research), and other critical areas such as capacity for research management, resource mobilization, infrastructure and utilization of research findings (e.g. research synthesis and the use of evidence in health policy development).

Another report indicated a significant improvement of a nearly 200% increase in research output in the last 5 years in developing countries more broadly (HINARI, 2009). The improvement is consistent with the increasing involvement and research capacity of some large, middle-income developing countries such as those in the BRIC group (Brazil, Russia, India, China). Developing countries are also boosting their spending on R&D from $134 billion in 2002 to $272 billion in 2007, with a corresponding increase in the number of researchers from 1.8 to 2.7 million in the same time frame (Nature, 2009a). Aside from publication outputs, there are also promising signs of better capacity on the ground: research excellence and institutional capacities appear to be improving in Africa where 11 centers across the continent are now conducting phase 3 trials of a potentially revolutionary and effective malaria vaccine (RTS,S) (Nature, 2009b).

Accountability and the ethics of research

Third, there are increasing concerns with lack of transparency and accountability and the unethical conduct of research in the developing world. As a result of a variety of factors, including lower costs and larger patient/participant "pools," more and more clinical research is being conducted in developing countries with countries like India, China and Russia seeing significant increases in clinical trials conducted within their borders in the past 5 years (Normile, 2008). Beyond the broader, well-known problems of publication bias and the non-reporting of adverse events or negative results, there have also been, worryingly, reports of unethical conduct in the performance of clinical trials in developing country settings (Wemos, 2008). Farrar (2007) has also highlighted that many developing countries feel disempowered and are

unable to be true participants in clinical trials being pursued within their national borders due to excessive regulatory and administrative demands and standards for the conduct of trials which are set by the developed world. In many developing countries (e.g. India), there are also concerns with illegal, dangerous and uncontrolled testing of new, unproven therapies, e.g. those associated with stem cell therapies for a whole range of conditions.

From research to policy and practice

Fourth, in the important area of knowledge utilization and translation there are weak linkages between research, and the evidence it generates, and health policy development. This is partly due to the lack of an adequate evidence base needed to make informed decisions. For example, a review of the Cochrane Collaboration systematic reviews database showed that, on average, less than 10% of systematic reviews in the Cochrane database are dealing with developing country health problems (McMichael *et al.*, 2005). A survey of systematic review production in 22 low- and middle-income countries in Asia, Africa and Latin America between 2004 and 2007 showed that some countries produced no systematic reviews and that only 10 unique reviews (out of a total of nearly 700) addressed governance, financial and delivery issues within health systems (Lavis, J., unpublished).

Governance of research

Finally, global health research is currently suffering from fragmented and confused governance arrangements which are resulting in gross inefficiencies in the research process as outlined above. In the past two decades many more players have entered the arena, each with their own priorities and agendas, often with a focus on short-term results in specific disease areas.

Indeed, the present state of fragmentation and confusion is reflected in a recent call for a rationalization of the global health research "architecture" through a merger of some of the key stakeholders (Rottingen *et al.*, 2009). At a higher political level, and as a follow-up to the G8 Summit in L'Aquila, Italy in July 2009, plans are underway to establish a Network of Centers of Health Innovation with the objective of increasing the impacts of health research investments into structures and institutions in sub-Saharan Africa. Specifically, the initiative aims to ensure that health research capacities are built on a sustainable basis and

Table 24.1. Key elements of a new health research agenda.

- Inclusiveness in defining priorities
- Appropriate balance between generation and utilization of knowledge, between new interventions and stronger health systems
- Ensure equitable access to the fruits of research
- Promote transparency, accountability and ethical behavior
- Emphasize evaluation of impact of research
- Greater willingness on the part of donors for better alignment and harmonization of activities
- Formal platform which ensures implementation, accountability and monitoring

that skills are transferred to ensure in-country research is translated into clinical and public health practice. A call was similarly issued that "we need a G8 for research (R8)" consisting of the major health research funding agencies (Lancet, 2008).

Ministers of health meeting in Bamako, Mali in November 2008 to discuss research for health also issued a call "to better align, coordinate and harmonize the global health research architecture and its governance through the rationalization of existing organizations, to improve coherence and impact, and to increase efficiencies and equity" (WHO, 2009a). The World Health Organization has similarly acknowledged the need for a more harmonized approach by developing a first-ever Organization-wide strategy on research for health (WHO, 2009b) which is focused around the four goals of priority setting, capacity building, setting of norms and standards and translation of knowledge into policy and practice. The implementation of this strategy is seen to be closely linked with the Global Strategy and Plan of Action emanating from the Inter-Governmental Working Group on Innovation, Public Health and Intellectual Property, endorsed by the World Health Assembly in 2009.

Although the true picture is undeniably complex and there are clearly multiple causes and factors responsible for the above challenges, global health research governance is arguably one of the key areas influencing and affecting the effectiveness and sustainability of global health research as a whole, and it is difficult to predict whether or not it will achieve its objectives.

Given the multitude of problems around global health research and its governance, what might be the way forward? What would elements of a new research agenda look like, and what would it take, from a governance perspective, to implement such an agenda effectively?

Elements of a new health research agenda

A new global health research agenda, developed through consultative and inclusive processes, and guided by a sustainable and equitable approach to good governance, should ideally strive to achieve several objectives and meet a set of key criteria (Table 24.1).

Efficiency and priority setting

First and foremost, it should aim to improve the efficiency of the research process as a whole by achieving the right balance of priorities, both in terms of priority research areas and types of research, promoting the open sharing of research results and ensuring good standards for both the conduct of research and access to its results. New, more objective, inclusive and quantitative approaches to priority setting in health research should be taken into account and evaluated more widely. The drive for new technologies and interventions must be balanced with appropriate attention to "implementation science" as a framework for translating research for the benefit of global health (Madon et al., 2007) by ensuring delivery of, and access to, the new and the existing interventions. It is time to reframe the debate and as expressed eloquently by Elias (2006) "only solutions that creatively integrate the need for new and culturally relevant technologies with stronger systems and substantial behaviour change have a chance of reducing the health inequity between rich and poor countries."

The increasing trend towards publication in open access journals is an encouraging development and has been recently suggested to be an important means to bridging health inequities (Chan et al., 2009). One analysis has indicated that open access to scientific publications increased developing world participation in global science (Evans & Reimer, 2009). Research efficiency and transparency will also be improved if the results of all clinical trials are available on a publicly accessible database or search portal. This is the objective of WHO's International Clinical Trials Registry Platform (ICTRP) which acts as a search portal across all major registers of clinical trials worldwide. The platform aims to register all clinical trials, even Phase I exploratory trials, and requests the submission of a 20-item minimum data set providing key information on the trial. Finally, improving efficiency also means evaluating the impact and benefits of research, as seen in several recent reports to assess the returns on investment in research (Lane, 2009; Frank & Nason, 2009).

The new agenda should also maximize the powers of information and communication technologies as a means to improve research efficiency. Unprecedented advances in the past decade can serve as a facilitator of better linkages and connectivity between researchers and how they access relevant data and information. A suggestion has been made, for example, to provide every researcher with a unique identification number, which would facilitate retrieval of publications, following career paths and the establishment of collaborations (Enserink, 2009). Infectious diseases research can also be facilitated by the earlier identification of potential epidemics of infectious disease through the use of internet search engines such as Yahoo and Google.

Targeted research

Second, the agenda should be seen primarily as research for health improvement, and not research for the sake of research. In this context, implementation research to maximize use of existing interventions should be given a much higher priority and support, as should efforts to develop urgently needed new interventions and ensuring that such interventions reach those who need them the most. In this regard, new approaches to improve access such as prizes (Travis, 2008) "patent pools" (Nature, 2009c) or "health impact funds" should be explored. The "patent pools idea" proposes to create a pool for companies to share patents in order to boost research into neglected diseases prevalent in developing countries. In contrast, a "health impact fund" is "an optional mechanism that offers pharmaceutical innovators a supplementary reward based on the health impact of their products, if they agree to sell those products at

cost. The proposed Fund is to be financed mainly by governments" (Incentives for Global Health, 2009).

Innovative ways to accelerate drug development should also be pursued, as exemplified by the Institute for One World Health which focuses on identifying and developing promising drugs and vaccine candidates and then partnering with developing country partners to conduct research, manufacture and distribute these new therapies. The Tropical Diseases Initiative is another innovative approach which aims to apply an open-source collaborative approach to biomedical research for tropical infectious diseases.

At the same time, health improvement depends on effective policies which are well informed by evidence. Efforts to strengthen linkages between researchers and policy- and decision-makers should therefore be vigorously pursued. WHO's Evidence-informed Policy Networks (EVIPNet) attempts to do so by working closely with national ministries of health to establish country teams which function to perform research syntheses, develop policy briefs, promote "safe harbor" country dialogs and strengthen needed capacity in relevant areas (e.g. performing systematic reviews). Other areas of related activity include the establishment of "rapid response" mechanisms to help policy makers in accessing the relevant evidence.

Building equitable and sustainable research capacity

Third, continued efforts must be made to develop research capacity in an equitable, effective and sustainable manner. Unlike previous models for "capacity building" which was often centered around a leading research institution in the developed world, new and innovative approaches must be explored as exemplified recently by the Wellcome Trust's African Institutions Initiative which aims to establish seven new international consortia, each led by an African institution (Lancet, 2009). In an encouraging new development, 13 African governments, the WHO and the US government have recently approved an accreditation system, which includes a rating scale, for medical laboratories across Africa to improve standards of research and care in the continent.

New models to attract back the overseas diaspora of scientific talent (Seguin *et al.*, 2006), as exemplified by China's recently launched Qianren Jihua program (Thousand Person Plan) (Hao Xin, 2009), should also be considered by other developing countries. Given the highly intersectoral and interdisciplinary nature of current global health problems, an "integrative expertise" approach to capacity building in developing countries would also greatly facilitate better research utilization through more evidence-based practices which cut across more traditional research disciplines and boundaries (MacLachlan, 2009). The efforts of the Council for Health Research and Development (COHRED) to strengthen national health research systems should be strongly supported by the funders of research (COHRED, 2008).

Translational and implementation work

Fourth, a new agenda must possess the capacity to utilize the latest scientific advances and, importantly, place the translation of such advances in the context of public health improvement. A good example in this regard are the unprecedented advances in the post-genomic era which have important implications for public health (Pang, 2009), and where developing countries are increasingly active participants (Sgaier *et al.*, 2007). Of particular importance is the potential of pharmacogenomics and "personalized medicine" to improve the efficiency and safety of drug use, and of genome-wide association studies to identify genetic risk factors for chronic diseases. Another critically important dimension is the need to have effective international research collaboration, taking into consideration different incidence of both disease and genetic risk factors in different population groups. Methodologies and strategic approaches in this area are still in their infancy and need to be developed further.

The way forward

What of the way forward? How would such an agenda be developed and implemented in reality? At the core of the answer to this question is the fundamental need for effective governance of global health research, and how it must be linked to global health initiatives more broadly.

First and foremost it would require a willingness and commitment on the part of the major supporters and funders of global health research to better harmonize, coordinate and align their activities. This is a difficult challenge given the diversity of donors, their differing agendas and *modus operandi*. An agreement, at least in principle, around a set of shared values would be an important starting point for future discussions. A good example of this is the Paris Declaration on Aid

Effectiveness which proposes five principles for more effective aid: ownership, alignment, harmonization, managing for results and mutual accountability.

Second, it would require the convening of an inclusive, neutral platform which has capabilities to perform critical secretariat functions and, importantly, possesses more formal processes and mechanisms to hold participating players accountable for their commitments and promises. Importantly, and as part of its terms of reference, it should include processes to evaluate the effectiveness of resource allocations and interventions in solving or alleviating health problems.

Third, it would seem strategically desirable that the putative new agenda for global health research be presented as part of an overall package and strategy for health improvement in the developing world more generally.

In terms of a possible mechanism to implement such an agenda, several have been mentioned previously (Rottingen *et al.*, 2009), but the establishment of a "Committee C" of the World Health Assembly (WHA) of the WHO could be a possible step towards achieving the stated objectives (Silberschmidt *et al.*, 2008).

Article 18 of the WHO constitution gives the organization a legitimate role to "ensure more transparency and debate between global health players." Committee C would complement the existing Committees A (which deals with programmatic-technical matters) and B (which deals with budget and managerial matters). The proposed committee would bring together WHO member states, major global health initiatives (GHIs), major funders of health research and other key stakeholders (e.g. civil society) in an annual, formal platform to strive for better coordination, alignment and harmonization according to the Paris declaration on Aid Effectiveness. It would, in the standard *modus operandi* of the WHA, operate through proposing resolutions for adoption but "to explicitly welcome within such resolutions commitments independently taken by other partners that would be annexed to the resolution" (Silberschmidt *et al.*, 2008). Critically, however, and to overcome major concerns over such a structure disempowering developing countries, the voting power to pass resolutions should be solely vested in the member states, thus preserving their autonomy and independence in the governance of WHO. While Committee C would not address the underlying problem of the WHO which is that it is heavily reliant on voluntary contributions and thus vulnerable to donor priorities, it would take a step at addressing the democratic deficit within the WHO, as well as provide a platform for the various global health and health research actors to meet annually. While the actual form of "Committee C" needs much more discussion and reflection, what it is ultimately attempting to address is the chaos in the global health and health research systems, and the leadership role the WHO could assume in linking them together to improve health in the developing world.

Conclusions

Health research pursued and judiciously applied on a global scale, and effectively coordinated and harmonized, could play a critical role in helping to alleviate the complex and diverse health problems facing the developing world today. However, the present governance arrangements for global health research, and an agenda which is fragmented and uncoordinated, represent formidable barriers to achieving this goal. New strategic thinking, more goodwill and innovative platforms are needed to overcome these barriers.

References

Black, R. E., Bhan, M. K., Chopra, M., Rudan, I. & Victora, C. G. (2009). Accelerating the health impact of the Gates Foundation. *Lancet* **373**, 1584–1585.

Chan L., Arunachalam S. & Kirsop, B. (2009). Open access: a giant step towards bridging health inequities. *Bulletin of the World Health Organization* **87**, 631–635.

Chirac, P. & Torreele, E. (2006). Global framework on essential health R&D. *Lancet* **367**, 1560–1561.

Council on Health Research for Development (COHRED) (2008). Annual Report 2008: Supporting national health research systems in low and middle income countries. Geneva: COHRED. www.cohred.org/how-we-work (Accessed January 24, 2010).

Coloma, J. & Harris, E. (2009). From construction workers to architects: developing scientific research capacity in low-income countries. *PLoS Biology* **7**, e1000156. doi:10.1371/journal.pbio1000156.

CPTech (2008). Consumer Project on Technology. A letter to the WHO proposing a medical R&D treaty. http://tacd.org/index2.php?option=com_docman&task=doc_view&gid=17&Itemid= (Accessed October 26, 2009).

Elias, C. J. (2006). Essay: can we ensure health is within reach for everyone? *Lancet* **368**, S40–1.

Enserink, M. (2009). Are you ready to become a number? *Science* **323**, 1662–1664.

Evans, J. A. & Reimer, J. (2009). Open access and global participation in science. *Science* **323**, 1025.

Farrar, J. (2007). Global health science: a threat and an opportunity for collaborative clinical science. *Nature Immunology* **8**, 1277–1279.

Frank, C. & Nason, E. (2009). Health research: measuring the social, health and economic benefits. *Canadian Medical Association Journal* **180**, 528–534.

Global Forum for Health Research (2008). *Monitoring Financial Flows for Health Research 2008: Prioritizing Research for Health Equity*. Geneva: Global Forum for Health Research.

Gostin, L. (2008). Global health law: a definition and grand challenges. *Public Health Ethics* **1**, 53–63.

Hao Xin (2009). Help wanted: 2000 leading lights to inject a spirit of innovation. *Science* **325**, 534–535.

HINARI (2009). Research output in developing countries reveals 194% increase in five years. Press release July 2, 2009. www.who.int/hinari/Increase_in_developing_country_research_output.pdf (Accessed July 29, 2009).

Hofman, K., Kanyego, C. W., Rapp, B. A. & Kotzin, S. (2009). Mapping the health research landscape in sub-Saharan Africa: a study of trends in biomedical publications. *Journal of the Medical Librarians Association* **97**, 41–44.

Hotez, P., Fenwick, A., Savioli, L. & Molyneux, D. (2009). Rescuing the bottom billion through control of neglected tropical diseases. *Lancet* **373**, 1570–1575.

Incentives for Global Health (IGH) (2009). *The Health Impact Fund: Making New Medicines Accessible to All*. www.yale.edu/macmillan/igh/ (Accessed October 26, 2009).

Lancet (2008). The state of health research worldwide. *Lancet* **372**, 1519.

Lancet (2009). Strengthening research capacity in Africa. *Lancet* **374**, 1.

Lane, J. (2009). Assessing the impact of science funding. *Science* **324**, 1273–1275.

Laurance, J. (2009). Peter Pronovost: champion of checklists in critical care. *Lancet* **374**, 443.

Leroy, J. L., Habicht, J. P., Pelto, G. & Bertozzi, S. M. (2007). Current priorities in health research funding and lack of impact on the number of child deaths per year. *American Journal of Public Health* **97**, 219–223.

MacLachlan, M. (2009). Rethinking global health research: towards integrative expertise. *Globalization and Health* **5**, doi:10.1186/1744–8603-5–6.

Madon, T., Hofman, K. J., Kupfer, L. & Glass, R. I. (2007). Implementation science. *Science* **318**, 1728–1729.

McCoy, D., Kembhavi, G., Patel, J. & Luintel, A. (2009). The Bill & Melinda Gates Foundation's grant-making programme for global health. *Lancet* **373**, 1645–1653.

McMichael, C., Waters, E. & Volmink, J. (2005). Evidence-based public health: what does it offer developing countries. *Journal of Public Health* **27**, 215–221.

Moran, M., Guzman, J., Ropars, A. L., McDonald, A. *et al.* (2009). Neglected disease research and development: how much are we really spending? *PLoS Medicine* **6**: e1000030. doi:10.1371/journal.pmed.1000030.

Nature (2009a). Funding watch. *Nature* **461**, 853.

Nature (2009b). Malaria vaccine enters phase III clinical trials. *Nature* **459**, 627.

Nature (2009c). Drug patent pools start to take shape. *Nature* **458**, 562.

Normile, D. (2008). The promise and pitfalls of clinical trials overseas. *Science* **322**, 214–216.

Pang, T. (2009). Pharmacogenomics and personalized medicine for the developing world-too soon or just-in-time? A personal view from the World Health Organization. *Current Pharmacogenomics and Personalized Medicine* **7**, 149–157.

Paraje, G., Sadana, R. & Karam, G. (2005). Increasing international gaps in health-related publications. *Science* **308**, 959–960.

Rothwell, P. M. (2006). Funding for practice-oriented clinical research. *Lancet* **368**, 262–266.

Rottingen, J. A., Buss, P., Davies, S. & Touré, O. (2009). Global health research architecture-time for mergers? *Lancet* **373**, 193–195.

Seguin, B., Singer, P. A. & Daar, A. S. (2006). Scientific diasporas. *Science* **312**, 1602–1603.

Sgaier, S. K., Jha, P., Mony, P. *et al.* (2007). Biobanks in developing countries: needs and feasibility. *Science* **318**, 1074–1075.

Silberschmidt, G., Matheson, D. & Kickbush, I. (2008). Creating a Committee C of the World Health Assembly. *Lancet* **371**, 1483–1486.

Travis J. (2008). Prizes eyed to spur medical innovation. *Science* **319**, 713.

Tucker, T. J. & Makgoba, M. W. (2008). Public-private partnerships and scientific imperialism. *Science* **320**, 1016–1017.

Wemos (2008). *SOMO Briefing Paper on Ethics in Clinical Trials, #1: Examples of Unethical Trials.* http://somo.nl/html/paginas/pdf/Examples_of_unethical_trials_dec_2006_NL.pdf (Accessed October 26, 2009).

World Health Organization (WHO) (2009a). *WHO's Role and Responsibilities in Health Research – Bamako Global Ministerial Forum on Research for Health.* Document EB124/12 Add 2. http://apps.who.int/gb/ebwha/pdf_files/EB124/B124_12Add2-en.pdf.

World Health Organization (WHO) (2009b). *WHO's Role and Responsibilities in Health Research – Draft WHO Strategy on Research for Health.* Document EB124/12. http://apps.who.int/gb/ebwha/pdf_files/EB124/B124_12-en.pdf.

25

Justice and research in developing countries

Alex John London

Clinical research is a morally complex activity. When properly conducted, it represents a powerful tool for generating information and knowledge that often cannot be obtained by other means. When properly oriented, this knowledge represents the key to advancing the standard of care and creating the policies, practices and interventions that can be used to improve the health of large populations of people.

For almost two decades now, clinical research has become an increasingly global enterprise. With the "outsourcing" or "off-shoring" of research, new ethical complexities have arisen that are not easily accommodated within frameworks that are primarily oriented to protecting research participants in a domestic context. In part this is because profound conditions of social, economic and political deprivation and inequality play a fundamental, and sometimes unique, role in cross-national research. Because of such deprivation and inequality, for instance, what is an unreasonable risk for someone in a high-income country (HIC) may represent a valuable opportunity for someone in a low- or middle-income country (LMIC). Similarly, information that has the potential to generate significant social benefits in HICs may be of little relevance to host communities that struggle with poverty and underdeveloped medical, public health and scientific infrastructures.

Although there is widespread agreement that international research should not take unfair advantage of the disease and deprivation in LMICs, there is significant disagreement about what conditions need to be met in order to ensure that research is fair and consistent with fundamental principles of justice (Angell, 1997; Lurie & Wolfe, 1997; Crouch & Arras, 1998; Glantz *et al.*, 1998). In the discussion that follows I argue that a desire to remain agnostic about controversial issues of justice and to rely instead on the values that constitute

the traditional pillars of research ethics, results in a way of framing central issues in international research that is essentially biased in favor of what Brian Barry calls "justice as mutual advantage" (Barry, 1982). As a result, someone who approaches this topic wanting to remain agnostic about controversial issues in global justice may find herself formulating the basic problem in a way that tacitly presupposes a particularly anemic theory of justice.

I begin by outlining how issues of justice or fairness may arise at a variety of levels in the process of international research. I then discuss a case that dramatizes a limited subset of these issues in order to illustrate the powerful intuitions and principled commitments that make justice as mutual advantage an attractive framework in this context.

After criticizing justice as mutual advantage, I outline what I call the Human Development Approach to international research. This view highlights the respect in which clinical research is a unique social good whose power to advance the health needs of large populations of people is predicated on its fitting into a particular social division of labor. This view also articulates the terms on which internationally sponsored research can satisfy claims that host community members have against one another to ensure that their basic social institutions advance the interests of all community members. It also sets out the conditions on which international research can contribute to a process of human development. This in turn, establishes conditions under which the conduct of research represents a means of discharging a duty to aid. Finally, this approach is more likely to sustain widespread support for international research because it fosters collaborations between HIC and LMIC on terms of mutual respect and moral equality.

An earlier version of this work appeared: London, A J. (2005). Justice and the human development approach to international research. *Hastings Center Report* **34** (1), 24–37.

Foci of concern in international research

It is often noted that the health problems of populations in HICs receive a disproportionate share of scientific attention. The so-called "10/90 research gap" refers to the fact that 90% of the world's medical research dollars are spent on diseases that affect just 10% of the world's population (Commission on Health Research for Development 1990; World Health Organization, 1996). This imbalance in research priorities raises concerns of fairness about the extent to which the scientific enterprise is systematically focusing on the health of populations that are already comparatively well off, to the exclusion of populations that bear the heaviest burdens of sickness and disease (Attaran, 1999).

Although the amount of international research has grown significantly over roughly the last decade, research priorities are still largely set by external sponsors. Because the priority health problems of LMICs differ from those of HICs, this creates the potential for a mismatch between the focus of specific initiatives and the health needs and priorities of the populations in which the research is carried out.

Additionally, many LMICs lack a robust infrastructure related to clinical research. As a result, there may not be an established system of research oversight and human-subjects protection at the local and regional level. Additionally, they frequently lack key elements in the social division of labor that operates in HICs to translate research findings into interventions, methods or policies, and to disseminate these through the medical and public health system so that they can ultimately be used to enhance the standard of care. As a result, even when research generates information or interventions that are relevant to the health needs of the host community it can be difficult to ensure that these are integrated into or provided within the health infrastructure in the host community.

Finally, the above concerns arise out of the range of social, economic and health inequalities that often divide HICs and LMICs. People in LMICs who live in poverty and toil under some of the world's poorest social conditions also bear some of the heaviest burdens of sickness and disease. Of the 3.5 million deaths from pneumonia each year, 99% take place in LMICs where pneumonia claims the lives of more children than any other infectious disease. To some degree, people in LMICs are more likely to die from pneumonia because they cannot afford the low-cost antibiotics that are widely available in HICs. Twenty-seven cents (US) for a five-day regimen of antibiotics is more than a day's income for roughly 1 billion people. Also, in rural communities and other places where the health-care infrastructure is not well entrenched, hospitals and clinics may be too far away to reach.

Poverty and poor social conditions also make those in LMICs more susceptible to a wider array of illnesses. Pneumonia is more common in LMICs, for example, because children are more likely to be malnourished and to suffer from medical conditions that weaken their immune systems. Where sanitation is poor and the drinking water is unsafe, diarrhea-related diseases such as cholera, dysentery, typhoid fever and rotavirus themselves claim the lives of nearly 2 million children under the age of 5. In HICs, in contrast, such infections are much less common and more easily treated when they occur. Similarly, of the roughly 1600 children infected with HIV every day, approximately 90% live in LMICs. Africa alone is home to some 70% of the world's HIV-positive individuals, even though the continent contains only about 10% of the world's population.

These dramatic differences between HICs and LMICs, and the toll that such social, economic and health burdens take on the welfare and opportunities of LMIC populations, provide the context for international research. To give a concrete illustration of some of these facets, consider what I will refer to as the "Surfaxin" case.

Extremely premature infants frequently suffer from a potentially life-threatening condition known as respiratory distress syndrome (RDS). Respiratory distress syndrome can be successfully treated with the use of surfactant replacement therapy. Surfactants are substances produced in the lungs that are essential to the lungs' ability to absorb oxygen and maintain proper airflow through the respiratory system. During the 1990s, several natural and artifical surfactant agents received FDA approval and were in widespread use in the USA and other high-income countries.

In 2001 the pharmaceutical firm Discovery Laboratories proposed a large-scale, placebo-controlled clinical trial of their new surfactant drug, Surfaxin. The trials would be carried out in impoverished Latin American communities where neonatal intensive care units were poorly equipped and where children did not at the time have access to surfactants. Discovery Laboratories would upgrade and modernize the intensive care units that participated in the clinical trial so that all of the children included in the research would receive improved medical care including ventilator support. Half of the children in the trial would then receive Surfaxin, and the other half, roughly 325 dangerously ill children, would receive a placebo.

Critics of this study argued that a placebo control would not have been permissible in the USA and that its use in a LMIC constituted an unfair double standard (Lurie & Wolfe, 2007). They argued that participants in the control arm were entitled to receive the established standard of care for treating RDS, namely, surfactant replacement therapy, and that the use of a placebo would result in roughly 17 preventable deaths. Moreover, they claimed that the relevant scientific question was whether Surfaxin was equivalent or superior to currently available therapy, not whether it was better than nothing. This claim was bolstered by the fact that Surfaxin did not have properties that made it especially well suited for use in LMICs and that it would be marketed primarily in HICs. Finally, some argued that it was unfair to conduct this study without plans to make Surfaxin available more broadly in the host community at the completion of the trial. To such critics, Discovery Laboratories was in effect leveraging the poverty and disease of LMIC communities as a mechanism to increase its profit margins.

Proponents of this study, such as Robert Temple of the Food and Drug Administration argued that, "If they did the trial, half of the people would get surfactant and better perinatal care, and the other half would get better perinatal care. It seems to me that all the people in the trial would have been better off" (Shah, 2002, p. 28). They also argued that providing roughly 325 dangerously ill newborns with a placebo does not violate the standard of care since newborns in these communities do not otherwise have access to surfactants.

Others have argued that requiring the provision of surfactant replacement therapy in the control group would eliminate the advantages associated with conducting the trial in a LMIC context. If the study were relocated with the USA, then approximately 17 infants whose lives might be saved by receiving Surfaxin would be consigned to death. Even though poverty and deprivation may have created the background conditions for this trial, that alone does not entail that the trial was taking unfair advantage of participants. As such, proponents argued that the trial should be permitted to go forward as designed.

Justice as mutual advantage

Powerful intuitions, as well as a desire not to hold pressing practical problems hostage to broad theoretical disputes about the requirements of social justice, support a variety of approaches that fall under the heading of justice as mutual advantage. In this view, the terms of a research collaboration are just if they are mutually beneficial and each of the parties freely accepts them without the interference of force, fraud or coercion, and with an adequate understanding of the relevant information.

Although some may hold this view explicitly and defend it on substantive grounds, others who wish to remain agnostic about substantive issues of global justice may nevertheless find themselves committed to this view. In part, this view fits very nicely within the existing regulatory structures in HICs. For instance, the relevant unit of concern in this view is the dyadic relationship between researchers and host communities. Issues of justice or fairness are a property of the relationship between researchers and the host communities with whom they interact.

Similarly, the central focus of this view accords nicely with values that stand as the traditional pillars of research ethics: non-maleficence, beneficence and respect for autonomy. It seems to satisfy a requirement of *non-maleficence* by prohibiting research agreements that would leave host communities worse off than they otherwise would have been. It seems to satisfy a requirement of *beneficence* because just agreements must provide a meaningful benefit to each of the parties. Finally, it seeks to respect the *autonomy* of host communities by leaving it to them to determine in light of their own values how much of which kind of benefits represent a sufficient return for hosting a particular research project.

If one views issues of justice in this context as primarily a property of the way that researchers treat host community members, and if one uses these traditional pillars of research ethics to provide the content for the value of justice, then any voluntary agreement that is mutually beneficial and grounded in an adequate understanding of the relevant information will be regarded as fair or morally permissible.

Perhaps the most explicit articulation of this position has come from proponents of the "fair benefits" approach to international research (Participants, 2002, 2004). The central focus of this view is avoiding exploitation, and its proponents follow Wertheimer in holding that party A exploits party B if party A receives "an unfair level of benefits as a result of B's interactions with A" (Participants, 2004, p. 19). They thus hold that the crucial issue is not "what" benefits host communities receive but "how much" and that host communities should be free to choose from a wide range of possible benefits – such as receiving access to vaccinations or other public health measures.

This approach is critical of the requirement, enshrined in the Declaration of Helsinki and elsewhere, that researchers must ensure that members of the host community can obtain interventions proven effective by a clinical trial. From the standpoint of the fair benefits approach, the "reasonable availability" requirement is overly restrictive both of important international research and of the ability of LMIC populations to receive a wide range of potential benefits that can come from hosting a research initiative.

Similarly, if the host community is not interested in the information or the interventions that the study is designed to generate, and if it is not obligatory to provide post-trial access to the study intervention, then it would seem to follow that international research initiatives would not need to target or to be aligned with the urgent health needs or priorities of the host community.

In order to ensure that host communities receive a fair level of benefits, researchers and community members are supposed to engage in a process of "collaborative partnership" in which the parties negotiate an agreement under conditions that approximate those of an ideal market. Because this view holds that "a fair distribution of benefits at the micro-level is based on the level of benefits that would occur in a market transaction devoid of fraud, deception, or force, in which the parties have full information" the outcomes of this process are regarded as fair as long as the transaction is free from the enumerated defects (Participants, 2004, p. 20). In order to ensure that these conditions are met, the proponents of this approach also propose a "principle of transparency" that would provide all parties with the information that they need in order to properly value participation in a clinical trial.

Shortcomings of justice as mutual advantage

One problem with justice as mutual advantage is that it is too parochial and conservative to capture the full range of concerns that are relevant in the context of international research.

The charge of parochialism relates to its narrow focus on the obligations of researchers and community members. For example, proponents of the fair benefits approach are explicit that as Wertheimer explicates the concept, exploitation is a micro-level concern that deals with the fairness of discrete exchanges between identifiable parties. Even if one assumes that Wertheimer's is the correct view of exploitation, one might legitimately question whether the most relevant and important ethical issues in this context occur at the micro-level. In particular, if there are issues of justice or fairness associated with the degree to which scientific inquiry targets the needs of those who are already comparatively well off, to the neglect of those who bear the most significant burdens of disease and disability, then those concerns could not be easily accommodated within a framework exclusively focused on the researcher-participant relationship.

Similarly, it may be true that researchers have special obligations in this context, but it is questionable whether they should be seen as the primary, or even the most important duty bearers. Other stakeholders play a powerful role in shaping the research agenda. As such, governments, NGOs, and the public and private entities that fund and support the research enterprise may have equally if not more important duties in this context.

Because Wertheimer's account of exploitation only applies to micro-level transactions between individual parties it does not apply directly to the operation of social systems that shape and coordinate the behavior of large numbers of people, often dispersed geographically and temporally. Concerns about whether the *social systems* of international clinical research make unfair use of the sick and the vulnerable would have to be articulated in a different framework.

Justice as mutual advantage may be regarded as too conservative because it only applies once some cooperative endeavor has been initiated; it cannot ground or generate an obligation to engage in cooperation where none exists. As Brian Barry notes, it does not "say that it is unfair for a practice that would, if it existed, be mutually beneficial, not to exist" (Barry, 1982, p. 231).

This is a conservative approach, therefore, to the extent that it presupposes that there are not broader moral obligations or requirements that should factor into: how funding for research programs is allocated, which research programs receive key social and economic support, how host communities are identified and selected, or how research should relate to the existing health-related social structures or infrastructure of the host community. These are substantive questions and if, in fact, researchers and their sponsors have complete discretion over these issues – if there are no larger moral obligations or requirements that must be reflected in their decisions about these issues – then the conservatism of justice as mutual advantage would be entirely justified. If, in contrast, there are larger moral obligations that are relevant to the determination of these issues, then the conservatism of justice as mutual advantage would be morally objectionable.

Those who think that there is a moral imperative to address the staggering health needs of LMIC populations can object to justice as mutual advantage on a number of grounds. In particular, it encourages a piecemeal and ad hoc approach to the needs of those in LMICs for two reasons. First, it allows decisions about which research should be carried out, and where it should be conducted, to be determined primarily by interests in HICs rather than by the health needs of LMICs. Second, without focusing on host community health needs and the social environment in which they arise, justice as mutual advantage does not differentiate health needs that require new advances in understanding from those that could be met through the application of existing knowledge or interventions. Nor does it give priority to addressing the root causes of disease in LMICs over symptomatic manifestations of deeper problems.

Finally, those who think that there are broader obligations to aid LMIC populations are likely to find the bargaining model embraced by the fair benefits approach to be both detrimental and demeaning to members of LMICs.

The use of a bargaining model in this context is likely to work to the disadvantage of LMIC communities because, whereas their needs are urgent and often time sensitive, sponsors can usually find alternative locations for a trial and they have less at stake if negotiations drag out. Whatever their individual preferences, researchers are also under pressure from funding agencies to use scarce resources only for research purposes, narrowly construed, which puts a cap on the kind of benefits that researchers can offer a host population even if they want to offer more. Given this significant imbalance in bargaining power, agreements may satisfy the requirement that each party receives a net benefit, but the distribution of those benefits is likely to be hugely disproportionate (London & Zollman, forthcoming).

This approach may be seen as disrespectful of the moral status of people in LMICs because it effectively treats the toll that morally problematic social structures exact from individuals in LMICs as a boon for research that addresses HIC health needs. In many LMICs medical problems are often widespread, and potential research participants frequently have few treatment alternatives. Such populations can be easily recruited, at considerable cost savings to sponsors, who can use their considerable influence and bargaining power to further advance their interests. Disease and lack of access to medical care come to function as valuable commodities whose use-value gives people a place at the bargaining table.

Those who lack the "good fortune" to suffer from a condition interesting to science are consigned to die in silence because the power differential in their case is so great that they cannot either help or harm potential collaborators. The result is a system in which, as Hobbes put it, "the value or worth of a man is, as for all other things, his price, that is to say, so much as would be given for the use of his power; and therefore is not absolute, but a thing dependent on the need and judgment of another" (Hobbes, 1985, chapter X, section 16). Within such a system there may be individuals and groups in LMICs who benefit from access to clinical trials. Although they may willingly accept succor where they can find it, this does not mean that they could not also feel disrespected, and even resentful of a system that wields tremendous knowledge resources, and confers the benefits of life and health, not out of a concern to improve the lives of specific individuals or enhance the capacities of local communities, but as a necessary means of advancing the profit motives of those who are already comparatively well off (Benatar, 2002).

Whether these objections hold, and how forceful they are, depends on the prior question of whether there are compelling reasons to believe that researchers, sponsors or other stakeholders in the research enterprise have duties or obligations to individuals in LMICs that are broader than, or that arise prior to, those recognized by justice as mutual advantage. In the next three sections I consider several possible grounds for such obligations.

Obligations within host communities

Whether members of a community have a justified claim on one another to something beyond the status quo depends crucially on whether they can endorse the terms of social cooperation set by their community's social structures as basically fair. As a minimal condition of fairness, it must be possible to see the fundamental structures of the community as organized around, and functioning in the service of, the common good of its members (London, 2003). In other words, a morally permissible division of labor must strive to secure for individuals what Rawls calls the "fair value" of their basic capacities for welfare and human agency – meaning that the division of social labor should be designed to give each person an effective opportunity to cultivate and use their basic intellectual, affective and social capacities to pursue a meaningful life plan (Rawls, 1971; Korsgaard, 1993). Social structures that do not meet this minimal requirement create conditions in which some are denied effective opportunities to develop their basic capacities while others enjoy a rich array of opportunities and benefits. In the most extreme cases, these are the social conditions in which starvation, sickness and disease flourish.

Consider some parallels between Amartya Sen's groundbreaking work on famine and the health needs of LMIC populations (Sen, 1981; Sen & Dreze, 1989). Famines are commonly viewed as natural disasters caused principally by a combination of poverty and poor food production. Sen showed, however, that these factors alone do not account for the occurrence of famines. For example, in 1979–1981 and 1983–1984, Sudan and Ethiopia experienced declines in food production of 11 or 12% and, like a number of other countries in sub-Saharan Africa, suffered massive famines. During the same period, however, food production declined by 17% in Botswana and by a precipitous 38% in Zimbabwe, yet these countries did not suffer the ravages of famine (Sen, 1999, pp. 178–180). According to Sen, the reason for this difference in outcomes can be traced to differences in the social and political structures of these countries. Botswana and Zimbabwe had rudimentary democratic social institutions that enabled them to stave off famine. They implemented a series of social support programs targeted at enhancing the economic purchasing power of affected groups while also supplementing food supplies. Mass starvation occurred in Sudan and Ethiopia because the dictatorial regimes in those nations failed to take such relatively simple social and economic steps to safeguard their citizens' interests.

These lessons should inform our view of sickness and disease in LMICs (Benatar, 1998, 2001). For example, HIV/AIDS is devastating many populations in sub-Saharan Africa. In some nations, as much as 30% of the population is HIV positive and infection rates continue to climb. In sharp contrast, Senegal has been able to limit both the prevalence of HIV/AIDS and the rate of new infections to about 1% of the population. The principal cause of Senegal's success lies not in advanced technology or great wealth, but in the government's longstanding, grass-roots investment in its human resources. In Senegal, information about HIV/AIDS, and many other sexually transmitted diseases has been disseminated through an assortment of educational programs. Empowering individuals with information and opportunities for activism enhances the public's capacities for communal interaction, free expression and political participation, and so creates a social context in which people can more effectively safeguard and secure their welfare.

This focus on education and activism has been further enhanced by the judicious use of scarce resources. Senegal closely monitors its blood supply and distributes millions of condoms free of charge. It invests in monitoring and treating many sexually transmitted diseases, especially in target populations such as commercial sex workers, young people, truck drivers and the spouses of migrant workers. Additionally, as part of a program of perinatal care, it has recently begun to offer antiretroviral drugs to pregnant women, although on a very limited basis. There remains room for improvement in Senegal. Still, the country's multisectoral approach to HIV/AIDS, and to public health in general, illustrates the positive health effects of policies that strive to protect citizens' basic capacities for agency and welfare.

These examples illustrate the profound impact that the basic political, legal, social and economic institutions of a community have on the health of community members. Because they determine the distribution of basic rights and liberties within a society, these structures set the terms on which individuals may access basic goods and resources such as food, shelter, education and productive employment, as well as more specialized health-care resources. They therefore determine the opportunities available to individuals to develop and exercise their basic human capacities.

When individuals lack access to the basic building blocks of social and economic opportunity and healthy living, the harms that result cannot be dismissed as accidents of nature or justified by reference to the common good. They represent a failure to use the state's monopoly on force and control over basic social structures to advance the interests of community members. Those who suffer in these cases can legitimately claim, as a strict obligation of justice, an entitlement to relief from such hardships.

In such cases, resources that domestic authorities may be willing to make available for research purposes may not be "available" in a more fundamental moral sense: those who control them may have a prior moral obligation to deploy them in the service of other ends. Moreover, although the use of monetary and material resources may be particularly important in this regard, there are other social resources that matter as well. For example, regimes can fail to serve the common good by neglecting basic social institutions altogether, by misappropriating or misdirecting the time and energies of their personnel, or by inappropriately restricting or occupying important institutional spaces. These failures can generate prior moral claims that community members have against their own authorities, and such claims might constrain the ways in which important social institutions can use or allocate social resources as well as the kind of agreements or cooperative activities that it might foster and support.

This might affect the liberties and duties of researchers in several ways. The right of community members to a social division of labor that advances their basic interests may entail that community members have a claim on their own leaders and social institutions to foster research that targets the priority health needs of their community. In the face of this claim, and the pressing needs of community members, community leaders and important social institutions may have a duty not to facilitate or cooperate in research that does not focus on or align with the priority health needs of that community. Because the rights, welfare and opportunities of community members are profoundly influenced by the way that their basic social institutions function, researchers may thus have a duty not to propose research projects to communities that would conflict with the claims of community members and the duties of their leaders and institutions.

Duties of rectification

If researchers, their sponsors or other stakeholders have acted in ways that have contributed to the conditions of deprivation and disease in LMICs, then they may have a special duty to aid those populations, grounded in a duty of rectification (Benatar, 1998; Crouch & Arras, 1998).

At the most general level, duties of rectification may attach to all citizens of democratic nations whose policies and international activities have contributed to the plight of those in LMICs. In a series of recent articles, Thomas Pogge has argued that western democratic nations have contributed greatly to the poverty and poor health of the global poor simply by recognizing and supporting two international privileges, namely the "international resource privilege" and the "international borrowing privilege." Any group that succeeds in wresting control of the national government in a LMIC is recognized as having the legitimate authority to dispose of a country's resources (the international resource privilege) and "to borrow in the name of its people and to confer legal ownership rights for the country's resources" (the international borrowing privilege) (Pogge, 2002b, p. 73). Both these privileges provide powerful incentives for the unscrupulous to seize power, and convenient mechanisms for consolidating power and then wielding it for the enrichment of a privileged few (Pogge, 2002a, chapters 4 and 6). Employing power in this way can saddle a LMIC with disastrous long-term debt and prevent most of the population from sharing in the benefits generated by their country's natural resources. Instead, the benefits are enjoyed primarily by a ruling elite and by governments and corporations of HICs.

A duty to aid grounded in this kind of pre-existing relationship would apply to medical researchers insofar as they are citizens of the basically democratic nations that have contributed to and benefited from such policies. Such obligations may be strengthened if researchers are employed or funded by governments or private entities that have actively supported such policies. For example, one reason drugs are so scarce in LMICs is their cost. Many pharmaceutical companies played an active role in the negotiation of the Trade Related Aspects of Intellectual Property Rights (TRIPS) Agreement at the World Trade Organization, and the pharmaceutical lobby has used its considerable influence on US and EU trade representatives to enforce the companies' patent rights. The TRIPS agreement allows countries to produce or import generic versions of beneficial medications in cases of national emergency, but the western pharmaceutical industry has aggressively pressed for trade sanctions or taken active legal action against countries that have tried to implement this emergency clause (Barry & Raworth, 2002; Schüklenk & Ashcroft, 2002). In doing so, it has blocked legitimate efforts to provide medicines to some of the populations that need them most.

Taking basic interests seriously

It is a fact of the contemporary world that even moderately affluent individuals and social entities have the ability to affect the lives of distant people. It is also a fact of the contemporary world that whether people are able to cultivate their most basic capacities for agency and welfare, and to live a life in which they find meaning and value, is too often determined by their place of birth rather than by any features of their individual character. These facts have led a variety of moral theorists to argue from within diverse and even competing conceptual frameworks that claims of justice cannot be limited to the boundaries of the contemporary nation state (Beitz, 1979; Cullity, 1994; Pogge, 1994; Ashford, 2003). Although these theorists' arguments may be controversial, they are both coherent and compelling. We should therefore be cautious of begging the question against such views by accepting, without defense, the assumption of justice as mutual advantage, that no such duties exist.

When we approach the problem of assessing potential collaborative research initiatives, therefore, we must at the very least leave conceptual room to consider whether the interests that are frustrated or defeated by less-than-decent social structures are so fundamental as to generate a duty on the part of others to assist them. This point is of special importance, not only for welfare consequentialist theories, but for any theory of rights that grounds the moral force of a right in the significance of the interest that it either protects or advances. For example, Raz (1984) argues that " 'X has a right' if and only if x can have rights, and other things being equal, an aspect of x's well-being (his interest) is a sufficient reason for holding some other person(s) to be under a duty." Such concerns will also be salient for theories of human rights that ground rights claims in the basic capabilities of agents (Nussbaum, 1999, p. 236).

The human development approach

The human development approach is a framework for evaluating international clinical and public health research that begins from a premise that has deep roots in liberal political theory – the idea that justice is properly *about* the basic social structures of society and the state and whether they work to advance the interests of community members. It uses this idea to define a particular vision of human development, to define a target for international aid, and to specify the conditions under which clinical or public health

research represents a permissible means of discharging that duty.

In this view, "human development" is understood as the project of establishing and fostering basic social structures that guarantee to community members the fair value of their basic human capacities. Perhaps the most important determinant of health within a community is the extent to which its basic social structures guarantee its members opportunities for education, access to productive employment, control over their person and their personal environment, access to the political process and the protection of their basic human rights (Sen, 1981, 1999; Sen & Dreze, 1989). More important than the sheer economic wealth of a community, is whether the community directs the available resources to creating and sustaining the right social conditions (Sen, 1999).

The human development approach holds that governments of HICs and the individuals they represent have a duty to aid people in LMICs and that this should be understood as a duty to engage our energies and resources in this project of human development. That is, the target of the duty to aid is helping LMICs to create and sustain basic social structures that secure individuals' capacities for welfare and human agency. This focus reflects the idea that because the duty to aid is owed equally to all with an equal claim, efforts to provide aid must give priority to responses that strive for what Henry Shue refers to as full coverage (Shue, 1998).

Decent social institutions play an essential role in providing full coverage to all with a claim to assistance because they involve a division of labor in which particular duties are assigned to individual agents or groups of agents who are given special resources, permissions and authority to discharge those duties. Social institutions provide a mechanism through which duty bearers can pool and magnify their efforts in order to accomplish more than individuals alone are capable.

What is required of different stakeholders to discharge the duty to aid depends on their ability to influence either social structures in LMICs, or those social structures in HICs that influence LMIC social structures. For example, the citizens of HICs have a duty to support efforts to make better use of existing knowledge, resources and interventions that could make a significant impact on the lives of those in LMICs.

The efforts of individuals and entities from HIC to advance the health of LMIC populations should therefore focus on what Prabhat Jha and colleagues refer to as the "close-to-client" health system in these countries (Jha *et al.*, 2002). Since 90% of the avoidable mortality in low and middle-income countries stems from a handful of causes for which effective interventions already exist, even a relatively modest increase in international aid targeted at expanding the physical, material and human capacity of local clinics, hospitals and the fundamental institutions of public health would transform the health needs of LMIC populations (Jha *et al.*, 2002; Pogge, 2002b, p. 79).

The human development approach recognizes, however, that even if a greater share of existing resources are directed toward providing LMICs with access to existing clinical and public health knowledge and interventions, scientific research still has an important role to play in the development process. This is because clinical and public health research play an invaluable role in an important social division of labor when they use scientific and statistical methods to generate information that will advance the ability of the health systems of a community to better meet the health needs of that community's members.

The human development approach thus holds that stakeholders who shape the direction and focus of scientific research have a duty to ensure that research targets the priority health needs of LMIC populations and that it is carried out in a way that is responsive to and aligned with those needs. The research enterprise represents a permissible use of a community's scarce public resources and is a permissible target of social support when it functions to expand the capacity of the basic social structures of that community to better serve the fundamental interests of that community's members. *Therefore, if clinical research is to be permissible, it must function in the host community as a part of a division of labor in which the distinctive scientific and statistical methods of the research enterprise target and investigate the means of filling the gaps between the most important health needs in a community and the capacity of its social structures to meet them.*

Once this necessary condition has been satisfied, the imperative to make the results of successful research available within the host community increases in inverse proportion to the capacity of that community's basic social structures to translate those results into sustainable benefits for community members. To the extent that the host community cannot translate the results into sustainable benefits for its population on its own, there is an imperative either to build partnerships with groups that are willing to augment the community's capacity to do so, or to locate the research within a community with similar health priorities and more appropriate health infrastructure.

Research like the Surfaxin study would not be permitted on the human development approach. In this regard, those who would have enrolled in this trial would be better off under the framework of fair benefits than under the human development approach. But the point of the human development approach is not to prohibit research – it is to foster more research that targets the health needs and priorities of LMICs. It is intended to provide a framework that informs the deliberations of researchers, research sponsors and governmental and private entities as they make decisions about what scientific questions should be explored, which research initiatives should be funded, where research should be carried out and how research can benefit those who most need aid. A much larger population of people, therefore, stands to benefit from the application of the human development approach.

At the institutional level, the human development approach requires changes in how international research is evaluated. Mechanisms need to be developed to facilitate reflection by various stakeholders, at various stages of research development, on how research might promote human development. This will require a proactive model in which issues of justice are considered much earlier in the research process.

For example, enhancing the basic capabilities and social opportunities of women is an important goal of development (Sen, 1999, p. 189–203; Ash & Jasny, 2002). Roughly half of the global burden of HIV/AIDS is borne by women, and in southern Africa more than one in five pregnant women are HIV-positive. The complications of HIV/AIDS are increasing maternal death rates during labor, and vertical or maternal–fetal transmission of HIV still accounts for roughly 90% of new pediatric HIV infections – 600 000 annually – the vast majority of which occur in LMICs. When used properly and consistently, condoms are good at preventing horizontal or partner-to-partner transmission of the HIV virus. But condoms are often not used consistently because men dislike them. As a result, the range of options available to women – who are already a disadvantaged social group and who are 1.2–2.5 times more likely to contract HIV from heterosexual intercourse than men (World Health Organization, 2003, p. 7) – may be further restricted by men's preferences and behavior.

International research aimed at developing a safe, effective and affordable vaginal microbicide would thus contribute to several important developmental goals. A microbicide is an agent delivered in gel form that would reduce the odds of HIV transmission, and perhaps secondary STI transmission, during heterosexual, vaginal intercourse (Stone, 2002). It would provide an intervention that expands the range of options available to women to safeguard their own health. Given the influence of gender inequalities on condom use, this positive effect would not necessarily be achieved just by emphasizing condom usage more strongly. Also, because it could help reduce the frequency of HIV transmission to women, it could contribute to a reduction in transmission to children. Finally, by targeting the needs of an often disadvantaged subpopulation, such research would contribute to social equity.

Similar arguments could be mounted on behalf of vaccine research and more effective treatments for a variety of tropical diseases (Flory & Kitcher, 2004). They cannot be marshaled in support of initiatives like the Surfaxin trial. Several effective surfactant agents are widely used in HICs, and there is nothing about Surfaxin that would make it particularly attractive to LMIC communities. Many Latin American countries need improved neonatal care but that need could be more effectively and efficiently addressed, for larger numbers of people and on a more sustainable basis, with existing medical knowledge and resources.

From the standpoint of justice as mutual advantage, this conclusion looks inefficient because it prevents Discovery Laboratories from expeditiously pursuing its research agenda and along the way benefiting people in LMICs. From the standpoint of the human development approach, justice as mutual advantage represents an inefficient means of trying to assist LMIC communities in meeting their priority health needs. Providing ad hoc benefits in exchange for participating in trials that are targeted at the health needs of HIC populations will not close the 10/90 gap or address the most pressing health priorities of communities that suffer the heaviest burdens of disease and deprivation.

Acknowledgment

This is a condensed version of: London, A. J. (2005). Justice and the human development approach to international research. *Hastings Center Report* **35**(1), 24–37.

References

Angell, M. (1997). The ethics of clinical research in the Third World. *New England Journal of Medicine* 337: 847–49.

Ash, C. & Jasny, B. (2002). Unmet needs in public health. *Science* **295**, 235.

Ashford, E. (2003). The demandingness of Scanlon's contractualism. *Ethics* **113**, 273–302.

Attaran, A. (1999). Human rights and biomedical research funding for the developing world: discovering state obligations under the right to health. *Health and Human Rights* **4**(1), 27–58.

Barry, B. (1982). Humanity and justice in global perspective. In J. R. Pennock & J. W. Chapman (Eds.), *NOMOS XXIV, Ethics, Economics, and the Law* (pp. 219–252). New York: New York University Press.

Barry, C. & Raworth K. (2002). Access to medicines and the rhetoric of responsibility. *Ethics and International Affairs* **16** (2), 57–70.

Beitz, C. (1979). *Political Theory and International Relations.* Princeton, NJ: Princeton University Press.

Benatar, S. R. (1998). Global disparities in health and human rights: a critical commentary. *American Journal of Public Health* **88** (2), 295–300.

Benatar, S. R. (2001). Justice and medical research: a global perspective. *Bioethics* **15**(4), 333–340.

Benatar, S. R. (2002). Reflections and recommendations on research ethics in developing countries. *Social Science and Medicine* **54**, 1131–1141.

Commission on Health Research for Development (1990). *Health Research: Essential Link to Equity in Development.* New York: Oxford University Press.

Crouch, R. A. & Arras, J. D. (1998). AZT trials and tribulations. *Hastings Center Report* **28**(6), 26–34.

Cullity, G. (1994). International aid and the scope of kindness. *Ethics* **105**(1), 99–127.

Flory, J. H. & Kitcher, P. (2004). Global health and the scientific research agenda. *Philosophy and Public Affairs* **32**, 36–65.

Glantz, L. H., Annas, G. J., Grodin, M. A. & Mariner, W. K. (1998). Research in developing countries: taking "benefit" seriously. *Hastings Center Report* **28**(6), 38–42.

Hobbes, T. (1985). *Leviathan.* C. B. Macpherson (Ed.). New York: Penguin Books.

Jha, P., Mills, A., Hanson, K. *et al.* (2002). Improving the health of the global poor. *Science* **295**, 2036–2039.

Korsgaard, C. M. (1993). Commentary: G. A. Cohen: Equality of what? on welfare, goods and capabilities. In M. C. Nussbaum & A. Sen (Eds.), *The Quality of Life* (pp. 54–61). Oxford: Oxford University Press.

London, A. J. (2003). Threats to the common good: biochemical weapons and human subjects research. *Hastings Center Report* **33**(5), 17–25.

London, A. J. & Zollman, K. J. S. (2010). Research at the auction block: problems for the fair benefits approach to international research. *Hastings Center Report* **40**, 34–45.

Lurie, P. & Wolfe, S. M. (1997). Unethical trials of interventions to reduce perinatal transmission of the human immunodeficiency virus in developing countries. *New England Journal of Medicine* **337**, 853–856.

Lurie, P. & Wolfe, S. M. (2007). The developing world as the "answer" to the dreams of pharmaceutical companies: the Surfaxin story. In J. V. Lavery, C. Grady, E. R. Wahl & E. J. Emanuel (Eds.), *Ethical Issues in International Biomedical Research: A Casebook* (pp. 159–170). New York: Oxford University Press.

Nussbaum, M. C. (1999). Women and equality: the capabilities approach. *International Labour Review* **138**(3), 227–245.

Participants in the 2001 Conference on Ethical Aspects of Research in Developing Countries (2002). Fair benefits for research in developing countries. *Science* **298**, 2133–2134.

Participants in the 2001 Conference on Ethical Aspects of Research in Developing Countries (2004). Moral standards for research in developing countries: from "reasonable availability" to "fair benefits". *Hastings Center Report* **34**(3), 17–27.

Pogge, T. W. (1994). An egalitarian law of peoples. *Philosophy and Public Affairs* **23**(3), 195–224.

Pogge, T. W. (2002a). *World Poverty and Human Rights*. Cambridge: Polity Press.

Pogge, T. W. (2002b). Responsibilities for poverty-related ill health. *Ethics and International Affairs* **16**(2), 71–79.

Rawls, J. (1971). *A Theory of Justice*. Cambridge, MA: Harvard University Press.

Raz, J. (1984). On the nature of rights. *Mind* **93**(370), 194–214.

Schüklenk, U. & Ashcroft, R. E. (2002). Affordable access to essential medications in developing countries: conflicts between ethical and economic imperatives. *Journal of Medicine and Philosophy* **27**(2), 179–195.

Sen, A. (1981). *Poverty and Famines*. Oxford: Clarendon Press.

Sen, A. (1999). *Development as Freedom*. New York: Anchor Books.

Sen, A. & Dreze, J. (1989). *Hunger and Public Action*. Oxford: Clarendon Press.

Shah, S. (2002). Globalizing clinical research. *The Nation* July 1, 23–28.

Shue, H. (1998). Mediating duties. *Ethics* **98**(4), 687–704.

Stone, A. (2002). Microbicides: a new approach to preventing HIV and other sexually transmitted infections. *Nature Review Drug Discovery* **1**(12), 977–985.

World Health Organization (WHO) (1996). *Investing in Health Research and Development: Report of the Ad Hoc Committee on Health Research Relating to Future Intervention Options*. Geneva: World Health Organization.

World Health Organization (WHO) (2003). *AIDS Epidemic Update: December 2003*. Geneva: World Health Organization.

Values in global health governance

Kearsley A. Stewart, Gerald T. Keusch and Arthur Kleinman

Introduction

Over the past several decades, political conflicts, economic volatility and large-scale cultural and social changes have strongly influenced not only global health problem and solution frameworks, but the very way we conceive of global health as a public good. As politicians, business people and cultural elites employ the language of global health to shape discourse and policies focused on displaced and migratory peoples, they have perhaps unwittingly broadened the classic public health agenda. As a consequence, that agenda now includes violence and its traumatic consequences, the health (and mental health) impact of natural and social catastrophes, other health-related problems from obesity to substance abuse, and the effect of pharmaceutical and digital technology innovations not previously considered to be core public health issues. They expand and reformulate the traditional spheres of public health, and challenge classic public health values.

As a result, debates shaping global health research, ethics, policy and programs have developed along two parallel tracks. One can be characterized as a neoliberal approach combining economics (liberalization of trade and financing; new mechanisms for product development for diseases of poverty involving public–private partnerships; cost-effectiveness analysis), disease-specific and biotechnology programs and security concerns. The other has focused on human rights, social justice and equity frameworks with a broader, more inclusive model of the determinants of health. This perspective calls for a transformation of the current fractured system of global health governance into a transparent and accountable system, better equipped to address the world's global health agendas. It embraces public health as one of the essential features of a new moral commitment to remake the world, similar to the environmental/climate change movement. In

fact, in 2002, the American Public Health Association explicitly affirmed in their professional code of ethics, *Principles of the Ethical Practice of Public Health*, that the pursuit of public health is an "inherently moral" obligation (APHA, 2002).

Very recently, the two approaches appear to be converging around a *values focus* to bolster arguments in favor of increased resource allocation for global health programs. By values, we mean the set of expressed qualities that guide behavior, for example, honesty, compassion, generosity, empathy, tolerance. What is new is an emerging recognition that the "social context" of values must be explored before we can begin to understand the meaning of any value, whether personal, political or invoked directly in reference to global health. This is so because values, while expressed as individual behaviors, are often rooted in cultural interests or shaped by accepted norms that can appear to be so natural as to be invisible. At times, closely related values may be in conflict. For example, within the notion of justice as fairness there are values such as equity, need, merit, solidarity, social worth and freedom, each of which could lie at the heart of a particular and somewhat distinctive theory of justice. Values are also so central to political life that policy makers freely admit that political discourse that appropriates values talk builds political support, consequently driving policy goals. The result is that values may be neither consistently applied nor shared across diverse policy sectors. Important global health policies and programs need the underpinning of values, broadly and deeply embedded, specifically to bolster arguments for increased resource allocation. These values can be hidden, in plain view in mission statements or remain unexamined. Where is the values debate in global health headed and what can public health, the social sciences and the humanities contribute to shaping and amplifying the discussion?

An earlier version of this work has appeared: Stewart, K. A., Kleinman, A. & Keuseh, G. T. (2010). Introduction: values and moral experiences in global health: bridging the local and the global. *Global Public Health* 5, 115–121.

Background

To address this issue, the authors jointly convened a workshop entitled, "Values and moral experiences in global health: bridging the local and the global." Drawing on an interdisciplinary and international group of scholars and practitioners, the workshop explored the emerging values discourse as it relates to global health priority-setting, policy, governance, practice and research. An innovative approach was to form working groups after the workshop in order to reflect new thinking on the subject informed by the debates and discussions at the workshop. The collection of papers recently appeared in a special issue of *Global Public Health* (Stewart *et al.*, 2010) and explore a variety of questions: What values are deeply embedded in the most important global health policies and programs? How do we combine moral philosophy, applied (empirical) bioethics, economics and public health and engage people in high-income countries to work to improve the health of people in resource-poor settings? How could we change this engagement from a charitable/humanitarian value to a fundamental shared value that could withstand the inevitable periodic global economic downturns or perhaps even prevent these? How do we balance multiple, often personalized values to find consensus for setting priorities in global health policy and research agendas? How do we translate insights from highly specific, local cultural contexts into theoretical frameworks for effective global health governance that could transcend local boundaries? What is the relevance of political, ethical and economic theories to global health governance or offered assessments, of specific global-acting entities, such as the UN agencies, World Bank and the World Health Organization?

Values and moral experiences in global health governance

Values are situated in two spheres: first, actual moral experiences of people in their local worlds whose practices regarding what really matters can, and often do, diverge from their ethical aspirations; and second, more disciplined professional articulations of ethical responsibilities. By ethics we mean aspirations for and deliberations about universal values such as justice, the good, etc. In contrast, we use the word moral to refer to actual local practices that demonstrate values that are partisan, self-interested and not necessarily "ethical." More recently, practicing public health professionals have drawn upon liberation theology and social justice frameworks to raise awareness and financial support for global health initiatives. For example, Paul Farmer and Jim Kim in their work in Haiti, Peru and Rwanda, clearly recognize the connection between political structures and health inequities and therefore focus their efforts on political will to improve health. Others, like former US Senator and physician Bill Frist, use evangelicalism to attempt to reduce health inequalities through the ideology of individual responsibility and sheer determination. Feierman *et al.* (2010) have addressed the implication for global health of values animated by individual and local commitment but routinized by institutionalization through macro-level health policies.

Whereas values are deeply embedded in the most important global health policies and programs, even when the dialog is highly pragmatic or political, there is little understanding of how values function as important rhetorical devices for global health decision makers. It is evident that values are neither consistently applied nor shared across the diverse policy sectors of the players in global health. Who should shape and influence so-called international values? For example, what were the deep value commitments of Halfdan Mahler in 1979, when, as the secretary general of the United Nations at Alma Ata, he pressed for an emphasis on primary health care and an institutional commitment to *Health for all by the Year 2000*? His Scandinavian origins and familiarity with the social democratic welfare state clearly influenced his emphasis on health and social equity. But did the deeper values of his Lutheran religious traditions or his own personal biography transform an idea into a commitment? Many public health policy makers today seem comfortable with the idea of a "right to health care," but less comfortable with the idea of a "right to health." Amongst those who have made the commitment to a right to health, to what extent is it liberation theology, commitment to religious values or philosophical notions of distributive justice that undergird their passions for the human rights and health domain?

We posed several questions to be addressed by the workshop participants: Do values change as a result of an unfolding developmental process in global health? What conflicts in values exist between program donors at the global level and recipients at the local level? How are these conflicts resolved? Who decides? Do we need consensus? If so, to what degree?

What should happen when these values, that shape global intervention, conflict with the local values of the intended beneficiaries of global health programs? No clear pathway exists to address or resolve these conflicts. How do we manage a plurality of values, especially in the context of the new public–private partnership paradigm for funding global health initiatives? How do we bridge local moral experiences with global health policies?

In response, Benatar *et al.* (2010) and Yang *et al.* (2010) contend that global health programs have failed to deliver better primary health care in resource-poor countries for three central reasons: a vertical rather than a combined vertical-horizontal system to reducing disease; a traditional disease-control model that focuses on preventing or treating individual illness while ignoring the broader social and cultural determinants of health; and the increasing inequity in access to basic health resources that are often available only to those who can afford them. Benatar *et al.* (2010) have argued that existing values in global health reflect the growth of global capitalism and a narrow commitment to scientific solutions delivered through large-scale programs. Therefore they advocate a new set of values that emphasize sustainability and global distributive justice. Yang *et al.* (2010) have offered an original analysis of the concept of sustainability in global health, arguing that the current donor-driven approach will never reach sustainability because the resulting narrow focus on disease control, combined with inconsistent funding, can have the paradoxical effect of sustaining the disease itself, rather than developing the broader assets and capabilities essential to preventing future outbreaks. They believe major opportunities exist right now to provide the right health services at the right prices where they are needed most.

Ethics and priority-setting in the governance of global health research

Awareness of the ethical challenges of conducting global health research in resource-poor settings emerged most famously in 1997 with the controversy over the use of a placebo-controlled study design in a clinical intervention to prevent perinatal HIV transmission in developing countries (Angell, 1997). The controversy sparked a decade of debate and research by bioethicists, public health practitioners, biomedical researchers and social scientists that focused primarily on the technicalities of health research study design,

the compliance in resource-poor settings with international research regulations, and the appropriateness of Western normative research ethics for health research in the developing world. Recently, the debate about global health research has moved beyond the technical and regulatory questions of study design to a reconsideration of health research itself as a means to achieve better health equity. In a 2002 paper, Benatar proposed engaging global health research ethics not only as a mechanism to improve health care, but as a means for promoting a broader approach to reducing global inequities. Noting that the public health tools to treat, and perhaps even to eradicate, TB have existed for decades, he argued that the persistence of TB is due to inadequate attention to the fundamental causes of poverty (Benatar, 2002). To remedy this, he suggests that global health research ethics demand not only a higher standard of care for research participants in resource-poor settings, but obligate the research sponsors to improve the health-care needs in the community as well (Shapiro & Benatar, 2005).

However, this raises new questions: What constitutes a need? Who will define it? Who should prioritize it and based on what principles and values? Who will pay for it? What is the role of the humanities and social sciences in this emerging debate? Global health research is a collaborative, multisectoral and multidisciplinary effort; how can we move forward in this interdisciplinary endeavor when there are multiple sets of principles competing to define social value and determine how to achieve social justice through global health research? Do we describe the social value of global health research from an individual or aggregate (and which aggregate) level? Can we build principles based on a conglomerate of evidence and arguments from ethnographic, empirical and philosophical/theoretical data?

To respond to such questions, IJsselmuiden *et al.* (2010) have focused on the principles of global justice and solidarity to argue for a new era in the ethics of international health research. They insist that research must be more responsive to local health systems and strive to enhance local capacity through equitable collaboration. Thus, they envision new approaches in the research review process to prompt funders from the North to consider the inclusion of local priorities as a condition for funding. Finally, they argue that researchers have an obligation to conduct research promoting health equity and linking results with future local development. In contrast, Stewart & Sewankambo (2010) have considered the process of global health research itself as a socially embedded activity. Their analysis of therapeutic misconception reveals that local expectations of research benefits are infinitely more complex than previously thought, while motivations for participating in research suggest an intricate calculus of responsibilities between researcher, participant and community. By studying the cultural value and social impact of global health research from the lived experience of the research participant, rather than from the operational perspective of the researchers, a more meaningful understanding of the social value of global health research should emerge.

Economic valuations in global health governance

Measurement is a core concern for economists, and so it is natural for economists to strive to measure the value of health in the context of economic theory. One way for this, whether on a national or global scale, is to assess the value of health in financial terms (the generation of wealth measured as Gross Domestic Product or GDP). A second measure to assess the value of an individual's health at the individual level is to calculate their total projected lifetime earning, which contrasts to assigning a cost to the extension of healthy years of life and the reduction of years lived with disability due to ill-health. A third approach to measuring the value of health recognizes that health status might be defined, acted on, rejected or narrated in quite distinct ways. For example, as an abstract normative principle in times of non-crisis, as a more "objective" or concrete assessment in times of crisis, or as a moral tale, explanation or regret when reflecting on or narrating the event. Moral positions on violence and trauma are often experienced in this manner. Yet however we assign value to health, we must find common ground for answering basic questions of assessing value in global health. To begin with, how do we measure the value of health and how do we scale it? How is new health-related value created and distributed? We suggest that by connecting the analytics of an economic model of evaluating health with the advocacy efforts of a social justice approach, the effort to measure value in the creation of global health programs will contribute to better outcomes in the implementation of those programs.

The international development community has elevated health as a central concern since the publication of the 1993 World Development Report, *Investing in Health* (World Bank, 1993). This report not only documented the importance of healthy populations in the creation of wealth, but also determined that the generation of new knowledge through health research was an essential factor. This has led to many initiatives from global intergovernmental institutions, bilateral assistance agencies, foundations and charities, religious and secular, that link programmatic interventions to knowledge generated largely through external support, both financial and intellectual. Investment in health research in high- and many middle-income countries which can afford the costs, has improved. The predominant investment has been on research on the problems of these more economically developed societies, characterized by the Global Forum for Health Research (GFHR) as the 10/90 gap, the reality that 90% of investments are directed towards the health problems of 10% of the world's population.

McGahan & Keusch (2010) have argued that the concept of value or valuations in economics represents something different than the concept of value in global health advocacy. For example, we have the knowledge and technology to prevent or treat most diseases, however those with the greatest need have the least access. This is the consequence of the interplay between the moral content we assign to equitable access to health resources and the reality of shortages in local health-care markets. Markets, the most common way of assigning value, fail to address these inequities, indicated by the inability of the 1994 Trade Related Aspects of Intellectual Property Rights (TRIPS) Agreement of the World Trade Organization (WTO) to significantly improve pharmaceutical innovation for diseases of the poor. They note there are several mechanisms to assign market value to health and the importance of the market mechanism for improving local access to health-care resources (McGahan & Keusch, 2010). However, the imperative is to use the method of economic valuation best suited to stimulating product and service development, and to insist on the relevance of the global public good perspective, if there is to be a real chance to reduce scarcity at the local level.

Anthropology as a bridge between the local and the global in global health

An empirically based ethnographic approach may be the best way to effectively bridge local narratives of health with the cosmopolitan global health values that shape macro-level health policies. Transparency and accountability have emerged as key values in the formulation and implementation of global health policy, necessitating a more direct and intimate relationship between those who control global health assets and those whose lives are shaped by the distribution of resources. For instance, the development of community advisory boards to act as translators between the language of research protocols and the idioms that resonate with the community and relay local concerns back to investigators. While this may facilitate more efficient and effective health research, it also raises local expectations of the power of community opinions to influence globally financed health interventions. This local–global interface can be a litmus test of the true worth of transparency and accountability as essential values for the funders and practitioners of global health. Feierman *et al.* (2010) consider the production of contextualized ethnographic knowledge about local experiences of global health programs (kinship, technologies, sources of power and authority) to be critical to the success of those programs. Equally important, but often overlooked, is how the new content and knowledge moves or "flows" amongst global health actors and defines the contours of the local–global interface. More than a lack of ethnographic description and analysis, the absence of a deep understanding of social action at all levels in the practice of global health is a serious barrier to effective program implementation at the local level (Feierman *et al.*, 2010).

A recent example of the unique value of empirically based anthropology to resolve a serious problem between a local community and a global intervention is the re-emergence of wild polio virus in northern Nigeria in 2003. Between 1988 and 2002, the WHO Global Polio Eradication Initiative, the world's single largest, internationally coordinated public health project, reduced the number of cases of wild polio virus worldwide by 99%. However, in August 2003, three states in northern Nigeria suspended polio immunization campaigns, following concerns by some public figures regarding the safety of the polio vaccine. Local political and religious leaders, and even physicians, called on parents to refuse the polio vaccine for their children. They accused western countries of deliberately contaminating the vaccine with anti-fertility agents, HIV, and/or cancer cells in a plot to sterilize or sicken African children, particularly Muslim children. Subsequently, a new outbreak occurred, originating in the northern state of Kano, re-infecting previously polio-free areas within Nigeria (including Lagos)

and eight previously polio-free countries across west and central Africa. As a result, for the first time since efforts to eradicate polio began, more countries suffered polio cases in 2003 due to importations than were themselves endemic for the disease. Resolution was achieved in July 2004 through dialog after the WHO and UNICEF consented to allow the vaccine to be tested in a Muslim country (Indonesia) with new suppliers of polio vaccine from Biopharma, an Indonesian company. Within 12 months, polio eradication campaigns resumed across northern Nigeria in July 2004. However, Nigeria continues to report wild polio virus. In 2006, 1124 cases were identified in Nigeria, accounting for well over two-thirds of the total number of cases worldwide. Wild polio virus, as well as cases of vaccine-related polio, continue to plague northern Nigeria as recently as mid 2009.

Local anxieties about the 2003 polio campaign in Nigeria reflect a difficult history of externally supervised public health projects. It is widely believed that the deaths of five children enrolled in a 1996 research study in northern Nigeria were caused by the unethical use of Trovafloxacin (Trovan), an antibiotic produced by Pfizer to combat meningitis. Even before this tragedy, aggressive anti-fertility campaigns sponsored by the southern-dominated Nigerian government in the 1980s generated mistrust of the public health system in the northern areas of the country. The significance of these facts was grossly underestimated by the implementers of the *Kick Polio out of Africa* campaign. However, anthropological analysis offers a clearer assessment of why parents refused an effective life-saving public health intervention while public health ethics outlines a more responsive, and ultimately effective, approach to mass vaccination conducted in an atmosphere of fear and mistrust. Several anthropologists cautioned that local suspicion of the polio eradication campaign was rooted in the stark contrast between the well-organized and free delivery of the polio vaccine and the chronically under-funded and dysfunctional primary health-care system (Renne, 2006). Furthermore, from the perspective of the local community, more pressing health issues, such as malnutrition or malaria, were consistently ignored by public health officials. Even the 2003 Nigerian government report that confirmed the safety of the polio vaccine was rejected by the northern states because the local Muslim community did not participate in the production of the government report. The impasse was finally broken after the government and external health agencies consulted with the local communities and fresh testing of the polio vaccine was commissioned in Muslim-operated biomedical facilities in Muslim countries. One of the primary principles of ethical public health decision-making is a respect for autonomy and human dignity; this is the opposite of the paternalism demonstrated by both the Nigerian government and the international sponsors of the immunization campaign. Understanding local cultural norms is a cornerstone for effective collaboration between public health workers and community leaders and members. Anthropologists can help public health workers anticipate when health intervention protocols may be at odds with local sentiments, thus avoiding these tragic breakdowns of communication between the community and the public health sector.

New approaches in global health practice

Given the critical role of research and new knowledge generation for the improvement of health status, it is surprising that academic values (for example scientific integrity, consistency, measured judgment, curiosity, intuition, creativity and data-driven decision-making) are generally ignored in the complex governance of global health. However, new directions in global health practice are beginning to appear. Kim *et al.* (2010) believe that twenty-first century global health programs must shift from a series of individual, disease-centric programs to a coordinated system of fully-functioning health-care delivery programs. They describe the Harvard Global Health Delivery Project, a partnership between the Harvard Medical and Business Schools, as a strategic road map towards the creation of a systematic framework for innovation in the infrastructure of global care-delivery programs. Application of the core business value of profitability to the core global health value of maximizing health in resource-poor settings, offers the opportunity to address one of the greatest constraints in medicine today, the delivery of health care. Kim *et al.* (2010) consider it essential to foster more effective partnerships between academic institutions, NGOs, private entities and the public sector in order to deliver real value through the effective delivery of health care in resource-poor settings. Sharing a similar vision, a group of biomedical, business and social science researchers at Northwestern University are combining industry, donors and academia to narrow the gap between supply and demand for HIV/AIDS

diagnostics (Palamountain *et al.*, 2010). Universities are uniquely positioned to catalyze a new type of partnership between non-profit global health donors and commercial diagnostic companies, build on the efficiency and creativity of the private sector, reduce industry risk by guaranteeing a low-margin, high-volume financial opportunity and provide medical goods to resource-constrained populations. Universities are increasingly engaged in implementation programs on the ground in global health settings, and yet at the same time, provide the academic milieu to advance critical reflection on value issues. Hence, they are engaged with practice as well as with reflection on that practice. The third unique qualification of the university is its role in the education and shaping of the values of its students, who represent the future for all endeavors. No other institution can claim a serious engagement in all three domains of teaching, research and service as strongly as universities.

Conclusion

New initiatives in global health, like biomedicine itself, display a striking inadequacy to examine the meanings, experiences and practices that so significantly shape the nature of their governance. By developing a robust, multidisciplinary discourse on values, and in particular, by connecting the local and the global, we can better understand the sources, frameworks and larger implications of the governance of global health entities. Local worlds and local lives anchor anthropological accounts of sickness, care and prevention in resource-poor and resource-rich societies. Without this focus, no bridge can effectively connect large-scale policies and programs with real people struggling to find solutions to their health problems. Without this focus, unintended social consequences, as with inequality itself, will continue to undermine the effectiveness of global programs to reduce unequal access to health care. Equity and justice cannot be understood apart from local realities. Hence the local must be recognized as a core value in all global health efforts, equivalent to equity, justice and human rights. We assert that this new dialog must take place among the broad range of stakeholders and participants in the ongoing global health revolution, and that social scientists must have an equal seat at the table, to ensure that decision making can reflect the concerns of those most in need of improvements in health status.

References

American Public Health Association (APHA) (2002). *Principles of the Ethical Practice of Public Health, Version 2.2.* Washington, DC: Public Health Leadership Society, APHA.

Angell, M. (1997). The ethics of clinical research in the Third World. *New England Journal of Medicine* **337**, 847–849.

Benatar, S. R. (2002). Some reflections and recommendations on research ethics in developing countries. *Social Science and Medicine* **54**(7), 1131–1141.

Benatar, S. R., Lister, G. & Thacker, S. C. (2010). Values in global health governance. *Global Public Health* **5**(2), 143–153.

Feierman, S., Kleinman, A., Stewart, K. A., Farmer, P. E. & Das, V. (2010). Anthropology, knowledge-flows, and global health. *Global Public Health* **5**(2), 122–128.

Global Forum for Health Research (GFHR) www.globalforumhealth.org/About/10–90-gap (Accessed January 21, 2010).

IJsselmuiden, C. B., Kass, N. E., Sewankambo, N. & Lavery, J. V. (2010). Evolving values in ethics and global health research. *Global Public Health* **5**(2), 154–163.

Kim, J., Rhatigan, J., Jain, S. & Porter, M. E. (2010). From a declaration of values to the creation of value in global health: a report from Harvard University's Global Health Delivery Project. *Global Public Health* **5**(2), 181–188.

McGahan, A. & Keusch, G. T. (2010). Economic valuations in global health. *Global Public Health* **5**(2), 136–142.

Palamountain, K., Stewart, K. A., Krauss, A., Diermeier, D. & Kelso D. (2010). University leadership in global health and HIV/AIDS diagnostics. *Global Public Health* **5**(2), 189–196.

Renne, E. (2006). Perspectives on polio and immunuization in northern Nigeria. *Social Science and Medicine* **63**(7), 1857–1869.

Shapiro, K. & Benatar, S. R. (2005). HIV prevention research and global inequality: towards improved standards of care. *Journal of Medical Ethics* **31**, 39–47.

Stewart, K. A. & Sewankambo, N. (2010). Okukkera Ng'omuzungu (lost in translation): understanding the social value of global health research for HIV/AIDS research participants in Uganda. *Global Public Health* **5**(2), 164–180.

Stewart, K. A., Kleinman, A. & Keusch, G. T. (2010). Introduction: values and moral experiences in global health: bridging the local and the global. *Global Public Health* **5**(2), 115–121.

World Bank (1993). *The World Development Report 1993: Investing in Health.* Washington, DC: World Bank.

World Trade Organization (WTO) www.wto.org/english/docs_e/legal_e/27-trips_01_e.htm (Accessed January 21, 2010).

Yang, A. T., Farmer, P. E. & McGahan, A. M. (2010) "Sustainability" in global health. *Global Public Health* **5**(2), 129–135.

Chapter

27

Poverty, distance and two dimensions of ethics

Jonathan Glover

In the rich countries, we are all vaguely aware that there is an appalling degree of poverty in the developing world. But, perhaps through wanting to avoid psychological discomfort, we usually manage to minimize the scale of its human devastation. In sub-Saharan Africa, the median age at death is less than 5 years. Amartya Sen, who quotes this figure from the 1993 *World Development Report* of the World Bank, understandably feels it necessary to point out that this astounding figure is not a typographical error (Sen, 2005). He goes on to say the figure has got worse since the AIDS epidemic hit hard.

We know that the poverty, the shortages of water and the lack of available medical care are not just natural phenomena. They come about through the interaction of the natural and the social. They are, at least partly, remediable by human action. So what moral claims do babies born in Africa with such a horrifyingly but avoidably low life expectancy have on us?

Oxfam at one time used a poster with a picture of a starving African child and a slogan that said something like "If he was here in front of you, you would buy him a meal. Is it really different because he is far away?"

The answer to that question has all sorts of qualifications about the effectiveness of acting at a distance, but on the central issue the suggestion on the poster is right. If we can act effectively to help people, whether they are near or far changes neither their needs nor their moral claims on us. The poster is also right in the implied comment on our psychology. Even if the moral claim is just as strong, we are much less stirred to act when the person needing help is far away rather than in front of us.

I will start by looking at our psychology. We all know that huge numbers of people have lives that are blighted and shortened by lack of food, lack of clean water and lack of medical care. Most of us know that this matters morally and that some of our wealth could make a great difference. Why do we help so much less than we could?

Then I will talk about the kinds of moral claims that poor people have on rich people. Are their claims based on appealing to our compassion and charity, or is what we owe them a matter of justice?

Finally I will ask how much is required of us. How do the claims of poor people compare to other moral claims on us? How should we weigh these moral claims against our own inclination to prefer things that contribute to our enjoyment of our own lives?

The sources of paralysis

According to one recent estimate, starvation and preventable diseases kill 30 000 children every day (Benatar, 1999). They cause a child's death roughly every three seconds, round the clock every day of the year. Suppose these deaths were not mainly far away from us, located in many different places. Suppose they all happened in one place. If any of us had to be in that place, we would be overwhelmed by the horror and sadness of it all, and overwhelmed by the moral urgency of putting a stop to these preventable deaths of children. But, not having had that experience, we are not in that way overwhelmed by the urgency. What is it about our psychology that protects us from this urgency? What are the sources of our moral paralysis on this matter?

We are influenced by distance. We are also inclined to paralysis by the vastness of the problem. This vastness sometimes makes it seem insoluble. It often prompts at least the thought that the problem is too big for me to make a significant difference to it. Some of these responses have a grain

Global Health and Global Health Ethics, ed. Solomon Benatar and Gillian Brock. Published by Cambridge University Press.
© Cambridge University Press 2011.

of reasonableness. But for the most part they rest on cognitive illusions.

Distance

It is a platitude that physical distance makes a great difference to our responses. The crime figures do not horrify us in the way that seeing someone being attacked or killed does. In war it is easier to kill people from a distance, by dropping bombs or firing missiles rather than with bayonets. This often holds for other atrocities. The Nazis did not murder millions of German Jews in Germany, but first sent them away to "the East," so that other Germans would be less acutely aware of what was being done. In Stanley Milgram's experiments on obedience, where people thought they were administering electric shocks to other people, it was easier to carry out the orders if the supposed victim could not be seen.

This same psychology makes us care less about a starving child who is in the Sudan or Bangladesh than one we could see. The fact that this psychology is so natural to us does not generate any very impressive moral justification or excuse for our inactivity. We would not be particularly won over if someone explained his lack of resistance in the Third Reich by saying, "but they were not killed here: all that took place a long way away." When our descendents ask how we could have acquiesced in the preventable deaths of 30 000 children each day, the explanation is partly about distance, but they may not be much won over by it.

As well as physical distance, there is what can be called "moral distance." Because of our tribalism, people physically close to us, but who have different ethnicity, religion and culture, can seem psychologically distant, while we care greatly about people we are "close to" even when they are on the other side of the world. The plight of people dying from preventable diseases in a far-off country may stir us less because of the great differences between them and us. As with physical distance, it is hard to defend this downgrading of people's claims because of psychological distance, but there is little doubt of its anesthetizing power.

"The problem is insoluble"

If a problem seems insoluble, that gives psychological support to the thought that any action we take is futile. We can be overwhelmed by the difficulties in the way of eliminating poverty in the world.

The difficulties come partly from the complexity of its causes. People may be starving because a drought has caused crops to fail. But, as Amartya Sen has taught us, famine often co-exists with there being enough food for people to eat, but those who are starving do not have access to it, sometimes through lack of money (Sen, 1982). Poverty and starvation may come from wars. Peasant farmers are driven away by invaders who take their land and crops. Or people may be trapped in poverty by cultural constraints. "The causes of her condition – Devki was born weighing 5 lb. but within six weeks her weight had fallen 3 lb. 8 oz – are as much cultural as they are because of the grinding poverty of Indian village life. Her twin brother, Rahul, sleeps contentedly, his limbs positively plump by comparison-stark evidence of the social preference for boys"(*Daily Telegraph*, May 2, 2006).

Other cultural constraints come from common features of the way of life of the huge numbers of urban poor people in the developing world. There will soon be more people living in Bombay than in Australia (Mehta, 2004). Films like *Salaam Bombay* and *City of God* portray this culture in India and in Brazil. In 1992, Mexico City had about 6.6 million poor people living in an extended shanty-town (Davis, 2006). Oscar Lewis used the term "culture of poverty" in his accounts of life in Mexico City. He said he used this term to emphasize that "poverty in modern nations is not only a state of economic deprivation … It has a structure, a rationale, and defence mechanisms without which the poor could hardly carry on … it is a way of life, remarkably stable and persistent, passed down from generation to generation along family lines … (with) its own modalities and distinctive psychological consequences for its members"(Lewis, 1961).

These complex economic and cultural causes can paralyse the willingness to give aid. The paralysis comes through the thought that tackling poverty means changing the whole social world: eliminating war, redistributing wealth, changing some very intractable cultural attitudes about gender, transforming the shanty towns and undoing the psychological distortions they have created in those growing up there.

It is interesting that, when we see people's lives being wrecked by some event that is not entangled in all these cultural and psychological complexities, the paralysis may not set in. The 2004 Tsunami and its effects were seen round the world. Sympathy was aroused and none of the economic and cultural complications intervened to make action seem useless.

The people who were its victims needed aid quickly in order to eat, to have shelter and to rebuild their houses. There were no insurmountable preliminaries like stopping a war or changing deeply entrenched cultural practices. Sympathy was not paralysed, and the response from people in the richer countries was on a scale that took their political leaders by surprise and put pressure on them to increase governmental contributions.

"The problem is too big for me to make a difference"

Even if the elimination of world poverty is not in principle impossible, it may still seem too huge a problem for any individual to affect it significantly. "My contribution would be only a drop in the ocean." This response has several components.

The elusiveness of the causal links

Even if a single person's contribution to famine relief does make a difference, the complexity of the causal links makes it hard to relate sending a cheque to saving someone's life. The role of the single contribution is obscured.

There are two kinds of life-saving. Relief agencies sometimes give handouts of food. But a lot of their work is enabling people to support themselves through such things as irrigation schemes, enabling the cultivation of previously barren land. The food handout saves someone's life on one day. Next day, without further aid, they will still be at risk. The irrigation scheme can rescue people from starvation permanently.

The irrigation scheme may save hundreds of lives, and may have been funded by the contributions of hundreds of people. But none of the contributors knows there is a particular person who was rescued by their contribution. Most donors do not know that this irrigation scheme, or even any irrigation scheme, is what their money went into. Particular donations are not usually tagged for particular projects. The only way of saying that one donation went to an identifiable project is if it is possible to work out which project would have been the one to be cut back if total funding had been slightly reduced. This lack of transparency of the causal connection makes the help given less vivid to the donor and may encourage the thought that the donation made no significant impact.

Cognitive illusions: size and imperceptibility

We are prone to our thinking being distorted by size illusions created by large numbers. It may be true that my contribution is only a drop in the ocean, but that drop may be the saving of someone's life, or even several people's lives. In a fire, if we are unable to rescue all the dozen or so people in danger, this does not mean we need not bother to rescue the one or two that we can. Undistorted thinking would take the same view when it is millions of people where we cannot save all of them.

And even where the contribution is not large enough to save someone's life, or even in itself to make a detectable difference, it may still do good. This point applies strikingly in the context of environmental issues. If I switch off my television instead of leaving it on standby, this may have no detectable impact on global warming. But real harm is done if millions of people conclude that it is not worth bothering. Increments individually below the threshold of detection make a difference, both in matters of the environment and in the response to poverty.

We are used to familiar visual illusions and are used to correcting for them. Psychologists have also mapped out some of the more widespread cognitive illusions and it is becoming more common to correct for them. In morality there are also common illusions. Those created by large numbers and by the imperceptibility of individual contributions help cause the paralysis about poverty relief. We should start correcting for them too.

The shift to collective action

The feeling that an individual's contribution will be dwarfed by the scale of the problem does not have to lead to paralysis. An alternative response is to shift the emphasis away from individual to collective action. One person's contribution may be tiny, but a change of a government's policy on aid or on developing countries' debt can make a big difference. The campaign started by the churches on debt relief, and the public pressure on the governments of the G8, are cases in point. Of course, campaigns and public pressure require action by individuals. And taking part in a campaign is something that can be done as well as making a donation to Oxfam. The donation may still save someone's life. But the contribution to the campaign, whether it is a financial contribution or one of time and work, may make a bigger difference. The power of collective action may be greater than the sum of uncoordinated individual actions.

The moral claims of poor people

Humanitarianism to the rescue

What are the moral claims of the poor on the rich? What is their basis? Start with people in one of the parts of Africa where the median age at death is less than 5 years. Take a child born there and that child's mother. Without help from outside, much of the child's very short life will be taken up with dying from starvation or disease. The mother will have the experience of trying and failing to save her child from extreme suffering and death. The claim that none of this matters at all is too callous and horrible to deserve the compliment of being argued with. Anyone who makes it either has no imagination or no concern for others. Because of the harm such an attitude does to others, we may try to change such people. But, until we succeed, they have at least a severely diminished claim to be participants in moral discussion.

I shall assume that we all think that, other things equal, people should be rescued from such horrors. (Of course a lot hangs on "other things equal," which different people will interpret differently. But I shall assume we all at least accept the absolute minimum interpretation that, if we could rescue the mother and child from starvation and disease simply by waving a wand, we should do so. To deny *this* is equivalent to saying their plight does not matter at all.)

Most of us would go beyond the view that rescue is morally obligatory when the means are as cost-free as waving a wand. Surely rescue is often obligatory even when there is some cost? I once argued this using the case of seeing a child (one for whom I have no special responsibility) drowning in a river. If I do nothing, this may be perfectly legal, at least under English law. If I drown the child, that is murder. But the English law sees no crime if I knowingly fail to rescue the child. But, morally, the distinction between act and omission may not bear this weight. Morally, the failure to rescue may be much closer to murder than it is legally. This claim about a moral obligation to rescue went (minimally) beyond the wand-waving case. There will be some small costs attached to the rescue: I may be late for an appointment; my clothes may need cleaning, and so on. I assume that nearly all those of us who think saving someone's life by waving a wand is morally obligatory will think saving life in this case is also obligatory. The

cost is so small that someone who refuses to accept this conclusion places on saving a child's life a value perilously close to zero. But, as the cost rises in different cases, when does rescue stop being obligatory?

One answer to this question has been given by Peter Singer. Taking up the discussion of rescuing the drowning child, he proposed a principle to explain why and when rescue is obligatory. He suggested that "if it is within our power to prevent something very bad happening, without thereby sacrificing anything of comparable moral significance, we ought to do it" (Singer, 1979). I agree that this principle is very plausible, although a lot will hang on what is "of comparable moral significance."

It seems clear that being late for the appointment and messing up my clothes do not come anywhere near being of comparable moral significance to the death of a child. Obviously, I should rescue the child.

It seems equally clear that a parallel argument can be made about saving the African child. The Oxfam poster I mentioned earlier also had a claim along the lines of "£10 from you could save this child's life." Let us suppose that a claim of this order is true. (And suppose the life-saving is not a one-off handout, but permanent rescue on the model of the irrigation scheme.) Every time I spend £10 on a DVD I could save someone's life instead. This suggests, very plausibly, that I ought to buy fewer DVDs and send the money to famine relief. Again, there are questions about how far this line of thinking can be extended before something of comparable moral importance is at stake. We will come back to that. But, wherever the boundary is best drawn, the claims of saving the child's life are very strong indeed. The humanitarian duty of rescue is a strong one and only very serious considerations will outweigh it.

Compensatory justice: "Some of their poverty comes from exploitation"

The people in developing countries who are poor also have claims based on compensatory justice. Some of their poverty comes from our exploitation. Part of the prosperity of those of us in the developed world comes from buying the raw materials and agricultural products of the developing world extremely cheaply. Part of it comes from protectionist policies designed to prevent their industries from competing successfully with ours. Part of it comes from the way corporations based in the developed world have so much muscle in negotiating with the weak governments of the developing world. Part of it comes from the way the rules governing international trade often tip the scales still further in favor of the corporations.

This broad picture is well known to many of us in the richer countries, but of course we do not experience the reality with anything like the vividness of those in the poor countries. The picture becomes a little more vivid when we focus on its details.

A recent report by Jeremy Laurance in *The Independent* focuses on a bag of salad or a bunch of cut flowers bought in a supermarket (Laurance, 2006) If the salad contains lettuce, rocket, baby leaf salad, mangetout, peas or broccoli, any of these may have come from Kenya. A small 50 g bag of salad uses almost 50 litres of water in countries like Kenya where water is in short supply. If the bag also includes tomatoes, celery and cucumber, the water used goes up to more than 300 litres. Washing and packaging increase the total further. Half of the cut flowers sold in British supermarkets come from Kenya, again using huge amounts of water badly needed locally.

Irrigation schemes for these crops sometimes cause farmers downstream to find that in the dry season their rivers have dried out. As one expert puts it, "We are exporting drought." Another expert is quoted as saying that these crops are drying out Lake Naivasha: "Almost everybody in Europe who has eaten Kenyan beans or Kenyan strawberries or gazed at Kenyan roses has bought Naivasha water. It is sucking the lake dry. It will become a turgid, smelly pond with impoverished communities eking out a living along bare shores" (Bruce Lankford and David Harper – quoted in Laurance, 2006).

The thought that we owe something to the people to whom we are doing this kind of thing is not easy to refute. Most of us who buy salad, flowers or the many other products about which a similar story could be told, are only inadvertently doing this harm. And it is not clear how we as individuals can alter these practices of exploitation. But as we do become aware of the general picture, it is hard to resist the thought that we owe *something* to the victims of these practices from which we benefit.

"The colonization of the natural by the just"

The claims of justice here do not have to depend on compensation. Compare the baby in sub-Saharan Africa with a typical baby born here in Europe, who may well have a life more than ten times as long. The African baby has done nothing to deserve such a cruelly

brief life and the African mother has done nothing to deserve having to watch her child die from hunger or preventable disease. There is a huge natural unfairness about this, even if the poverty is not caused by human agency.

One response to this is to say, "life *is* unfair." It is true that life is in many ways unfair. People vary in their beauty, their gifts and their temperament. Some catch fatal or debilitating diseases while others are healthy. Some live in countries at peace while others live in countries at war. Some are born into happy families while others are not. And so on. But the fact that life contains a lot of good and bad luck does not mean that all "bad luck" has to be put up with. There is what – in another context – Allen Buchanan has called "the colonization of the natural by the just" (Buchanan *et al.*, 2000). Illness not brought about by human agency was once seen as a "natural" piece of bad luck about which nothing could be done. But with the development of cures and of preventive medicine, we now see it as unjust if someone is denied available treatment. To the extent that devastating "bad luck" can be remedied, it moves away from being accepted as "natural" and enters the realm of justice and injustice.

If the "naturally caused" starvation and disease of southern Africa were unavoidable, they would still be a horror, but moral criticism would have no place. Because they are avoidable, they are both a horror and an injustice.

The moral scandal of extreme poverty

All the moral claims of the poor are rooted in the fact that most of their misery is preventable. This creates a humanitarian imperative. It also creates a claim of justice, which is then further strengthened by the fact that much of their misery is actually caused by economic conditions from which those of us in rich countries benefit. Humanitarianism and justice unite in seeing the continuation of extreme poverty as a moral scandal.

Competing claims: how much is required of us?

If the Oxfam poster is right, the price of a DVD can save someone's life.

Obviously I can't say that my having a DVD is morally more important than someone's life being saved.

But how far does this go? Applying this each time will mean that buying a DVD is never justified. And, of course, it is not just DVDs. A holiday in France is not more important than someone's life. Most of what we buy is going to fail this test. And most of what we own is going to fail the test too: selling a house and moving somewhere cheaper might enable us to save large numbers of lives. It starts to look as though the argument is going to require giving away most of our income and selling most of our possessions. And then there is our time. Having given away income and possessions, we could save more lives if we spent all our free time raising money for famine relief. This conclusion is so demanding that virtually none of us comes anywhere near it.

This upshot can be called a "life at the moral maximum." It is often taken to be a *reductio ad absurdum* of those moral theories, such as many forms of utilitarianism or egalitarianism, that at some level give equal weight to the interests of everyone. Our intuitions are that saints and heroes may adopt this extreme self-sacrifice, but that there is something absurd about saying that everyone has a *duty* to act in this way. Isn't such a morality utterly unrealistic?

I believe this dismissal of the demanding morality is much too easy. The dismissal is comfortable, but harder to defend than is generally supposed. We should be much more discomforted by the question than most of us are. Yet, at the same time, the demanding morality as so far described is too simple. I will start by filling in some of the necessary complications.

Poverty is not the only public evil

There are many moral claims that compete with those of relieving poverty. Someone who gives money to medical research or to the care of victims of torture instead of to famine relief should not be criticized for this. Nor should we criticize someone who devotes time (which could have been spent raising money for Oxfam) to campaigning about global warming or to running a party in a children's hospital. Obviously some causes are more important than others. But there is room for debate about this and it is a good thing not everyone adopts the same cause. This line of thought does not absolve us from living life at the moral maximum, but rather shows that its content may vary for different people.

Psychological sustainability

For nearly all of us, life at the moral maximum is likely to be unsustainable. After a time, our motivation

would collapse and we would abandon the whole project. In the long run, we do more good in the world by taking on something more modest that we are able to keep up.

This point about life at the moral maximum being too hard to sustain seems obviously true and at the same time obviously open to abuse. It is easy to duck out of any moral commitment that is at all difficult by saying that it is not psychologically sustainable. The scope for self-deception is enormous. Yet we do have to take some account of sustainability if we are to avoid officially subscribing to the idea of life at the moral maximum and while in practice ignoring the official policy.

There is a worry about going for a "sustainable" policy. Suppose you say that you need some time and money for things you enjoy and so you depart from living at the moral maximum. Part of this might be spending money on a concert. You are in Africa on business. In the evening you queue to buy the concert ticket. You are holding the note needed to buy the ticket, when the wind blows it out of your hand. It is caught by a young girl, who is delighted, saying, "Now I will be able to afford the medicine needed to stop me going blind." Would you take the money back, saying, "No, sorry, you can't have that, I am already close enough to the moral maximum and need this concert to keep my moral efforts sustainable"? If not, does that suggest that the apparent permissibility of giving yourself a break depends on illusions created by distance?

The issue of psychological sustainability raises the question of the balance to be struck between moral demands and living lives of our own, with space to pursue our own interests and pleasures. It seems a strange psychological distortion to say that living our own lives as we want to is *only* justified as a means to avoid the collapse of our commitment to doing good in the world. Some space and means to live our own lives is important in itself. But there is no very obvious higher principle or set of principles to adjudicate between the claims of morality and of living our own life.

Two dimensions of ethics

Within morality too, there are different kinds of claims which it is hard to weigh against each other. We owe things to spouses, partners, lovers, children, parents and friends who are close to us. How should we weigh their claims against the claims of making the world a better place?

There are two polarities. At one extreme is the person who says that personal relationships are everything, and that the claims of humanitarianism and of justice count for nothing. This outlook can be called one of "strictly circumscribed warmth." It is fairly obviously narrow and unattractive. It probably needs either great hardness of heart or else the support of distance and other defense mechanisms.

The other extreme is taking public-spirited good works to be everything.

In *Bleak House* the visit to Mrs. Jellyby is a vivid portrait of how someone's concern with the general good at a distance can be the ruin of dependent people close at hand. Mrs. Jellyby was "a lady of very remarkable strength of character, who devotes herself entirely to the public" and was "devoted to the subject of Africa." Her filthy house was swarming with her neglected children, who were always getting their heads stuck between railings and falling downstairs. There was no hot water as the boiler was broken and the kettle was missing. At the meal, the meat and fish were almost raw and the potatoes had been mislaid in the coal scuttle. Mrs. Jellyby herself "had very good hair, but was too much occupied with her African duties to brush it." Her secretary was her exploited oldest daughter, who privately said she wished Africa and herself and the rest of the family were all dead. The chapter heading Dickens gives to this devastating portrait is "telescopic philanthropy."

Perhaps most of us would like to avoid both strictly circumscribed warmth and telescopic philanthropy. People occupy a huge range of positions on the continuum between the two. And, once again, there seems no obvious way of saying that one point on the continuum is the right one. It may be that there is a right balance to strike between the two kinds of claim and we just have not found out how to be sure where it is. But, perhaps more plausibly, there may be no such thing as *the* right balance to strike.

The need to work with the grain of our nature

Alternative strategies

One problem with thinking of helping to reduce poverty in terms of life at the moral maximum is that it may make us blind to other strategies. Sending money – while good in itself – may not be the best strategy. Contributions that do not involve great sacrifices of money and time sometimes make more difference than those that do. The "war on terror" has rather put me off the metaphor of the war on poverty. But, relenting about this for a moment, the most effective war on poverty may not be costly attrition modeled on the First World War. The most effective contributions may need our intelligence, as we try to match what we like doing and what we are good at with what will help the problem.

For instance – as I assume the audience contains a fair proportion of students and academics – those of us of an academic disposition are often better at thinking and campaigning than we are at raising money. So perhaps we should be thinking creatively about strategies against poverty and then should campaign to get them implemented. Let me mention just a few areas where we could contribute.

In Africa – and elsewhere – local wars are a major exacerbation of poverty. Why do the major powers think it right to campaign against the drug trade but acceptable to profit from the arms trade? The arms trade and the assumptions underlying its supposed justifications cry out for the analysis and criticism needed for a campaign to have it stopped.

The lives of many are made shorter and far worse by lack of decent water. Recently, I noticed that the British government plans to develop a rapid reaction military force to intervene in likely future conflicts caused by water shortages. Would it not be better to invest in research and development of affordable technologies of desalination? Living on a planet mainly covered by sea, it should not be impossible to have enough water.

Then there is the question of the unavailability in developing countries of affordable medications. The pharmaceutical companies say they cannot afford to sell them at a cost that would make them affordable and that the development of generic versions breaching their patents would make research no longer economic. Perhaps this is bluff. If so, could we not work out ways of using the purchasing power of the NHS as leverage to bring about a change of attitude?

Perhaps it is not bluff and research really would be uneconomic without the patents being respected. If so, could we not work out some alternative to patents as a way to fund research? For instance, we could give companies subsidies to fund research based on the medical benefits (*not* the profitability) of their recent research (Pogge, 2008). Or we could encourage development of particular kinds of medication by guaranteeing to buy a lot if they are produced.

I am not an economist and do not know what the best schemes for solving these problems would be. The point is that intelligent thought by competent people about issues like these is likely to contribute on a different scale from those same people giving most of their income away.

Grounds for cautious optimism

Finally, the need to avoid the paralysis that comes from thinking the problem is too big for us to make any impact on it. Poverty is a daunting problem, but there are grounds for optimism about the possibility of progress. The key is collective action. The public campaign against the debt burden started by the churches has changed public opinion and brought pressure on governments. The agreement to cancel the debts of the poorest countries has already brought results. Zambia has been able to make basic health care free. The Tanzanian government has bought food for millions hit by drought. Nigeria has been able to employ 150 000 more teachers. There are transparent causal links between the campaign, the debt relief and these benefits.

It is true that much more is needed. And it is true that money is not enough because there are cultural constraints, such as the attitudes to women and the patterns of behavior encouraged by the huge urban shanty-towns. Although cultural change is slow, it does happen. Those depressed by the entrenched attitudes to women in India and China should draw some encouragement from what happened to entrenched attitudes 50 years ago towards gay people. Prejudices that stifle people lead to protest, and over time prejudices that are indefensible sometimes stop being defended.

The culture of the shanty-towns is obviously going to be changed only gradually. But I take some comfort from this description of the culture of urban poverty: "The filth and tottering ruin surpass all description. Scarcely a whole window pane can be found, the walls are crumbling, doors of old boards nailed together, or altogether wanting in this thieves' quarter … Heaps of garbage and ashes … the foul liquids emptied before the doors gather in stinking pools. Here live the poorest of the poor, the worst paid workers with thieves and

the victims of prostitution. Those who have not yet sunk in the whirlpool of moral ruin which surrounds them, sinking daily deeper, losing daily more of their power to resist the demoralizing influence of want, filth and evil surroundings." That was Engels in the 1840s on the courts and alleyways near the Strand and Covent Garden (Engels, 1969). I teach in the Strand. It is not like that round here now. One day it will not be like that in Mexico City and Bombay. Let us try to make the time-lag less long.

References

Benatar, S. R. (1999). A perspective from Africa on human rights and genetic engineering. In J. Burley (Ed.), *The Genetic Revolution and Human Rights*. Oxford: Oxford University Press.

Buchanan, A., Brock, D. W., Daniels, N. & Wikler, D. (2000). *From Chance to Choice: Genetics and Justice*. Cambridge: Cambridge University Press.

Daily Telegraph (2006). The forgotten victims of India's drive to success. May 2, 2006. www.telegraph.co.uk/news/uknews/1517215/The-forgotten-victims-of-Indias-drive-to-success.html (Accessed September 4, 2010).

Davis, M. (2006) *Planet of Slums*. Brooklyn: Verso.

Engels, F. (1969). *The Condition of the Working Class in England*. London: Panther.

Laurance, J. (2006). The real cost of a bag of salad: you pay 99p, Africa pays 50 litres of fresh water. *The Independent*, April 29, 2006. www.independent.co.uk/environment/the-real-cost-of-a-bag-of-salad-you-pay-99p-africa-pays-50-litres-of-fresh-water-476030.html

Lewis, O. (1961). *The Children of Sanchez*. New York: Random House.

Mehta, S. (2004). *Maximum City, Bombay Lost and Found*. New York, NY: Vintage Books

Pogge, T. (2008). *World Poverty and Human Rights*. (2nd edition). Cambridge: Polity Press.

Sen, A. (1982). *Poverty and Famines: an Essay on Entitlement and Deprivation*. Oxford: Oxford University Press.

Sen, A. (2005). Foreword. In P. Farmer (Ed.), *Pathologies of Power: Health, Human Rights and the New War on the Poor* (page xi). Berkeley, CA: University of California Press.

Singer, P. (1979). *Practical Ethics* (p. 168). Cambridge: Cambridge University Press.

Chapter

28

Teaching global health ethics[1]

James Dwyer

In Japan, Switzerland and Australia, the average life expectancy is about 82 years. But in Sierra Leone, Angola and Afghanistan, it is about 41 years. Within the USA, people in some social groups can expect to live 20 years longer than people in other social groups. What are we to make of a world with such unequal health prospects? What does justice demand in terms of global health? And what is our moral responsibility?

I have thought about those questions for many years. In fact, I have fallen into a pattern that is both commendable and deplorable. I grow concerned about global health, study the causes of poor population health, think about the moral implications, and take some action. Then, gradually, I slip back into my daily concerns and work. These concerns and work are not without merit, but they don't provide much space for activities that promote global health and justice.

But over the last 15 years, I have done at least one thing consistently: I have integrated ethical issues about global health into my teaching. In courses for medical students, I have tried to address fundamental issues about global health, justice and responsibility. And I have done the same in courses attended by students from other fields – nursing, biology, engineering, philosophy and drama. I have also reached out beyond the university to discuss global health ethics with high school students, religious groups, professional associations and the general public.

Now is a good time to reflect on my experience teaching global health ethics. In this chapter, I shall describe how I address some key issues, comment on how students react and speculate about what needs to be done. To begin, I shall describe health prospects in the world. Then I shall frame these prospects

in terms of justice. After a brief discussion of theories of justice, I turn to issues about responsibility and responsiveness. To conclude the chapter, I shall reflect on engagement in the world and hope for a better world.

Health prospects in the world

Most people are aware, at least vaguely, of the large inequalities in health that exist in the world, but they do not reflect very often on the extent, nature and implications of these inequalities. So I describe in my classes some measures of population health that illustrate these inequalities. One measure is average life expectancy (World Health Organization, 2008). This is simply the number of years that people who are born now can expect to live. In about 15 countries, people can now expect to live more than 80 years. While people born in countries like Japan, Switzerland, Australia, Sweden, Canada and Norway can expect to live long and relatively healthy lives, people born in other countries cannot. Life expectancy in Sierra Leone is 40 years; in Angola, 41 years; in Afghanistan, 42 years; in Zimbabwe, 43 years. In about 20 countries the average life expectancy is less than 50 years.

Another measure of population health is the under-5 mortality rate. This is simply the number of children, per 1000 live births, who will die before they are 5 years old (World Health Organization, 2008). In about 20 countries, the under-5 mortality rate is less than 5. In countries like Finland, Singapore, Austria, Ireland and Sweden, less than 0.5% of children will die before they are 5 years old. But in other countries, children die at a high rate. In Sierra Leone, the under-5 mortality rate is 269; in Angola, 260; in Afghanistan, 257; in Niger, 253. In these countries, a quarter of all children will die before they reach their fifth birthday.

---

[1] This chapter draws on two previously published papers (Dwyer, 2003a, 2005).

Global Health and Global Health Ethics, ed. Solomon Benatar and Gillian Brock. Published by Cambridge University Press.
© Cambridge University Press 2011.

Even after studying health prospects in low-income countries, I find one statistic particularly shocking: the number of women who die of causes related to pregnancy. In about 20 countries, the maternal mortality rate is less than 7 per 100 000. In countries like Ireland, Denmark, Italy, German, Spain and Slovenia, pregnancy and childbirth are relatively safe experiences. But in some countries, pregnant women face grave risks. In about 15 countries, the maternal mortality rate is greater than 1000. In countries like Sierra Leone, Afghanistan, Niger, Somalia, Rwanda and Cameroon, more than 1% of pregnant women die of causes related to their pregnancies. This risk of death is repeated with each pregnancy.

In a sea of statistics, we sometimes lose sight of the human meaning of the numbers. So I give students a few comparisons. I compare the risk of live liver donation in the USA with the risk of pregnancy in some other countries. Here is a prospective donor reflecting on the risks of liver donation (Dwyer, 2003b):

> To make things work, they need a living donor with a good liver, a recipient with a bad liver, two adjacent operating rooms, and two sets of transplant surgeons. While the surgeons in one room are cutting out half of your liver, the surgeons in the next room are cutting out the recipient's liver. Then your surgeons pass the good piece over to the other surgeons, who hook it up in the recipient. Each operation takes about 8 hr.
>
> If things go well, you recover. Slowly. When you wake up, you have a ventilator tube in your mouth, a catheter in your bladder, a feeding tube in your stomach, some kind of drain in your abdomen, and several intravenous lines stuck here and there. If there are no complications, you need 6 days in the hospital, 3 months off work, and lots of home care.
>
> If things don't go well, you die.
>
> "How often does that happen?" I asked the surgeon.
>
> "Although we have to quote a mortality rate of 1%," he told me, "we think the actual rate may be as low as 1 in 200."
>
> "As low as?" I wanted to say. Think about it. Two hundred people are sitting in a theatre watching a movie. One of them doesn't go home.

This prospective donor accurately describes the risks and fears associated with liver donation. But the risk of death to the donor (1 in 200) is less than the risk that a pregnant woman faces in 40 countries!

The health prospects for many people are actually worse than I have described because national averages tend to mask inequalities within nations. The poor and marginalized within a country often have shorter life expectancies, higher mortality rates and more illness than average. Inequalities vary from country to country, but measures of health inequalities within the USA illustrate the problem. Chris Murray and his colleagues divided Americans into eight epidemiological groups (Murray, 2005). They found that life expectancy among Asian–American women was almost 21 years greater than life expectancy among urban African–American men. Even if we confine comparisons within one gender, the gap is huge. Asian–American men can expect to live 15 years longer than urban African–American men. That is roughly the difference in life expectancy between Sweden and Mongolia! Studies like this one actually complicate the ethical picture: Should we focus more attention on the inequalities between countries or the inequalities within our own country?

All the measures that I have cited are based on mortality. They ignore morbidity, and the suffering, impairment and lost opportunity that come with it. Measures that do take these factors into account – measures that use healthy life expectancy or disability adjusted life years – suggest a grimmer picture. Rather than cite more statistics, I give my students one example. In low-income countries, pregnant women who have protracted labor sometimes survive but are left with a fistula that causes urine and feces to leak out of them. The medical consequences of an obstetrical fistula are bad, but the social consequences are often worse: loss of job, loss of spouse and loss of community.

A matter of justice

When we learn that so many people in the world have such poor health prospects, most of us react with concern. I have never had a student who was really indifferent to the suffering and ill health of millions of people. But our initial reactions do not take us very far. They do not lead automatically to ethical understanding and action. Without education and effort, they rarely lead to active personal habits, just social institutions, and responsive international arrangements.

Although most students react with concern, many of them see poor health prospects as a matter of misfortune. I try to show them that the poor health prospects of populations are often a matter of justice. Toward the end of his life, John Rawls wrote an account of international justice (Rawls, 1999). Because he did not want to presuppose traditional views about the sovereignty of states, he referred to his work as the law of peoples. He made explicit the ideas that motivate this work:

Two main ideas motivate the Law of Peoples. One is that the great evils of human history – unjust war and oppression, religious persecution and the denial of liberty of conscience, starvation and poverty, not to mention genocide and mass murder – follow from political injustice, with its own cruelties and callousness. … The other main idea, obviously connected with the first, is that, once the gravest forms of political injustice are eliminated by following just (or at least decent) social policies and establishing just (or at least decent) basic institutions, these great evils will eventually disappear. (Rawls, 1999, pp. 6–7)

In his work, Rawls tries to specify a conception of justice that will address the great evils in the world.

To the list of evils that destroy lives and plague human history, I want to add two: ill health and premature death. That seems plausible enough. But I also want to suggest that these evils follow from political injustice. That seems implausible at first. Don't people die of diseases and accidents, caused by microbes and mishaps? Yes and no. Health depends on exposure to risks, susceptibility to illness, access to health care, the social consequences of ill health, and many other factors. But all these factors are influenced by the justice of the social environment. Whereas the health of an individual may depend on particular exposures or susceptibilities, the health of a population often depends on justice. Or so I argue.

One way to shift the perspective from misfortune to injustice is to examine the root causes of poor health. I ask medical students to list the leading causes of death among children in countries with high mortality rates. Most students place AIDS at the top of their lists. But in fact, in many of these countries, the leading causes of death are respiratory infections and diarrhea. Some students do include these immediate causes, but few students list poor sanitation, malnutrition, lack of access to medicines and shortages of health-care workers. And even fewer students list poverty, corruption, war and international arrangements.

To illuminate the role of social structures and contexts, it helps to examine a problem like malnutrition. Since malnutrition renders people more susceptible to many diseases, it contributes to poor health prospects. *The World Health Report 2002* estimates that, in countries with high mortality rates, 14.9% of the burden of disease is due to being underweight, 3.2% to zinc deficiency, 3.1% to iron deficiency and 3.0% to vitamin A deficiency (World Health Organization, 2002). In total, almost 25% of the burden of disease is due to malnutrition.

Chronic malnutrition and outright starvation are rarely due to a lack of resources or to declines in food production within a country. Amartya Sen and others have shown that famines and malnutrition are often due to the way land, food, entitlements and power are distributed (Sen, 1981; Lappé & Collins, 1986). The real problem is that governments and privileged groups don't care enough to create systems of entitlements to supplement the food supplies that marginalized groups have.

A careful study of malnutrition shows that what looks at first to be a matter of misfortune is also a matter of justice because some of the causes of malnutrition are embedded in social and international structures. What is true of malnutrition is also true, to a greater or lesser degree, of many health problems. For example, one could look at the role that social structures and gender inequalities play in the HIV epidemic. With all health problems, it is important to consider a full range of causes: biological, behavioral, cultural, social, international and environmental. It is too easy to focus on the biological and behavioral factors and to ignore the social and international structures that form the context. Yet these structures profoundly affect health prospects. Because these structures are human constructs that can be changed, they raise questions about justice.

Theories of justice

Since poor health prospects often raise questions about justice, it is natural and important to consider theories of justice when teaching global health ethics. A theory of justice might serve many roles. It could orient us in experience by helping to focus our attention in needed ways. It could conceptualize problems in ways that guide action and reform. And it could work, by the way it is reflected in public discourse, to shape institutions. For the most part, I shall focus on the first function: the way a theory might direct our attention and help us to focus on key features. I shall show how one theory focuses our attention. Then I shall consider, more briefly, important features that receive too little attention in that theory.

The work of John Rawls is an example of a political theory of justice. Rawls notes how issues of justice arise at three levels: at the local level (about associations like families and civil groups); at the societal level (about basic institutions like constitutions and economies); and at the international level (about interactions like war, aid and trade). But he cautions us not to assume that the same principles apply to all levels. Since the arrangements at different levels have different natures and serve somewhat different purposes, they may call for different principles and duties. In Rawls' view, the duties we have to family members are different from the duties we have to fellow citizens, which in turn are different from the duties we have to people in other countries.

So Rawls' account is political in this sense: he attaches moral significance to political boundaries. But his view is political in a deeper sense. When he wrote *A Theory of Justice*, he suggested that his account of justice was part of a comprehensive moral view (Rawls, 1971). Later he emphasized that his account of justice is a political view that appeals to the idea of public reason and that recognizes the fact that a democratic culture will be marked by a plurality of reasonable comprehensive moral views. His work on global justice continues in this vein. It recognizes a plurality of reasonably just and decent societies, gives a prominent place to political autonomy, looks for an overlapping consensus, and appeals to the idea of public reason.

In his work on justice, Rawls begins with and emphasizes the role of *societal* justice in shaping people's life prospects. Rawls believes that poor life prospects rarely reflect an absolute lack of resources; more often they reflect problems with political traditions, rule of law, respect for rights, division of property, class structures and the status of women. The two principles of justice that Rawls formulates address these points. The principle of equal liberty and the difference principle are meant to secure equal liberties, ensure the fair value of political liberty, promote fair equality of opportunity and improve the situation of the least advantaged. To do these things will require certain background institutions and conditions. Rawls says that

> background institutions must work to keep property and wealth evenly enough shared over time to preserve the fair value of the political liberties and fair equality of opportunity over generations. They do this by laws regulating bequest and inheritance of property, and other devices such as taxes, to prevent excessive concentrations of private power. (Rawls, 2001, p. 51)

Because concentrations of private power often lead to political domination and grossly unequal opportunities, a society needs to frame and regulate economic structures and conditions in order to ensure fair value of political liberty and to promote fair equality of opportunity. A commitment to justice that ignores background conditions is naïve or hypocritical.

Although societal justice is crucially important, modern societies are not isolated, closed and self-contained. They are interrelated by the influence that they have in many areas: the natural environment; war and peace; legitimacy and human rights; trade and finance; migration and travel; disease and public health; communication and culture; and forms of aid. Because interactions in these areas often raise questions of justice – indeed, because interactions between societies can support or undermine justice within a society – Rawls needs to formulate an account of international or global justice.

In *The Law of Peoples*, Rawls tries to articulate principles that specify just relations between societies (Rawls, 1999). These principles aim to set out basic terms for guiding cooperation and regulating conflict among peoples. To begin, Rawls explains that peoples should respect the freedom, independence and political autonomy of other peoples. This principle of respect recognizes a reasonable pluralism among peoples, but it does not entail that peoples or states have unlimited sovereignty. The traditional view of sovereignty is limited in important ways.

In their internal affairs, peoples may not treat their own members and minorities in any way they please. Internally, they must adhere to certain standards, such as respecting human rights and engaging in consultation with representatives from all groups. In their external affairs, peoples should recognize limits on both the right to wage war and the way war is conducted. Peoples may only go to war in self-defense or to stop very grave violations of human rights (like genocide). And in conducting war, peoples should recognize constraints that aim to protect rights and achieve a just peace. Inspired by Kant's discussion in *Perpetual Peace*, Rawls tries to specify principles, structures, and conditions that would promote a stable peace for the right reasons.

The last principle that Rawls articulates deals with the duty to assist. Rawls believes that societies have a duty to assist other societies when unfavorable conditions (economic, social or historical) make it difficult for those societies to achieve a reasonably just social and political order (Rawls, 1999, pp. 5, 37). The principal aim of this duty is not to aid individuals or small groups who are in dire straits. Nor is it to implement a principle of distributive justice that would operate between societies. In Rawls' account, the aim of the duty to assist is to help societies to create and maintain reasonably just institutions so that the assisted societies become autonomous and good members of a just federation of peoples. The duty to assist is complex because it combines different ideas: the importance of societal justice, a recognition of reasonable pluralism, the ideal of meaningful autonomy (but not unlimited sovereignty), and the hope that internally just societies will be more peaceful and fair in their foreign affairs. The duty to assist does aim to benefit people, but in an indirect way.

What is the best way to fulfill the duty to assist? In general, the means should be chosen to further the aims. Assistance should not aim to promote the narrow interests of the assisting country, but to promote just and decent conditions in the assisted countries. Well-designed assistance would avoid the ignorance, arrogance and narrow self-interest that so often characterize aid. And it would involve the right combination of short-term and long-term projects. To do all that in practice requires knowledge of particular situations, good political judgment and a willingness to experiment. In some situations, assistance to organizations in civil society may prove worthwhile since these organizations are often working to fight injustices, increase community involvement and give voice to marginalized people.

Rawls' work on justice focuses attention on vitally important matters: societal justice, international relations, war, assistance, and the need to create a confederation of reasonably just societies. But other important matters do not receive enough attention. As everyone must, Rawls starts with some simplifying assumptions. He assumes that a society is a closed and self-contained unit. Only after he specifies principles of justice for such a society, does he consider how such a society should relate to other societies. Following the social contract model, he starts with individual units and builds up relationships, structures and conditions. Although he notes that the economic background conditions for international justice "have a role analogous to that of the basic structure in domestic society" (Rawls, 1999, p. 42), he does not emphasize this point. Hence some scholars have worried that Rawls' way of proceeding does not focus enough critical attention on the background conditions and transnational structures that characterize the world in the twenty-first century.

Whereas Rawls tries to develop a conception of international justice, other scholars try to develop a conception of transnational justice (Cohen & Sabel, 2006; Young, 2006). They begin by characterizing

some of the existing and emerging features of globalization: the patterns and structures that surround trade, consumption, manufacturing, labor markets, capital flows, corporations and so on. To these patterns, I would add carbon emissions and ecological footprints (Dwyer, 2008, 2009). This characterization of globalization includes the fact that organizations like the World Trade Organization (WTO) come to acquire considerable power and independence in making rules that profoundly affect people and the environment (Cohen & Sabel, 2006, pp. 164–173). The point is not merely that people are causally linked across borders, but that they are connected by structures and rules shaped by transnational groups and organizations.

What moral norms are appropriate for the transnational relations and associations that have emerged? Although this question is debated and contested in global civil society, it receives too little attention in accounts of justice that start with separate national units. It may be that the norms of justice appropriate for transnational relations are closer in substance to principles of societal justice than to traditional principles of international justice. By focusing our attention on important features, an account of transnational justice may help to make sense of demands for alternative forms of globalization – forms that are more inclusive and more responsive to basic needs.

Both the view of transnational justice that I mentioned and Rawls' view of international justice assume that the appropriate norms of justice depend on the relations that exist among people and the nature of their association (family, society, transnational organization, confederation of societies). But this assumption may lead us to overlook some important ethical features. Peter Singer avoids this assumption and starts with the idea that ethics requires us to give equal consideration to other persons' fundamental interests, quite apart from the connections between them and us (Singer, 1993, 2002).

Although he recognizes an increased responsibility to care for family members, he views national boundaries as morally arbitrary, and he remarks on the contingency of being born into a rich or poor country. So he argues that people in relatively affluent circumstances – most people in Europe, North America, Japan, Australia and so on – have a strong duty to assist those who are worse off. In specifying this duty, he sees no moral justification for taking into account distance, community membership or citizenship (Singer, 2002, pp. 150–95). This view focuses our attention – whether appropriately or excessively – on the fundamental needs and interests of other human beings.

Responsibility and responsiveness

When I first began teaching global health ethics, I devoted a lot of time to explaining, contrasting and evaluating theories of justice. I spent time analyzing Rawls' account of international justice, two accounts of transnational justice and Singer's account of cosmopolitan justice. But I noticed that most of the students grew impatient with my detailed analysis. When I came to understand why they were impatient, an unexpected thing happened: I too grew impatient. What the students sensed, in a somewhat inarticulate way, was that the points of agreement among various accounts of justice are more important than the points of disagreement.

The accounts of justice that I discussed tend to focus our attention in different ways and to emphasize different features: the importance of societal justice in determining life prospects, the role of transnational organizations in shaping the context and the needs of unrelated people, for example. But they all agree that our world is marked by severe and persistent injustice. And they all agree that we need to reconstruct institutions and practices so as to meet basic human needs. They also believe that change is possible. If they didn't believe that change was possible, that humans could construct a better social world, then they would view the current state of affairs as a misfortune, not as an injustice.

Once the students learned basic ideas about population health, they were able, with some help, to see how poor health prospects raise issues of justice. And once they used theories of justice to focus their attention on key features, they were quick to see some of the underlying injustices, including structural injustices. But what they really wanted to know was how they should respond, what they should do to change institutions and practices. But at this crucial point, philosophical accounts of justice do not provide much guidance.

What the students wanted was a less detailed analysis of justice and a more detailed discussion of responsiveness. The idea of responsiveness is related to, but not the same as, responsibility. It is certainly not the same as legal responsibility. Legal responsibility tends to be backward looking. When a particular harm has already occurred, an individual person can be held liable if a clear causal chain connects the harm to that person's actions, and if that person was at fault (acted intentionally or negligently). This form of responsibility is an important feature of social life. And it applies to some actors in the realm of global health: soldiers who rape women, people who sell counterfeit drugs, pharmaceutical companies that conduct research without informed consent and so on.

But a legalistic account of responsibility does not apply to many of the underlying problems in global health. Many of the harms are ongoing or in the future. Some are not harms in the literal sense, but general risks that are spread across populations. The causes are rarely chains linked to particular actions or omissions. They are structural, diffuse, and overlapping. And the faults of the actors are not usually intentional. They are often unintended consequences or embedded features of complex practices. The notion of legal responsibility does not capture the breadth and depth of moral concern in the realm of global health. It does not adequately articulate the idea of responsiveness.

The idea of responsiveness is more closely related to what Iris Young calls the social connection model of responsibility (Young, 2006). In her work on responsibility and global justice, she notes the need to address injustices that arise from social structures, processes and norms. Since these structures are often embedded in the background conditions that shape and constrain individual conduct, we need to look beyond individual acts. We need to focus on the background conditions that are hard to see because they are simply assumed or accepted as given. Our responsibility for these background conditions is not a backward-looking responsibility based on a clear causal chain and an intentional moral fault. Rather, our responsibility arises because, by acting and pursing projects, we participate in and contribute to the social processes and structures, even though we don't intend any injustice.

Our responsibility is to work to change these structures in order to remedy the injustice. Young says that this

> responsibility can be discharged only by joining with others in collective action. This feature follows from the essentially shared nature of the responsibility. Thousands or even millions of agents contribute by their actions in particular institutional contexts

to the processes that produce unjust outcomes. Our forward-looking responsibility consists in changing the institutions and processes so that their outcomes will be less unjust. No one of us can do this on our own. … The structural processes can be altered only if many actors in diverse social positions work together to intervene in these processes to produce different outcomes.

(Young, 2006, p. 123)

In most cases of structural injustice, an adequate response calls for action that is collective and political.

But even when we work with others, we cannot be responsible for remedying all the structural injustices in the world. Nor is it workable to assign partial responsibility based on a calculation of how much we participate in and contribute to various social structures. At some point, we simply need to *take responsibility* for addressing some injustices. This selective taking of responsibility comes closest to the idea of responsiveness. Based on our situation and ability, we need to respond appropriately. To find an appropriate response, we may need to take many factors into account: the nature of the injustice, the effectiveness of action, possible partners, our abilities, our roles, our histories and so on. In matters like these, appropriate moral responses will often involve creativity and discretion. But discretion in responding does not mean that responses are exempt from all questions, examination and criticism.

More and more medical students from North America and Europe respond by going abroad to work. Their intentions are good: to benefit people in underserved areas. They go to places like Guatemala, Haiti, Mali and South Africa to work in clinics and hospitals or to work on public health projects and campaigns. These sojourns abroad are enormously educational but morally problematic. First, consider some of the ways that these sojourns are educational. Students often learn about and see a wide range of diseases and medical conditions. And they learn to practice medicine in a way that is less reliant on tests and more reliant on clinical skills and reasoning. Sometimes the learning goes deeper. The students observe how underlying social conditions and structures affect people's health. And they learn from experience what poor health prospects mean in human terms. And sometimes the learning goes even deeper. In their work abroad, students see forms of relationships, solidarity and community that are underdeveloped in their own society. And when they return, they see troubling aspects of their own society: the hyper-individualism, the consumer

mentality, the wasteful medical system and the ecological costs.

If these experiences abroad are so educational, why are they morally problematic? They are morally problematic because they do little to remedy injustice. Indeed, in some cases they perpetuate unjust patterns. Because many students go abroad without adequate preparation and at an early stage in their training, they require considerable supervision or end up working without adequate supervision. They stay for a short time, disrupt local systems of care and leave no sustainable benefits. Many projects and countries extract more benefits from the host countries than they provide: while relatively wealthy and healthy societies are sending medical students abroad to work for 4 weeks, they are hiring away foreign doctors and nurses to work for 40 years (Dwyer, 2007). In sum, too many experiences and projects provide little sustainable benefit, lack forms of reciprocity and even embody elements of paternalism.

What is to be done? People need to develop projects that provide educational benefits while more adequately addressing problems of sustainability, reciprocity, respect and justice. Recall that morally appropriate responses to problems of global health involve creativity and discretion, but are open to criticisms and questions. So before going abroad, a student might consider the following questions.

1. *Have I studied adequately the language of the people I will be working with?* Students should consider how much help they can provide, and how much burden they will be to bilingual staff, if they don't have an adequate command of the local language. They should reconsider going to Honduras without a fair grasp of Spanish or going to Mali without a fair grasp of French. If the aim is really to provide benefits, then an adequate study of the relevant language seems like a reasonable prerequisite.

2. *Have I prepared by studying the history, culture and social structures of the society I will be working in?* Students need to learn important things about the context in which they will be working. For example, before going to Guatemala, students should learn about the treatment of the indigenous peoples, the history of American involvement in the country, the human rights movements and so on. A study that is equivalent to a college course does not seem too much to ask.

3. *Have I committed adequate time for my work abroad?* Students need to consider how much time is needed to understand the setting, adapt their skills and provide some significant benefit. Four-week electives seem more suited to the medical students' schedules than the needs of projects. Even short stays by experienced physicians can reinforce bad attitudes and patterns. People need to consider longer commitments to projects that are continuous and sustainable.

4. *Am I going at an appropriate stage in my training?* Students need to think about the best time in their careers to go abroad. The point is not to delay forever going abroad, but to choose a time that is good not only for the student, but also for the project. Too many experiences abroad reflect a troubling pattern: students learn and develop their clinical skills on poor people and then move on to apply those skills for the benefit of rich people (Dwyer, 1993).

5. *Is the project that I am considering part of a meaningful partnership that is based on respect?* Students need to consider whether a project is based on mutual respect and meaningful collaboration. Too many projects embody a problematic pattern: they aim to benefit people without consulting and collaborating with those people. The local people and institutions should have a leading voice in a dialogue about how to define needs, develop capacities and provide care.

6. *Are the benefits and burdens of the project fairly distributed?* The host institution and country should benefit as much as, or more than, the sending institution. After all, that is the principal point of the project. To meet this requirement, experienced faculty and senior doctors, as well as medical students, should devote substantial time to the project. And the sending institution should devote enough resources to cover the true costs of the project.

7. *In addition to providing clinical care, am I working with people to remedy structural injustices?* Everyone needs to take some responsibility for working with others to remedy structural injustices. Of course, not every clinical encounter needs to address structural injustices, but all projects and work abroad should keep this aim in mind because these injustices are the big impediments to improving health prospects.

8. *Do I want to go abroad primarily for the adventure and feeling of altruism, or am I concerned enough about health and justice to also work in my own country to change patterns that impede better global health?* Students should consider not only their motives, but also the opportunities to work in their own country to improve global health. Everyone could learn a lot and do some good by working on campaigns to change foreign aid, agricultural subsidies, the brain drain, violations of human rights, labor conditions, human trafficking, environmental degradation and so on.

Reflecting on questions like these could lead to more appropriate responses.

Engagement and hope

I want to conclude by describing two issues that I have struggled with. The first issue concerns engagement. Is it appropriate for teachers, as teachers, to depart from a detached stance of reflection, and to adopt an engaged stance of working to improve health prospects? The question suggests that the ideal, at least for a teacher, is to maintain a detached and theoretical stance in order to understand the world and to convey that understanding to students. The question also suggests that a move away from this ideal toward a more active engagement needs to be justified. This issue is often tied to a series of contrasts: between detachment and engagement, understanding and change, ethics and politics, teacher and activist. Although I recognize the concerns behind this issue, I have come to question the view that it presupposes.

The view that is operating here sees human beings as detached observers who function best by representing the world in the form of theoretical knowledge. But as Dewey, Heidegger and Wittgenstein point out (in different ways and with different political sympathies), we human beings are practical, interested, engaged participants in the world. We come to know our way in the world because we grow up, actively engaged with people and equipment, in social practices and forms of life. We don't need to justify engagement in the world. Engagement, action and practice are primary. They allow us to make sense of and find meaning in the world.

Detached reflection and theoretical understanding are secondary. But that does not mean they are unimportant. We can adopt a detached attitude in order to better understand a conflict, situation, course of action or aspect of the world. But this detachment is only a relative disengagement that serves particular purposes. It is not the paradigm of human experience. One purpose of detachment and reflection is to render our active engagement more intelligent, coherent and ethical. And one purpose of teaching global health ethics is to render our activities to address health prospects more intelligent, coherent and ethical. The problem that I now struggle with is not how to justify engagement, but how to connect engagement and reflection in a better way.

To take engagement, action and practice as primary does not turn a teacher into a crude partisan. There are still virtues that all teachers should strive to embody: a sense of humility about the limits of their own views and activities; a respect for students' views and experiences; a willingness to consider many perspectives; a recognition of the role of creativity and discretion in ethical life; a concern to better integrate engagement and reflection; and so on. But detachment is not one of these virtues. It is a phase in a learning process that must and should include engagement.

The second issue that I have struggled with concerns hope. Each year I used to teach a semester-long course on global health ethics, and by the end of the course, I often felt tired and depressed. There might have been many reasons for my depression: biological, psychological and social. But one reason seemed philosophical. I was entangled in a false picture of hope.

Can we reasonably hope for a more just and healthier world? In trying to respond to this question, I made two mistakes. First, I assumed that reasonable hope is grounded in probabilities. I studied the reasons to be optimistic: developments in science, renewed interest in global public health, a recognition of health disparities, developments in global civil society, courageous activists, the role of education and so on. But I also examined reasons to be pessimistic: unmitigated climate change, environmental degradation, continued marginalization of people, the persistence of war, powerful economic interests, social structures resistant to change and so on. I must admit that the difficulty of changing social structures weighed most heavily on my mind; it even seemed to be the root cause of climate change and environmental degradation. After considering the reasons to be optimistic and the reasons to be pessimistic, I tried to come up with an algebraic sum. The result was not always positive.

But my mistake was to think of hope in terms of probability. Reasonable hope depends not on the probability of future developments, but on the possibility of a better world. Better health prospects are possible, given the natural world we live in, the state of science that we have attained, and the kinds of social organization that we can realize. Indeed, some societies have achieved relatively good measures of population health at relatively low environmental costs (Dwyer, 2009). So there are good grounds for hope.

My second mistake was to think of hope as a belief, based on thought and reflection, about the future of the world. But hope is more like an attitude, stance or quality of engagement in the world. It contrasts with passivity, resignation and cynicism. It connects with striving, perseverance, resilience and readjustment. Reasonable hope requires a skillful combination of traits. In adopting forms of engagement, reasonable people take into account difficulties and probabilities; in trying to address problems of global health, reasonable people learn from failures and adjust their approaches and aims. But hopeful people do not tie their continued engagement, their striving to improve situations, to particular results in particular time frames. This is a lesson that I am still struggling to learn.

References

Cohen, J. & Sabel, C. (2006). Extra republicam nulla justitia? *Philosophy and Public Affairs* **34**(2), 147–175.

Dwyer, J. (1993). Case study: one more pelvic exam. *Hastings Center Report* **23**(6), 27–28.

Dwyer, J. (2003a). Teaching global bioethics. *Bioethics* **17**, 432–446.

Dwyer, J. (2003b). Part of my liver. *Transplantation* **76**, 1266–1267.

Dwyer, J. (2005). Global health and justice. *Bioethics* **19**, 460–475.

Dwyer, J. (2007). What's wrong with the global migration of health care professionals? Individual rights and international justice. *Hastings Center Report* **37**(5), 36–43.

Dwyer, J. (2008). The century of biology: three views. *Sustainability Science* **3**(2), 283–285.

Dwyer, J. (2009). How to connect bioethics and environmental ethics: health, sustainability, and justice. *Bioethics* **23**, 497–502.

Lappé, F. & Collins, J. (1986). *World Hunger: Twelve Myths*. New York: Grove Press.

Murray, C. J. L., Kularni, S. & Ezzati, M. (2005). Eight Americas: new perspectives on U.S. health disparities.

American Journal of Preventive Medicine **29**(5S1), 4–10.

Rawls, J. (1971). *A Theory of Justice*. Cambridge, MA: Harvard University Press.

Rawls, J. (1999). *The Law of Peoples*. Cambridge, MA: Harvard University Press.

Rawls, J. (2001). *Justice as Fairness*. Cambridge, MA: Harvard University Press.

Sen, A. (1981). *Poverty and Famines*. Oxford: Clarendon Press.

Singer, P. (1993). *Practical Ethics*. Cambridge: Cambridge University Press.

Singer, P. (2002). *One World*. (2nd edn.) New Haven, CT: Yale University Press.

World Health Organization (WHO) (2002). *The World Health Report 2002*, p. 162. Geneva: World Health Organization.

World Health Organization (WHO) (2008). *Life Table for WHO Member States, 2006*. www.who.int/whosis/en/ (Accessed June 15, 2009).

Young, I. M. (2006). Responsibility and global justice: a social connection model. *Social Philosophy and Policy* **23**(1), 102–130.

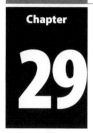

Chapter

29

Towards a new common sense: the need for new paradigms of global health

Isabella Bakker and Stephen Gill

Tax struggle is the oldest form of class struggle.

(Karl Marx, 1967, cited in O'Connor 1973, p. 10)

Introduction

In our earlier chapter we outlined a reading of the present global conjuncture which we characterized as one of "organic crisis." The term was meant to invoke a paradoxical situation, one pregnant with possibilities for alternative ways in which global health might be improved, yet nevertheless a situation in which new alternatives have yet to emerge, or indeed to be born.

We also noted how the broad-ranging nature of the organic crisis was characterized by a number of "morbid symptoms" such as deterioration in global health and global nutrition associated with the way in which capitalist social forces have come to determine increasingly not only whether we have access to useful and affordable health care, but also what we eat and whether we are actually able to eat. More broadly the deepening and extension of the power of capital – since capitalism is a system of power relations and power structures – has come to determine increasing aspects of social reproduction, our health and indeed the very means of survival for a large proportion of the inhabitants of the planet.

We noted therefore that the global organic crisis involves a global crisis of accumulation, the dominant governmental responses to that crisis which have so far been one-sided, lean in favor of financial interests and big corporations, and how capitalism in crisis and its mode of relentless accumulation intersect with deepening and long-term threats to our social and ecological reproduction.

To address the global organic crisis in both theory and practice, we need, in effect, a new paradigm of global political economy – one based on a new "common sense" concerning the nature and potentials of the world that can address global health challenges in a progressive way that connects to the fundamental bases of social reproduction and human security as people face them in their everyday lives. A new paradigm therefore requires new modes of thought ("epistemological perspectives") as well as the means to be able to re-conceptualize our most fundamental objects of analysis ("ontological depth") that help explain the deeper and broader material and political determinants of global health – issues that we have initially addressed elsewhere in our earlier work (Bakker & Gill, 2003). In particular we believe that a critical feminist political economy analysis can shed light on the necessary proposals, such as those associated with public finance and taxation, and the governance of the social commons, assuming they can be combined with political pressure to implement them.

We think therefore, that many of the well-meaning solutions proposed by liberal cosmopolitans fail to touch the most fundamental structures and relations of power which ultimately determine questions of livelihood, life chances and indeed life or death for billions of people. The structures of global exploitation and injustice are not simply in need of "moderate" reforms; these structures require radical surgery and transformation. As the G20 responses to the financial and economic meltdown of 2008–09 have demonstrated conclusively, unless there is massive democratic pressure placed on the dominant governments of the world, all that can be expected is a minor tinkering with the exploitative structures of global capitalism. G20 policies – with or without Tobin or carbon taxes – will continue to be responsive to and underwrite the priorities and needs of large corporations and investors, or more broadly what we have called the power of capital. Only by taming and democratizing the power of capital will it be possible to

---

produce a different type of world economic order, one in which the right to a decent livelihood, to social justice, and to appropriate nutrition and health will become possible, not just for a privileged few but for a majority.

With this in mind, the rest of this short chapter outlines a few measures that would need to be made as first steps in this process – understood as practical aspects of the development of a new paradigm to adequately address global health challenges.

Measures needed to bolster the social commons

As we noted in our earlier chapter in this collection, new measures are needed to provide adequate financing to rebuild and extend the social commons and these must rest upon a more equitable and broad-based tax system where capital and ecologically unsustainable resource consumption are taxed more than labor. Progressive principles of taxation also suggest less reliance on value added taxes which are regressive and a burden on the poor (especially on basic needs such as fuel and food). Developing world countries need help with strengthening tax administration and public financial management and many of the loopholes associated with the offshore world, and the accounting innovations noted in chapter 19, such as transfer pricing need to be closed. Feminists also point out that a more progressive and equitable tax system needs to not only be inclusive, involving tax compliance for all, it also needs to be gender-sensitive, particularly since taxation regimes affect men and women across the social spectrum in very different ways.[1]

Stepping back from these exigencies, we see at least three sets of measures, interconnected and overlapping, which are needed to both support and to finance a broadening of the social commons in ways that are consistent with greater democracy, social justice and social and ecological sustainability.

Address our interdependencies with each other and with nature

This involves both questions of epistemology and questions of political economy and public policies. Our prevailing systems of knowledge in political economy

---

[1] The latter requires support for expanding existing efforts to improve the collection of sex-disaggregated data and data on the gender bias in indirect taxes such as VAT, consumption and trade taxes.

and social science have rendered certain problems invisible, such as the ways in which mainstream public policies and systems of governance associated with market civilization have obscured issues of inequality as well as ecological and social sustainability. In other words we need to break what has been called the "strategic silence," associated with mainstream economic and political thinking, which has rendered invisible or unknowable all of these key components of social and ecological life (Bakker, 1994). This presupposes new knowledge in the fields of political economy and the social sciences in ways that are linked to:

(a) A shift in the nature of agricultural and food production systems away from petroleum and chemical-based agricultural methods towards more organic, localized methods of production, distribution and provisioning – here the example of the Brazilian Landless Workers Movement, with its 1.5 million members, is instructive.

(b) A shift in thinking and practice to take more fundamental account of what feminist economists call the care economy, which involves both paid and unpaid work relating to caring for people. The concept of the care economy recognizes that all people need, give and receive care. Often policies assume this work will continue no matter what, or that as in the case of structural adjustment and responses to economic crisis, shift the burden of adjustment to the care economy and its unpaid work in households, which is normally carried out by women. Implicit in the orthodox view of economic adjustment therefore, women become the social safety net, by default.

(c) A need for rethinking the nature of health inequities in spending and entitlements and outcomes – all of which are connected to inequalities of life chances. This is therefore not simply an issue of public policy but also a fundamental ethical question.

Socialize the risks of the global majority whilst enhancing the social commons

One of the key characteristics of capitalism in general, and neo-liberal capitalism in particular, is the way in which it tends to socialize the risks of powerful corporations and investors (whilst allowing them to privatize profits), while subjecting the majority of the population to the discipline of market forces, in effect privatizing risks for the majority of the world's population – as they are forced to become part of the so-called "self-help society." In this way, neo-liberal capitalism has involved greater human and economic insecurity for the majority of people. Progressive policies must completely overhaul the regulation of finance, and in so doing protect the life savings and pensions of the vast majority of people – it should not simply be capital that receives government guarantees. This requires not only prudential regulation of banks and other financial firms to prevent them taking risks with depositors funds but also, more generally, making finance the servant, rather than the master of production and of wider social purposes.

One way to address this problem is through the public sector, which needs to be made much more accountable to the needs of the public as a whole, and this should be connected to policies that make private corporations more socially accountable and more willing to pay their rightful costs for the social commons and the social goods and infrastructure from which many of their activities benefit.

For this to be possible requires not only new systems of governance but also new systems of taxation, for example to institute steeply progressive taxation on the wealth and income of the top 20% of the world's population who have been the primary beneficiaries of neo-liberal globalization. This should be coupled to measures that provide guaranteed annual income for a majority, well above existing poverty lines, as well as substantially raised minimum wages, for the majority of people. Such a shift would still allow the wealthy to be able to live comfortable lives.

In addition markets can be reshaped to serve more socially useful ends and to contribute to public goods and the global commons. Indeed, Albritton (2009) has argued that we should not simply accept market prices but reshape them by placing surcharges on commodities or services that generate high social costs, while subsidizing those that generate social benefits. He points out that this is already done, for example education is already subsidized whereas cigarettes have a surtax placed upon them. Building on existing practices and extending them, we can therefore radically rethink how things are priced in order to create different incentive structures across society, and with respect to the effects of certain activities on the environment, e.g. by placing high taxes on carbon emissions.

However, any shift in the taxation regime needs to take full account of its redistributive consequences: Carbon taxes have to be combined with policies to redistribute wealth so that those on lower incomes are not forced into further economic difficulties because of the higher prices which result from the new taxes. Finally, with respect to government expenditures, there need to be innovations in the way in which we consider the appropriate mix of provisioning between private and public for social reproduction, both now and in the future. Policies should no longer be based upon a generic, ahistorical possessive individual, as with the conventional economic discourse, but instead should be based on concepts that take full account of the inequalities across social classes and across gender, as well as those caused by racialized policies.

Create a new "common sense" by nurturing alternative and progressive values

What we mean by the creation of the new "common sense" is a transformation in the way in which people conceive of the nature and potentials of the world in which they actually live. Market civilization has brought with it a bombardment of symbols, images and structures associated with ever-increasing consumption and the commodification of desire. The logic of market civilization is, however, ultimately destructive of conceptions of social solidarity and of social and ecological sustainability (Gill, 1995). In short we need new paradigms from which we can gauge the potential for progress in our civilization, in ways that put people before profits. One way in which we can begin to therefore foster a new common sense is through the education and media systems.

For example, in Chapter 19, we have alluded to the way in which many of the problems that led up to the global economic and financial crisis have been linked to the relatively unreflective application of orthodox economic thinking – thinking that has become more abstract and increasingly divorced from real economic processes and needs. Therefore we believe this calls for a revolution in the way in which economics is both taught in schools and universities and discussed in political discourse and particularly in the media, in ways that encourage a variety of different viewpoints and policy prescriptions.

For this to be possible requires new means of financing so that a media that is truly responsive to the diversity of public opinion begins to emerge. Indeed the diversity of public opinion and innovations in thought itself requires a vibrant education system, one that is premised upon education as a collective social good, and not as a private commodity. This requires that we build upon fiscal systems of the type alluded to above, and in particular to provide people with sufficient income so that they actually have the time to develop their knowledge and capacity for reflection under conditions where they do not feel insecure concerning the future.

References

Albritton, R. (2009). *Let Them Eat Junk: How Capitalism Creates Hunger and Obesity*. London: Pluto Press.

Bakker, I. (Ed.) (1994). *The Strategic Silence: Gender and Economic Policy*. London: Zed Books.

Bakker, I. & Gill, S. (2003). *Power, Production, and Social Reproduction: Human In/Security in the Global Political Economy*. Basingstoke: Palgrave Macmillan.

Gill, S. (1995). Globalisation, market civilisation, and disciplinary neoliberalism. *Millennium* **23**(3), 399–423.

O'Connor, J. (1973). *The Fiscal Crisis of The State*. New York, NY: St. Martin's Press.

Index

37124928R00197

Made in the USA
San Bernardino, CA
27 May 2019